The supplementary optical videodisc was developed by Frank D. Allan, Ph.D., Professor of Anatomy, George Washington University, in collaboration with staff of the Lister Hill National Center for Biomedical Communications, National Library of Medicine.

Sponsoring Editor: Sally Cheney
Project Editor: Lenore Bonnie Biller
Art Direction: Kathie Vaccaro
Text and Cover Design: Delgado Design, Inc.
Cover Photo: Exocrine gland—a specialization of epithelium. Courtesy of T. Nagato.
Text Art and Photo Research: Charles F. Bridgman
Production Manager: Kewal K. Sharma
Compositor: Ruttle, Shaw & Wetherill, Inc.
Printer and Binder: The Murray Printing Company
Cover Printer: Phoenix Color Corp.

Library of Congress Cataloging in Publication Data

Telford, Ira Rockwood
    Introduction to functional histology   /   Ira R. Telford, Charles F. Bridgman.
        p.   cm.
    Bibliography: p.
    Includes index.
    ISBN 0-06-046579-4
    1. Histology. I. Bridgman, Charles F.   II. Title.
QM551.T43   1989
611'.018—dc 19   88-32509
                                                                              CIP

89   90   91   92   9 8 7 6 5 4 3 2 1

INTRODUCTION TO FUNCTIONAL HISTOLOGY

IRA R. TELFORD, Ph.D.

Visiting Professor of Anatomy,
Uniformed Services University of the Health Sciences

CHARLES F. BRIDGMAN, Ph.D.

Formerly Senior Scientist,
Lister Hill National Center for Biomedical Communications,
National Library of Medicine

1817

HARPER & ROW, PUBLISHERS, New York
Grand Rapids, Philadelphia, St. Louis, San Francisco,
London, Singapore, Sydney, Tokyo

To our wives, Thelma and Amy, our families, and our students

CONTENTS

Chapter 4   *Epithelium*   59

Chapter 5   *Specializations of Epithelia— Glands, Serous and Mucous Membranes*   77

Chapter 6   *Connective Tissue*   89

Chapter 17   *Digestive System I—Oral Cavity and Pharynx*   325

Chapter 18   *Digestive System II—Alimentary Canal*   345

Chapter 26   *Organs of Special Sense—Eye and Ear*   527

Part IV   TOOLS FOR LEARNING   559

Chapter 27   *Microscopy*   561

PREFACE

Microscopic anatomy is undergoing a fundamental reconstruction, a modest revolution, especially at the molecular levels of organization and interaction. New morphological details and functions are constantly being discovered. In keeping with this spirit of discovery and change, we have written a unique, somewhat revolutionary textbook in histology. Not only do we explore subjects on the cutting edge of histophysiological research, we present concepts and data in a new, singularly unparalleled vehicle, a computer-enhanced textbook.

For the first time with a textbook, a computer-activated laser videodisc will be available. This instrument utilizes barcodes and other technologies to display a large series of full-color images on a graphics monitor. Video images from a data base of over 2500 histologic slides supplement the already exceptionally well-illustrated textbook and may replace conventional atlases in histology. Even without the optical videodisc, the textbook is complete in itself, enabling the student to achieve the educational objectives defined at the beginning of each chapter. For purchasing information on the optical videodisc, information systems, and hardware and software, see "A Visual Data Base on Optical Videodisc" on page 574.

The distinguishing features are:

1. A uniform picture-text continuity exists throughout the book. Practically every structure and concept is illustrated on the same page as the text. Rarely is the reader required to turn the page to view a figure. Such pictorial-text synthesis is accomplished by hundreds of original illustrations, photographs, and light and electron micrographs. (The illustrations were executed by one of us [C.F.B.].) Also, color is extensively used for content emphasis and contrast.
2. To help the student organize, review, and retain pertinent information, summarizing tables are placed at the end of most chapters. Such extensive summaries enable rapid and accurate retrieval of essentially all of the pertinent information covered in the text.
3. Most histological structures are tied to their origins, gross anatomical relationships, and functions. To enhance the student's comprehension of the importance of these relationships, each chapter has a clear and concise introductory statement.
4. Historical perspective is provided by identification of events and personalities that were critical in the discovery and development of important concepts. Clinical comments of special interest to the student are scattered throughout the text.
5. There is a mini full-color atlas of histological structures that look alike. Each of the 40 plates has photomicrographs of cells, tissues, or organs that closely resemble each other. These are the structures that are most commonly confused in histology. Careful study of these "look-alike" plates (referred to in the text as "L–A plates") will greatly facilitate the student's ability to distinguish quickly and accurately between similar structures. Because only the diagnostic differences, not similarities, are listed, the differentiating features between structures are immediately apparent, even to the beginning student.

The subject matter is divided into four parts: Part I—The Cell, Part II—Tissues (histology), Part III—Organ Systems (organology), and Part IV—Tools for Learning (microscopy). Basically this is a textbook of histology and organology, with limited coverage of cytology, which is usually a prerequisite to the study of microscopic anatomy. Terms used throughout the text are based on the nomenclature of the fifth edition of *Nomina Anatomica*.

Since we have taken a functional approach to microscopic anatomy, considerable space is devoted to physiological considerations. We hold with the Dutch neuroanatomist, J. Boeke, that "Histology still remains the basis for all our physiological deductions and theories. . . ." We have tried to find a balance between the morphological and physiological aspects of histology. Such a synthesis of ideas should lighten the burden for the student of histology, a prime purpose of this book.

Since another objective of the text is to provide the student with a concise yet fully illustrated account of normal histology, detailed experimental data are omitted, theoretical and controversial topics are largely avoided, and only a few references are cited. To complement the text, illustrations are frequently used to convey complicated information or concepts.

This highly pictorial, computer-assisted textbook meets the needs of students of mammalian biology and related disciplines, as well as medicine, dentistry, histopathology, and most paramedical sciences. We believe we have fulfilled our objective to present an extensively illustrated, yet succinct, synoptic version of histology, where function and structure are inextricably entwined. Furthermore, an understanding of the subject matter is greatly enhanced by the introduction of new, computerized techniques to dramatize and elucidate an already fascinating subject.

ACKNOWLEDGMENTS

We acknowledge our deep appreciation to our many colleagues for their advice and constructive criticism of the several drafts of the text. They include many faculty members of the Uniformed Services University of the Health Sciences; M. R. Adelman, R. C. Borke, M. B. Carpenter, D. S. Forman, C. H. Latker, R. P. C. Liu, D. B. Newman, M. D. Rollag, M. N. Sheridan, and especially K. J. Lynch, who, in addition to reading and evaluating several chapters, contributed to the text of Chapter 27. Also to the departmental chairman, Dr. D. C. Beebe, who has been very supportive, we express our gratitude.

We are grateful for the generosity of Dr. Martin Dym, Chairman, Department of Anatomy and Cell Biology, Georgetown University, who permitted us to draw heavily on their excellent collection of micrographs. We are also greatly indebted to Dr. F. D. Allan, Professor of Anatomy and Director of Audiovisual Services, George Washington University, School of Medicine, who, in collaboration with the staff of the Lister Hill National Center for Biomedical Communications, National Library of Medicine, accomplished the remarkable task of assembling over 2,500 superb, full-color microscopic images for an ancillary optical videodisc, a vital adjunct to our text. Most of the photomicrographs for the text were taken by Barbara Neuberger of Dr. Allan's staff.

Occasionally assisting Dr. Bridgman in the execution of the hundreds of original illustrations were Daniel Bridgman, Robin Bridgman, John A. Konstanzer, Paul Melloni, and Martin E. Nau.

We express our sincere thanks to David S. Lyons, University of Illinois, a graduate student in Mathematics and Computer Sciences, who developed the extensive barcodes found throughout the text to retrieve histologic images (except in Chapters 1 and 2).

To our secretaries, Margaret S. Grunewald, Brenda A. Perciballi, and especially Linda A. Porter, who typed most of the final copy, we express our sincerest thanks and appreciation.

Through the courtesy of The Upjohn Company, we have reproduced their full-color atlas of *Look-alikes in Histology*, which one of us (I.R.T.) prepared earlier. We would also like to acknowledge the Audiovisual Services, George Washington University Medical Center, for plates 1-30; Thomas M. Crisp, for plates 31, 32, 36a, 39, and 40; Frank Denys, for plates 37a and 37d; Joan Blanchette-Mackie, for plate 38, and the Department of Anatomy, Georgetown University Schools of Medicine and Dentistry, plates 33–36, 37b, and 37c.

Finally, we wish to acknowledge Claudia M. Wilson and Bonnie Biller for the constant guidance, interest, and total dedication to our common goals and to thank the entire book team at Harper & Row.

Ira R. Telford
Charles F. Bridgman

CREDITS

To the following individuals and publishers we are deeply appreciative for the excellent illustrative materials they so generously provided us.

Allan FD: pp. 94, 95, 105, 123, 211, 289, 311, 352, 356, 385, 494, 521.

Anders JJ: pp. 97, 573.

Andrews PM: pp. 19, 60, 64, 145, 149, 180, 291, 298, 300, 358, 362, 383, 401, 408, 410, 415, 477. -p. 316, The respiratory system. *In* Biomed. Res. Applications of SEM, GM Hodges, RC Hallows (eds.), 1979, with permission from Academic Press, San Diego, CA. -p. 404, J Electron Micros Techniques, 9:115, 1983, with permission from Alan R. Liss, Inc. -p. 413, Three Dimensional Microanatomy of Cells and Tissue Surfaces, DJ Allen, PM Motta, LJA DiDio (eds.), 1981, with permission from Elsevier/North Holland.

Banker BQ: p. 179, J Neuropath and Experi Neurology, 26:259, 1967, with permission from American Association of Neuropathologists.

Barberine F et al.: p. 513.

Bessis MC: pp. 141, 142, 151, 169, 280, Living Cells and Their Ultrastructure, 1973, with permission from Springer-Verlag, New York.

Blandau RJ: p. 496.

Borke RC: pp. 232, 233, 234, 235.

Boshell JL et al.: pp. 331, 332, Scanning Electron Microsc. III:505, 1980, with permission from Scanning Electron Microscopy.

Bourgery MJ: pp. 224, 244, 306, 326, 396, 468, 490, 528.

Brenner RM: pp. 67, 511, 564, Research Resources Reporter, p. 6, June 1980, with permission from Research Resources Information Center.

Bridgman PC, Reese TS: p. 72, J Cell Biol 99:1655, 1984, with permission from Journal of Cell Biology.

Brooks SM, Bernstein IL, Gallagher J: p. 321, Research Resources Reporter, p. 6, October 1981, with permission from Research Resources Information Center.

Claman HN: p. 280, *In* Immunology, Cellular Immunology, 1975, with permission from The Upjohn Company, Kalamazoo.

Clark R: pp. 532, 535.

Clarkson TB: p. 248, Research Resources Reporter, p. 8, September 1980, with permission of Research Resources Information Center.

Cline MJ: p. 23, Atlas of Blood Cells, Vol. I, eds. D Zucker-Franklin et al., 1981, with permission from Edi Ermes, s.r.l., Milano.

Correr S, Motta PM: pp. 434, 438, Cell and Tissue Res 215:515, 1981, with permission from Springer-Verlag.

Crisp TM: pp. 16, 17, 93.

DeSantis ME: pp. 97, 197.

Diggs LW et al.: p. 162, The Morphology of Human Blood Cells, 4/e, 1984, with permission from Abbott Laboratories, Abbott Park, IL.

Dubois FA: p. 351.

Edelson PJ: p. 106.

Engler W, Patterson RM: p. 42, Research Resources Reporter, p. 6, September 1982, with permission from Research Resources Information Center.

Engström H, Engström B: pp. 545, 546, Acta Otolaryngol 83:66–77, 1977, with permission from Acta Otolaryngologica. -p. 546, Hearing Res 1:52, 1978, with permission from Elsevier/North Holland Biomedical Press.

Fahim MA et al.: p. 204, J Neurocytology 23:13, 1983, with permission from Chapman and Hall, Ltd.

Fajer AB: p. 570.

Fawcett DW: p. 34, The Cell, 2/e, 1981, with permission from WB Saunders Co, Philadelphia.

Fazd A: p. 246.

Fujita T. Tanaka K, Tokunaga J: pp. 63, 141, 273, 275, 311, 315, 349, 510, SEM Atlas of Cells and Tissue, 1981, with permission from Igaku-Shoin, Tokyo.

Georgetown University Anatomical Collection: pp. 7, 9, 14, 20, 21, 22, 23, 35, 66, 68, 69, 85, 94, 101, 114, 129, 147,

148, 172, 178, 179, 181, 183, 184, 206, 252, 258 293, 298, 336, 337, 357, 374, 435, 436, 455, 498, 513, 564.

Gould KG: p. 514, Research Resources Reporter, p. 9, December 1980, with permission from Research Resources Information Center.

Henkart M: p. 150, Research Resources Reporter, April 1983, with permission from Research Resources Information Center.

Hirokawa N: pp. 47, 358, J Cell Biol, 94:425, 1982, with permission from Rockefeller University Press.

Hodson WA, Luchtel D: pp. 317, 319, Research Resources Reporter, p. 6, October 1981, with permission from Research Resources Information Center.

Hruban Z: p. 19.

Jacobson CB: pp. 36, 37.

Jerome WG: pp. 16, 20, 384.

Johnson RS: p. 41.

Kachar B, Behar T, Dubois-Dalcq M: pp. 236, 566, Cell and Tissue Res, 244:27, 1986, with permission from Springer-Verlag.

Kapur SP: pp. 354, 365, Acta Anat 112:224, 1982, with permission from S. Karger AG.

Keene SC: p. 175.

Koering MJ: pp. 65, 84, 85, 118, 178, 237, 253, 258, 310, 313, 315, 356, 360, 362, 381, 386, 402, 403, 405, 473, 478, 511, 567.

Leak LV: pp. 83, 96, 107, 145, 254, Bibliotheca Anatomica 17:115–135, 1979, with permission from S. Karger AG.

Lederberg EM: p. 36, Research Resources Reporter, p. 13, June 1983, with permission from Research Resources Information Center.

Lessin LS: pp. 138, 140, 142, 143, 146, 148, 158, 164, 280.

Lynch KJ: pp. 6, 10, 12.

Matsuda S, Uehara Y: pp. 190, 195, 210, J Electron Microsc 30:136, 1981, with permission from J Electron Microscopy.

McQuarrie IG: p. 199, J Comp Neurol 231:239, 1985, with permission from Alan R. Liss, Inc.

Merrill TG: pp. 66, 86, 267, 355, 362.

Motta PM: pp. 104, 383, 496.

Motta PM: pp. 387, 388, Three Dimensional Microanatomy of Cells and Tissue Surfaces, DJ Allen, PM Motta, LJA DiDio (eds.), 1981, with permission from Elsevier–North Holland.

Motta PM, Porter KR: p. 107, Cell Tissue Res 148:111, 1974, with permission from Springer-Verlag.

Motta PM, Van Blerkom J: p. 512, Cell Tissue Res 163:34, 1975, with permission from Springer-Verlag.

Nagato T et al.: pp. 60, 78, 81, 523, Cells and Tissue Res 209:1, 1980, with permission from Springer-Verlag.

Newman DB: pp. 193, 299, 230, 231, 334, 565.

Niederkorn JY: p. 317, Research Resources Reporter, p. 13, October 1982, with permission from Research Resources Information Center.

Nonomura Y: p. 10, J Mol Biol 60:303, 1971, with permission from Academic Press.

Okagaki T, Clark B, Fisch RO: p. 473, Scan Elect Micro (3):413, 1980, with permission from Scanning Electron Microscopy.

Pappas GD: p. 197.

Parsons DF: p. 39, Research Resources Reporter, p. 13, June 1982, with permission from Research Resources Information Center.

Payer AF: pp. 23, 475.

Phillips DM: pp. 41, 514, Research Resources Reporter, p. 3, May 1983, with permission from Research Resources Information Center.

Porter KR: p. 11, In DW Fawcett's The Cell, 1966, with permission from WB Saunders Company, Philadelphia.

Porter KR, Anderson KL: p. 70.

Porter KR, Tucker JB: p. 71, Sci Am 244:59, 1981, with permission from Scientific American, Inc.

Robison WG, Jr.: pp. 535, 536.

Russell TE, Kapur SP: p. 121, Oral Implantation, Vol VII, No. 3, 1977, with permission from the American Academy of Implant Dentistry.

Sappey MPC: p. 264.

Seegmiller JE: p. 15.

Sheridan MN: p. 464.

Siew S: p. 363.

Simionescu N: p. 247, In Histology, L. Weiss, RO Greep, 4/e, with permission from Elsevier Science Publishing Company, New York.

Tanaka K et al.: pp. 457, 519, SEM Atlas of Cells and Tissues, 1981, with permission from Igaku-Shoin, Tokyo.

Tortora GJ, Anagnostakos NP: p. 161, Principles of Human Anatomy and Physiology, 5/e, 1986, with permission from Harper & Row, New York.

Van Blerkom J, Motta P: pp. 496, 500, 503,
    Cellular Basis of Mammalian
    Reproduction, 1979, with permission
    from Urban and Schwarzenberg,
    Baltimore.
Van de Spiegel A: pp. 286, 508.
Willingham MC, Pastan I: p. 565, An Atlas
    of Immunofluorescence in Cultured
    Cells, 1985, with permission from

Academic Press, Orlando, FL.
Wright GM, Leblond CP: p. 127, J.
    Histochem and Cytochem, 29:791, 1981,
    with permission from the Histochemical
    Society.
Zucker-Franklin D et al.: pp. 32, 147, 280,
    281, Atlas of Blood Cells, Vol. I, 1981,
    with permission from Edi Ermes, s.r.l.,
    Milano.

Equivalent Lengths

10 angstroms (Å)	=	1 nanometer (nm)
1,000 nanometers	=	1 micron (μm)
1,000 microns	=	1 millimeter (mm)
10 millimeters	=	1 centimeter (cm)
100 centimeters	=	1 meter (m)

ABBREVIATIONS

Å	Angstrom (1/10 of nanometer)
ACTH	Adrenocorticotropic hormone
ADH	Antidiuretic hormone (vasopressin)
ADP	Adenosine diphosphate
AMP	Adenosine monophosphate
ANS	Autonomic nervous system
APUD	Cells with the capability of an *amine precursor uptake* and *decarboxylation*
ATP	Adenosine triphosphate
A-V	Arteriovenous
AVB or AVN	Atrioventricular bundle or node
BMR	Basal metabolic rate
CHO	Carbohydrates
CNS	Central nervous system
CRF	Corticotropin-releasing factor
CSF	Cerebral spinal fluid
ct	Connective tissue
CV	Cardiovascular
DCT	Distal convoluted tubule
DNA	Deoxyribonucleic acid
DOPA	Dihydroxyphenylalanine
EM	Electron microscope
ER	Endoplasmic reticulum
Fr.	French
FSH	Follicle-stimulating hormone
FSHRF	Follicle-stimulating hormone releasing factor
G	Ganglia
GAG	Glycosaminoglycans
Ger.	German
GI	Gastrointestinal
GH	Growth hormone
GHRF	Growth hormone releasing factor
GHRIF	Growth hormone release-inhibiting factor
GU	Genitourinary
H&E	Hematoxylin and eosin stain
HCG	Human chorionic gonadotrophin
HCS	Human chorionic somatomammotropin
ICSH	Interstitial cell stimulating hormone
IgG	Gamma-G globulin (immunoglobin G)
JGC	Juxtaglomerular cells or complexes
L.	Latin
L-A	Look-alike structures
LH	Luteinizing hormone
LHRF	Luteinizing hormone releasing factor
LM	Light microscope
LTH	Lactogenic or luteotropic hormone
mm	Millimeter (1000 μm)
mOsm	Milliosmols
MRF	Melanocyte-releasing factor
mRNA	Messenger RNA (transfer RNA)
MS	Multiple sclerosis
MSH	Melanocyte-stimulating hormone
MW	Molecular weight
nm	Nanometer (10 Angstroms)
PAS	Periodic acid-Schiff's reaction
PCT	Proximal convoluted tubule
PIF or PIH	Prolactin-inhibiting factor or hormone
pH	Hydrogen ion concentration
PNS	Peripheral nervous system
PRF	Prolactin-releasing factor
PTH	Parathyroid hormone
RBC	Red blood cell(s)
REF	Renal erythropoietic factor
RER or rER	Rough endoplasmic reticulum
RES	Reticuloendothelial system
RNA	Ribonucleic acid
rRNA	Ribosomal RNA
SAN	Sinoauricular node
SEM	Scanning electron microscope
SER or sER	Smooth endoplasmic reticulum
SRF	Somatotropin-releasing factor
STH	Somatotropin (growth hormone)
T$_3$	Triiodotryronine
T$_4$	Tetraiodothyronine (thyroxin)
TEM	Transmission electron microscope
TRF	Thyrotropin-releasing factor
tRNA	Transfer RNA (messenger RNA)
TSH	Thyroid-stimulating hormone
μm	Micrometer (1000 nm)
μ	Micron; older synonym for micrometer
WBC	White blood cell(s)

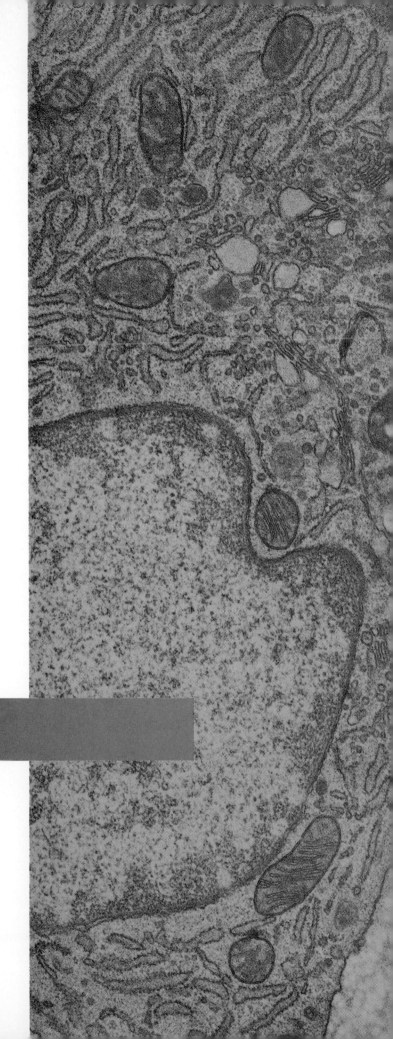

Part

I

THE CELL

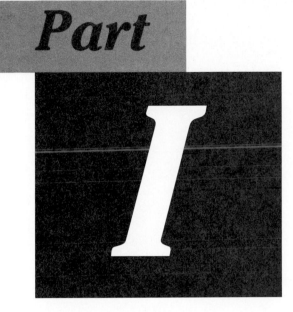

Chapter

1

CYTOPLASMIC ORGANELLES AND INCLUSIONS

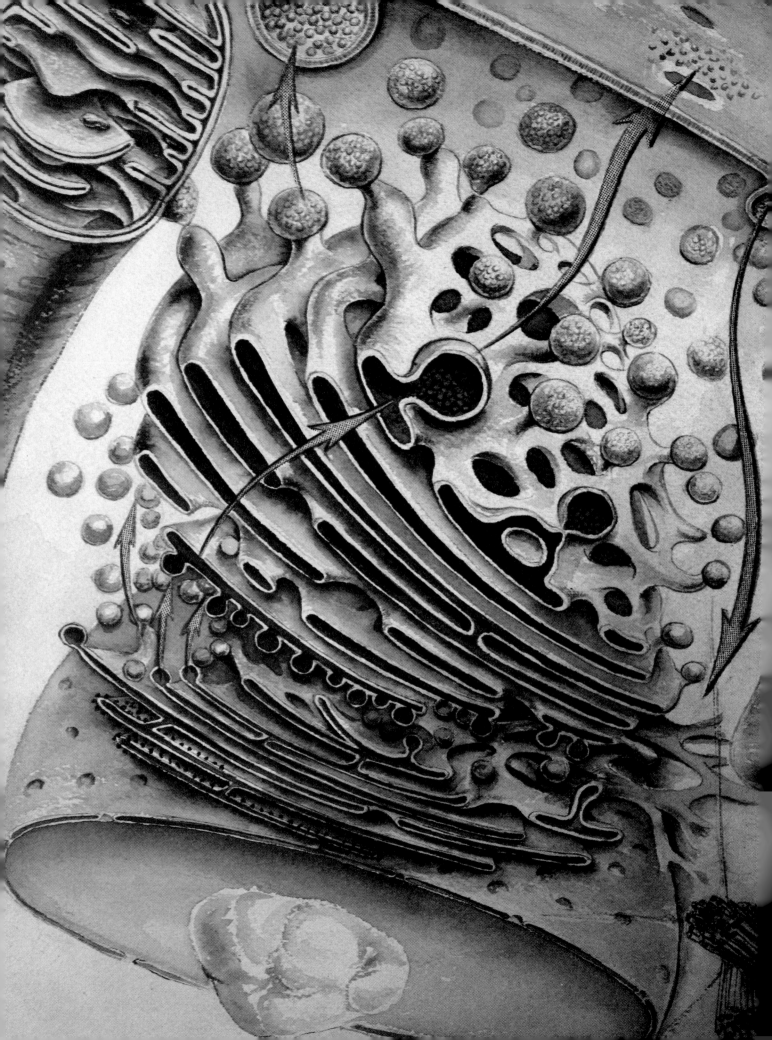

OBJECTIVES

FROM READING THIS CHAPTER, ONE SHOULD BE ABLE TO:

1. Identify various cellular organelles and inclusions by relative size and distinctive morphology, as seen with the light and electron microscopes.

2. Analyze how the characteristic structural detail of each organelle enables it to perform essential functions within the cell.

3. Follow sequential steps in the synthesis of various cellular products and know the function of each structure involved in a specific process.

4. Classify intracellular components into various categories as to their importance for the proper functioning of a cell, e.g., essential, nonessential, facilitative but not necessary, harmful, etc.

5. Gain a perspective of size relationships of objects and the range of magnification with various types of microscopes.

In 1665, Robert Hooke, curator of the Royal Society of London, examined razor-thin slices of cork under his very simple microscope. He discovered small, boxlike spaces which he named **cells.** A few years later, the Italian anatomist, M. Malpighi, described similar structures in animal tissues which he called vesicles or utricles. In 1672, the English botanist N. Grew published two extensively illustrated volumes greatly extending Hooke's findings. Thus, the concept of the cell as a **unit of structure** in the plant and animal kingdoms was launched.

However, it was two centuries later before scientists generally accepted the idea that the cell is the fundamental structural unit of living organisms, analogous to the atom as the fundamental unit in chemical structures. It also became widely accepted that the cell may remain separate as a complete organism, for example, as a protozoan, or cells may join together to produce tissues and organs which form a complex multicellular organism.

Today, the cell is recognized as a microcosm of the organism it populates. It usually has a complete complement of essential organelles whose functions are similar to the organs of the body the cell occupies. This intriguing concept will be a recurring theme in this chapter.

THE CELL

The cell, as the structural and functional unit of the body, is a mass of protoplasm divided into two compartments, the cytoplasm and the nucleus. The extensive **cytoplasm,** a complex, aqueous, colloidal gel, is limited by the cell membrane (plasmalemma). Within the cytoplasm are sequestered carbohydrates, proteins, fats, inorganic salts, and water. The **nucleus** is limited by two nuclear membranes, i.e., the nuclear envelope, and is filled with nucleoplasm that contains genetic information encoded in the deoxyribonucleic acid (DNA) molecules. The DNA is the principal component of chromatin in the nucleus that condenses into chromosomes.

Suspended in the cytoplasm are essential **organelles** (L., small organs), e.g., the mitochondria, Golgi apparatus, lysosomes, and others; these may be analogous to certain organs of the body. Also free in the cytoplasm are nonliving **inclusions,** which are usually transitory structures, such as pigments and stored food vacuoles. Many of these inert bodies are quite as necessary for the normal functioning of the cell as the living organelles. While the intact cell can usually perpetuate its individual existence, neither the organelles nor inclusions can maintain their entities outside the cell. Hence, the endowment of life is a characteristic of the intact cell and not of its parts.

CYTOPLASMIC ORGANELLES

Organelles, vital subunits of the cell, include mitochondria, endoplasmic reticulum (rough and smooth), ribosomes, the Golgi apparatus, lysosomes, centrioles, microbodies (peroxisomes), microtubules, microfilaments, annulate lamellae, and the very important plasmalemma, including its derivatives. (See Table 1.1.)

Plasmalemma

The **plasmalemma** (cell membrane) is a thin (8–10 nm), flexible, dynamic barrier between the organized, living particles within the cell and the nonliving disorder without. As a **selective barrier,** it is responsible for generating and maintaining the difference between the external and internal environment of the cell. It is the site of **transport** of molecules and particles in and out of the living cell. For example, hormone receptors are sites in the plasmalemma that allow a certain hormone to enter or prevent the entrance of another hormone. Also, the transmission of nervous impulses occurs along the length of a cell membrane. Furthermore, the exchange of information between cells occurs through their cell membranes.

The plasmalemma cannot be seen with the light microscope (LM) but can be resolved, in section, with the transmission electron microscope (TEM). It reveals an apparent **trilaminar structure** consisting of two electron-dense layers and a central electron-lucent layer. The earlier researchers called this structure the **unit membrane** since it surrounds all cells as well as membrane-bound particles within the cell. This trilaminar structure was viewed as being static, reflecting the arrangement of phospholipids into a bilayer. The central portion contains phospholipid side chains, while the outer layers contain the polar head groups of the phospholipids and most of the protein of the membrane.

Later, dissatisfaction with this model arose largely because it views all membranes as similar and static. However, membranes vary considerably in thickness, show some asymmetry, and their proteinaceous elements can move about in the plane of the membrane. Therefore, in the early 1970s, Singer and Nicolson proposed a **fluid mosaic model** for the structure of the unit membrane which is now generally accepted. They postulated that the lipids, proteins, and carbohydrates that comprise the unit membrane are arranged in the following patterns:

1. The **lipids,** mostly phospholipids, form a **central bimolecular layer** where the long hydrophobic (lipid-soluble) hydrocarbon chains (tails) are attached to the hydrophilic (lipid-insoluble) globular polar portions of the molecule. These head portions are directed outward, while the nonpolar chains project towards the center of the membrane where they interact with the tails of

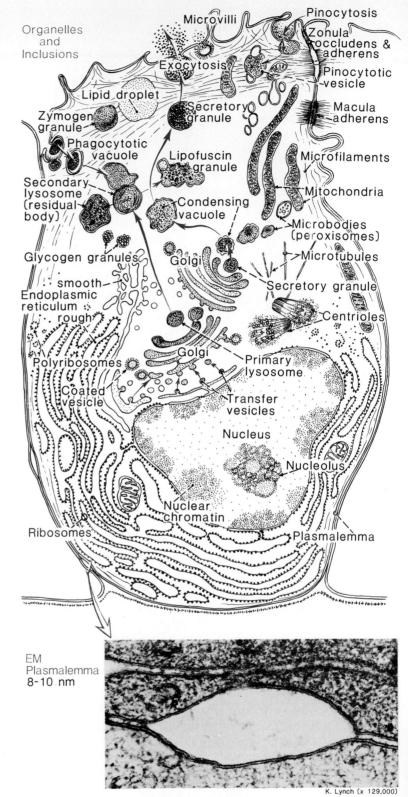

EM Plasmalemma 8-10 nm

K. Lynch (x 129,000)

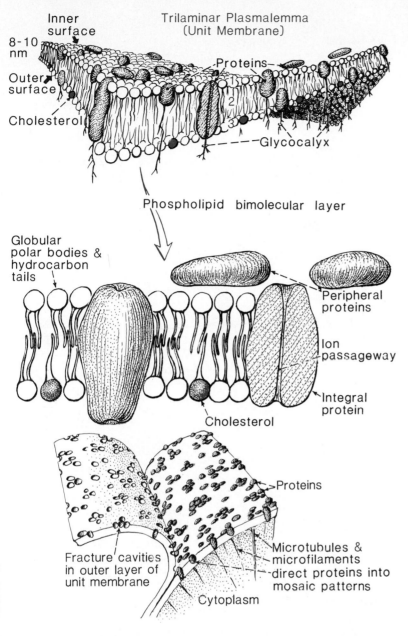

Inner surface

8-10 nm

Outer surface

Cholesterol

Trilaminar Plasmalemma (Unit Membrane)

Proteins

Glycocalyx

Phospholipid bimolecular layer

Globular polar bodies & hydrocarbon tails

Peripheral proteins

Ion passageway

Integral protein

Cholesterol

Proteins

Fracture cavities in outer layer of unit membrane

Microtubules & microfilaments direct proteins into mosaic patterns

Cytoplasm

EM Glycocalyx of polysaccharides -site of immune responses

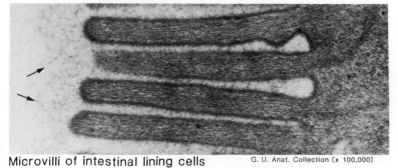

Microvilli of intestinal lining cells

G. U. Anat. Collection (x 100,000)

the opposite phospholipid layer, thus creating a **hydrophobic milieu** within the membrane.

The molecular forces holding components of the bilayer together are quite weak in the plane of the membrane, and therefore the phospholipid molecules can move freely within the layer. Hence, the plasmalemma has considerable lateral fluidity since the hydrocarbon tails are freely mobile.

2. Many **protein molecules** are associated with the phospholipid layer. In fact, they may represent 60–70% of the total mass of the membrane. Depending on their position in the membrane, they are identified as **peripheral proteins**, which loosely associate with the globular polar heads of the phospholipid layer, or integral membrane proteins, which are more tightly associated with the bilayer. These peripheral proteins may lie outside the bilayer or interdigitate somewhat between the lipid molecules. The integral membrane proteins may extend across the entire bilayer (**transmembrane proteins**). They have been described as "icebergs in a lipid sea." Those that extend completely through the lipid bilayer may provide a passageway for ions and other water-soluble materials to pass in and out of the cell. It also has been proposed that these integral protein molecules function as pores for the transfer of hydrophilic molecules.

With the acceptance of these two concepts, (1) that the plasmalemma is a quasi-fluid structure and (2) that it allows some movement of the integral proteins to occur, the idea of a **mosaic fluid structure** was established. However, the movement of these proteins is not random but controlled by intracellular organelles, such as microtubules and microfilaments, which may cause the proteins to congregate at certain locations or sites, suggesting a mosaic pattern.

3. On the exterior surface, another component of the cell membrane is located. It is composed of short chains of **polysaccharides** that are linked either to lipids as **glycolipids** or to proteins as **glycoproteins**. These delicate strands project from the external surfaces of the plasmalemma as an amorphous filmy covering called the **glycocalyx**, originally given the prosaic name "fuzz."

In addition to being a protective covering, this nondescript fuzzy layer has important functions in specific reactions between cells. It is the **site for the binding** of certain molecules, such as hormones. The glycocalyx is also the **site for immunological responses** and is involved in cell recognition. It may vary with each cell type. For example, it is thick on intestinal lining cells and thin on myelin sheaths.

The glycocalyx also functions as an **adhesive** to hold cells together and to **aid cells in recognizing each other** during development so that normal synchronous growth results. When it is removed or damaged, the cell is recognized as foreign and is destroyed by the body's immune system. Since malignant cells have an abnormal cell coat, they are usually destroyed before the cancer develops. However, if a breakdown of the immune system occurs, the damaged cells may multiply rapidly to form a life-threatening cancerous tumor.

4. **Cholesterol** is a prominent constituent of the cell membrane. It is present in nearly the same molar concentration as the phospholipids. Being a lipid, it readily associates with the long phospholipid chains, which changes their molecular configuration and movement. Therefore, cholesterol may determine how fluid or static the membrane will be under given conditions.

The contour of the plasma membrane varies greatly in the various cells. For example, it may project outward as minute finger-like folds, the microvilli, or project inward as pinocytotic vesicles, which become detached from the membrane as cytoplasmic vesicles or vacuoles. Other cells have an extensive network of irregular, membrane-bound, fluid-filled canals, the endoplasmic reticulum.

Endoplasmic Reticulum (ER)

This delicate network is (1) a series of hollow, flattened, anastomosing tubules; and (2) membranous, bladder-like structures called **vesicles** (L. vesicula, a small bladder). When flattened, the vesicles are termed **cisternae** (L. cisterna, cistern). Two types of ER are usually distinguishable: (1) **agranular or smooth** (sER), a delicate, branching network of tubules free of ribosomes; and (2) **granular or rough** (rER), a complex system of branching canals and tubules and flattened sacs or cisternae richly studded with **ribosomes** on their cytoplasmic face. (L-A, plate 31)

The rough endoplasmic reticulum (rER) appears granular in electron micrographs because much of its outer surface is covered by **ribosomes**. The rER consists of a series of interlocking membrane-bound canals in a pattern of flattened cisternae and long, branching tubules. The thickness of the membranes of the endoplasmic reticulum is about 6–7 nm, considerably thinner than the plasmalemma (8–10 nm). In addition to the network of canals, some cisternae have openings called **fenestrae** (L., windows). The potential for protein synthesis is directly related to the number of ribosomes attached to the reticulum. It is this system of tubules and ribosomes that forms the mechanism for the **synthesis and distribution of proteins.**

The smooth endoplasmic reticulum (sER) is a tubular network **free of ribosomes.** It is a membrane-bound, organized system with several enzyme sites. A major function is the **synthesis of steroids**, especially steroid hormones, while the sER of the liver functions primarily in the **degradation of hormones and drugs.**

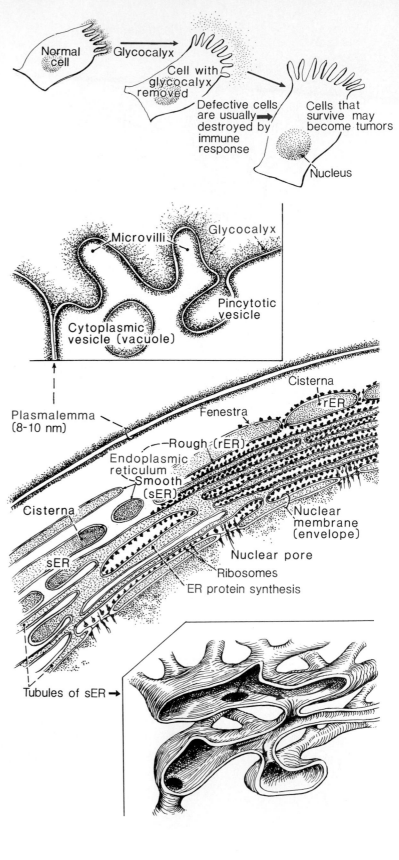

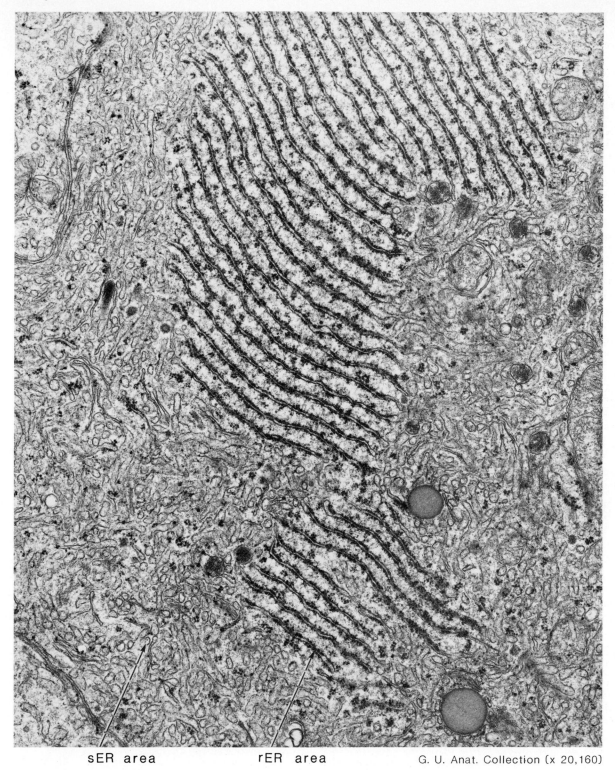

sER area   rER area   G. U. Anat. Collection (x 20,160)

In this EM micrograph of a secretory (liver) cell, the dominant organelles are the rough and smooth endoplasmic reticulum. The rER has many flattened cisterna with dilated extremities. Myriad ribosomes are embedded in the outer surface of the cisternal membranes. In H&E staining, the intense basophilia of the cell is due to the strong affinity for basic dyes of the RNA located in the ribosomes. Within the cisternae, the translation of messenger RNA into secretory proteins occurs. In contrast, the sER is a discontinuous, tubular network, free of ribosomes and possessing no specific staining reaction.

Ribosomes

Ribosomes are small, roughly spherical particles about 15–25 nm in diameter that participate in the **synthesis of protein.** They are found in all cells except mature red blood cells. They cannot be visualized with the light microscope but, when present in sufficient numbers, they stain deeply with basic dyes and were earlier called chromidial substance or **ergastoplasm.** With the EM, ribosomes can be seen to consist of **two subunits;** the larger unit is about twice the size of the smaller.

About 85% of the RNA is classified **ribosomal RNA (rRNA).** The remainder is either messenger RNA (mRNA) or transfer RNA (tRNA). Each type has unique functions in the **synthesis of peptides and proteins** in a cell. The process begins when RNA becomes associated with other proteins in the nucleolus to form the subunits of ribosomes which pass through the pores of the nuclear envelope to enter the cytoplasm, where they are assembled. Ribosomes in the cytoplasm, with the assistance of the other RNA types, bring about the **assembly of specific amino acids into polypeptides.**

Simultaneous with the assembly of ribosomes within the nucleus, **mRNA is formed on a template** of an uncoiled strand of deoxyribonucleic acid (DNA). Here it receives the replica or information (message) for the correct sequence of the specific amino acids required for the synthesis of new proteins. Similarly, **tRNA** is entering the cytoplasm from the nucleus. It is coupled by appropriate enzymes (synthetases) to the specific amino acid for which the tRNA has a **codon** (a triplet of nucleotides that specifies a particular amino acid in proteins). The interaction of tRNA and an amino acid complex with a corresponding codon in the mRNA sequence occurs on the ribosome, and a **specific protein is formed.**

Thus the ribosome acts as a **support scaffolding** for amino acids that are picked up and transferred by tRNA to the ribosome. Here the amino acids are inserted into the forming polypeptide chain in a sequence dictated by the message translated from the mRNA.

These ribosomes are arranged in linear groups along a strand of mRNA like beads on a string. Each ribosome is released from the string when the synthesis is completed.

Ribosomes are of two types. The **free ribosomes** are not attached to the rER, i.e., they are free floating in the cytoplasm and are primarily involved in synthesis of **protein for internal use** in the cell. The other type, attached to the rER, is involved in **protein production for export** or external use, e.g., secretion of enzymes.

Ribosomes, whether free or attached, may exist singly or in clusters. The latter are arranged in a beadlike fashion in a **rosette** or in helical configurations called **polyribosomes.** The lifespan of ribosomes is probably quite short, for when protein synthesis ceases, they disappear.

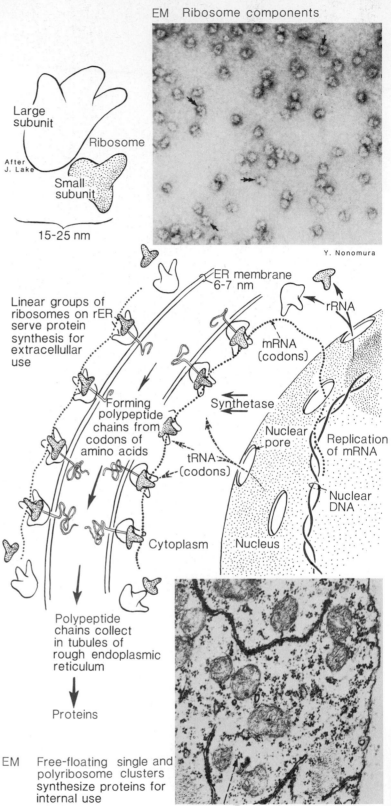

EM Ribosome components

Y. Nonomura

Linear groups of ribosomes on rER serve protein synthesis for extracellullar use

ER membrane 6-7 nm

rRNA

mRNA (codons)

Synthetase

Forming polypeptide chains from codons of amino acids

Nuclear pore

Replication of mRNA

tRNA (codons)

Nuclear DNA

Cytoplasm

Nucleus

Polypeptide chains collect in tubules of rough endoplasmic reticulum

Proteins

EM Free-floating single and polyribosome clusters synthesize proteins for internal use

Rosettes   K. Lynch (x 51,680)

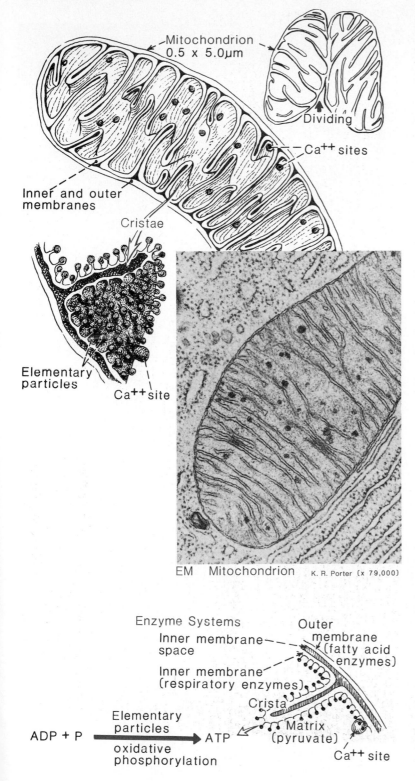

Mitochondrion
0.5 x 5.0μm

Dividing

Ca⁺⁺ sites

Inner and outer membranes

Cristae

Elementary particles

Ca⁺⁺ site

EM   Mitochondrion   K. R. Porter (x 79,000)

Enzyme Systems

Inner membrane space

Inner membrane (respiratory enzymes)

Outer membrane (fatty acid enzymes)

Crista

Matrix (pyruvate)

Ca⁺⁺ site

Elementary particles

oxidative phosphorylation

ADP + P → ATP

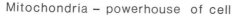

Mitochondria – powerhouse of cell

Mitochondria

Under the light microscope **mitochondria** appear as small, threadlike or ovoid bodies about 0.2–1.0 μm $\times$ 0.3–5.0 μm. They vary greatly in number depending on the function and metabolic state of the cell, ranging from a few in lymphocytes to several thousand in liver cells. With the phase-contrast microscope, mitochondria in living cells can be observed constantly moving, changing their shape, and dividing.

Electron micrographs reveal most mitochondria to be **rod-shaped or ovoid membranous structures.** They have an outer investing membrane and an inner, extensively folded membrane whose deep folds, extending to the center or beyond, are called **cristae.** The space between the cristae is filled with an amorphous matrix containing **electron-dense granules** that may be **binding sites for calcium** ions. All of these membranes are smooth, trilaminar unit membranes.

The membrane of the crista is modified by minute disk- or ball-shaped, repeating units projecting on slender stalks from its surface. These are the **elementary particles** which contain some of the enzymes involved in oxidative phosphorylation. The extensive folding of the inner membrane greatly increases the surface area available for the action of the respiratory enzymes involved in **adenosine triphosphate (ATP)** production. The ATP thus synthesized is the high-energy compound that **sustains aerobic life processes.** To accomplish this function, mitochondria contain at least the following **three enzyme chains** or systems:

1. **Glucose** is broken down by enzymes in the cytoplasm to **pyruvate,** with the formation of some ATP, which is sequestered in the matrix of the mitochondria. Through a series of enzymatic processes, called **the Krebs** (citric acid) **cycle,** the pyruvate is eventually converted to CO_2 and H_2O with the production of more ATP. The H_2O forms from H^+ and OH^- ions after a series of intermediate reactions.

2. The liberated hydrogen is fed into another enzyme system, the electron-transport system or **respiratory chain.** For each pair of hydrogen ions in the system, three ATP molecules are produced. The enzymes, flavoproteins, and cytochromes involved in the process are located on the inner mitochondrial membrane that forms the cristae.

3. The **oxidative phosphorylation** of adenosine diphosphate (ADP) to ATP occurs in the **elementary particles.** These are multiprotein complexes that form part of the inner mitochondrial membrane.

Thus mitochondria obtain energy from food by enzymatic action, then convert it into a form readily usable by all cells. Mitochondria are truly the powerhouse of the cell.

Golgi Complex

The Golgi apparatus (complex) was first described, by Camillo Golgi in 1898, as a network of filaments and granules near the nucleus of nerve cells. Considerable controversy arose about its reality because it could not be demonstrated in routine preparations. In fact, it was seen only in cells impregnated with silver salts or osmium and even then with only erratic success. Yet, in conventional staining procedures its location was indicated by a clear, unstained area near the nucleus, the so-called **negative Golgi.** Only with the advent of the electron microscope was its ubiquitous presence established in all living cells, except erythrocytes and keratinized epithelial cells.

From electron micrographs the **Golgi apparatus** is visualized as a series of six to eight **smooth-surfaced membranes,** each about 6 nm thick. They are arranged as **curved flattened saccules** (cisternae) stacked on one another like plates about 30 nm apart. Their cavities are filled with fluid and greatly expand during active secretory activity. (L-A, plate 32)

The **cisternae** are compressed at their centers to resemble a stack of shallow bowls—producing a **convex or forming (cis) face,** and a **concave or maturing (trans) face.** The peripheries of the cisternae are somewhat dilated to form rounded **vesicles** ranging from 40 to 80 nm in diameter, many containing electron-dense lipoidal material. Most of these vesicles are smooth surfaced; however, a few are covered by short filaments, the so-called **coated vesicles.**

The functions of the Golgi apparatus and associated structures are summarized as follows:

1. Ribosomes on the rER synthesize **polypeptides,** which are collected in the lumen of the rER.

2. Polypeptides are incorporated into small **transfer vesicles** that bud off the ribosome-free surface of the margins of the rER. These "shuttle" vesicles may be smooth surfaced or "coated."

3. The **shuttle vesicles** migrate and fuse to the cis surface of the Golgi apparatus where the polypeptides are released into the lumen of the cisternae (saccules).

4. In the **saccules,** carbohydrates are added to form **glycoproteins,** which condense the "package."

5. The newly formed protein is enclosed in a membranous sac that buds off the maturing (concave) Golgi face as the **primary storage granule.**

6. The "packaged" protein is concentrated by dehydration in a condensing vacuole. The membrane-bound protein is later recognized as a **secretory granule** awaiting release from the apical end of the cell.

LM   Golgi Apparatus

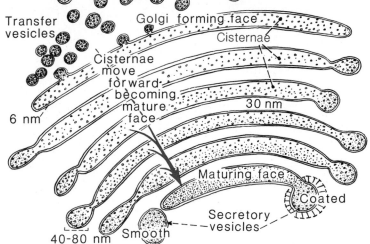

Negative   Positive

EM   Golgi Apparatus

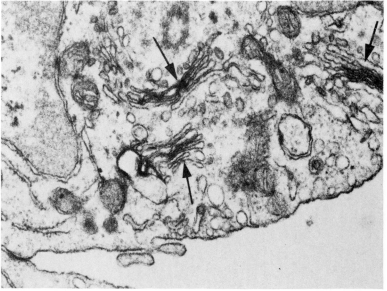

K. Lynch (x 37,400)

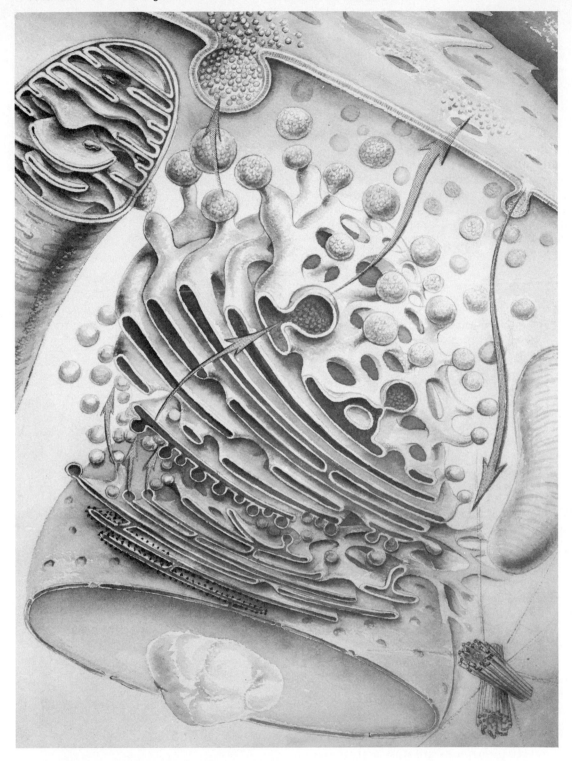

At the base of the sketch, superimposed on the nucleus, are several cisternae of rER which bud off transfer vesicles filled with proteins. These vesicles migrate to and fuse with the forming face of the Golgi apparatus. The synthesized proteins within the vesicles enter the lumen of the Golgi saccules (cisternae). Here the proteins are modified and become the secretory (zymogen) granules which are released from the secretory face of the Golgi. Most of the carbohydrate component of the secretory granules is added in the Golgi saccules. The zymogen granules move towards and fuse with the plasmalemma at the apex of the cell to discharge their contents (upper left) by the process of exocytosis. At upper right, the reverse process is occurring, namely, endocytosis (pinocytosis), where materials, mostly water, are brought into the cell.

7. **Primary lysosomes** also arise from the Golgi maturing face. Their enzymes are produced in the rER, which then collect in the Golgi complex. Here a carbohydrate component is added before the enzyme-rich, membrane-bound vacuoles are released from the Golgi as primary lysosomes.

It is convenient to visualize that the membrane of the forming face of the Golgi is constantly being added to by the transfer vesicles, while membrane of the maturing face is being lost by the production of secretory granules and lysosomes. Thus a **dynamic balance** is maintained between the **rate of accretion** of new membrane on the convex (forming) surface and the **loss of membrane** on the concave (maturing) surface. This activity waxes and wanes during the secretory cycle.

Lysosomes

Lysosomes are the **digestive and excretory systems** of the cell. They are heterogeneous organelles enclosed within a unit membrane, varying greatly in size from 25–50 nm for primary lysosomes, to 0.3 μm in secondary types. They may contain 30 to 40 **digestive (hydrolytic) enzymes** capable of breaking down intracellular substances, such as proteins, polysaccharides, etc. The most constant and characteristic enzyme is **acid phosphatase.** It is important to realize that these are bags of enzymes that must be kept separated from the other cellular constituents by their intact unit membranes, otherwise cell autolysis will result.

Their shape and density vary greatly depending on the type of cell and its function. Thus, lysosomes cannot always be accurately identified; however, they may be **classified** functionally and morphologically as follows:

1. The **primary lysosome,** or storage body, is produced by the budding-off of a vesicle on the maturing face of the Golgi body. Its matrix has a homogeneous, granular appearance and contains only latent enzymes. It is in a resting or storage state.

2. A **secondary lysosome** is formed when the limiting membrane of one or more primary lysosomes fuses with a **phagosome** (a membrane-bound vesicle brought into the cell by endocytosis). Digestive enzymes are now activated and proceed to break down the ingested material. Digestion of worn-out organelles and other intracellular substances also occurs. Both processes may leave behind remnants of undigested material often arranged as electron-dense whorls, the so-called **myelin figures.**

Functions of Golgi and Associated Structures:

- Peptides synthesized by ribosomes on rER
- Peptides form polypeptides by peptide bonds
- Transfer vesicles containing polypeptides fuse with Golgi
- Enzymes convert polypeptides into proteins
- Proteins "packaged" into sacs which bud off Golgi
- Proteins released from cell as secretory granules
- Primary lysosomes released from Golgi

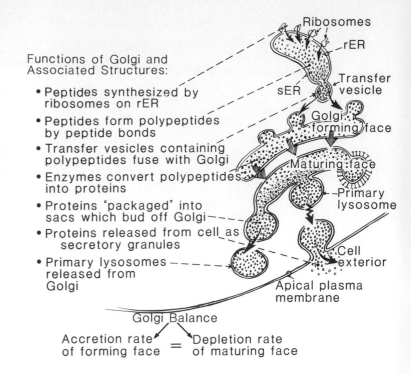

Golgi Balance

Accretion rate of forming face = Depletion rate of maturing face

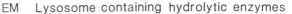
EM   Lysosome containing hydrolytic enzymes

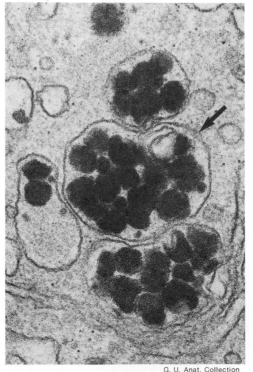

Intact unit membranes of enzyme packets prevent cell lysis

G. U. Anat. Collection

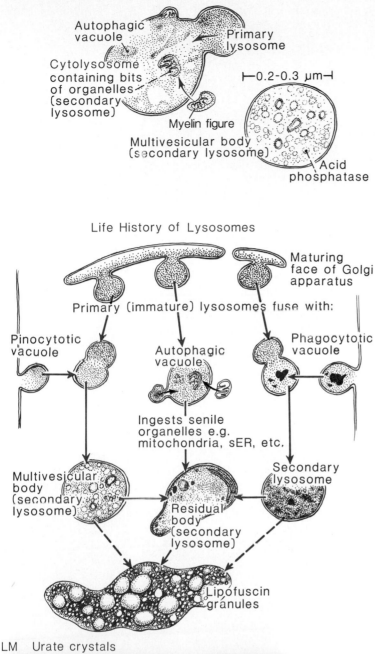

Autophagic vacuole

Primary lysosome

Cytolysosome containing bits of organelles (secondary lysosome)

├─0.2-0.3 μm─┤

Myelin figure

Multivesicular body (secondary lysosome)

Acid phosphatase

Life History of Lysosomes

Maturing face of Golgi apparatus

Primary (immature) lysosomes fuse with:

Pinocytotic vacuole

Autophagic vacuole

Phagocytotic vacuole

Ingests senile organelles e.g. mitochondria, sER, etc.

Multivesicular body (secondary lysosome)

Residual body (secondary lysosome)

Secondary lysosome

Lipofuscin granules

LM   Urate crystals

Gout - precipitation of urate crystals in joints results in leaking of lysosomal enzymes from leukocytes that have phagocytized crystals

J. E. Seegmiller

3. **A residual body** is a senile, exhausted secondary lysosome packed with the insoluble dregs of cellular metabolism, e.g., lipid pigments, myelin figures, perhaps bits of asbestos and silica, and cellular debris. These residues may accumulate until they can be seen with the light microscope as the yellowish-gold, fluorescent pigment, **lipofuscin.** It is also called old age or wear-and-tear pigment because it represents the end products of lysosomal activity that are sequestered in the cell during the aging process.

4. Another type of secondary lysosome is the **autophagocytic vacuole**, which arises from bits of functionless organelles, e.g., mitochondria, ribosomes, and rER that coalesce into membrane-bound vacuoles. Like phagosomes, they may fuse with primary lysosomes to form secondary lysosomes. They increase in number after tissue trauma, in starvation, and with aging. Often one can distinguish within them fragments of various organelles, especially mitochondria.

5. **Multivesicular bodies** are membrane-bound vacuoles about 0.2–0.3 μm in diameter, containing numerous **vesicles with acid phosphatase** in their matrix. The source of these vesicles is probably from fusion of pinocytotic vesicles. They apparently act as secondary lysosomes.

The normal functioning of lysosomes is largely dependent upon the integrity of their membranes, which must remain impermeable to the enclosed enzymes. If the membrane ruptures, as may occur in exposure to radiation, bacterial toxins, and anoxia, the hydrolytic enzymes are released into the cytoplasm and the cell is destroyed by autolysis.

In summary, the functions of lysosomes are (1) digestion of phagocytized material, e.g., bacteria and fungi; (2) digestion of worn out cell organelles (autophagy); (3) in cell death, the dissolution of the cell itself; and (4) resorption of tissues no longer needed by the body, for example, regression of the gravid uterus to its normal size following parturition, loss of the glandular epithelium of mammary tissue upon cessation of lactation, and loss of larval organs during metamorphosis, as in the resorption of the tail as the tadpole develops into an adult frog.

LYSOSOMAL DISEASES Since lysosomes have many metabolic functions, it is not unexpected that certain diseases would have their etiology in the absence or deficiency of one or more lysosomal enzymes. These inborn lysosomal diseases include:

1. Gout is indirectly the result of congenital lysosomal dysfunction. In the gout-disposed

individual, tiny thin, urate crystals are precipitated from saturated plasma in synovial cavities of certain joints, especially the big toe. The microcrystals attract leukocytes, especially neutrophils. The crystals are phagocytosed by the leukocytes and become incorporated into the secondary lysosomes. Eventually the leukocyte dies and ruptures, releasing the toxic lysosomal enzymes that cause the inflammation and searing pain so characteristic of gouty arthritis. A vicious cycle is now set up because the released enzymes cause increased acidity which further reduces the solubility of the crystals and more crystals are formed. The process is repeated ad infinitum.

2. Lysosomes are also involved in the degradation of glycogen to glucose. Absence of the enzyme α-glucosidase causes an excessive storage of glycogen, called Pompe's disease. It usually occurs during childhood and is characterized by marked liver enlargement (hepatomegaly).

3. Other storage diseases, e.g., Tay-Sachs, Fabry's, Niemann-Pick, and Gaucher's all have one etiological feature in common, the **congenital absence of a lysosomal enzyme.** Its absence causes an abnormal amassing of the enzyme's intracellular substrate, namely, ganglioside GM_2, ceramide trihexoside, sphingomyelin, or glucocerebroside, respectively.

Microfilaments

Essentially all cells, except red blood cells, have thin filamentous cytoplasmic structures whose diameters vary from 5 to 15 nm. These **microfilaments** are involved either in **contraction or support.**

The two most common contractile microfilaments are found in all muscle cells, namely **actin** and **myosin** filaments. They are most highly organized and concentrated in striated muscle. **Actin filaments** are about 6–7 nm in diameter, while **myosin filaments** are much thicker, about 10–15 nm. Both are in close association with each other and are involved in muscle contraction, discussed in detail in Chapter 10.

Actin filaments are also found in other cell types, e.g., epithelia. Here, they are in the cores of the microvilli, which are tiny finger-like projections on the apical surface of epithelial cells involved in absorption. Contraction of these actin filaments cause the microvilli to shorten or bend.

Another type, the intermediate filaments, e.g., the **neurofilaments,** are perhaps the most ubiquitous organelle in the neuron. They extend throughout the cytoplasm and into the dendrites and axon. They are best developed in larger neurons and stain selectively with silver salts. Under the EM, the neurofibrils consist of bundles of much smaller neurofilaments, about 10 nm in diameter. Another example are the tonofibrils in epithelia.

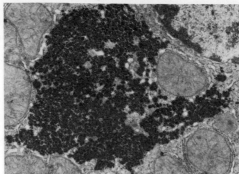

EM Glycogen granules

W. G. Jerome (x 30,000)

Excessive glycogen storage in liver cells as in Pompe's disease

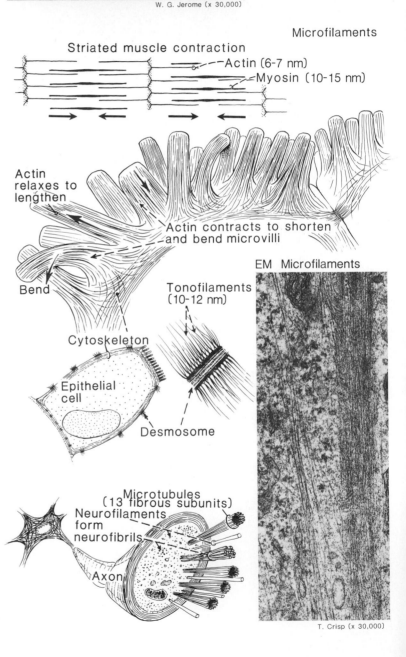

Microfilaments

Striated muscle contraction
- Actin (6-7 nm)
- Myosin (10-15 nm)

Actin relaxes to lengthen

Actin contracts to shorten and bend microvilli

Bend

Cytoskeleton

Epithelial cell

Desmosome

Tonofilaments (10-12 nm)

EM Microfilaments

Microtubules (13 fibrous subunits)
Neurofilaments form neurofibrils

Axon

T. Crisp (x 30,000)

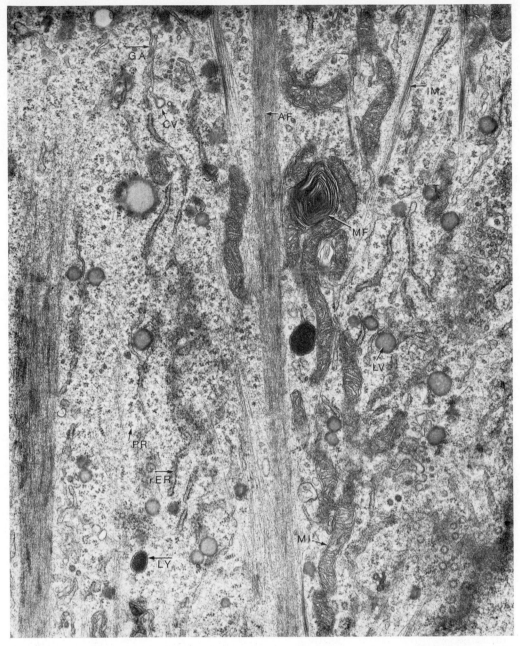

T. Crisp (x 30,000)

(GA) Golgi apparatus
(CV) Coated vesicle
(PR) Polyribosomes
(rER) Rough endoplasmic
       reticulum
(LY) Lysosome

(IM) Intermediate microfilaments
(AF) Actin filaments
(MF) Myelin figure
(LV) Lipid vesicle
(MI) Mitochondria

This EM micrograph of a fibroblast in tissue culture is of special interest because it reveals several longitudinal bundles of filaments. Two types are shown: actin filaments (AF), about 6 nm in diameter; and intermediate microfilaments (IM), with a constant diameter of 10 nm. The actin filaments are involved in cellular motility, such as locomotion, and ruffling and invagination of cell membranes. The larger, intermediate microfilaments do not appear to be involved in cellular movement but are an important component of the cytoskeleton of many cell types. The large lamellated myelin figure (MF) is an inclusion of cellular debris.

Annulate Lamellae

Annulate lamellae are a membranous system of parallel, double membranes with many regularly spaced **pores (annuli)**, which resemble the pores of the nuclear envelope. Both the lamellae and the nuclear envelope contain ATP. This organelle is a **modified type of sER** with direct connections with the endoplasmic reticulum. Its function is unknown but may have something to do with carrying information from the nucleus to the cytoplasm, thus influencing the control of the nucleus over cytoplasmic functions.

Microtubules

Formed from precursor proteins, called **tubulins, microtubules** are very important nonmembranous cellular organelles. They are slender, hollow, cylindrical structures about 24 nm in diameter and of indefinite length, often extending the length of the cell (as in the mitotic spindle). Each tubule is composed of 13 filamentous protein subunits (**protofilaments**), 4–5 nm in diameter. One function of microtubules is to act as a portion of the **cytoskeleton** that maintains the shape of the cell. They are also involved in various movements. For example, in the neuron they participate in the transport of proteins along the axon (**axoplasmic transport system**). During mitosis the microtubules greatly increase in number to form the **mitotic spindle**. Units of **triplet tubules** form the framework of the centrioles and the basal bodies of cilia. They are also arranged into nine doublets surrounding two central microtubules to form the central cores of cilia and flagella.

Centrioles

When observed under the light microscope, centrioles appear as small rods located near the center of the resting (interphase) cell. Under the TEM these granules can be resolved into two cylinders oriented at 90° to each other. The hollow, blind-ending cylinders are about 160–230 nm in diameter and range in length from 160 to 560 nm. In cross section each centriole has **nine sets of triplets** representing the open ends of three fused, longitudinal microtubules. Because these tubules are oriented about 30° to each other, they often present a pinwheel appearance.

During mitosis, centrioles replicate with 13 protofilaments and move as pairs to the opposite poles. Here they serve as the **organizing centers** for the microtubules that form the spindle apparatus of the dividing cell. Centrioles may also migrate to the cell surface where, as **basal bodies**, they are the sites of origin of **motile cilia or flagella**.

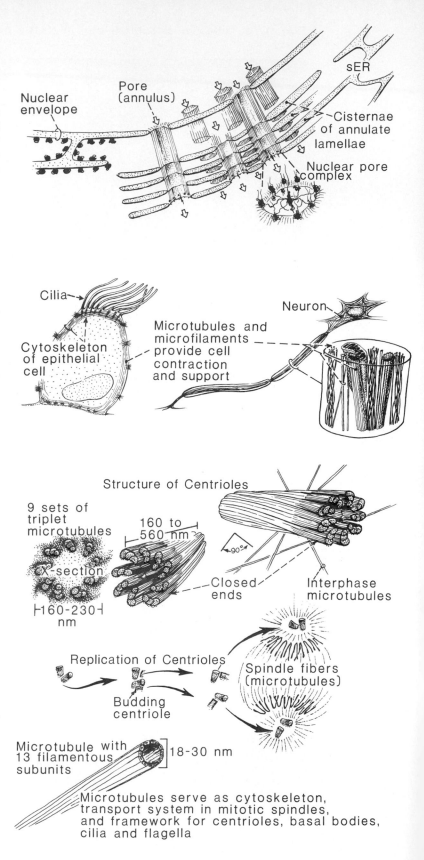

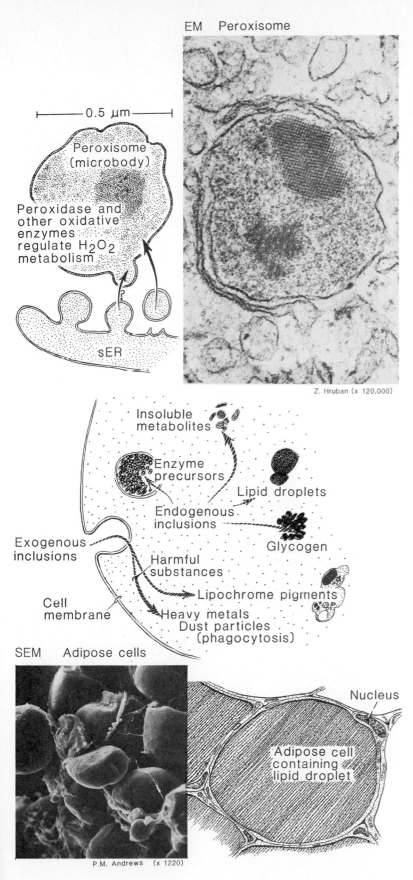

EM   Peroxisome

Peroxisome (microbody)

Peroxidase and other oxidative enzymes regulate H_2O_2 metabolism

sER

├── 0.5 μm ──┤

Z. Hruban (x 120,000)

Insoluble metabolites

Enzyme precursors

Lipid droplets

Endogenous inclusions

Glycogen

Exogenous inclusions

Harmful substances

Lipochrome pigments

Cell membrane

Heavy metals

Dust particles (phagocytosis)

SEM   Adipose cells

Nucleus

Adipose cell containing lipid droplet

P.M. Andrews   (x 1220)

Peroxisomes

Peroxisomes were originally called **microbodies** to designate membrane-bound spherical bodies found in the proximal convoluted tubules of the kidney. They are about the same size as lysosomes and frequently contain an electron-dense crystalline core within their granular matrix. Each peroxisome always contains the enzyme **peroxidase**, in addition to other oxidative enzymes. Its most important function is probably the regulation of H_2O_2 metabolism—hence its name peroxisome.

The origin of peroxisomes is obscure, but they are thought to arise from rER and sER. They are found principally in macrophages and several other cell types.

CYTOPLASMIC INCLUSIONS

In addition to organelles, there is a wide variety of cellular inclusions (see Table 1.2). They may be accumulations of **insoluble metabolites**, various food storage vacuoles, or substances ingested by phagocytosis. While these inclusions may be largely inert and transitory, they are nonetheless usually essential to the life and well-being of the cell. They are not in all cells but may be present in only specific cells during certain physiological activities.

All of the **beneficial inclusions are endogenous**, i.e., they arise from within the cell. They include lipid droplets, glycogen, enzyme precursors, and some pigments and crystalloids. Other inclusions are **exogenous**, i.e., generated outside the cell and later incorporated into it by phagocytosis, pinocytosis, absorption, or other methods. Among these **dispensable, transitory, and often harmful** exogenous inclusions are lipochrome pigments, such as carotene; heavy metals, as found in lead and silver poisoning; asbestos, silicon, carbon, and other dust particles ingested by phagocytic cells.

Lipid Droplets

Of the beneficial inclusions, **lipid droplets** are perhaps the most common. In the cytoplasm they are **storage sites for energy** sources. A mature, white **adipose cell** contains a single, large, lipid vacuole that essentially fills the cell. Since lipids are readily removed by organic solvents during routine histological procedures, the fat droplets cannot be seen, only an empty, clear space remains. However, if the tissue is preserved and specially stained without exposure to lipid solvents, fat droplets are easily identified. For LM studies the tissue is treated with osmic acid, which preserves the lipid droplets as black, spherical bodies, not membrane-bound.

Glycogen

Glycogen is the principal **storage form of carbohydrates.** It is present in the cytoplasm of a wide variety of cells, e.g., liver, muscle, and adrenal cortex. Unless specifically preserved and stained, it will be dissolved by water during most histological methods, giving the interior of the cells an irregular, fuzzy appearance. With special stains, such as Best's carmine, the glycogen granules are stained red; with periodic acid–Schiff (PAS) reagent—a magenta or crimson color.

TEM studies reveal **glycogen granules** to be electron-dense, irregular bodies of two types. The **larger (alpha) particles** are complexes of granules about 90 nm in diameter arranged in **rosettes or clusters.** The **smaller (beta) particles** (about 30 nm) occur **singly.** Glycogen granules are not enclosed by membrane nor do they attach to any membrane within the cell. (L-A, plate 34)

The organism cannot use glycogen per se, but when **converted to glucose**, it becomes the main **energy source** for the body. In starvation the glycogen storage is first depleted, then the fat and protein reserves. A congenital absence of the lysosomal enzyme, 1, 4-glucosidase (**acid maltase**), permits accumulation of glycogen within cells rendering them nonfunctional. Structures most involved are skeletal and cardiac muscles, and the liver. This disorder is called **glycogen storage disease** or Pompe's disease, as noted previously.

Zymogen

Zymogen granules are secretory products rich in **inactive enzymes.** They are found primarily in epithelial cells of the stomach, pancreas, and parotid gland. Under the light microscope, they appear as minute, spherical, **refractile granules** (0.1–1.5 μm) crowded into the **apical end** of the cell. Electron microscopic observations reveal that the granules have homogeneous, electron-dense cores **enclosed by a unit membrane.** However, one should be cognizant of the fact that these structures are viewed as granules only because their various proteins have been precipitated during fixation. In the living state, zymogen granules are really bags of fluid, rich in enzyme precursors. When the granules escape from the cell, their enzymatic proteins are activated by an appropriate chemical to produce various **digestive enzymes.**

Mucigen

Mucigen granules or droplets are characteristic of all mucous cells. Upon release from the cell, the granules absorb water to form **mucus,** a very excellent lubricant to aid, for example, passage of food and feces along the alimentary canal. As viewed with the LM, the granules are pale, indistinct, nonrefractile particles in the apex of the cell. EM studies show the **membrane-limited**

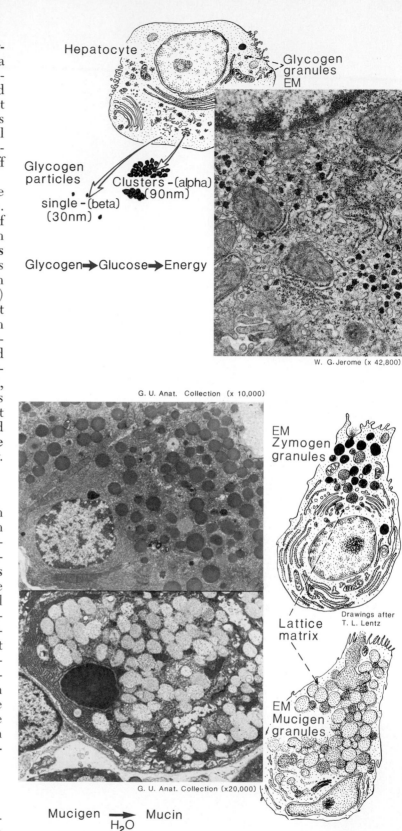

Hepatocyte

Glycogen granules EM

Glycogen particles

single - (beta) (30nm)

Clusters - (alpha) (90nm)

Glycogen → Glucose → Energy

W. G. Jerome (x 42,800)

G. U. Anat. Collection (x 10,000)

EM Zymogen granules

Drawings after T. L. Lentz

Lattice matrix

EM Mucigen granules

G. U. Anat. Collection (x20,000)

Mucigen $\xrightarrow{H_2O}$ Mucin

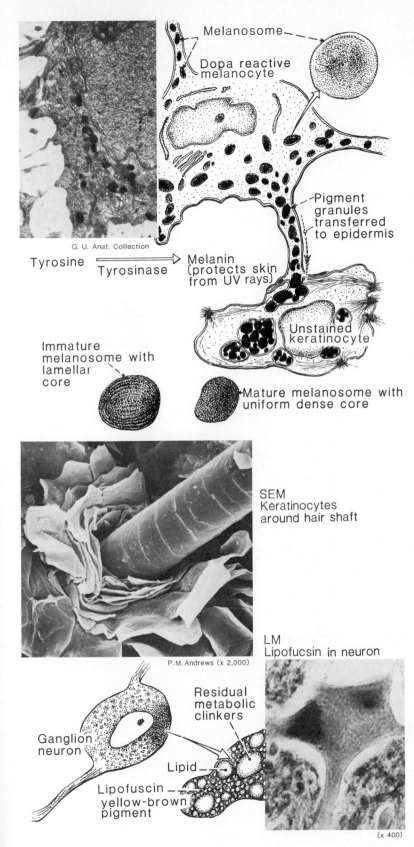

Melanosome

Dopa reactive melanocyte

Pigment granules transferred to epidermis

G. U. Anat. Collection

Tyrosine $\xrightarrow[\text{Tyrosinase}]{}$ Melanin (protects skin from UV rays)

Unstained keratinocyte

Immature melanosome with lamellar core

Mature melanosome with uniform dense core

SEM Keratinocytes around hair shaft

P.M. Andrews (x 2,000)

Ganglion neuron

Residual metabolic clinkers

Lipid

Lipofuscin yellow-brown pigment

LM Lipofuscin in neuron

(x 400)

granules to have an electron-lucent, lattice-like matrix. They are **poor in enzymes** but rich in **mucoproteins.** Since the droplets tend to fuse together during histological procedures, one seldom sees discrete mucigen granules in prepared slides, only the poorly defined remnants of the lattice matrix.

Melanin

Melanin is, by far, the most abundant and important **pigment** in the body. There are two major classes: (1) the black–brown eumelanin, and (2) the yellow-to-red pheomelanin, both formed by the action of the enzyme tyrosinase. The color of the skin, hair, and iris of the eye is dependent on the amount and distribution of these two types of melanin. The granules are usually unstained with conventional methods and retain their natural color. They are of **neural crest origin,** produced by specialized cells, called **melanocytes.** Melanin is formed by the action of the enzyme **tyrosinase** on the amino acid **tyrosine.** The synthesized melanin collects in membrane-bound granules called **melanosomes.** The pigment-bearing **melanocytes,** located largely in the basal layer of the skin, are interspersed with the epithelial cells. Much of the pigment produced and stored in the melanocytes is transferred by dendritic processes of the melanocytes to the cytoplasm of the basal epidermal cells (**keratinocytes**). The latter cells are now capable of screening out the harmful overexposure to ultraviolet light.

In most histological slides the melanocytes are difficult to distinguish from the keratinocytes because both contain melanin. However, **melanocytes** can be identified by their positive response to the **DOPA reagent** (dihydroxyphenylalanine) which stains melanocytes black due to the presence of tyrosinase in their cytoplasm. With the TEM one can distinguish between immature and mature melanosomes. Both are membrane-limited but the immature granules have variations in their **electron-dense cores.** The cores are composed of extended **lamellae,** some with helical configurations and others with marked striations. The mature granules have very dense cores of uniform density but no lamellae. (L-A, plate 34)

Lipofuscin

Lipofuscin is a yellow–brown, **fluorescent pigment** very different from melanin. It is also called old age or wear-and-tear pigment because it **accumulates with age,** especially in cells that do not undergo mitosis in the adult, e.g., muscle and nerve cells. Lipofuscin is mostly contained in the **residual bodies,** the end point of lysosomal digestive processes. It is the accumulation of all of the indigestible, intracellular "clinkers" or "ashes" left over from metabolic activity. From the EM viewpoint, lipofuscin has a very heterogeneous

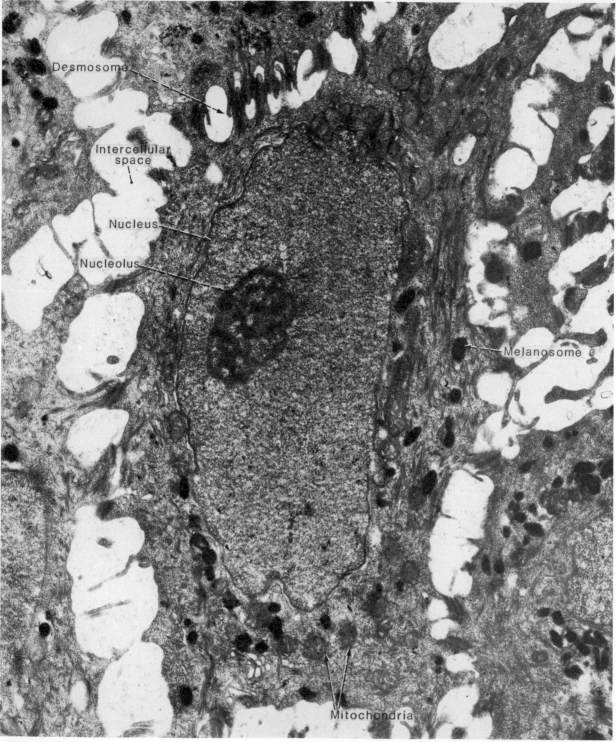

Desmosome

Intercellular
space

Nucleus

Nucleolus

Melanosome

Mitochondria

G. U. Anat. Collection

This is an electron micrograph of a melanocyte of the skin, characterized by many oval, dense, pigment granules called melanosomes. These are membrane-bound bodies that contain the enzyme tyrosinase, which is synthesized in ribosomes and packaged in the Golgi apparatus. Immature melanosomes have clusters of protein lamellae which often have a beaded appearance. As the melanosome matures, increasing deposits of melanin obscure the lamellar pattern and the mature melanosomes, as seen here, are dense, homogenous, dark-staining bodies. Other fine structural features include an ovoid or irregularly shaped nucleus with a prominent nucleolus, abundant mitochondria, considerable rER, and free ribosomes.

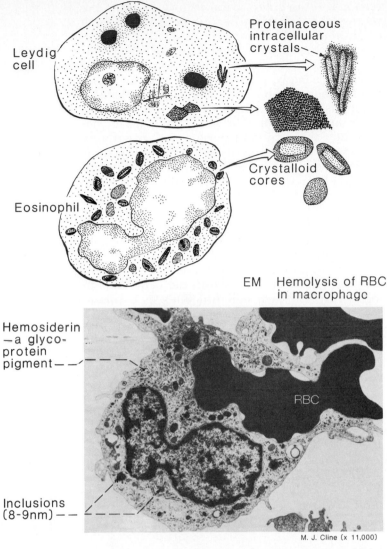

Leydig cell

Proteinaceous intracellular crystals

Eosinophil

Crystalloid cores

EM   Hemolysis of RBC in macrophage

Hemosiderin —a glyco- protein pigment

RBC

Inclusions (8-9nm)

M. J. Cline (x 11,000)

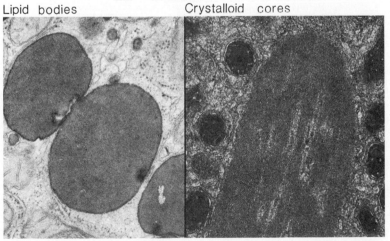

Lipid bodies

EM   Inclusions
Crystalloid   cores

G. U. Anat. Collection (x 36,000)

A. F. Payer (x 86,000)

appearance. The membrane-bound granules are irregular in shape and contain a variety of thin, dense, wavy lines often interposed between lipid vacuoles. Deposits of lipofuscin are known to have hydrolase activity, probably a holdover from the ingested lysosomes.

Crystals

Crystals are occasionally found in certain cells of the **testis** and **leukocytes.** In the testis they are usually rod-shaped bodies but may present a variety of shapes and sizes. Their composition is uncertain, but it may be proteinaceous. They lie free in the cytoplasm, void of a membrane. Their function is unknown.

Upon maturation the specific granules of the **eosinophilic leukocyte** have highly lamellated, dense, angular, **crystalloid cores.** These granules appear to function as **lysosomes.** Smaller crystals have been reported in the specific granules of neutrophils. Mitochondria and peroxisomes may also harbor minute crystalline bodies. The origin and function of these crystals are unknown.

Hemosiderin

Hemosiderin is a yellowish-brown **glycopro-tein pigment** derived from the degrading of the **hemoglobin** of senile, red blood cells. As its name suggests (Gk. haima, blood; sideros, iron), it is a compound rich in **iron,** especially the iron protein, **ferritin.** It can be identified under the TEM by the presence of electron-dense particles of uniform size (8–9 nm). Because it is a break-down product of hemolysis, hemosiderin is found as a cytoplasmic **inclusion in macrophages** in the spleen, bone marrow, liver, lungs, and at sites of blood clotting and destruction.

AN ANALOGY

It may be helpful to use the analogy of the cell as a factory to summarize its functions. In operation, cells and factories have many features in common. For example, they each have walls for support and protection, doors and gates for movement of raw materials in and finished materials out, and specialized equipment for the production, packaging, and storage of their manufactured products. An ample energy source must be available to produce these products. From these processes, waste materials are produced that must be disposed of. At the same time, all of these various functions must be continually coordinated and controlled from an administrative area.

A hypothetical factory sketch and a schematic diagram of a typical cell are shown to illustrate this concept. Here the organelles are arranged to correspond to the location occupied by analogous factory areas. Observe that the cell membrane serves as the protecting wall of the cell factory, while openings or pores in the membrane correspond to the gates of the factory to allow the ingress of nutrients and egress of products, such as enzymes and hormones.

In this hypothetical model, the rER performs the function of synthesizing specific cellular products, namely, proteins, while sER manufactures primarily steroids. The Golgi apparatus functions as the packaging mechanism. Products are temporarily stored as secretory granules before they are expelled from the cell, usually by exocytosis. The energy for all of these functions is provided by the mitochondria, the power plant of the cell. Lysosomes are the cell's garbage disposal units, which degrade and dispose of waste products.

Most of these functions are under the control of the nucleus, the administrative area of the cell. The DNA, providing blueprints and templates, functions to initiate and maintain the biochemical processes occurring within the cell. Thus in many respects each cell functions as a microscopic factory, complete in itself to accomplish its specific function.

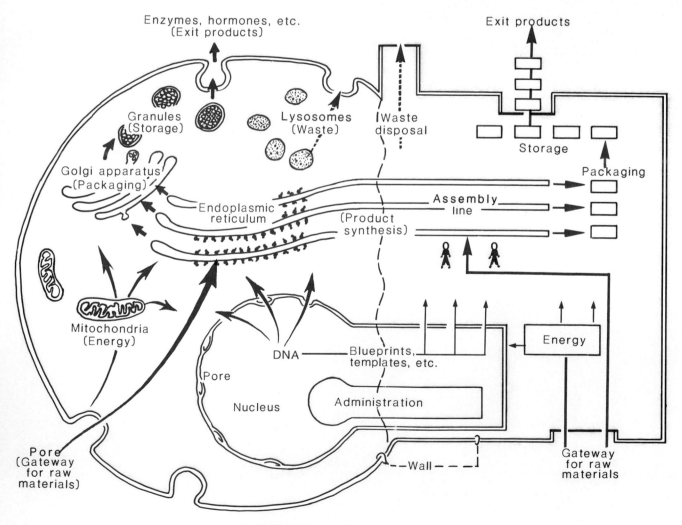

COMPARISON OF CELL TO FACTORY

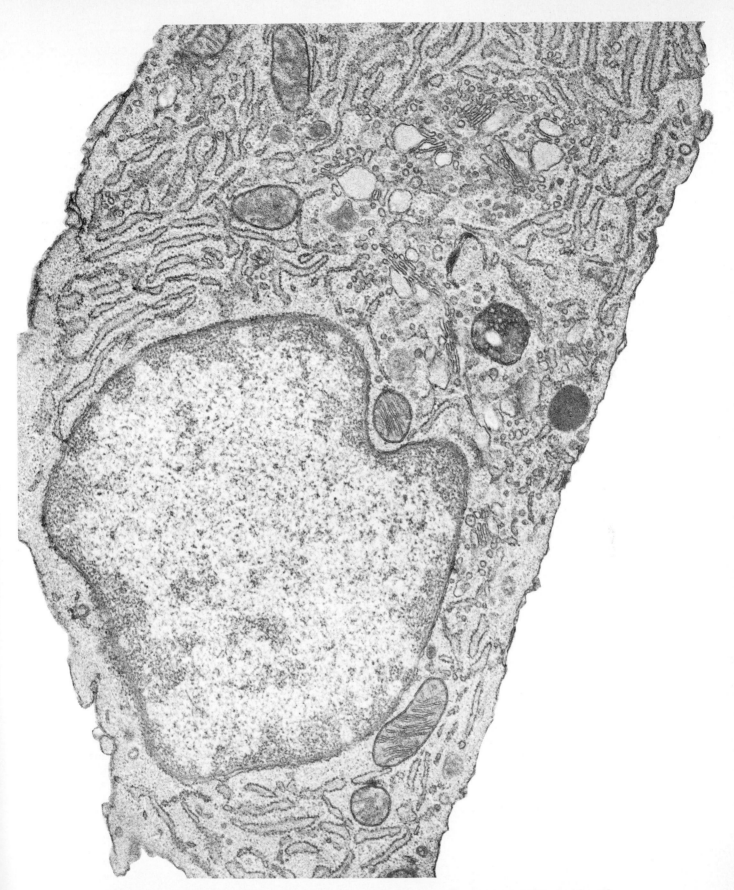

In this unlabeled EM micrograph of a connective tissue cell, test your ability to identify specifically the cell and the cellular organelles that dominate the field. If you have difficulty, a brief review of the illustrations in Chapter 1 may furnish you with the clues you need.

Table 1.1 CYTOPLASMIC ORGANELLES

	MORPHOLOGY		SIZE AND LOCATION
	LM	EM	
Plasmalemma	Not seen unless viewed obliquely	Trilaminar, quasi-fluid structure of lipids, CHO + proteins arranged in mosaic patterns	About 9–10 nm thick. Surrounds all animal cells
Endoplasmic reticulum (ER)	Discrete tubules or sheets cannot be seen, only the deeply baso-philic chromidial substance (er-gastoplasm)	Branching network of tubules (membranes) and cisternae. Two types: (1) smooth or agranular (sER) and (2) rough or granular (rER), studded with ribosomes	Tubule diameter about 6.0 nm; tubules extend throughout cyto-plasm and may connect with plas-malemma and nuclear membrane
Ribosome	Cannot be seen singly; in groups may appear as fine granules	Spherical, angular, or flattened particles; clusters called polyribo-somes or polysomes	12–20 nm in diameter; may be free in cytoplasm or attached to cytoplasmic surface of ER
Mitochondria	Very small spherical granules, rods, or filaments distributed in cytoplasm	Typically an oval or tubular struc-ture bounded by two trilaminar (unit) membranes about 6 nm thick. Inner membrane infolded to form cristae with small elementary particles attached. Finely granular dense matrix with DNA, RNA, ri-bosomes, and various enzymes	About 0.5×2.5 μm in size; pres-ent in all animal cells; vary greatly in number depending on the cell and its function, e.g., only few in lymphocytes to about 3000 in liver cell
Golgi apparatus	Shape varies from a small reticu-lar network to a solid body; if un-stained the clear, pale area at the Golgi site is called the negative Golgi	Flattened plates (cisternae) of unit membranes arranged in parallel stacks, compressed at their cen-ters, and dilated peripherally as saccules	Located usually between nucleus and apical end; very variable in size depending on activity of cell
Lysosomes	Not seen, except as granules in certain leukocytes	Single membrane-bound, oval or round bodies with sacs of en-zymes; have granular, uneven ap-pearance; often contain lamellar, stacked membranes (myelin fig-ures)	0.25–0.5 μm in diameter; in most animal cells except RBCs; found most often near the Golgi appara-tus in region called the "cytocen-ter"
Centrioles	Appear as two ovoid or rod shaped bodies near nucleus; dur-ing mitosis migrate to opposite poles of cell	Two compact cylinders at right angles to each other; their walls consist of nine longitudinal units (blades) each composed of three fused microtubules	About 0.3×0.15 μm in size; lie adjacent to and may indent nu-cleus
Peroxisomes (microbodies)	Not seen	Spherical or ovoid, single mem-brane-bound granules; often have crystalline cores	0.3–0.5 μm in diameter; widely distributed in most cells
Microtubules	Not seen (except as clusters in the mitotic spindle)	Usually stained, slender, cylindri-cal structures with a central ap-parently hollow core	About 25 nm in diameter; indeter-minate length; scattered through-out cell in parallel groups, or fused to form doublets or trip-lets in certain organelles (cilia, centrioles)
Fibrils • Collagenous	Not usually seen as discrete struc-tures; found outside the cell	Have unique cross-banding pat-tern of 64 nm; arranged in parallel rows	Average about 0.3 μm in width which increases with age; length indeterminate; found in nearly all types of connective tissue
• Myofibrils	Cylindrical columns	Each myofibril has about 1000–2000 myofilaments of two types; (1) thick myosin about 1.5 μm in length and 1.0 nm wide, and (2) thin actin about 1.0 μm long and 5.0 nm in width	1–2 μm wide, indeterminate length. Prominent in skeletal and cardiac muscle; scanty in smooth muscle
• Neurofibrils	Seen as delicate threadlike struc-tures in nerve cells	Bundles of microtubules and neu-rofilaments	Found in perikaryon, dendrites, and axon; about 0.2 μm in diame-ter

HISTOCHEMICAL REACTION(S)	FUNCTION(S)	OBSERVATIONS
PAS positive, largely due to glyco-calyx	Controls movement of materials in and out of cell	Is selectively permeable to certain substances
Basophilic staining which is removed by pretreatment with ribonuclease (RNase)	RER involved in synthesis of certain enzymes; sER associated with cells that produce steroid hormones and HCl; transports these substances and fluids throughout the cell	Provides an internal membrane surface for many complex biochemical reactions, e.g., protein and lipid syntheses; is an intracellular circulatory system for distributing reaction products throughout cytoplasm
Stain with toluidine blue, pyronin, or other RNA indicators; digested with RNase	Site of protein synthesis	Probably has short life-span; with cessation of protein synthesis they disappear
Positive reaction with Janus green B vital stain; also positive for various dehydogenases and other oxidative enzymes; stains red with acid fuchsin	Major energy source; site of synthesis of ATP; contain three enzyme systems: (1) glycolytic enzymes, (2) Krebs or citric acid cycle, and (3) respiratory chain with oxidative phosphorylating enzymes	Self-duplicating; can divide and join together; contain DNA and RNA; are the "powerhouse" of the cell
Stains by reducing silver and osmium salts; also PAS positive	Packages secretory products and transports them to cell surface for release; synthesizes carbohydrate portion of some glycoproteins; also forms lysosomes	Especially well developed in secretory cells; appears to be polarized, i.e., certain cisternae have specific function.
Take up vital dyes, e.g., acridine orange; stain positive for acid phosphatase	Intracellular digestion by reducing large molecules to smaller units; destroy bacteria and foreign substances	Contain many hydrolytic enzymes; if fixation is delayed after death, the enzymes are released into cell and autolysis follows
Stain black with iron hematoxylin	Important in mitotic spindle formation; in some cells they migrate to cell periphery and give rise to basal bodies in the formation of cilia and flagella	Replicate during mitosis and migrate to opposite poles of cell; not present in mature neurons; essential for mitosis in animal cells
Localize peroxidase activity with positive diaminobenzidine reaction	Has oxidative function of regulating H_2O_2 metabolism; perhaps also involved in lipid metabolism and gluconeogenesis	Resemble small lysosomes but do not contain acid hydrolases but peroxidases
	Serve as a cytoskeleton for cells; assist in intracellular movements to alter cell shape; form the mitotic spindle; act as a guidance system in intracellular transport	Colchicine blocks formation; formed from the protein, tubulin
Stain with acid dyes, e.g., eosin, aniline blue, picrofuscin, etc.	Many structural and mechanical functions, e.g., skeletal support, investments, bindings, etc.	Do not branch; held together by cement substance (microprotein); positive birefringence under polarized light; relatively inelastic with high tensile strength; yield gelatin in boiling water
	Contractile units	Cross-striations are not simply surface markings but reflect a regular alignment or register pattern of myofibrils; the thin actin filaments, extending from the Z line are in register as the I band, while interposed as the A band are the thicker myosin filament
Stain selectively with silver and gold salts	As support in cytoskeleton; may have an intracellular transport function	Best developed in large neurons; do not branch; with injury to cell they disintegrate

Table 1.2 *CYTOPLASMIC INCLUSIONS*

| | MORPHOLOGY | | SIZE AND LOCATION |
	LM	EM	
Lipid droplets	In adult—single large droplet fills cell; in fetus—several droplets in cell which later coalesce into one	Spherical body with homogeneous electron-dense core; periphery of droplet more dense; probably not membrane-bound	Size varies from a few nm to the diameter of cell; random distribution
Glycogen granules	With special stains appear as coarse clusters of granules	Appear either as electron-dense, uneven granules, the β particle, or as clusters (rosettes), the α particle; are not membrane-bound or attached to membranes	α particles, 90 nm; β particles, 30 nm; random distribution; abundant in liver, muscle, and adrenal cortex
Zymogen granules	Many small, round, highly refractile granules in apical portion of cell	Membrane-bound granules with very electron-dense, homogeneous matrix	Granules collect in apex of cell; variable in size, largest 1.5 μm; abundant in pancreas, chief cells of stomach and salivary glands
Mucigen droplets	Rather large, pale-staining droplets in apex of cell	Cytoplasm filled with large electron-lucent bodies with reticular matrix	Quite uniform in size; distributed throughout respiratory and digestive systems in isolated goblet cells, or in mucous glands
Melanin	Brown or black colored fine granules	Immature granules have several membrane-bound electron-dense, elongated lamellae with density variations; mature granules have spherical, very dense, uniform cores	Variable in size and distribution; found in melanocytes of epidermis of skin, pigmented layers of retina and iris, and some cells of the brain
Lipofuscin	Tan to light brown colored granules; has brownish fluorescence with ultraviolet light	Very heterogeneous appearance; variable amount of electron-dense, membrane-bound particles; granules contain lysosomes, residual bodies, and lipid-filled vacuoles	Granules are variable in size and distribution; found largely in CNS, muscle, adrenals, heart, and liver, of the elderly
Crystals	Variety of crystalline configurations; usually rod-shaped with sharp or rounded angles	Not membrane-bound; have closely packed parallel filaments with dense granules; regularly repeating pattern forming a lattice	In spermatogonia 1.0×7.0 μm in size, in Leydig cells about 2.0×20.0 μm; these latter crystals have macromolecules about 5 nm in diameter and spaced about 19 nm apart
Hemosiderin	Unstained are golden brown granules	Masses of electron-dense particles 8–9 nm in diameter	Collects mostly in macrophages in the spleen, bone marrow, liver, blood clots, and at sites of pathological RBC destruction

CHEMICAL CONSTITUENT(S)	STAINING PROPERTIES	FUNCTIONS	COMMENTS
Mostly triglycerides and cholesterol	Black with osmic acid or Sudan black B. Red with oil red O or Scharlach R, etc.	Storage of triglycerides; important energy reserves, membrane and hormone precursors	Reserves not static, constantly being replenished; can be used directly by cell when CHO reserves are exhausted
A large polymer of glucose; a polysaccharide (animal starch)	Red with Best's carmine, or magenta with PAS	Upon conversion to glucose is the prime energy source for the organism	Greatly depleted by fasting; tends to be associated with sER but not attached to it; is water soluble and therefore removed in most histological preparations, giving cells a spongy, "washed out" appearance
Contain many enzymatic proteins	With H&E are mostly acidophilic, refractile granules	Precursors of digestive enzymes, e.g., pepsin, amylase, trypsin, etc.	Produce a clear, watery secretion with high enzyme content; each granule may contain several enzymes synthesized by ribosomes on rER
Rich in mucoproteins	Stain selectively with Alcian blue, mucicarmine, and PAS; essentially unstained with H&E	Precursor of mucin which upon hydration forms mucus, an excellent lubricant	Droplets tend to swell and coalesce during specimen preparation, therefore are rarely seen as discrete bodies; form a thick, viscous, enzyme-poor secretion
A high-molecular-weight polymer produced by the action of tyrosinase on tyrosine	Stains with some fat stains, basic fuchsin, and PAS; its natural brown or black color is unaffected by H&E	Prevents sunburn by scattering light rays and absorbing ultraviolet radiation; imparts various color tones to skin, hair, eyes, etc.	Skin and hair color due to number, size, and distribution of granules (melanosomes), in the different types of melanin (eumelanin and pheomelanin)
Has prominent lipid component	Same as melanin	Unknown; represents accumulations of insoluble intracellular debris remaining after lysosomal activities	Increases with age, especially in neurons; may occupy half of cell volume
Unknown	In Leydig cells stain light red with Malloryazan	Unknown	Regularly seen only in testis; occasionally elaborated by adrenal cortex; granules of eosinophils have a central crystalloid core; considered to be lysosomes
An iron protein complex, contains the protein, ferritin	Intense positive reaction to Prussian-blue test	Storage of Fe for RBC production	Fe stored as ferritin or hemosiderin; collects in alveolar macrophages of the lung in cardiac valvular deficiences

Chapter

2

THE NUCLEUS AND ITS ORGANELLES

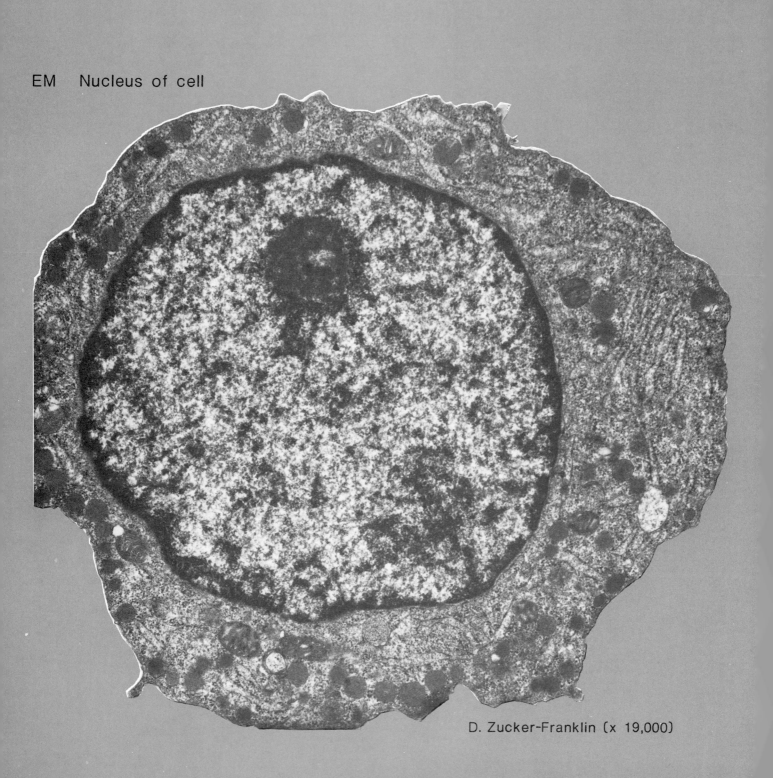

D. Zucker-Franklin (x 19,000)

OBJECTIVES

THE INFORMED STUDENT WILL BE ABLE TO DESCRIBE HOW THE NUCLEUS CONTROLS THE REPRODUCTION AND VITAL BIOCHEMICAL PROCESSES OF THE CELL, SUCH AS:

1. The rationale for the need for two types of chromatin, a nucleolus and a limiting membrane, in the nucleus

2. How it acts as the staging area for the formation of chromosomes which are formed from chromatin-containing coils of DNA and protein

3. Its role in mitosis and meiosis

4. The need for the various types of RNA synthesized in the nucleus

5. How chromosomal abnormalities cause certain clinical disorders, e.g., Down syndrome

The most conspicuous and important membrane-bound compartment of the cell is the **nucleus.** It is found in all eukaryotic (Gk. eu, true + karyon, nucleus) cells, except mature erythrocytes and possibly other senile, moribund cells. The nucleus is essential to the life of the cell. If it is experimentally removed, protein synthesis in the cell is arrested and the cell dies.

The nucleus of each cell of the body has the same genetic information stored in its **chromatin,** mostly DNA bound to proteins (largely histones). It is from this encoded information that the structure, function, and metabolic activities of the organism are determined and regulated. Although each cell contains the same genetic information (**genes**), cells vary greatly in their shape, functions, and metabolic products. It is the nucleus that has the decisive influence on these factors by **activating or repressing** the action of certain genes.

Some genes in the chromosomes contain coded information for the synthesis of proteins that act like enzymes in the cytoplasm. Other genes code for proteins that have a regulatory function. They may organize the activity of whole groups of genes, such as those that control the **replication of DNA,** which is passed on to the daughter cells during mitosis.

The interphase nucleus typically contains several distinctive organelles. They can be readily seen with the EM, and except for the nuclear envelope, they are also visible under the LM. They include the nuclear membrane or **envelope, nucleolus,** and **chromatin.**

NUCLEAR ORGANELLES

Nuclear Envelope

The **nuclear envelope** separates the nucleus from the cytoplasm. Under the EM it can be resolved into **two unit membranes,** each about 7–8 nm in thickness with a lucent, perinuclear cisterna (space) between them about 25 nm wide. The **outer membrane** may be studded with ribosomes and may be continuous with both the sER and rER. The **inner membrane** is smooth, i.e., free of ribosomes, but has clumps of heterochromatin (Gk. hetero, different) attached to its inner surface. In early mitosis, the nuclear envelope breaks up into small vesicles, releasing the chromosomes into the cytoplasm. It is significant that during the telophase of mitosis, the nuclear envelope re-forms from segments of endoplasmic reticulum and the vesicles of the residual nuclear envelope.

Nuclear pores are perhaps the most characteristic feature of the nuclear envelope. They are formed by fusion of the two nuclear membranes, which form an annulus or ring around each pore. Their circular openings are quite uniform in size (70–75 nm), are essentially the same distance apart, and may occupy a fourth of the surface of

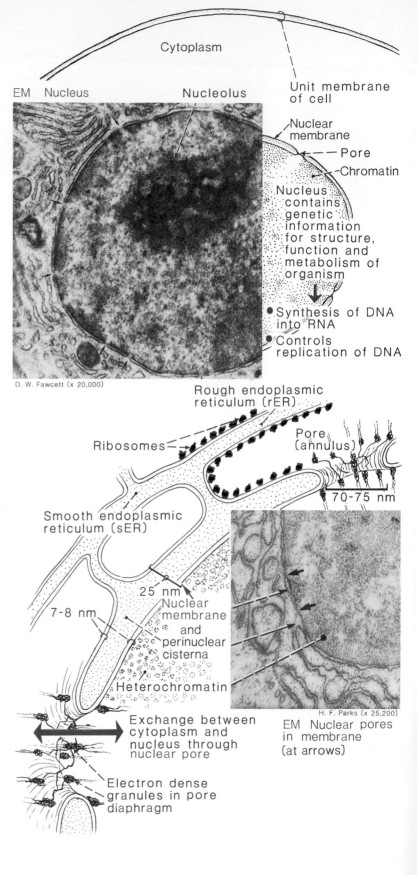

Cytoplasm

EM Nucleus   Nucleolus   Unit membrane of cell

Nuclear membrane

Pore

Chromatin

Nucleus contains genetic information for structure, function and metabolism of organism

• Synthesis of DNA into RNA
• Controls replication of DNA

D. W. Fawcett (x 20,000)

Rough endoplasmic reticulum (rER)

Ribosomes

Pore (annulus)

70-75 nm

Smooth endoplasmic reticulum (sER)

25 nm
Nuclear membrane and perinuclear cisterna

7-8 nm

Heterochromatin

Exchange between cytoplasm and nucleus through nuclear pore

Electron dense granules in pore diaphragm

H. F. Parks (x 25,200)

EM Nuclear pores in membrane (at arrows)

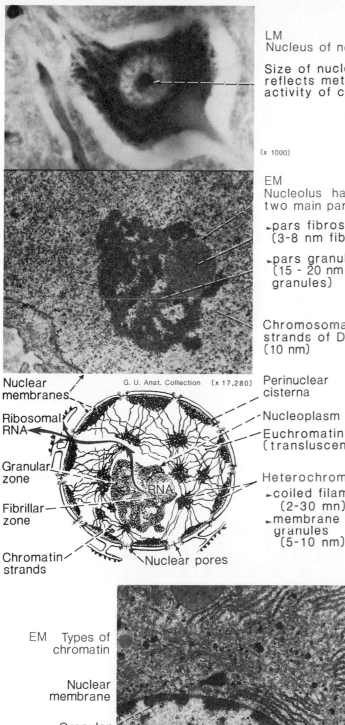

LM
Nucleus of neuron

Size of nucleolus reflects metabolic activity of cell

(x 1000)

EM
Nucleolus has two main parts:

►pars fibrosa (3-8 nm fibrils)

►pars granulosa (15 - 20 nm granules)

Chromosomal strands of DNA (10 nm)

G. U. Anat. Collection   (x 17,280)

Nuclear membranes

Ribosomal RNA

Granular zone

Fibrillar zone

Chromatin strands

Nuclear pores

RNA

Perinuclear cisterna

Nucleoplasm

Euchromatin (transluscent)

Heterochromatin:
►coiled filaments (2-30 mn)
►membrane free granules (5-10 nm)

EM   Types of chromatin

Nuclear membrane

Granular heterochromatin

Euchromatin

G. U. Anat. Collection (x 20,000)

the nuclear envelope. Stretching across each pore is a thin, diffuse **diaphragm,** which may contain a central electron-dense granule. These pores are potential **passageways for exchange of materials** (e.g., mRNA) between the nucleus and cytoplasm. It is probably the permeability characteristics of the pore diaphragm that determine the types of molecules that cross the nuclear envelope.

Nucleolus

With hematoxylin and eosin (H&E) stain, the **nucleolus** of the interphase nucleus is a discrete, **spherical,** highly **basophilic** body. Its size and staining intensity **reflect its metabolic activity.** The nucleoli are large (>1 µm) in cells with active protein synthesis, e.g., pancreatic, embryonic, and neoplastic cells; and are smaller (<1 µm) or absent in cells with limited protein production, such as muscle cells and male sex cells. They disperse during early mitosis and reappear during telophase.

As viewed under the LM, the nucleolus does not have a limiting membrane, as do many cell organelles, but rather a densely **coiled, fibrillar region,** the nucleolonema, and an amorphous, **granular, lighter area,** the pars amorpha. However, under the EM, it is obvious that these terms are not valid as both zones contain granules intertwined with fibrils. From EM micrographs of nucleoli, **four regions** or components emerge:

1. The granular region (pars granulosa)—an ovoid spherical mass of **electron-dense, poorly defined granules** about 15–20 nm in diameter with some fibrils interspersed (formally called the pars amorpha).

2. The fibrillar region (pars fibrosa)—a serpentine-like network consisting mostly of **fibrils** (3–8 nm in diameter) with some **granules** (formally the nucleolonema).

3. A structured matrix that suspends the two regions.

4. The nucleolar chromatin component of **delicate strands** (10 nm in diameter) of dispersed DNA which penetrate and link the granular and fibrillar zones. The strands extend into the nucleoplasm to adhere either to the inner surface of the nuclear envelope or to the granules of the granular region. It is within the nuclear chromatin component that **ribosomal RNA (rRNA)** is synthesized. When formed, the RNA is transported first to the fibrillar zone, then to the granular region, and finally through the nuclear pores into the cytoplasm of the cell.

Chromatin

Chromatin is the **chromosomal DNA** containing substance, the carrier of the genes in inheritance. **A strand of chromatin,** in an interphase nucleus, is formed from a number of **DNA molecules** combined with a large amount of **protein**, primarily histones, and limited RNA. Two types of chromatin are present in the nucleus of resting, eukaryotic cells: (1) irregular, densely basophilic clusters of granular **heterochromatin**, and (2) translucent, clear areas composed of **euchromatin**.

Heterochromatin or condensed chromatin is found in clumps attached to the inner membrane of the nucleus but leaves the pores unobstructed. Moribund cells have very dense heterochromatin within the nucleus, a condition known as **pyknosis**.

With the EM, **heterochromatin** is seen to consist of many membrane-free chromatin **granules** about 5–10 nm, and delicate, coiled **fibrils**. The untreated fibrils are 20–30 nm thick, but when treated with chelating agents, they unravel into **filaments** about 10 nm in diameter. When exposed to urea these filaments disrupt further into **microfilaments** 2–4 nm wide. Each microfilament probably represents a single DNA helix wrapped around clusters of histones. Each DNA-histone cluster is called a **nucleosome**, the fundamental structural unit of chromatin. Early in mitosis, heterochromatin and euchromatin are condensed and organized into the chromosomes.

Euchromatin is arranged in extended, uncoiled, **delicate strands of DNA** that occupy the large, electron-lucent areas of the nucleus. In the interphase nucleus it is very active in the **synthesis of messenger RNA**.

Only in early mitosis do both types of chromatin become so condensed that **chromosomes** can be recognized. This is not a haphazard phenomenon but a precise, exactly recurring process where chromosomes are molded from these entangled threads and granules of chromatin.

HUMAN CHROMOSOMES

Each human nucleus contains **46 chromosomes**, divided into 23 pairs. Twenty-two pairs are **homologous autosomes** (Gk. auto, self + soma, body) while the other pair are **sex chromosomes**. In the female, the sex chromosomes consist of two X chromosomes, while the male has one X and one Y chromosome.

Chromosomes replicate during the S period of interphase, but it is the metaphase stage of mitosis where the equal, longitudinal separation of the duplicated DNA strands is evident under the LM. These parallel chromosomal halves are called **chromatids**. The production of two chromatids results from the doubling of each chromosome by DNA synthesis during interphase.

The chromatids are attached to each other at a constriction along their length called the **centromere**. This attachment site provides a means for dividing chromosomes into three groups, namely, **metacentric**, if the centromere is central in position and divides the chromosome into

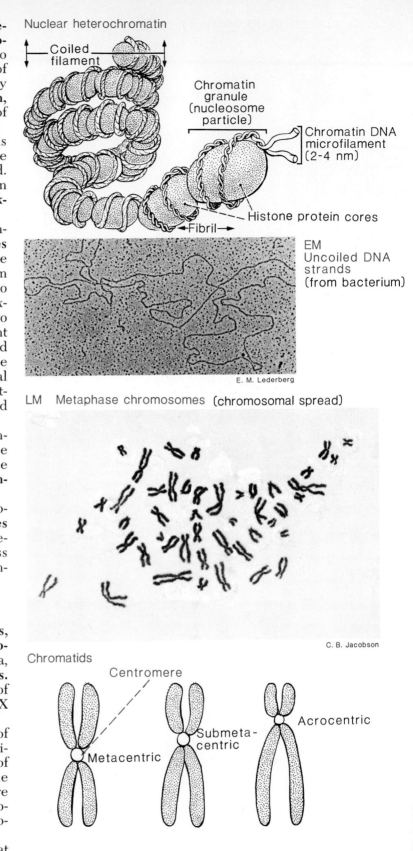

Nuclear heterochromatin

Coiled filament

Chromatin granule (nucleosome particle)

Chromatin DNA microfilament (2-4 nm)

Histone protein cores

Fibril

EM
Uncoiled DNA strands
(from bacterium)

E. M. Lederberg

LM   Metaphase chromosomes   (chromosomal spread)

C. B. Jacobson

Chromatids

Centromere

Metacentric

Submetacentric

Acrocentric

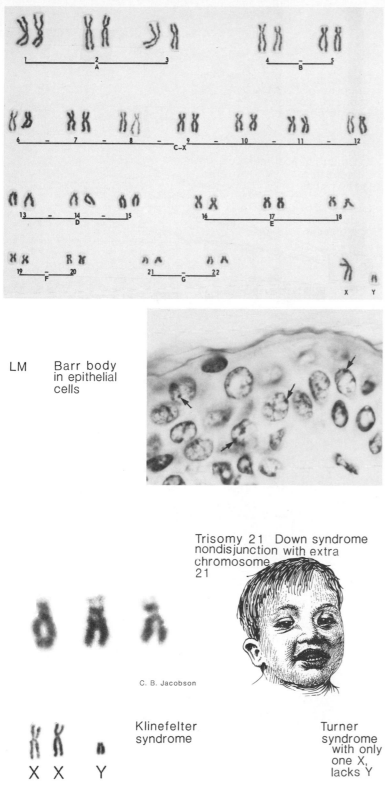

LM   Barr body
in epithelial
cells

Trisomy 21 Down syndrome
nondisjunction with extra
chromosome
21

C. B. Jacobson

Klinefelter
syndrome

X X   Y

Turner
syndrome
with only
one X,
lacks Y

equal segments (arms); **submetacentric,** if the centromere lies between the midpoint and the end of the chromosome; and **acrocentric,** if it is close to one end.

Variations in morphology and number of chromosomes can be determined from a **karyotype,** a photographic display of the individual chromosomes. It is prepared by cutting out each chromosome from a photograph of a **chromosomal spread** of metaphase chromosomes. The homologous pairs of chromosomes are matched and placed in groups depending on their length and the position of the centromere on the chromosome.

In the human, eight groups of autosomal chromosomes are identified. **Group A** comprises three pairs of the largest metacentric chromosomes (1–3). **Group B** has two pairs (4 and 5) of large submetacentric chromosomes. **Group C** has medium-sized metacentric chromosomes. This is the largest group and includes seven pairs (6–12). **Group D** has three pairs (13–15) of medium-sized acrocentrics. **Group E** has three smaller pairs (16–18), number 16 is metacentric while 17 and 18 are submetacentrics. **Group F** has two (19 and 20) short metacentrics, while **group G** consists of two pairs (21 and 22) of small acrocentric chromosomes. The small sex chromosome **group H** includes, in the male, a large submetacentric X chromosome and a very small acrocentric Y chromosome. In the female, two small X metacentric chromosomes are present.

A modification of the heterochromatin in the interphase nucleus is the **sex chromatin or Barr body.** It is one of the two X chromosomes found in cells of the female. It is **functionally inactive** and remains tightly coiled during interphase, therefore it stains deeply with basic dyes. Usually it is seen as an oval or flat, dark body, about 1 μm in diameter, lying against the inner nuclear membrane.

The presence of the Barr body indicates that the cell contains a second X chromosome and therefore permits the **determination of the genetic sex** of an individual. While all somatic cells in the female are believed to have a Barr body, only about 20–70% test positive, probably due to the plane of sectioning of the tissue. Nevertheless, genetic sex can be ascertained, since in the male only 0–5% of the somatic cells show sex chromatin.

Chromosomal Anomalies

Several clinical disorders are due to **chromosomal abnormalities.** These conditions may arise from extra chromosomes, e.g., in **Down syndrome** there are 47 instead of 46 chromosomes. There is an extra chromosome 21, called trisomy 21. It probably results from a failure of the two homologous chromosomes 21 to move to opposite poles during meiosis, instead they both migrate to the same pole. This condition is called

nondisjunction because the chromosomes stayed together. Therefore when fertilization occurs the zygote has one 21 from one parent and two 21 chromosomes from the other parent. Their off-spring will be born with the typical "mongoloid features" characteristic of Down syndrome.

Other conditions, such as **Klinefelter syndrome,** are caused by the presence of an **extra X chromosome in the male (XXY).** The resulting tall individual has extra long extremities, especially arms; probably is sterile from the hypogonadism; and has enlarged breasts. Females lacking an X chromosome (X0) develop **Turner syndrome,** characterized by sterility and lack of development of the ovaries, which causes a suppression of primary and secondary sexual characteristics.

CELL CYCLE

Each cell of the body arises from a preexisting cell. Although many neurons and perhaps some lymphocytes may live as long as the individual, other cells have a limited life-span. These cell lineages survive only if they continue to reproduce their genetically identical kind. This is done by cell division (**mitosis**). In this process each new daughter cell receives all of the genetic information (genes) carried in the DNA molecules of the parent cell.

Before cell division can occur, the parent nucleus must exactly double its DNA content for equal distribution to the two daughter cells. The process of duplicating the DNA molecules is called **replication.** The act of equally dividing the nuclear DNA between the newly created cells is mitosis. Thus cell division has two separate and distinct processes: (1) **biochemical,** through replication of genetic information in the parent cells; and (2) **morphological,** through mitosis.

Replication of DNA can be divided into two stages: (1) The **DNA molecule,** a double helix composed of **two helical strands** wrapped around the same axis, unwinds or "opens up" to become a template for the creation of two **new, complementary chains of DNA.** (2) Each chain becomes half of another double helix, an **exact replica** of the preexisting strand. Thus a normal, constant, linear relationship of genes is established in the newly constituted DNA molecule.

Mitosis

The process of mitosis consists of four active stages and one interphase. Highlights of these phases follow:

1. **Prophase.** In the first stage, **prophase,** the chromatin condenses into pairs of **coiled chromosomes.** There is a characteristic number of chromosomes in each body cell for each species. In man this number is 46. During prophase each **chromosome splits longitudinally** and each half

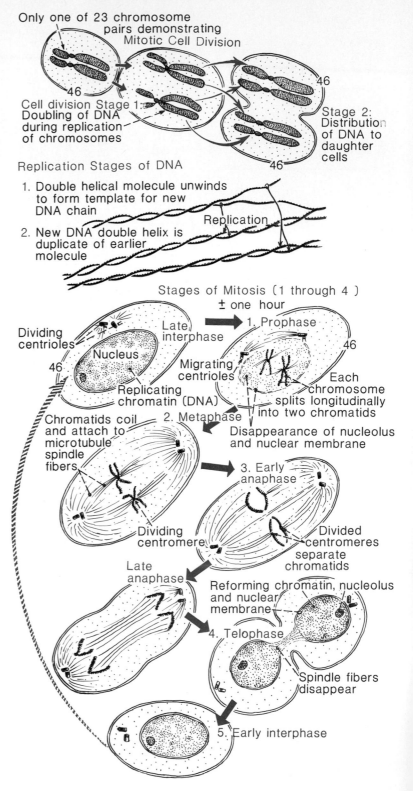

Only one of 23 chromosome pairs demonstrating Mitotic Cell Division

Cell division Stage 1: Doubling of DNA during replication of chromosomes

Stage 2: Distribution of DNA to daughter cells

Replication Stages of DNA

1. Double helical molecule unwinds to form template for new DNA chain

2. New DNA double helix is duplicate of earlier molecule

Replication

Stages of Mitosis (1 through 4) ± one hour

Late interphase

1. Prophase

Dividing centrioles

Nucleus

Migrating centrioles

Each chromosome splits longitudinally into two chromatids

Replicating chromatin (DNA)

2. Metaphase

Disappearance of nucleolus and nuclear membrane

Chromatids coil and attach to microtubule spindle fibers

3. Early anaphase

Dividing centromere

Divided centromeres separate chromatids

Late anaphase

Reforming chromatin, nucleolus and nuclear membrane

4. Telophase

Spindle fibers disappear

5. Early interphase

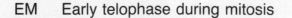

D. F. Parsons

In this EM micrograph of a cell in the early mitotic stage of telophase, the chromatids have separated and, under control of the spindle fibers (microtubules), approach the poles. As the paired centromeres on each chromosome separate, each chromosome is split into two identical chromatids, which immediately move towards a pole. During the process the fibers (microtubules) of the centromere shorten, the spindle fibers lengthen, and the two poles move apart. Upon reaching their respective poles (in late telophase), the chromatids, now called chromosomes, are equally distributed among the two newly formed daughter cells.

is called a **chromatid.** At this point, near the end of prophase, the **nuclear envelope** and the nucleolus disappear and each of the **two centrioles** move to the opposite poles of the cell, trailing after them delicate **astral fibers** (microtubules) that eventually form the spindle between the poles.

2. **Metaphase.** In the next stage, **metaphase,** the chromatids align themselves across the equator of the cell. Each chromatid is attached to the spindle fibers (microtubules) at a central point or region, the **centromere.**

3. **Anaphase.** During the third stage, or **anaphase,** the two chromatids of each chromosome become detached from each other and start moving to opposite poles along the spindle microtubules, led by the centrioles.

4. **Telophase.** In the telophase the chromatids have reached the poles. **Nuclear envelopes reform** and enclose each new set of chromatids, now called **chromosomes.** The spindle microtubules disappear, a **nucleolus reappears** in each nucleus, and the chromosomes uncoil and reform into a long chromosomal thread. Finally, the cell membrane is drawn inward by a band of microfilaments to form a complete constriction between the newly formed nuclei. Thus, **two new cells are formed,** each with the normal complement of 46 chromosomes.

These four phases proceed as a continuous process, each blending with the next phase. The whole process may take about one hour in rapidly dividing cells, such as liver cells in tissue culture.

5. **Interphase.** The interval between mitoses is often called the resting stage but is more correctly termed the **interphase.** The cell is not really resting. In fact, during interphase the cell is **most active** in the synthesis of new products, organelles, and DNA required for the next mitosis.

The interphase is divided into three distinct stages: (1) G_1 is the initial **time gap** which follows mitosis and usually lasts for about ten hours. During this time the new daughter cell grows in size and actively **synthesizes RNA** and proteins but not DNA. (2) The S stage is the period of **active DNA and histone synthesis** and probably replication of the two centrioles. It continues for about nine hours. (3) G_2 is the **second gap period** or the time between DNA synthesis and the resumption of mitosis. It persists for about four hours. (All time intervals are for liver cells in tissue culture and may vary for other cell types.)

Meiosis

Meiosis is a **type of cell division** that occurs during **gametogenesis,** i.e., the formation of ma-

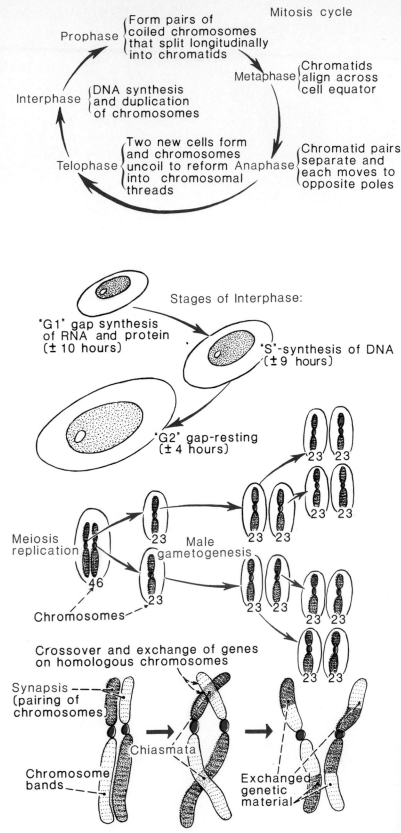

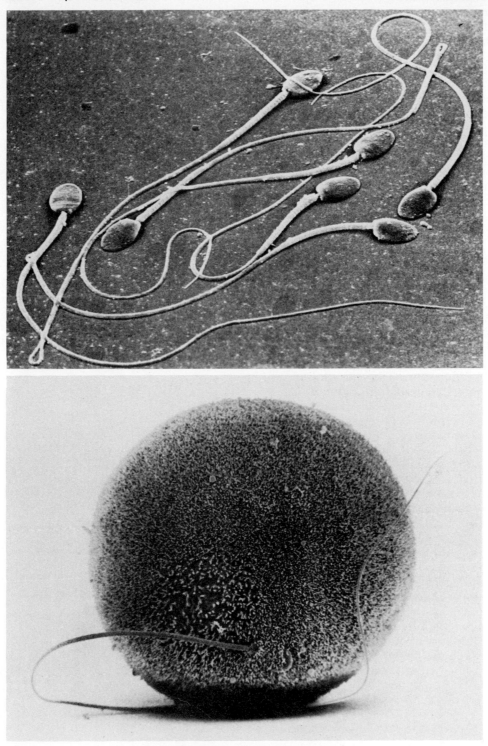

SEM   Ovum being fertilized by one **spermatozoon**   D. M. Phillips

The upper SEM micrograph of human spermatozoa reveals three distinct regions on each sperm, i.e., a large oval head, a narrow neck, and a long tapering tail or flagellum. The head is composed largely of a dense nucleus.

The lower micrograph shows a single spermatozoon penetrating the outer covering of the ovum (zona pellucida). Once the sperm head has pierced the zona pellucida, the whipping action of the tail ceases, the entire spermatozoon is drawn inward and is engulfed by the cytoplasm of the ovum.

ture gametes, spermatozoa, and ova. The word meiosis means "to diminish," which accurately describes this process in which the **number of chromosomes is halved** in the mature gamete. While in mitosis each somatic cell has the full complement of 46 chromosomes, after meiosis each gamete contains only 23. Then, in fertilization the 23 chromosomes of the ovum are joined by the 23 chromosomes of the spermatozoon, giving the offspring the normal complement of 46 chromosomes.

The other function of meiosis is the production of **genetic variations in offspring.** One way this is accomplished is by the exchange of segments of homologous chromosomes by a process called "**crossing over.**" A reciprocal exchange of genes occurs during the prolonged prophase, while the paired homologous paternal and maternal chromosomes lie touching each other, paired gene for gene, a condition known as **synapsis.** The contact points where the chromosomes adhere or overlap are called **chiasmata.** During synapsis breaks in the DNA chains appear and an **exchange of genetic material occurs** between the two contiguous chromosomes. In other words, some genes have crossed over between the paired chromosomes. Thus an infinite number of chromosomal combinations can occur and the uniqueness of each individual is assured.

The role of the chromosomes in the reproductive processes is discussed in more detail in Chapters 23 and 24. Now to reiterate salient facts, recall that the largest cell organelle, the nucleus, is present in all normal cells except erythrocytes. It is the repository for the genetic information (DNA) that is present in chromosomes. The nucleus is the source of three types of RNA: ribosomal, messenger, and transfer RNA. These macromolecules initiate and control the protein synthesis that occurs in the cytoplasm.

By a clumping and coiling of the chromatin in the nucleus, the chromosomes are fashioned into their typical hairpin or rod shapes during prophase. In late prophase the nuclear envelope and nucleolus disappear, later to be reconstructed into two identical nuclei in late telophase. When cell division is complete, with the creation of two identical daughter cells, each new cell contains a nucleus that is an exact replica of the nucleus of the parent cell, endowed with all of the genetic information needed for the development of a new individual.

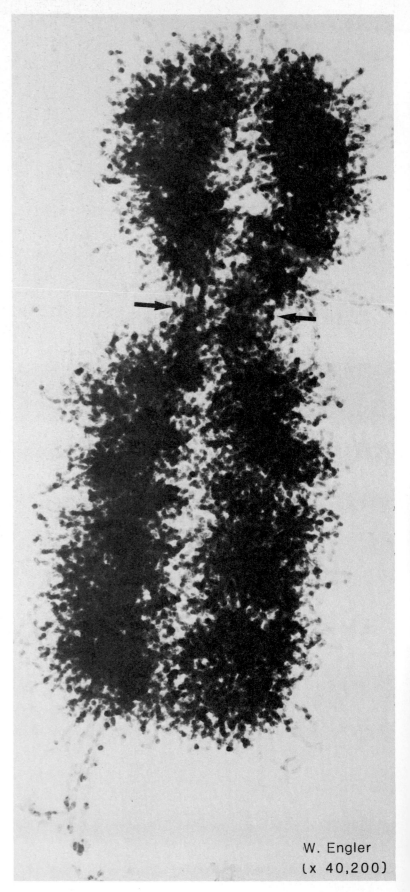

EM   Human chromosome composed of sister chromatids joined by the centromere

W. Engler
(x 40,200)

Part

II

TISSUES

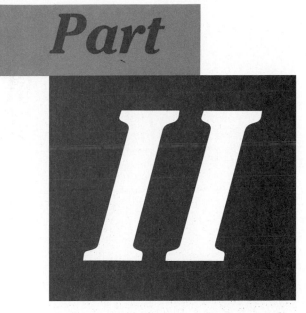

Chapter

3

PRIMARY TISSUES

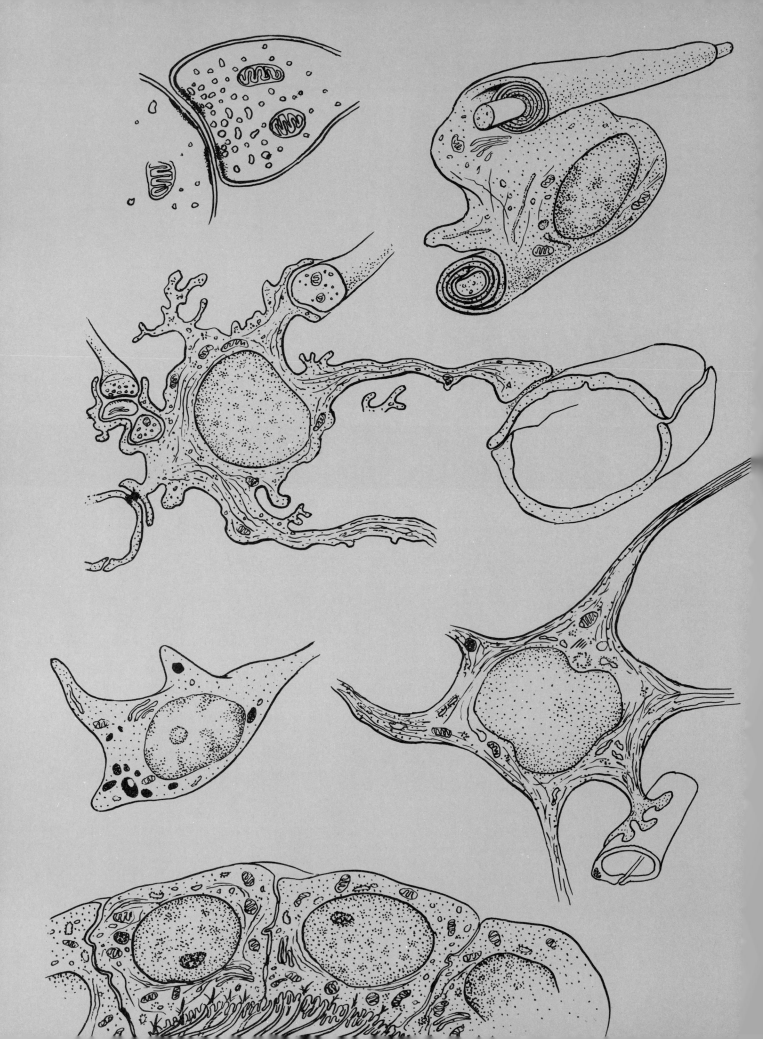

AFTER STUDYING THIS CHAPTER, THE STUDENT SHOULD BE ABLE TO:

1. Categorize the morphological features of the four primary tissues and recognize their interplay in forming organs.

2. Recall the development and distribution of various epithelial tissues, including structural differences and their roles in bodily functions.

3. Prepare a classification of connective tissues, ranging from bone and cartilage to lymph and blood.

4. Explain how the contractile units of muscle fibers are "ingenious contrivances to facilitate motion." Also distinguish histologically between smooth, cardiac, and skeletal muscles.

5. Identify the nerve cells and fibers that propagate, transmit, and/or respond to various stimuli.

By definition a **tissue** (L. texere, to weave) is a functional aggregation of similar cells and their intercellular materials that combine to perform a common function. Through tissues an effective division of labor between cells is established so that specific functional needs of the organism can be quickly and efficiently provided.

Tissues are the building blocks for the formation of **organs**, the next higher order of organization of the body. Four tissues are considered basic or primary, namely, **epithelial, connective, muscular,** and **nervous.** They are classified in Table 3.1.

EPITHELIUM

Distribution and Origin

For the most part, **epithelium** (Gk. epi, upon; thele, nipple) forms continuous layers that **cover surfaces** (skin) and **line cavities** of the body. These cavities include the closed peritoneal, pleural, and pericardial cavities, where the epithelium is called **mesothelium,** and open organ cavities, i.e., the digestive, respiratory and urogenital organs, which connect with the outside. In addition, epithelium lines the cardiovascular and lymph passageways as **endothelium.** The parenchymal (the essential or secretory) cells of **glands** are also epithelium.

Epithelial cells are derived from all three germ-cell layers. Those cells lining the digestive and respiratory systems arise from **endoderm.** Those lining the oral and nasal cavities, and the anus are derived from **ectoderm.** The lining cells of the pleural, pericardial, and peritoneal cavities and of the vascular system are **mesodermal** cells. Some epithelial organs also are derived from **mesoderm** and include the kidneys, gonads and their ducts, plus the liver and pancreas.

Functions

The importance of epithelium to our well-being, even our very existence, cannot be overemphasized. Epithelium, as epidermis, covering the exterior of our bodies, **protects** us from mechanical trauma, loss of moisture, and noxious substances in our environment. We receive our nourishment by the **absorptive** action of the epithelium that lines the digestive tract. We **digest** our food by the action of enzymes synthesized by glandular epithelium. Hormones that **regulate** our endocrine functions are epithelial secretions. Without the **excretory** function of certain epithelial cells of the kidney, we would die of uremic poisoning. Through **neuroepithelium** we smell, taste, see, and hear. The very survival of the species is dependent on the integrity of the epithelial **sex cells,** i.e., ova and spermatozoa.

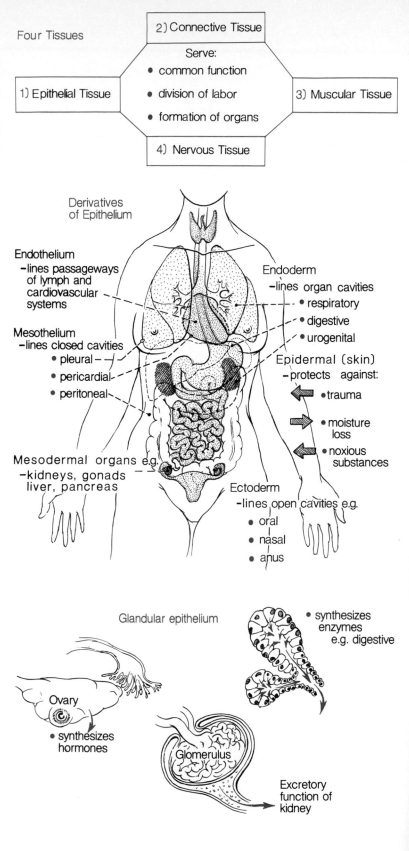

8630

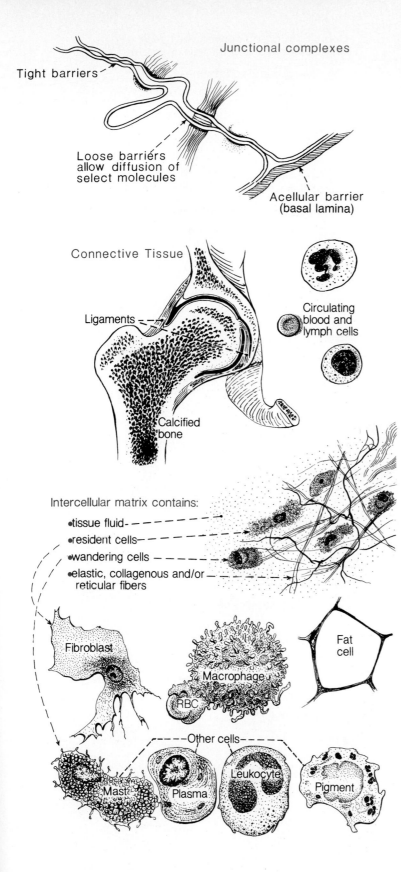

Junctional complexes

Tight barriers

Loose barriers allow diffusion of select molecules

Acellular barrier (basal lamina)

Connective Tissue

Ligaments

Calcified bone

Circulating blood and lymph cells

Intercellular matrix contains:

• tissue fluid
• resident cells
• wandering cells
• elastic, collagenous and/or reticular fibers

Fibroblast

Macrophage

RBC

Fat cell

Other cells

Mast

Plasma

Leukocyte

Pigment

To stay alive we are dependent on the integrity and normal functioning of a wide variety of **epithelial tissues.** To form a compact, continuous sheet, the epithelial cells are firmly attached to each other by a variety of junctional complexes (discussed in Chapter 4). Many are very tight junctions which prevent free passage of materials between epithelial cells. Other cell junctions fit less snugly and allow molecules of a certain size to pass.

Essentially all epithelia are **avascular.** Therefore, if nutrients and oxygen reach the epithelial cells, they must diffuse through the matrix that lies between the capillaries and the epithelial cell membrane. Molded against the bases of the epithelial cells is a thin, acellular barrier, the **basal lamina,** which limits the types of materials entering the cells (see Chapter 4).

When we look at ourselves or others, most of the beauty we see is epithelium, usually the **epidermis** and **derivatives of the skin,** such as hair and nails. The **coverings** of the cornea, the conjunctiva of the eye, and the **linings** of the oral and nasal cavities are all epithelia. Finally, most of our **diseases,** including many types of cancer, usually result from the malfunctioning of epithelia.

CONNECTIVE TISSUE

Components

Connective tissues are the **supporting framework** for all tissues and organs of the body. In addition to support, they provide the means of **anchoring and binding** organs together as well as providing the packing tissue between them. Connective tissue varies in structure and character, from hard, calcified bone to the circulating blood and lymph. In spite of this wide range of morphological variation, all connective tissues have an **intercellular matrix.** Usually it is composed of an **amorphous ground substance** in which are embedded **cells,** and one or more types of **extracellular fibers,** e.g., elastic, collagenous, or reticular. In blood and lymph the fibers are strands of fibrin, which are seen only during clotting.

Except in blood and lymph, the predominant cell type is the **fibroblast,** or one of its derivatives, followed by the **macrophage** and the **fat cell,** either singly or in groups. Other cells may be regarded as wandering cells or visitants, since they appear only erratically. Such cells include mast cells, plasma cells, various leukocytes, and pigment cells.

Classification

Connective tissue is classified according to the nature of its **intercellular material,** e.g., the characteristics of the ground substance; the type, arrangement, and abundance of its fibers; and the type of cells present (Table 3.1). In contrast, recall that epithelium is classified by the type and the orderly **arrangement of the cells.** Also its intercellular material (matrix) is very scarce and inconspicuous. The abundance of matrix is a very prominent feature of connective tissue.

Functions

The importance of connective tissue to our well-being can be best appreciated by considering its various functions. (1) It provides a supporting bony or cartilagenous **framework** for all our organs and tissues. Without this rigid skeleton, we would literally have no definitive shape or form. We would be amorphous blobs of cells and fibers spread out as misshapened mounds, crowned perhaps with a central thatch of hair. (2) Blood, as a fluid connective tissue, **transports O_2 and nutrients** throughout the body and removes CO_2 and metabolites from the tissues. Both are life-sustaining functions. (3) Adipose cells act particularly to provide **storage** of energy-rich lipids. Other connective tissue cells store vital water and electrolytes. (4) Fat cells also provide an excellent **insulation barrier** against heat loss. (5) Certain connective tissue cells provide an effective **defense** against pathogenic organisms, e.g., ingestion of bacteria by phagocytes. (6) Plasma cells are the principal **source of antibodies** that are essential for combating infectious diseases. (7) Through the proliferation of connective fibers, called fibrosis, our bodies **repair** fractures, sprains, wounds, abrasions, etc. This built-in, self-repairing mechanism enables us, during our entire life spans, to survive the almost continuous onslaught of a hostile environment against our somewhat fragile bodies.

MUSCULAR TISSUE

Function

Contractility is an inherent property of protoplasm. At some stage in their development all animal cells possess it to some extent. Without it neither ameboid movement nor cell division would be possible. It is, however, the **muscle cells** that retain and develop to the highest degree the ability to **contract,** while all other cells essentially lose it. Muscle remains as the primary tissue of action and motion because its fibers contain contractile units called **myofibrils.**

Classification of connective tissue by characteristics of intercellular material

➤ ground substance

➤ fiber content

➤ cell types

Functions

- Support
- Transport
- Defense
- Storage
- Binding

- Anchoring
- Insulation
- Tissue repair
- Antibody production
- Packing

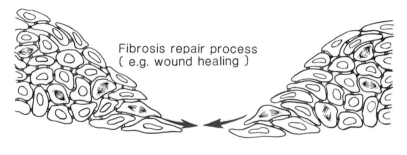

Fibrosis repair process (e.g. wound healing)

Contractile cells

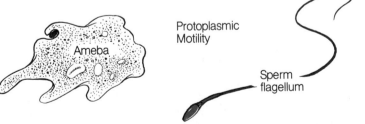

Ameba

Protoplasmic Motility

Sperm flagellum

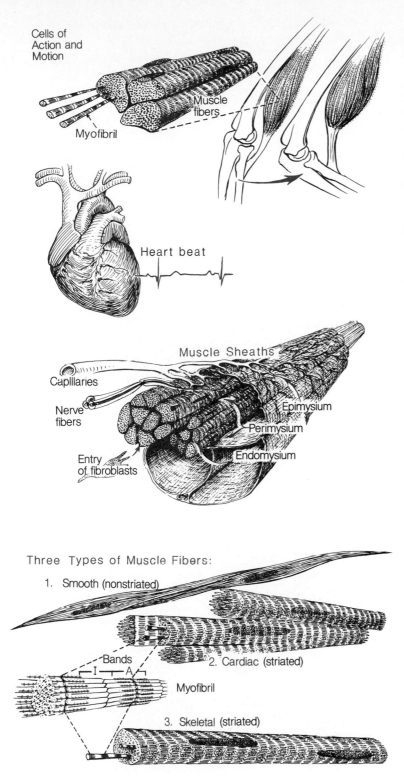

Cells of Action and Motion

Muscle fibers

Myofibril

Heart beat

Muscle Sheaths

Capillaries

Nerve fibers

Entry of fibroblasts

Epimysium

Perimysium

Endomysium

Three Types of Muscle Fibers:

1. Smooth (nonstriated)

Bands

I — A

2. Cardiac (striated)

Myofibril

3. Skeletal (striated)

To accomplish movement a muscle cell must shorten, i.e., its ends must be brought closer together by **contraction** of the myofibrils. Obviously a muscle cell that is long and narrow has a much greater capacity to shorten than a spherical or ovoid cell. It is precisely the elongated, threadlike morphology of the muscle cell that enables it to contract so vigorously and also justifies calling it a muscle fiber instead of a muscle cell.

There are all degrees of movement. For example, in expressing anger the movement may be as gross and violent as striking a blow with the fist, or as delicate and subtle as the slight flaring of the nostrils. **Muscular movement** is the external manifestation of life. If something moves, we assume it is alive. Not only are our outward movements dependent on muscle action but also our heartbeat, respiration, digestion, elimination, and other bodily functions.

Muscle tissue is really a composite. In addition to muscle cells, it consists of several **other cells** and **connective tissue fibers**. Between each muscle fiber is a thin, connective tissue sheath, called the **endomysium**. Within this investment are fibroblasts, collagenous fibers, nerves, and a rich plexus of blood capillaries lined with endothelial cells. In addition to the endomysium, a more robust sheath, the **perimysium**, envelops each bundle of fibers, and finally, a strong, fibrous, tendinous covering, the **epimysium** surrounds the entire muscle. These sheaths form a harness to channel the muscular energy towards the site of insertion of the muscle causing movement, usually on a bone, a cartilage, or the skin.

Types of Fibers

There are three types of **muscle fibers**, i.e., **smooth** (involuntary, nonstriated), found in the walls of viscera; **cardiac** (involuntary, striated), in the walls and septa of the heart; and **skeletal** (voluntary, striated), which is usually attached to bones or skin. Cardiac and skeletal muscle fibers appear striated or cross-banded because each fiber is packed with longitudinally arranged subunits, **myofibrils**, which have light (I) bands and dark (A) bands lying side by side in near perfect register. Under the microscope the alternating light and dark disks are seen as **striations**. In contrast, smooth muscle fibers contain fewer myofibrils that are uneven in diameter and length and are not in register. Therefore, no striations are visible. These muscle types are discussed in detail in Chapter 10.

NERVOUS TISSUE

All primitive cells respond to their environment. They react because they possess the physiological property of **irritability**, i.e., they have the capacity to generate nervous impulses. They also have the property of **conductivity**, or the ability to transmit these impulses along processes arising from their cell bodies. However, it is the **neuron** (nerve cell) that develops these attributes to the highest level of expression. It is the nervous tissue that alerts us to changes in both our external and internal environment. Nerve cells function to coordinate and integrate the functions of all tissues and organs of the body so that the organism is in harmony with its environment.

Organization

Nervous tissue is divided into three systems. The two major systems are: (1) the **central nervous system (CNS)**, which includes the spinal cord and brain, and (2) the **peripheral nervous system (PNS)**, formed by the nerves that arise in pairs from the brain and spinal cord, as well as ganglia (clusters of nerve cells) associated with the nerves.

The third, minor system is the **autonomic nervous system (ANS)**. It is composed of many small ganglia and nerve fibers. They are arranged either in long chains on either side of the vertebral columm, as the **sympathetic ganglion cells**, or as **parasympathetic ganglion cells** embedded within, or closely associated with, the various organs of the body. The ANS carries nerve impulses to smooth muscles, e.g., gastrointestinal tract and blood vessels, to cardiac muscle, and to glands.

Neuron

The neuron is the nerve cell body with all of its processes. It is the structural and functional **unit** of the nervous system. The typical neuron consists of three characteristic parts: (1) a cell body (**perikaryon**) containing a large nucleus with a conspicuous nucleolus; (2) usually several short processes, called **dendrites**, which respond to stimuli and convey impulses *toward* the cell body; and (3) a single, long process, the **axon**, that transmits impulses *away* from the cell body to terminate on a muscle, gland, or another neuron. Nissl bodies (ribosomes) fill the cell.

Neurons may be classified by the number of their **cell processes.** For example, a neuron with a single emerging process (the axon) is called **unipolar.** This is a common cell type in the mammalian embryo but is rare in the adult, found only in the sensory (spinal) ganglia. **Bipolar** cells have a single dendrite and an axon. Such cells are found in the organs of the special senses, e.g., eye, ear, and nose. By far the most common neuron is the **multipolar** cell having a single, long

Properties of Neurons (irritability and conductivity)

- Generate signals
- Conduct signals as impulses
- Coordinate interactions of tissues and organs

Three systems of nervous tissue:

1) central (CNS)
    spinal cord & brain

2) peripheral (PNS)
    paired nerves from brain, spinal cord and ganglia

3) autonomic (ANS)
    sympathetic and parasympatic ganglia and nerve fibers

Classification of Neurons

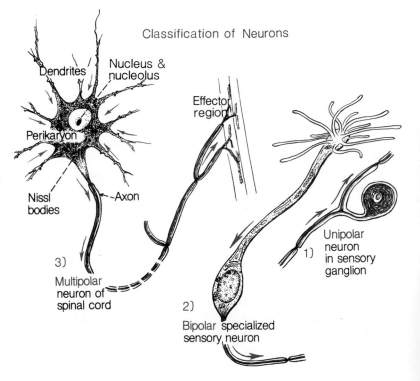

Dendrites

Nucleus & nucleolus

Perikaryon

Nissl bodies

Axon

Effector region

3) Multipolar neuron of spinal cord

2) Bipolar specialized sensory neuron

1) Unipolar neuron in sensory ganglion

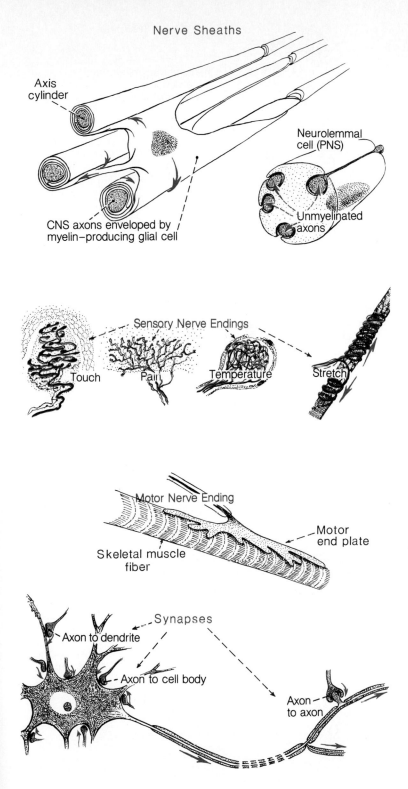

Nerve Sheaths

Axis cylinder

Neurolemmal cell (PNS)

CNS axons enveloped by myelin–producing glial cell

Unmyelinated axons

Sensory Nerve Endings

Touch   Pain   Temperature   Stretch

Motor Nerve Ending

Skeletal muscle fiber

Motor end plate

Synapses

Axon to dendrite

Axon to cell body

Axon to axon

axon and many shorter dendrites. Most neurons of the brain and spinal cord are of this type.

Fibers

Nerve processes (fibers) are covered by one or more sheaths. In the peripheral nervous system all fibers have a thin covering, the **neurolemma,** also called the **sheath of Schwann.** Most of these fibers have a second investment, the **myelin sheath,** interposed between the neurolemma and the central core of the axon, the axis cylinder. These are the **myelinated fibers** which are capable of rapid transfer of impulses. In the central nervous system, the large fibers are myelinated but do not possess a sheath of Schwann. **Unmyelinated fibers** are common in the smaller axons of both the PNS and CNS. However, they are the predominant nerve fibers in the autonomic nervous system. (L–A, plates 5 and 6)

Nerve Endings

Nerve fibers convey impulses to and from nonnervous structures, such as the skin and muscles, where they terminate in **peripheral nerve endings.** These terminations may be **sensory receptors** responding to the sensation of touch, pain, temperature, etc., or **motor endings,** which activate the heart, smooth muscle, glands, and skeletal muscle. The latter is activated by a more complex ending called a **motor end plate,** which lies at the junction between the motor nerve fiber and the skeletal muscle fiber. In small muscles that perform very delicate movements, such as the muscles of the eye, a nerve fiber may supply only a single muscle fiber. In massive muscles that execute gross movements, a profusely branching neuron may innervate 100 or more muscle fibers, each possessing a motor end plate.

Synapse

There is a constant, dynamic flow of information (impulses) along complex chains of neurons throughout the nervous system. The juncture between two neurons is a **synapse.** The cell membranes of the two neurons involved, e.g., axon to dendrite, axon to axon, or axon to cell body, are separated by a space called the **synaptic cleft,** about 20 nm wide. Therefore, the membranes are not fused or in direct physical contact with each other. There is contiguity without continuity of neurons at a synapse. In vertebrate synapses, chemical transmission occurs. The **chemical transmitters** that are released at synapses are usually acetylcholine and norepinephrine.

These chemicals are stored in small vesicles, called **presynaptic vesicles,** within the bulbous end of the axon at the synapse. The vesicles fuse with the presynaptic membrane of the axon where they discharge the chemical transmitters into the synaptic cleft by the process of **exocytosis.** The binding of the transmitter to the postsynaptic membrane initiates a **nervous impulse** which activates a muscle fiber, a gland, or another neuron. Structurally, synapses may end in a variety of shapes. However, they most often terminate in club-shaped expansions, called, boutons terminaux (Fr. end feet).

Neuroglia

The other cell type in nervous tissue is the **neuroglia** (glia, a Greek word meaning glue), aptly named because it binds or glues together all elements of nervous tissue within the central nervous system. There are four types of glial cells.

1. The large, star-shaped **astrocytes,** with extensive branching processes, are subdivided into two categories depending on the morphology of the cytoplasmic processes. **Protoplasmic astrocytes** (mossy cells) have rather long, branching, thick processes and are located principally in the gray matter of the brain and spinal cord. The **fibrous astrocytes** (spider cells) are found mostly in the white matter and have much longer, less branching, more filamentous processes.

2. **Oligodendroglia** (Gk. oligo, few) are glial cells with only a few processes. They are smaller cells than astrocytes but much more numerous. They synthesize myelin for nerve fibers in the CNS.

3. **Microglia** are small, angular cells resembling inactive fibroblasts. They are phagocytic cells of mesodermal origin. All other glial cells are derived from the ectoderm.

4. **Ependymal cells** are cuboidal glial cells that line the cavities of the CNS. In the adult some of these cells are ciliated—a holdover from the embryo when all of them were ciliated.

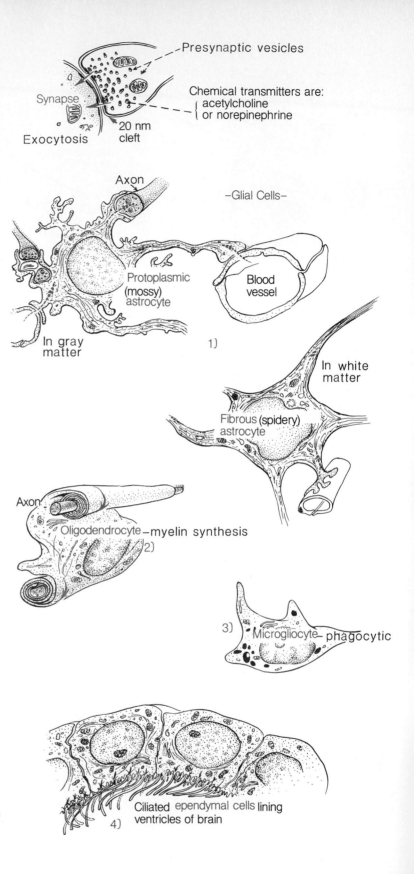

CLASSIFICATION OF TISSUES

A tissue is a group of similar cells modified to perform a common function or functions. Although there are many specialized types of tissues, there are only four primary or basic types, namely, epithelial, connective, muscular, and nervous.

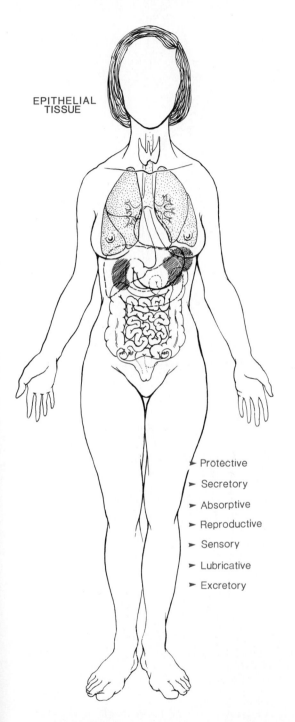

EPITHELIAL
TISSUE

▶ Protective

▶ Secretory

▶ Absorptive

▶ Reproductive

▶ Sensory

▶ Lubricative

▶ Excretory

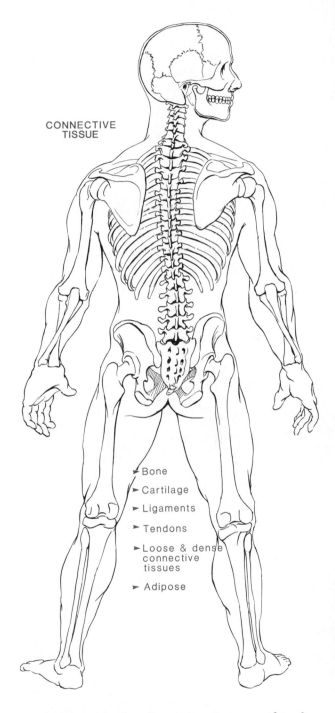

CONNECTIVE
TISSUE

▶ Bone

▶ Cartilage

▶ Ligaments

▶ Tendons

▶ Loose & dense
connective
tissues

▶ Adipose

Epithelial cells primarily cover surfaces and line cavities. The cells are close together with very little intercellular material. Epithelia are chiefly avascular structures that receive oxygen and nutrients by diffusion from nearby blood capillaries. Epithelial cells have great regenerative capacities. Their many functions range from a passive, protective, flat layer to an active, secretory gland synthesizing hormones or enzymes.

Connective tissues function in support and in the binding of parts of the body together. The principal cells (fibroblasts) are widely spaced with large amounts of intercellular matrix. The type and quantity of the fibers, e.g., collagenous, elastic, or reticular, determine the morphology and function. Connective tissues include a wide variety of specialized tissues, ranging from blood and lymph to cartilage and bone.

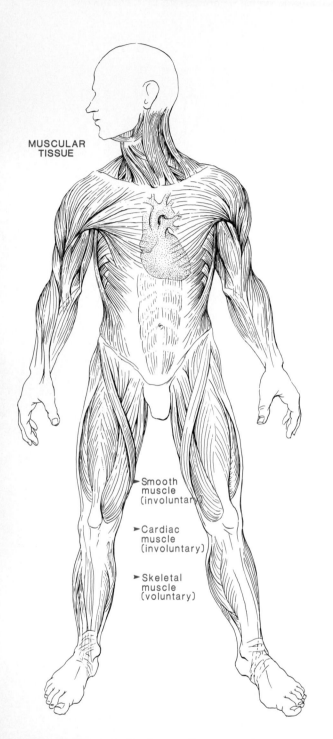

MUSCULAR
TISSUE

Smooth
muscle
(involuntary)

Cardiac
muscle
(involuntary)

Skeletal
muscle
(voluntary)

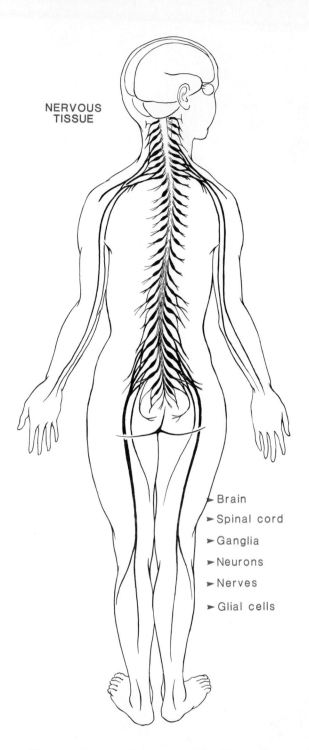

NERVOUS
TISSUE

Brain

Spinal cord

Ganglia

Neurons

Nerves

Glial cells

Muscle tissue is the tissue of action and movement since it has the capacity to contract because of the presence of many myofibrils within the muscle fiber. There are three general types of muscle: smooth (nonstriated), found in the walls of organs and blood vessels; cardiac (striated), found in the walls of the heart; and skeletal (striated), muscle that is usually attached to bones or skin.

Nervous tissue consists of cell bodies, cell processes (nerves), and glia (connective tissue cells). Neurons possess the physiological properties of generating impulses (irritability) and of conductivity (the ability to transmit these impulses). The brain and spinal cord comprise the central nervous system. The nerves that emerge from the spinal cord and brain to pass to parts of the body are the peripheral nervous system, while the organs of the body are innervated by the autonomic nervous system.

Table 3.1 *CLASSIFICATION OF PRIMARY TISSUES*

TYPE	MORPHOLOGY	TYPICAL EXAMPLES	EMBRYONIC ORIGIN
EPITHELIAL TISSUE			
Simple	Squamous cells Cuboidal cells Columnar cells	Endothelium Kidney collecting tubules Lining intestines	Mesoderm Mesoderm Endoderm
Stratified	Squamous cells Cuboidal cells Columnar cells Transitional cells	Epidermis Excretory sweat ducts Part of male urethra Urinary bladder	Ectoderm Ectoderm Endoderm Endoderm
Pseudostratified	Columnar cells (usually ciliated)	Trachea	Endoderm
CONNECTIVE TISSUE			
Connective tissue proper	Loose	In subcutaneous areas	All mesodermal derivatives
	Dense		
	• Irregular	Dermis of skin	
	• Regular	Ligaments and tendons	
Hard	Bone		
	• Spongy (cancellous)	Ends at long bones	
	• Compact (cortical)	Shafts of long bones	
	Cartilage		
	• Hyaline	Tracheal rings	
	• Fibrous	Intervertebral disks	
	• Elastic	External ear	
Fluid	Blood Lymph		
MUSCULAR TISSUE			
Smooth (non-striated, involuntary)	Spindle shaped, mononucleated cells	Wall of gastrointestinal tract and blood vessels	All mesodermal derivatives
Cardiac (striated, involuntary)	Mononucleated cells in branching, cylindrical fibers	Walls and septa of heart	
Skeletal (striated, voluntary)	Long, cylindrical, multi-nucleated fibers	Usually attached to skeleton or skin	
NERVOUS TISSUE			
Cells	Neurons		All ectodermal derivatives except microglia which are mesodermal
	• Unipolar	Spinal (sensory) ganglion	
	• Bipolar	Olfactory cells	
	• Multipolar	Motor cells of spinal cord	
	Neuroglia		
	• Astrocytes	Large star-shaped connective tissue cells in CNS	
	• Oligodendrocytes	Small ovoid connective tissue cell in CNS	
	• Microglia	Small phagocytic cells in CNS	
	• Ependyma	Cuboidal cells lining cavities of CNS	
Neuronal processes	Myelinated	Most fibers of the central and peripheral nervous systems	
	Nonmyelinated	Most fibers of the ANS	
Receptors (nerve endings)	Free (naked) Encapsulated, e.g.,	In cornea and skin	
	• Pacinian	In dermis	
	• Meissner's	In dermal papillae	

Chapter

4

EPITHELIUM

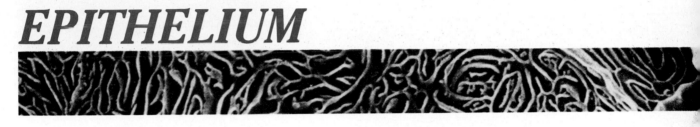

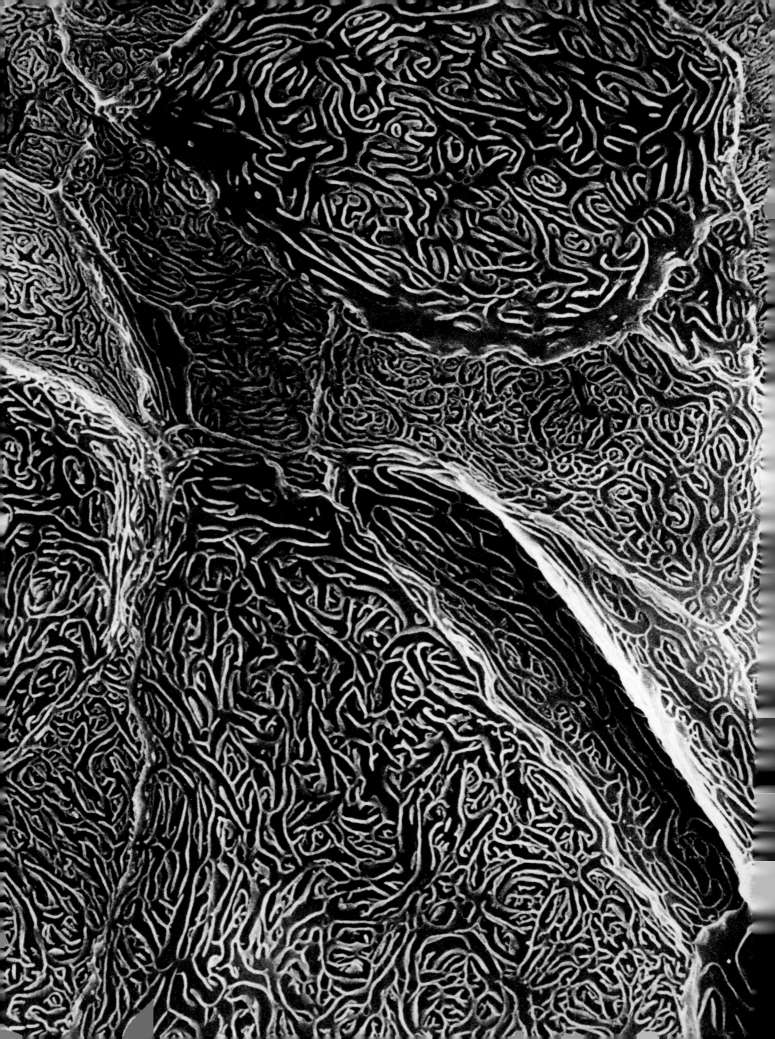

FROM THIS CHAPTER, THE PERCEPTIVE STUDENT WILL BE ABLE TO DEMONSTRATE:

1. Knowledge of the general and specific characteristic features of the various epithelia of the body

2. The ability to distinguish and compare the functions of eight or more morphologically different types of epithelium and where they are located in the body

3. An understanding of the important functions and a visualization of the fine structure of various modifications of the apical, basal, and lateral surfaces of epithelial cells

4. An ability to make judgments on how the many functions of epithelia, including protective, secretory, excretory, lubrication, absorptive, and reproductive, contribute to the health and well-being of the individual

5. An awareness of the concept that if the great capacity for growth and regeneration of epithelial cells becomes uncontrolled, cancer often results

Typically **epithelium** is a layer or layers of closely packed cells that **line cavities** of the body or **cover free surfaces,** as the epidermis of the skin. One surface of the epithelial cell is free (apical), i.e., it is exposed directly to fluid, as in the gastrointestinal (GI) tract; or to air, as in the respiratory system. The opposite or basal surface is fixed, attached to a rather delicate structure, the **basal lamina,** which rests on a vascular bed within the underlying connective tissue. Since epithelium is nearly always **avascular,** it derives its nutrients by diffusion from this vascular plexus. Because epithelial cells have an apical and a basal surface, they are said to be **polarized.**

Epithelium is the most cellular tissue in the body. Its cells are always in close apposition to each other, with only a small amount of **intercellular material,** formerly called cement substance. The intercellular substance often allows cells to glide over each other and offers only minimal resistance to the migration of leukocytes and other connective tissue cells through the epithelial layers. Even when the intercellular space is modified by the presence of junctional complexes between adjacent cell walls, the movement of cells is not entirely blocked.

SPECIAL FEATURES (TABLE 4.1)

Distinctive features of epithelium include: (1) It is the **most distinguishing tissue** of most organs and the cardinal clue for microscopic identification of a structure. It is the **parenchyma,** i.e., the secretory part of a gland or organ, as contrasted to the stroma, which is the supporting connective tissue framework. (2) Practically everything, such as, cells, fluids, and molecules that enter or leave the body at some point in their journey, **pass through an epithelial layer** where these substances may be modified or even synthesized. (3) Epithelial cells have a tremendous capacity for **regeneration,** e.g., in skin wound healing, in the renewal of the lining cells of the uterus following menstruation, and in the replacement of cells lining the GI tract. (4) Some epithelia have the capacity to change from one type of epithelium to another, a transformation called **metaplasia,** as in heavy smokers where the ciliated pseudostratified columnar epithelium may become stratified squamous in type. Other primary tissues are less plastic and usually do not undergo this change. (5) An epithelium usually has **modifications** on its **free surface,** e.g., cilia, microplicae, or microvilli; on its basal surface, **hemidesmosomes,** and **flagella** in sperm cells; and on its lateral surfaces, **junctional complexes.** (6) Epithelia have **many diverse functions,** including protection, digestion, secretion, excretion, and others. (7) Glandular epithelia produce many **secretory products,** e.g., enzymes, hormones, mucus, milk, sweat, oil, and others.

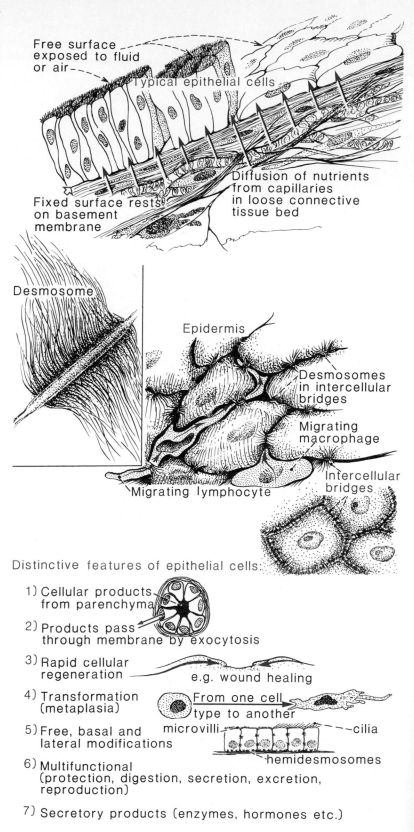

Free surface exposed to fluid or air

Typical epithelial cells

Diffusion of nutrients from capillaries in loose connective tissue bed

Fixed surface rests on basement membrane

Desmosome

Epidermis

Desmosomes in intercellular bridges

Migrating macrophage

Intercellular bridges

Migrating lymphocyte

Distinctive features of epithelial cells:

1) Cellular products from parenchyma

2) Products pass through membrane by exocytosis

3) Rapid cellular regeneration — e.g. wound healing

4) Transformation (metaplasia) — From one cell type to another

5) Free, basal and lateral modifications — microvilli — cilia — hemidesmosomes

6) Multifunctional (protection, digestion, secretion, excretion, reproduction)

7) Secretory products (enzymes, hormones etc.)

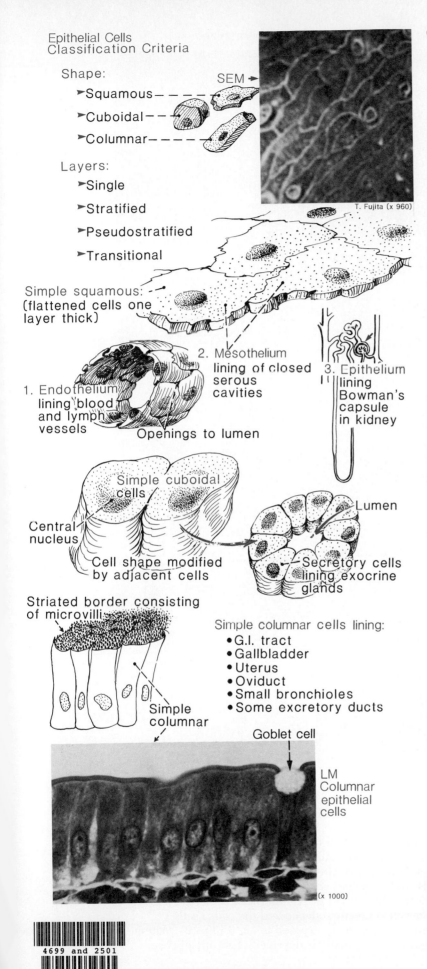

Epithelial Cells Classification Criteria

Shape:
➤Squamous
➤Cuboidal
➤Columnar

SEM ➤

T. Fujita (x 960)

Layers:
➤Single
➤Stratified
➤Pseudostratified
➤Transitional

Simple squamous:
(flattened cells one layer thick)

1. Endothelium lining blood and lymph vessels

2. Mesothelium lining of closed serous cavities

Openings to lumen

3. Epithelium lining Bowman's capsule in kidney

Simple cuboidal cells

Central nucleus

Cell shape modified by adjacent cells

Lumen

Secretory cells lining exocrine glands

Striated border consisting of microvilli

Simple columnar cells lining:
• G.I. tract
• Gallbladder
• Uterus
• Oviduct
• Small bronchioles
• Some excretory ducts

Simple columnar

Goblet cell

LM Columnar epithelial cells

(x 1000)

GENERAL CLASSIFICATION OF EPITHELIA

Epithelium is **classified morphologically** according to (1) the **shape** of the individual cells and (2) the **arrangement** of the cells into one or more layers. The shape of the cells may be **squamous** (flattened), **cuboidal** (about equal dimensions), or **columnar** (taller than it is wide). Epithelial cells are arranged in a **single layer** (simple) or in more than one layer (**stratified**). Based on the shape of the cell and the arrangement of cells into layers, most epithelia are classified as simple squamous, simple cuboidal, or simple columnar. The other types are stratified squamous, stratified cuboidal, or stratified columnar. In addition, some epithelia may be **pseudostratified,** while others are **transitional.**

GENERAL FEATURES OF THE TYPES OF EPITHELIA

Simple Squamous Epithelium

Simple squamous (L., scaly) epithelium consists of **flattened cells** joined together in a sheet, **one cell layer thick.** Centrally each cell may be somewhat thicker due to the presence of a nucleus. In certain structures, the epithelium has special names. For example, simple squamous cells lining the heart, and blood and lymph vessels are called **endothelium**; while the cells lining the closed serous cavities of the body, i.e., peritoneal, pleural, and pericardial, are named **mesothelium.** Because of its thinness, simple squamous epithelium **functions** primarily wherever an **exchange of gases, fluids, nutrients, or metabolites** occurs.

Simple Cuboidal Epithelium

A simple cuboidal epithelium is a sheet of polygonal cells whose **dimensions are essentially equal,** typically forming a cube. However, compacting of the cells may force them into a pyramidal shape. The rounded nucleus is centrally located and does not bulge the cell walls. This type epithelium is found principally (1) lining the ducts of many exocrine glands, (2) as the parenchyma of most glands, and (3) lining most of the larger kidney tubules. In addition to lining various ducts, simple cuboidal epithelia function in vital **secretory activities,** e.g., hormone and enzyme production.

Simple Columnar Epithelium

The cells of simple columnar epithelium resemble the polygonal cuboidal cells except that they are considerably **taller than they are wide.** When seen **in profile the cells resemble columns,** not cubes. The rounded, basal nuclei are usually arranged in a single row. However, crowding of the cells may displace the nuclei into a staggered row or into two rows. Simple columnar epithelia

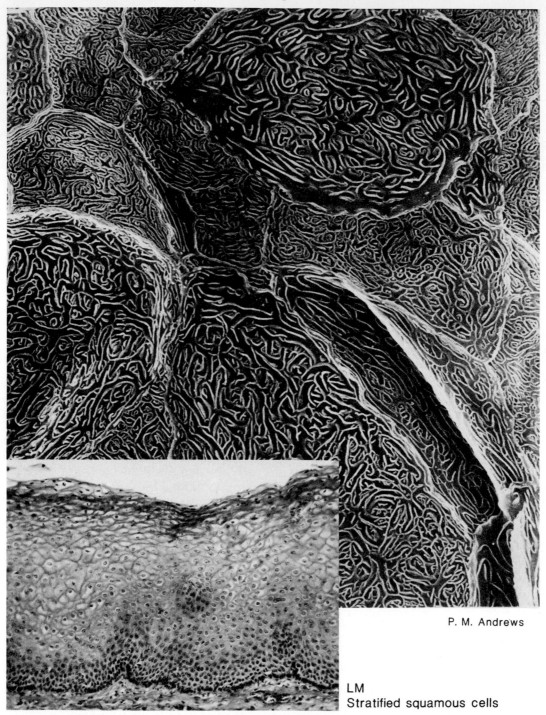

P. M. Andrews

LM
Stratified squamous cells

The exposed, outer surface of certain moist stratified squamous epithelial cells displays a labyrinthine pattern of microscopic ridges, called microplicae. Only moist epithelia exposed to considerable abrasion, such as in the oral cavity, develop these ridges. The microplicae are about 0.1–0.2 μm wide and 0.2–0.8 μm in height, may be straight or curved and often branched. Continuous, circumferential ridgelike elevations demarcate the boundaries of the cells. In the deeper cell layers, desmosomes are associated with many of the microplicae, while in the more superficial cells only a few such junctions are found. Hence, adhesion is greatly reduced and the cells easily desquamate. When the moist epithelium is repeatedly exposed to air, it loses its coating of mucin, becomes dehydrated, keratinized, and finally is deprived of all microplicae.

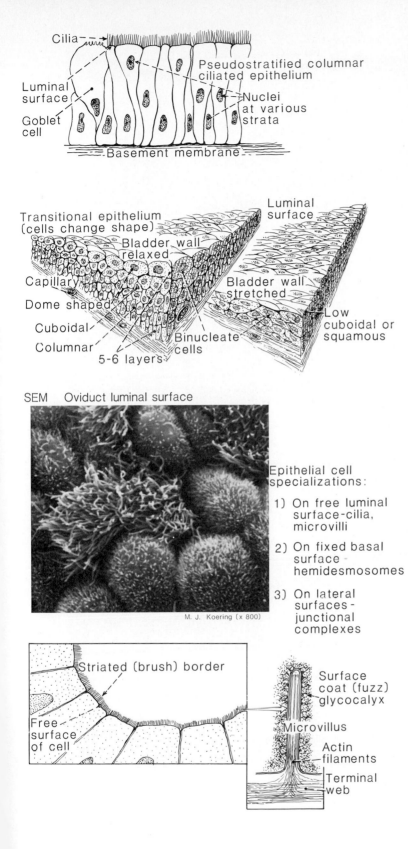

Cilia

Luminal surface

Goblet cell

Pseudostratified columnar ciliated epithelium

Nuclei at various strata

Basement membrane

Transitional epithelium (cells change shape)

Luminal surface

Bladder wall relaxed

Capillary

Dome shaped

Cuboidal

Columnar

5-6 layers

Bladder wall stretched

Binucleate cells

Low cuboidal or squamous

SEM   Oviduct luminal surface

M. J. Koering (x 800)

Epithelial cell specializations:

1) On free luminal surface-cilia, microvilli

2) On fixed basal surface - hemidesmosomes

3) On lateral surfaces - junctional complexes

Striated (brush) border

Free surface of cell

Surface coat (fuzz) glycocalyx

Microvillus

Actin filaments

Terminal web

are widely distributed in the body, especially **lining** the **GI tract, gallbladder, uterus, oviducts,** large excretory **ducts of glands,** and small **bronchioles.** As suggested by their diverse locations, these epithelial cells function principally in **secretion of enzymes and mucus,** and **absorption of nutrients and fluids.** Note that all three types of epithelium look alike in surface view. Only in a profile (vertical) section can they be identified as either squamous, cuboidal, or columnar.

Stratified Epithelium

Where cells form **more than one layer,** they are classified **stratified.** For example, stratified squamous epithelium forms the **epidermis,** stratified columnar cells line large excretory ducts, and the rare stratified cuboidal epithelium lines sweat ducts.

Pseudostratified and Transitional Epithelium

Two additional types of epithelium, which do not fit the above categories, are pseudostratified and transitional. In **pseudostratified epithelium,** a single layer of cells appears to be more than one layer because the **nuclei lie at various levels,** suggesting the presence of several layers of cells. The cells are tightly packed and rest on a common basal lamina. However, some of the cells do not project to the luminal surface. Those that reach the surface are usually **ciliated,** as found in the passageways of the **respiratory system,** and are usually associated with goblet cells.

In **transitional epithelium,** the cells can actually **change their shape,** as observed in cells lining the **ureters and urinary bladder.** For example, when the **bladder is distended** with urine, cells are **reduced to two to three layers** and the surface cells are typically squamous or low cuboidal. In the **empty bladder,** the epithelium may be **five or more layers thick** with the luminal surface cells modified into rounded, **dome-shaped cells, a distinctive feature** of transitional epithelium. Also, many of the surface cells are binucleate. Cells in the relaxed bladder are of all three shapes. (L-A, plate 1)

EPITHELIAL SURFACE MODIFICATIONS

To accommodate the wide variety of functions performed by epithelial cells, their **cell membranes** are frequently **specialized** to enhance these functions and to maintain cellular integrity.

Specializations have been identified on all surfaces of the cells, namely, (1) on the **free luminal surface,** (2) on the **basal fixed surface** next to the compact basal lamina, and (3) on the **lateral surfaces** of adjacent epithelial cells. Also, certain intracellular specializations of the cytoskeleton are adapted to lend support to some of these surface structures.

T. Merrill (x 1200)

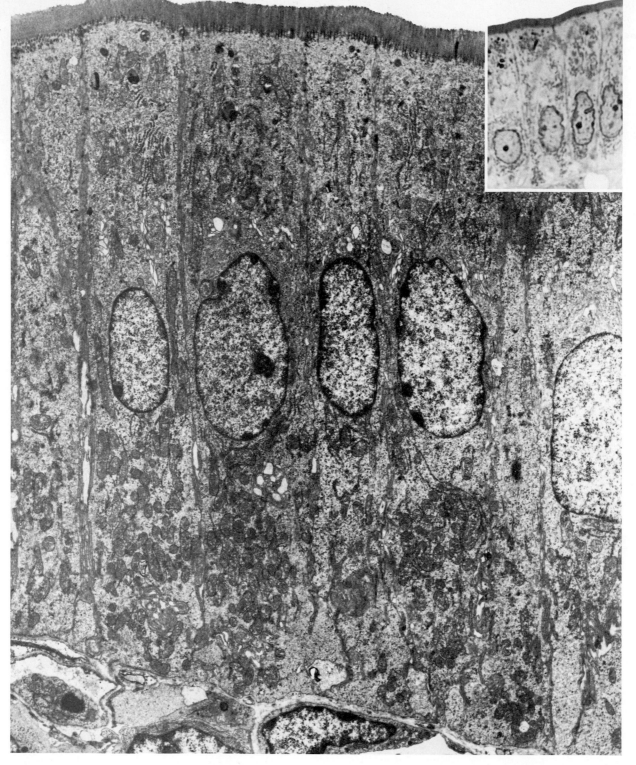

G. U. Anat. Collection (x 2200)

The simple columnar surface epithelial cells covering an intestinal villus demonstrate polarity by marked differences between the free and attached surfaces. The luminal (free) surface is covered by closely packed, uniform microvilli. The subjacent, clear zone is the terminal web (TW), which is relatively free of organelles. The basal lamina separates the basal cell boundary from the underlying capillary bed. Numerous junctional complexes attach adjacent cells. The upper right insert is a LM view of a similar region. The thin, wavy structures are mitochondria, and the small, dark spheres are lipid droplets.

SEM Microvilli and terminal web

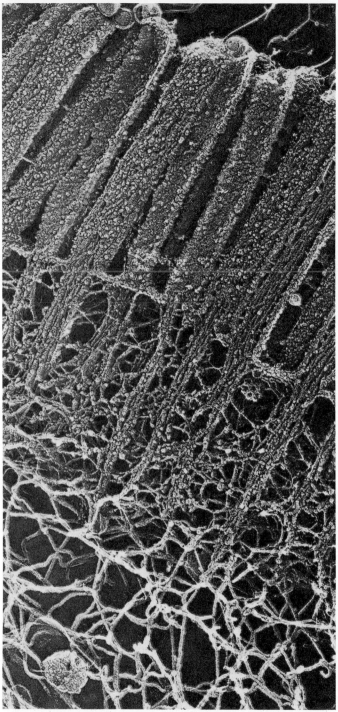

N. Hirokawa, et al. (x 97,000)

EM Cilia

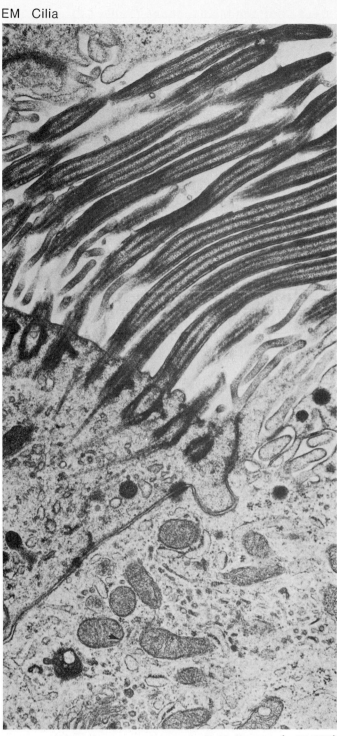

R. M. Brenner (x 24,000)

This figure is a rapid-freeze, deep-etch fracture replica of the striated (brush) border of the mouse intestine, revealing a filamentous cytoskeleton. From this EM micrograph, the cytoskeleton of the terminal web consists of: (1) prominent bundles of actin filaments (rootlets) that extend from the core of the microvillus into the terminal web; (2) an extensive bed of intermediate filaments beneath the rootlets; and (3) a population of well-defined, thinner filaments that run horizontally among the rootlets, and between the rootlets and the deeper intermediate filaments.

This figure is an electron micrograph of a ciliated epithelial cell of the oviduct. Numerous cilia, in longitudinal section, project into the lumen. The shaft (axoneme) of each cilium consists of nine pairs of peripheral and two single microtubules enclosed in the plasmalemma. This arrangement is the so-called 9 + 2 pattern seen in cross-sections of cilia. Each cilium is anchored to the terminal web by a basal body which has a ring of nine triplets of microtubules, identical with centrioles.

Free Surface Modifications (Table 4.2)

MICROVILLI Specialized structures, **microvilli,** appear on the free surface of some epithelial cells. These submicroscopic, fingerlike projections enormously increase, up to 30-fold, the absorptive surface area (see Chapter 1). The light microscope discloses only delicate vertical lines, or striations, in a thin border along the free surface, called the **striated border.** Electron microscopic studies reveal that an irregular **amorphous layer,** the **glycocalyx,** is superimposed on the distal ends of microvilli.

CILIA In the **air passages,** the free surfaces of most of the epithelial lining cells have tiny mobile cilia (5–15 μm in length) **that beat in a rhythmic, wavelike fashion.** In their rapid forward motion (stroke), the cilia are quite rigid yet bend slightly forward. On the slower recovery stroke, each cilium becomes less rigid and curves backward, then becomes stiff again. The rigidity begins first at the base and then proceeds towards the tip of the cilium. The cilia propel mucus and entrapped foreign particles toward the mouth.

TEM studies reveal that the internal structure of a **cilium resembles a centriole.** The central core of a cilium consists of microtubules arranged in **nine pairs (doublets)** of fused microtubules that surround **two central tubules,** forming an **axoneme,** a 9 + 2 microtubular complex. The axoneme is characteristic of cilia and flagella.

Cilia have their origin from **basal bodies** located in the apical cytoplasm of epithelial cells. Basal bodies are hollow cylinders, **identical to centrioles,** with **nine triplets** of microtubules forming their walls. Since they have no central microtubules, they form a **9 + 0 complex.**

STEREOCILIA Cilialike processes can be seen on free ends of epithelial cells lining portions of the male reproductive tract and parts of the inner ear, but here they are matted into tufts and are nonmobile. Their resemblance to cilia has caused them to be named **stereocilia,** but the electron microscope reveals them as unusually long, often branched **microvilli** which do not contain microtubules.

FLAGELLA Flagella resemble cilia but are longer and wider, and usually occur singly on free, unattached cells, such as **spermatozoa.** Through a vigorous whiplike action, they aid in propelling the spermatozoa forward.

Lateral Surface Modifications

JUNCTIONAL COMPLEXES With the electron microscope it is possible to recognize spe-

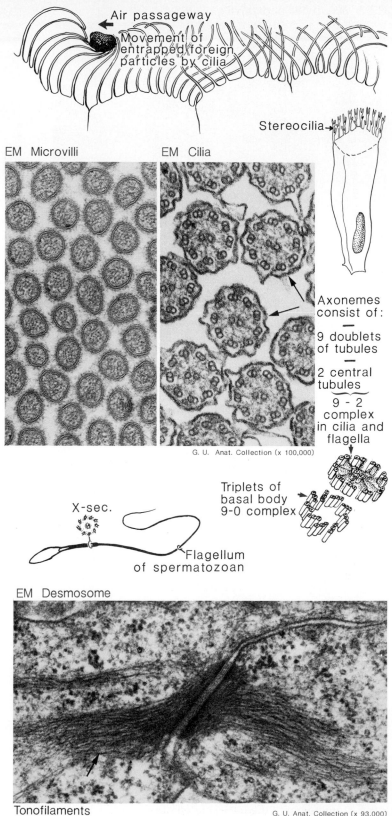

Air passageway

Movement of entrapped foreign particles by cilia

Stereocilia

EM Microvilli

EM Cilia

Axonemes consist of:

— 9 doublets of tubules

— 2 central tubules

9 - 2 complex in cilia and flagella

G. U. Anat. Collection (x 100,000)

Triplets of basal body 9-0 complex

X-sec.

Flagellum of spermatozoan

EM Desmosome

Tonofilaments

G. U. Anat. Collection (x 93,000)

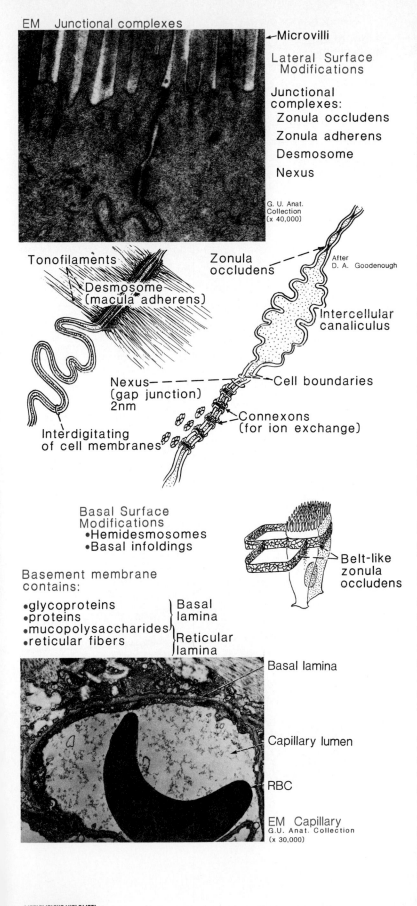

EM Junctional complexes

← Microvilli

Lateral Surface
Modifications

Junctional
complexes:
  Zonula occludens
  Zonula adherens
  Desmosome
  Nexus

G. U. Anat.
Collection
(x 40,000)

After
D. A. Goodenough

Tonofilaments

Desmosome
(macula adherens)

Zonula
occludens

Intercellular
canaliculus

Nexus—
(gap junction)
2nm

Cell boundaries

Interdigitating
of cell membranes

Connexons
(for ion exchange)

Basal Surface
Modifications
  •Hemidesmosomes
  •Basal infoldings

Basement membrane
contains:

•glycoproteins
•proteins
•mucopolysaccharides
•reticular fibers

Basal
lamina

Reticular
lamina

Belt-like
zonula
occludens

Basal lamina

Capillary lumen

RBC

EM Capillary
G.U. Anat. Collection
(x 30,000)

cialized structures, the **junctional complexes**, that link adjacent cells on their lateral surfaces. The most numerous and prominent of these is the **desmosome** (Gk. desmo, bond + soma, body) or **macula adherens**, which resembles an elongated disk split into halves that are separated by a space about 25 nm wide. Each half, derived from contiguous cells, is firmly fixed in place by fine, hairpin loops of **tonofilaments** extending into the cytoplasm of the cell. Desmosomes are the most basal of the cell junctions and may occur wherever two epithelial, or some other cells, are apposed.

The **zonula adherens, or close junction**, has a space about 20 nm wide between apposing cell membranes. It is a **beltlike attachment zone** that encircles the distal ends of epithelial cells and binds them to each other. The **zonula occludens, or tight junction**, appears to seal the channel between adjacent cells, limiting extracellular material from entering or leaving the lumen of an organ lined by epithelium. It is also **a beltlike zone** encircling the distal ends of epithelial cells, distal to the zonula adherens.

The **gap junction, or nexus**, is common to many cells, especially **epithelial, cardiac, and smooth muscle cells,** and some **nerve cells.** Tiny channels termed **connexons** extend across a 2 nm gap between cell membranes like small pipes, permitting an **exchange of ions and small molecules (1000–1200 MW)** between the cytoplasm of cells. In this way, gap junctions provide a means of intercellular communication.

Clinical Comment Most cancer cells do not have gap junctions. Therefore, these cells probably cannot communicate freely with each other. That causes the uncontrolled cell division, which results in tumor growth. In contrast, normal cells "are informed" by neighboring cells of their mitotic activity through interconnecting gap junctions. When a developing tissue mass reaches its "normal" or predetermined size, its mitotic cycle is drastically curtailed and cellular growth is reduced to match approximately cellular death. Hence the tissue remains at its normal volume and, unlike malignant cells, does not invade surrounding tissues.

INTERCELLULAR CANALICULI Intercellular canaliculi are small, irregular **spaces separating the lateral walls** of adjacent epithelial cells. One type extends from the **lateral apical surfaces** to the zonula occludens, which seals off the rest of the intercellular compartment. Another variety is located near the middle of the cell wall, **deep to the junctional complex,** e.g., the bile canaliculus, which is situated between the walls of two adjacent liver cells. A third type may extend as a narrow, often branched, **blind-ending passageway** that ends before reaching the basal lamina. Microvilli of various lengths project into these canaliculi, greatly increasing the absorptive surface of the cell.

Basal Surface Modifications

BASEMENT MEMBRANE Nearly all epithelia rest on a **basement membrane,** which is interposed between the basal surface of epithelial cells and the underlying loose connective tissue layer.

Under the EM the basement membrane is resolved into two distinct layers: (1) A thin, flocculent zone next to the epithelium is called the **basal lamina.** It is rich in carbohydrates, especially **mucopolysaccharides,** which stain deeply with periodic acid-Schiff (PAS) reagent. (2) The deeper layer closer to the connective tissue, the **reticular lamina,** is composed mostly of **reticular fibers** and condensed ground substance.

After considerable controversy, it is now generally agreed that the **reticular lamina** is derived from **connective tissue,** while the **basal lamina** is a product of the **epithelium.** Keep in mind that the basement membrane is a distinct, separate entity and should not be confused with the basal segment of the plasmalemma of the epithelial cell that lies upon or attaches to the basal lamina of the basement membrane. One may question the accuracy of describing the basement membrane as a modification of the basal surface of an epithelial cell, since it is not actually a part of the cell. However, long-established usage dictates its inclusion here.

HEMIDESMOSOMES Electron micrographs, especially of the epidermis (the epithelial layer of the skin), reveal basal attachment plates that help **anchor the epithelial cells to the basal lamina.** They are called **hemidesmosomes** because they are only half desmosomes. There is no matching half of the structure in the underlying connective tissue, as in adjacent epithelial cells.

BASAL INFOLDINGS Basal infoldings of the plasma membrane are another type of basal surface specialization of epithelial cells. These infoldings are especially prominent in the cells lining certain of the tubules of the kidney. Such infolding of the cell membrane greatly **increases the surface area** of the cell, thus markedly augmenting its absorption capacity.

Cytoskeleton Modifications

TONOFILAMENTS In epithelial cells, especially adapted for protection, e.g., stratified squamous (epidermis), there develops a system of cytoplasmic reinforcements, a **modification of the cytoskeleton.** It consists of submicroscopic **tonofilaments,** about 10 nm in diameter, which are arranged in bundles to form tonofibrils that can be seen with the light microscope. Most of the fine tonofilaments **attach** to the **desmosomes and hemidesmosomes** that provide support to these structures.

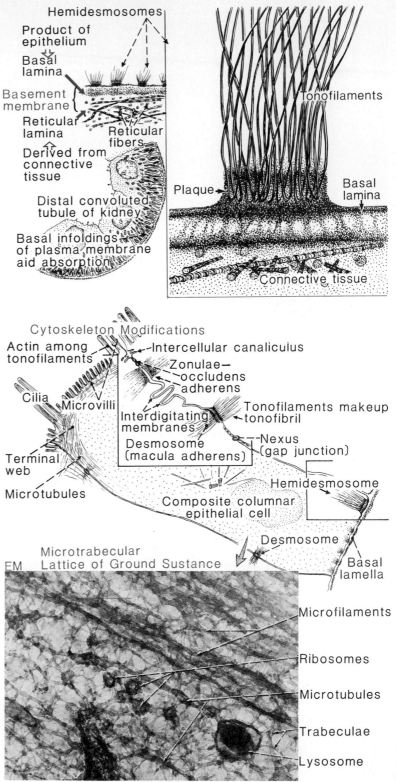

K. R. Porter and K. L. Anderson (x120,000)

Microtrabecular Lattice of Ground Substance

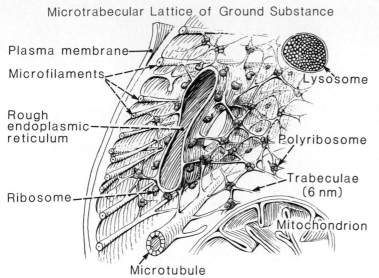

Plasma membrane

Microfilaments

Rough endoplasmic reticulum

Ribosome

Lysosome

Polyribosome

Trabeculae (6 nm)

Mitochondrion

Microtubule

Adapted from K.R. Porter & J.B. Tucker

Functions of Epithelial Cells of Mucous Membranes

➤ Protection from:
- mechanical trauma
- dehydration
- pathogens

➤ Secretion of:
- hormones, milk, sweat
- enzymes, HCL, glycoproteins
- mucous and serous products

➤ Lubrication of:
- contents of GI tract
- fetus in birth canal
- joints

➤ Filtration of wastes

➤ Absorption of foods

➤ Taste

➤ Smell ⎱ neuro-epithelium

➤ Hearing

➤ Reproduction

LM Mesothelium

(x 400)

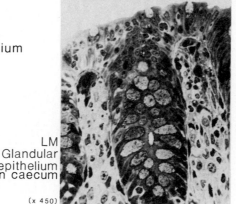

LM Glandular epithelium in caecum

(x 450)

TERMINAL WEB The terminal web, a poorly defined zone **adjacent to the apical free cell surface,** is another modification of the cytoskeleton. It is found in epithelial cells with apical appendages, either microvilli or cilia. It is essentially free of cell organelles and contains clusters of tonofilaments that lie parallel to the apical surface. Thus the terminal web supplies **support** for the microvilli or cilia located on the apical surface. These filaments also form a support core for each microvillus to give it slight rigidity and may possibly contract the microvilli since some tonofilaments contain the **contractile protein, actin.**

INTRACELLULAR GROUND SUBSTANCE In the 1980s, Porter et al., using the high-voltage EM, discovered a new **cytoplasmic support network within the matrix** (ground substance) of several strains of cultured epithelial and connective tissue cells. Their conclusions on this newly discovered structure are that:

. . . the **cytoplasmic ground substance,** long assumed to be a homogeneous, protein-rich solution is now believed to possess a highly intricate structure and behaviour of its own. The **microtrabecular lattice** organizes the diverse components of the cell into a functional unity—the **cytoplast**—and mediates regulated and directed transport within the cell. It is also becoming increasingly apparent that the control of cell shape and of cell movement depends on the integrated functioning of the microtubules, the microfilaments, the microtubule-organizing centers and microtrabecular lattice.

A somewhat different concept of the intracellular ground substance has been reported by Bridgman and Reese (1984). Also using a high-voltage electron microscope, they found that the cytoplasm of fibroblasts and epithelial cells consists of a meshwork of electron-dense, interwoven filaments, some ending free, while others make junctions with adjacent filaments. Large, very electron-dense granules (ribosomes?) adhere randomly to the filaments. Extended processes of these cells contain mitochondria, large stress fibers, and a matrix containing fine granular material.

FUNCTIONS

Epithelia have many functions. Among them are:

1. **Protection.** Some cells, such as the epithelium of the skin, protect the body against mechanical damage. Also the cornified cellular layers of the epidermis protect the body from dehydration and the invasion of harmful bacteria.

2. **Secretory.** Certain epithelial cells secrete products that are expelled into the bloodstream (hormones), into ducts and hollow organs (acids and enzymes), or onto the skin (sweat, sebum, and oil).

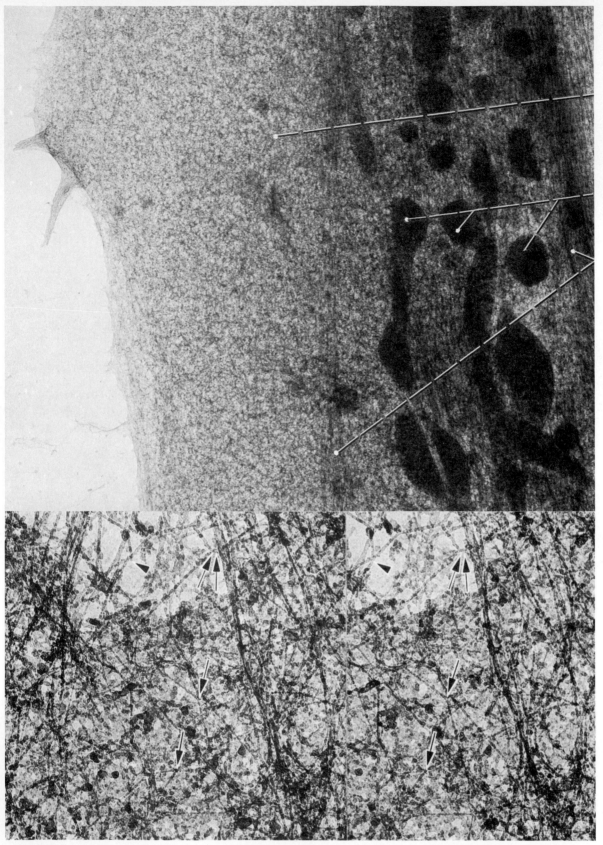

Filamentous
meshwork
containing
cytoplasmic
ground
substance

Mitochondria

Stress fibers

P.C. Bridgman
and
T.S. Reese
(x 16,500)

EM

Stereo view
of lysed cell

Filamentous
meshwork

Fiber junctions
at arrows

Cytoplasmic
ground
substance

P.C. Bridgman
and
T.S. Reese
(x 54,000)

Cell filamentous meshwork and cytoplasmic ground substance as seen with the hi-voltage electron microscope. The cytoskeleton consists of discrete interwoven filaments as seen in cultured fibroblasts from the frog. Numerous finer filaments (as seen in the lower figure at higher magnification) interconnect with the larger filaments. Fiber junctions (in the bottom figure) are indicated by arrows; pseudo junctions by double arrows; free endings by arrowheads. The granular ground substance represents aggregates of cytoplasmic proteins when freeze substitution methods are utilized.

3. **Lubrication.** Various types of glandular epithelial cells secrete copious amounts of **mucus,** a viscous product rich in mucopolysaccharides and mucoproteins but poor in enzymes. It is an excellent lubricant and functions in such dissimilar ways as aiding the movement of food along the alimentary tract and facilitating the passage of the newborn through the birth canal. Mesothelial cells, lining the closed body cavities, secrete a thin **serous fluid** that prevents friction of organs rubbing against each other.

4. **Excretion.** Other epithelial cells filter waste products from the blood which are then excreted as urine or sweat.

5. **Absorption.** We are nourished by the food we eat because of the absorptive function of the epithelial cells lining the digestive tract.

6. **Special sensations.** We taste, smell, and hear with specialized neuroepithelia.

7. **Reproduction.** Even the perpetuation of the species is accomplished by unique epithelial cells, the sex cells, of the ovaries and testes.

Epithelia produce a legion of **diverse products,** as varied as milk and mucus, sebum and sweat, enzymes and hormones, bile and hydrochloric acid, and sex cells and neuroepithelial cells. Epithelia may function in **protection,** e.g., against dehydration, invasion of pathogenic organisms, and mechanical trauma; in **secretion,** both exocrine and endocrine; in **excretion** of organic wastes; in **absorption** of nutrients, and oxygen and carbon dioxide; in **lubrication** with mucus and serous fluids; in **sensory reception** through neuroepithelium located in the nose, ears, and mouth; and in **reproduction,** since ova and spermatozoa are epithelial cells.

Epithelia have a variety of **surface specializations** to aid in their varied functions. They include microvilli, intercellular canaliculi, and basal infoldings which greatly **increase the cell surface area** for the transport and absorption of nutrients into or out of cells. Cilia, covering the free surface of some cells, sweep debris-laden mucus along the cell surface, while a basal flagellum propels each sperm cell along the reproductive tract. Modifications of lateral surfaces into specialized **junctional complexes** link adjacent cells together to form continuous sheets of cells. Gap junctions provide communication between cells by the exchange of ions and small molecules.

Epithelium is usually the most characteristic tissue of any organ. Its morphology is the best clue for the differentiation of normal from abnormal growth. Most cancers are essentially uncontrolled proliferation of epithelial cells that invade and destroy adjacent tissues.

Table 4.1 *DISTINGUISHING FEATURES OF EPITHELIA*

MORPHOLOGICAL TYPES	SHAPE OF CELLS	NUMBER OF LAYERS	SPECIALIZATIONS OF FREE SURFACE	SPECIALIZATIONS OF BASAL SURFACE
SQUAMOUS				
● Simple	Flat plates	One	Microvilli and microplicae	Hemidesmosomes
● Stratified (nonkeratinized)	Surface cells flat; deeper cells irregular polyhedral	Two or more	Microplicae	Hemidesmosomes
● Stratified (keratinized)	Same	Same	Superficial cells markedly keratinized; deeper cells much less	Same
CUBOIDAL				
● Simple	About same height as width, a cube	One	May have microvilli with fuzzy coat superimposed (brush border); some cilia in small bronchioles	Extensive basal infoldings in convoluted tubules of kidney
● Stratified	Cuboidal	Usually 2–3	None	None
COLUMNAR				
● Simple	Of various heights which are always greater than widths	One	Microvilli (striated border) prominent; has fuzzy coat (glycocalyx)	Hemidesmosomes
● Stratified	Surface cells columnar; deeper cells more cuboidal	2–6	A few short microvilli present in urethras	Same
● Pseudostratified (ciliated)	Cells varying in height but all rest on basal lamina	Only one but appears to be several because of different levels of nuclei	Abundant motile cilia; some microvilli interposed	Same
● Transitional (stratified)	Surface cells dome-shaped in empty bladder; flat in distended organ; basal cells polyhedral	2–4 in full bladder; 6 or more in relaxed state	None	None

SPECIALIZATIONS OF LATERAL SURFACES	EXAMPLES OF LOCATIONS	FUNCTION(S)	EMBRYONIC ORIGIN	COMMENTS
SQUAMOUS				
Gap junctions (in endothelium); interdigitations of cell boundaries	Thin kidney tubules; lines closed body cavities (mesothelium); lining of vessels (endothelium)	Absorption of H_2O; protection; diffusion of O_2 and CO_2	Mesoderm	Mesothelium facilitates movements of viscera; may regenerate from adjacent connective tissue cells
Desmosomes numerous, especially between basal and intermediate cell layers	Lines oral cavity, esophagus, vagina, and anus	Protection	Endoderm and ectoderm	Often confused with transitional epithelium
Same	Epidermis	Prevents dehydration; protection; synthesis of vitamin D	Ectoderm	Effective barrier against noxious substances in environment
CUBOIDAL				
Some desmosomes	Thyroid follicles; kidney tubules; covering ovary (germinal epithelium)	Secretion; protection	Endoderm and mesoderm	Very common in kidney, salivary glands and pancreas
Same	Sweat gland ducts; developing ovarian follicle	Protection; secretion	Ectoderm and mesoderm	Rare type
COLUMNAR				
Abundant desmosomes, zonula occludens, zonula adherens, nexus, and interdigitations of adjacent plasmalemmae	Lines GI tract	Secretion; protection; absorption; lubrication	Endoderm	Number of goblet mucous cells increases distally along GI tube; largely replace epithelial cells in colon
Same junctional complexes as above, but fewer in number	Parts of male and female urethras and large excretory ducts, e.g., salivary and mammary glands	Protection	Endoderm	Rare type
Same	Respiratory passageways	Protection; elimination of airborne particulate matter entrapped in mucus which is moved towards mouth by ciliary action	Endoderm	Also called respiratory epithelium
Only a few, small desmosomes; numerous interdigitations and projections which disappear during distension	Lines urinary passageways, except distal parts of urethras	Protection	Mesoderm and endoderm	Adapts to distension by cells sliding over each other to reduce height of epithelium and number of layers

Table 4.2   SPECIALIZATIONS OF FREE SURFACE OF EPITHELIA

	MICROVILLI OF STRIATED BORDER	MICROVILLI OF BRUSH BORDER	STEREOCILIA (MICROVILLI)	CILIA	FLAGELLA
Location	GI tract, gallbladder	Proximal convoluted tubule of kidney, choroid plexus, placenta	Epididymis, ductus deferens, internal ear	Respiratory system, oviduct, uterus, ependyma	Spermatozoa
Morphology	Even rows of short, narrow, nonbranching cytoplasmic processes	Longer, uneven in length, closely packed, nonbranching processes	Longest, uneven in length, branching, matted together as tufts	Hairlike cytoplasmic extensions anchored by basal bodies	Similar to cilia but much longer
Size	0.5–1.0 μm × 0.1 μm	1–2 μm × 0.1 μm	2–3 μm × 0.1 μm	5–15 μm × 0.2 μm	30–60 μm × 1.0–0.2 μm
Number per cell	About 2000	Same	Less than 2000	About 250	One
Cytoskeleton	Straight, parallel actin filaments anchored into terminal web and extend to apex	Same	Same	Two central microtubules surrounded by nine doublet tubules that extend from tip of cilium into basal body	Same as cilia
Mobility	May shorten producing a "pumping" action	Same	None	Continuous, vibratory, metachronous, beating rhythm	Regular, lashing, whiplike movements
Function	Absorption	Absorption	Absorption and perhaps secretion	Movement of surface mucus and particulate matter	Propel sperm forward
Histochemical reaction	Stains with PAS (due to glycocalyx)	Same	Same		

Chapter

5

SPECIALIZATIONS OF EPITHELIA—GLANDS, SEROUS AND MUCOUS MEMBRANES

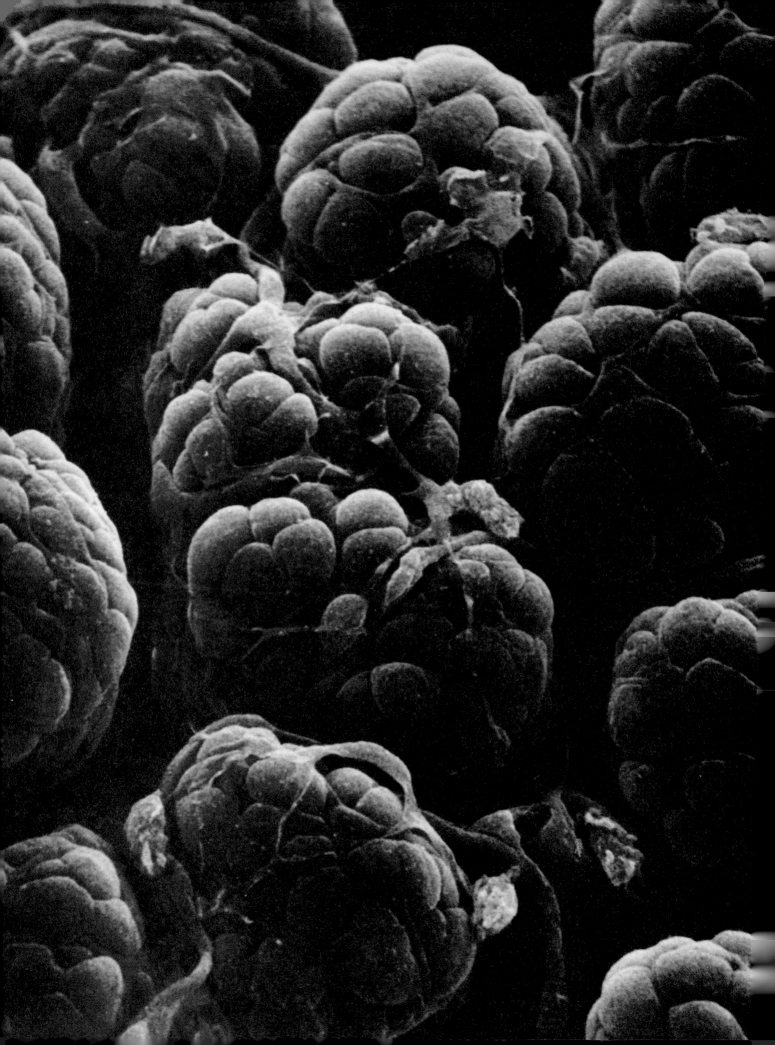

THE READER SHOULD BE ABLE TO:

1. Accept the concept that glands are largely masses of epithelial cells clustered together to perform a specific function.

2. Realize that exocrine multicellular glands have an elaborate duct system that discharges secretions, while endocrine glands are free of ducts and secrete hormones eventually into the circulatory system.

3. Understand the functional and structural differences between mucous and serous membranes.

4. Discuss the different modes of secretion of exocrine glands, i.e., merocrine, apocrine, and holocrine.

5. Demonstrate that glandular secretions, aided by the nervous system, participate in the regulation of the vital functions of the body.

GLANDS

Glands are aggregates of epithelial cells clustered together to perform a specific secretory or excretory function. These cells, called **glandular epithelium,** synthesize and secrete products peculiar to their metabolism, e.g., hormones, enzymes, milk, mucus, sweat, and oil. Glandular epithelium is also specialized to **remove metabolic wastes** from the blood stream and to eliminate them from the body. For example, urea is a metabolic by-product, eliminated from the blood stream by the kidney, and bile is excreted by liver cells into ducts that eventually empty into the duodenum.

Glands are classified into two main functional types: exocrine and endocrine. **Exocrine** glands pour their products into ducts that open into the lumen of an organ or onto the skin. **Endocrine** glands have no duct system, therefore, they are also called ductless glands. Their secretions eventually empty into the lymph or bloodstream.

Exocrine Glands

UNICELLULAR GLANDS Individual cells may function as exocrine glands, such as the **mucous goblet cells** in the lining epithelium of the intestines, or air passageways. These cells act as **unicellular glands.** The mucus they release **lubricates** the passage of materials along the intestinal tract, and, in the respiratory system, it **moistens** the air and **entraps** inhaled dust and carbon particles. However, most exocrine glands are multicellular.

MULTICELLULAR GLANDS Certain simple exocrine glands do not have a discrete duct system but are entirely **intraepithelial,** that is, they lie wholly within the epithelial layer, where the lumen of the structure acts as the duct. Examples of this type of gland are **mucous crypts** found in the urethral and nasal epithelia. They are quite rare and may be transitory structures.

If glandular epithelial cells extend from an epithelial layer into the underlying connective tissue, they develop a duct system and are called **intramural glands** because they remain within the wall (L. murus) of an organ, e.g., deep esophageal and duodenal glands. During development, certain internal glandular epithelia penetrate the organ wall to migrate to some distant area where they proliferate into definitive secretory structures with an extensive duct pattern. They are the **extramural glands,** e.g., pancreas, liver, and salivary glands.

The pancreas has two major functions. As an exocrine gland, it secretes digestive enzymes that react primarily in the small intestine. As an endocrine gland, it synthesizes the hormones insulin and glucagon, which regulate the level of blood sugar in the circulating blood.

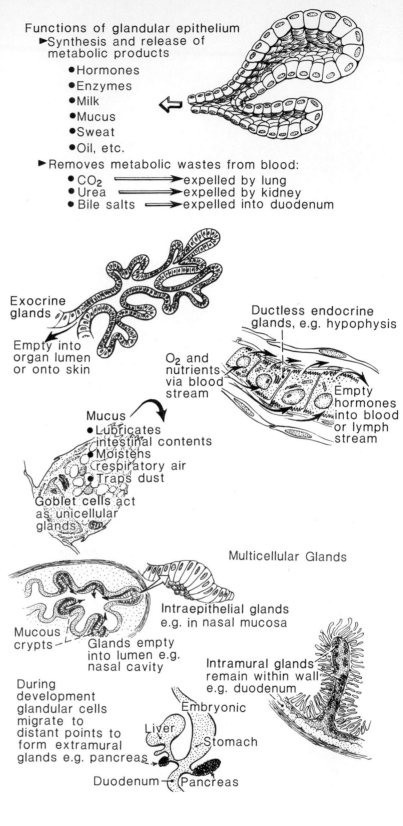

Functions of glandular epithelium
► Synthesis and release of metabolic products
- Hormones
- Enzymes
- Milk
- Mucus
- Sweat
- Oil, etc.

► Removes metabolic wastes from blood:
- CO_2 ⟹ expelled by lung
- Urea ⟹ expelled by kidney
- Bile salts ⟹ expelled into duodenum

Exocrine glands
Empty into organ lumen or onto skin

Ductless endocrine glands, e.g. hypophysis

O_2 and nutrients via blood stream

Empty hormones into blood or lymph stream

Mucus
- Lubricates intestinal contents
- Moistens respiratory air
- Traps dust

Goblet cells act as unicellular glands

Multicellular Glands

Intraepithelial glands e.g. in nasal mucosa

Mucous crypts

Glands empty into lumen e.g. nasal cavity

Intramural glands remain within wall e.g. duodenum

During development glandular cells migrate to distant points to form extramural glands e.g. pancreas

Embryonic
Liver
Stomach
Duodenum
Pancreas

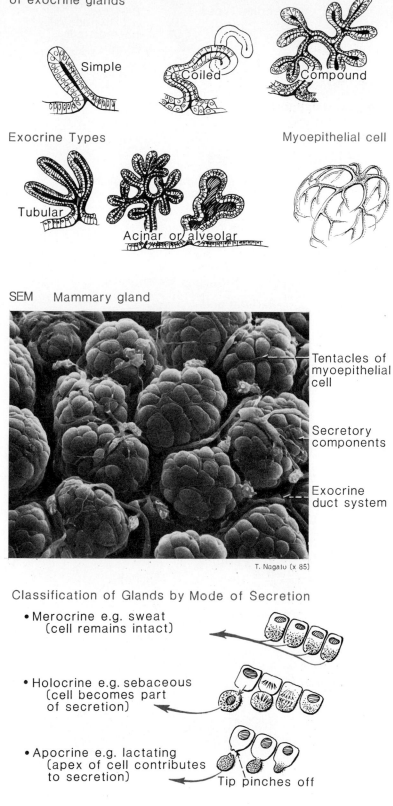

Morphological classification of exocrine glands

Simple   Coiled   Compound

Exocrine Types   Myoepithelial cell

Tubular

Acinar or alveolar

SEM   Mammary gland

Tentacles of myoepithelial cell

Secretory components

Exocrine duct system

T. Nagato (x 85)

Classification of Glands by Mode of Secretion

- Merocrine e.g. sweat (cell remains intact)

- Holocrine e.g. sebaceous (cell becomes part of secretion)

- Apocrine e.g. lactating (apex of cell contributes to secretion)   Tip pinches off

MORPHOLOGICAL CLASSIFICATION

(Table 5.1) Morphologically, some exocrine glands are **simple**, i.e., they consist of a single, straight or coiled tube, or a single saclike structure called an acinus or alveolus. Others are **compound glands**, with very complex, multiple branchings of their excretory ducts and a variety of secretory endpieces. By definition, a compound gland has a branched, excretory duct system, while a simple gland has a single, unbranched duct.

The secretory terminations may be **tubular**, **acinar** (grapelike), **alveolar** (tublike), or **saccular** (pouchlike). In transverse sections these latter three types closely resemble each other and their distinctive features become indistinct and more arbitrary than real. Therefore, the terms alveolar, acinar, and saccular are often used as synonyms.

Often associated with these secretory endpieces are **myoepithelial (basket) cells.** As their name implies, they contract like muscle cells, yet they have the appearance of epithelial cells. They lie within the **basal lamina** of the glandular cells. Their long, branching, cytoplasmic tentacles or processes surround and attach, by desmosomes, to the secretory cells. These processes are richly supplied with microfilaments, mostly **actin microfilaments.** Contraction of the processes aids in the **discharge** of the exocrine secretions.

Both the duct system and the secretory components are surrounded by loose connective tissue laced with many blood capillaries. These vessels supply the gland with oxygen and nutrients essential for the production of specific secretory products.

MODE OF SECRETION Exocrine glands are also classified by their **manner of secretion**, i.e., merocrine (Gk. meros, part; krinein, to separate) or eccrine; holocrine (Gk. holos, all), or apocrine (Gk. apo, from). In the **merocrine type,** e.g., salivary glands, the secretion passes from the cell without damage to the plasma membrane or loss of cytoplasm, by the process of exocytosis. In **holocrine** glands the cells rupture, die, and become part of the secretory product, as in the sebaceous glands of the skin. In **apocrine** glands characteristics of both of the other types are present. For example, in the lactating mammary gland, the apical end of the glandular cell is pinched off with a portion of the cytoplasm, which becomes part of the secretory product. However, the remainder of the cell is still functional, for it repairs itself and continues to secrete milk.

The major exocrine glands, e.g., salivary, pancreas, and liver, are discussed in detail in Chapters 17 and 19.

Endocrine Glands

Table 5.1 is a morphological classification of glands. The **ductless or endocrine glands** include pituitary, pineal, thyroid, parathyroid, adrenal, pancreas, testis, ovary, and others. Their cells may be arranged as **cords** (in adrenal cortex), **follicles** (in thyroid), or **clusters** (in pituitary). Their **profuse blood supply** ensures ample oxygen and raw materials for the **synthesis** of their various **hormones** and for the transport of the hormones to target cells elsewhere in the body. These glands will be discussed in detail in Chapters 19, 21, and 22.

EPITHELIAL MEMBRANES

In the larger sense, there are two kinds of epithelial membranes, **serous and mucous**, present in the body. Each type contains both epithelial and connective tissue components. These membranes are kept moist by secretions of epithelial cells and fluid extruded from underlying capillaries. Because of their wet surfaces, they are also called **moist membranes.**

Serous Membrane or Serosa

The surface epithelium of a **serous membrane** consists of a sheet of simple squamous cells, the **mesothelium,** resting on a thin layer of loose connective tissue, collectively called the serosa. Mesothelial cells line the closed body cavities. Through these cells pass a clear, watery secretion, the **serous fluid,** which is essentially free of enzymes. The fluid spreads as a thin, moist film over the organs and walls of the serous cavities. Since it is an excellent **lubricant,** the viscera glide freely over each other without perceptive friction.

The serous membrane is also a highly **absorptive** structure. It can rapidly transfer solutions (drugs, glucose, etc.) from its surface into the blood stream. Absorption is facilitated by the presence of scattered, uneven **microvilli** that project from the flat, **mesothelial cells. Wandering phagocytic cells,** e.g., macrophages and neutrophils, act as scavengers as they move over the serous membrane (page 106).

SEROUS CAVITIES In addition to lining the large closed cavities in the body, serous membranes form small closed sacs, or **bursae,** associated with certain muscles and joints, and also surround some tendons as **synovial sheaths.** Examples of closed serous cavities are: (1) the **peritoneal cavity** of the abdomen and pelvis, (2) the **pleural cavities** surrounding the lungs, (3) the **pericardial cavity** around the heart, and (4) the **synovial cavities** of joints. The serous membranes in these specific regions are called the peritoneum, pleura, pericardium, and synovial membranes, respectively.

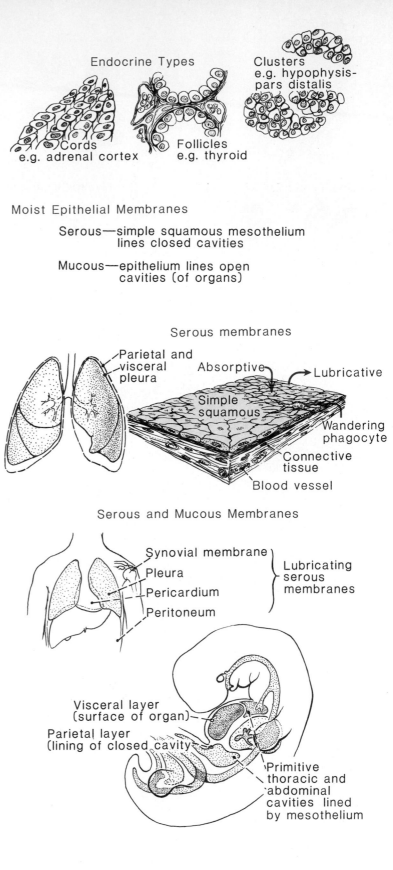

Endocrine Types

Clusters e.g. hypophysis-pars distalis

Cords e.g. adrenal cortex

Follicles e.g. thyroid

Moist Epithelial Membranes

Serous—simple squamous mesothelium lines closed cavities

Mucous—epithelium lines open cavities (of organs)

Serous membranes

Parietal and visceral pleura

Absorptive

Lubricative

Simple squamous

Wandering phagocyte

Connective tissue

Blood vessel

Serous and Mucous Membranes

Synovial membrane

Pleura

Pericardium

Peritoneum

Lubricating serous membranes

Visceral layer (surface of organ)

Parietal layer (lining of closed cavity)

Primitive thoracic and abdominal cavities lined by mesothelium

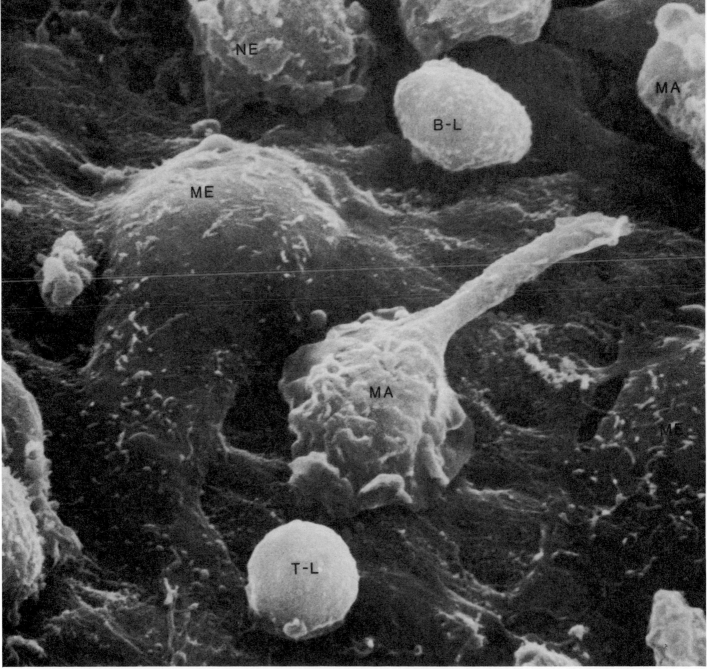

(NE) Neutrophil
(T-L) T-Lymphocyte

(B-L) B-Lymphocyte
(MA) Macrophage
(ME) Mesothelium cell

L. V. Leak (x 4,750)

This is a SEM micrograph of the inferior surface of the mouse diaphragm. It is covered with the peritoneal (serous) membrane that lines the abdominal cavity. This view shows two distinct populations of cells. The deeper, intact layer is composed of pleomorphic, dome-shaped mesothelial cells (ME) with many broad, interlocking cytoplasmic processes. The other cell group consists of various cell visitants that rest superficially upon the mesothelial cells. These various cells can be identified by characteristic surface markings. For example, in addition to its large size, the macrophage (MA) has extensive, deep surface ruffles and several pseudopodia. The small T-lymphocyte (T-L) has a relatively smooth surface, except for a few short microvilli, while the B-lymphocyte (B-L) has a roughened surface with many microvilli. The neutrophil (NE) is intermediate in size and is covered by shallow surface folds. Usually it does not show pseudopodia in fixed specimens.

Mucous Membrane or Mucosa

Mucous membranes line the cavities of most organs of the body that **open to the outside**, such as the lumens of the **respiratory, digestive, reproductive,** and **urogenital** organs. However, the term mucous membrane is slightly misleading because it implies that only mucous cells or glands are present. This is not always true. For example, in the mucous membrane of the respiratory and digestive tracts, both serous and mucous glands coexist; while in the urinary tract the mucous membrane has no glands.

A typical mucous membrane (mucosa) consists of **four layers:**

1. A free, moist, **inner layer** may be formed by many types of **epithelium.** These cells vary in morphology and function depending on their location. For example, interspersed among the simple columnar cells lining the digestive tract are many **goblet cells** whose mucoid secretion protects the intestinal lining cells and aids in the movement of the intestinal contents. Also the apical ends of the columnar cells are completely covered by even, closely packed **microvilli** that greatly increase the absorptive area of the gut. The adjacent SEM micrograph shows rounded, globular goblet cells projecting above the heavy mat of microvilli that covers the distal ends of the columnar cells. At higher magnification, the heavily packed, uniform microvilli of an intact goblet cell are seen projecting above the surface of the lining cells, while an exhausted goblet cell has receded below the cell surface.

In contrast, the **mucous membrane** of the **respiratory system** has many **ciliated cells** but sparse microvilli. Cells of some mucous membranes of the **urinary system,** such as certain tubules of the kidney, have no cilia but very long, uneven **microvilli,** called the **brush border.** However, the urinary passageways have no cilia or microvilli, and the lining cells are usually of the **transitional** variety. Functions of the lining cells may be protective, secretory, absorptive, excretory, or combinations of these actions.

2. The next layer is the very **thin basement membrane** that, under the EM, reveals two layers. The inner layer is the **basal lamina,** a homogeneous, electron-dense, PAS-positive layer, 50–100 nm thick, located next to the bases of the epithelial cells. The outer layer is the **reticular lamina,** a tangle of fine, **reticular fibers** interposed between the basal lamina and the underlying loose connective tissue layer, the tunica propria (see next page). The basement membrane serves two vital functions: (a) It acts as a two-way **filter** or diffusion barrier to protect the body from the entrance of harmful, macromolecular substances into the bloodstream; and (b) it provides an elastic support for **protection** against the trauma from hard, rough materials as they pass through the lumen of an organ.

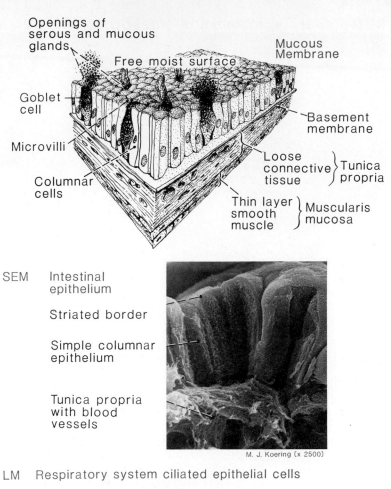

Openings of serous and mucous glands

Free moist surface

Mucous Membrane

Goblet cell

Basement membrane

Microvilli

Loose connective tissue } Tunica propria

Columnar cells

Thin layer smooth muscle } Muscularis mucosa

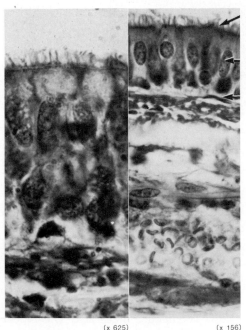

SEM Intestinal epithelium

Striated border

Simple columnar epithelium

Tunica propria with blood vessels

M. J. Koering (x 2500)

LM   Respiratory system ciliated epithelial cells

Ciliated border

Goblet and columnar epithelial cells

Basement membrane

Lamina propria with blood and lymph capillaries

(x 625)   (x 156)

SEM
Goblet
cells

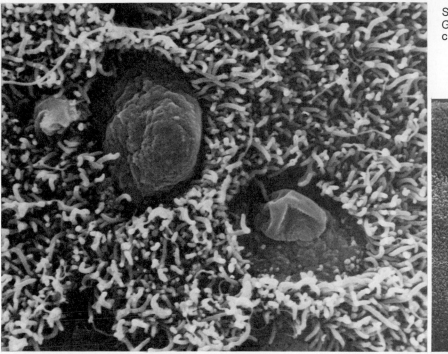

SEM   Mucus extruding
goblet cell
M. J. Koering (x 220)

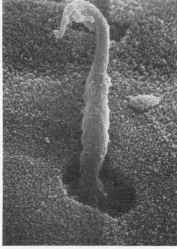

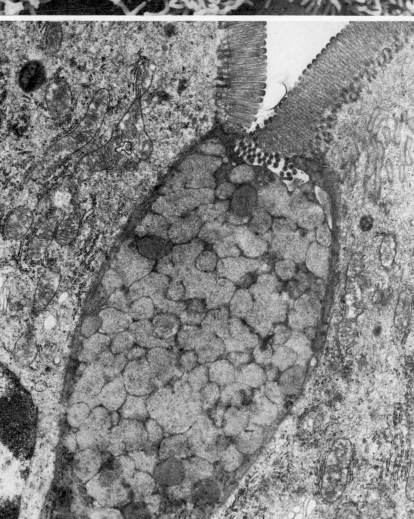

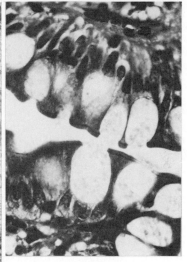

LM   Goblet cells (x 1000)

The lower left view is a TEM micrograph of
a mature goblet cell. Its apex opens onto
microvilli of the striated border of the
intestine.

The upper left figure is a SEM
micrograph of two goblet cells embedded in
a mat of cilia of respiratory epithelium lining
the trachea. Observe that the lower cell is
collapsed after expelling its contents and
microvilli are scattered over its base.

The upper right SEM micrograph is a
dynamic view of a goblet cell caught in the
act of discharging a column of mucus. In the
background a goblet cell is poised to release
its contents.

The lower right photomicrograph is a LM
view of several, light-staining goblet cells
lining an intestinal gland.

EM Goblet cell

G. U. Anat. Collection (x 10,000)

2144

3. The third layer of a mucous membrane is the **tunica or lamina propria.** This is the thickest layer, consisting of **loose connective tissue** in which **lymphoid nodules** are often located. Its loose, spongy structure provides an effective **shock absorber** for the passage of bulky materials, especially through the GI tract. It has a rather large population of lymphocytes and plasma cells that are important in the body's defense against pathogenic bacteria and viruses, and other foreign substances. Within the lamina propria are also abundant **blood and lymph capillaries,** which lie close to the basal surfaces of the epithelial cells. Thus the exchange of nutrients and gases (O_2 and CO_2) across the capillary wall and the cell membrane is greatly facilitated by their close approximation.

4. The **muscularis mucosae** is the outermost component of the mucous membrane. As its name implies, it is a layer of muscle surrounding the mucosa. It usually consists of a few **smooth muscle fibers** which may course in circular and/ or longitudinal directions. Upon contraction, it modifies the shape of the mucous membrane into **folds or rugae** and may also contribute slightly to the peristaltic action of the gut.

Mucous membranes may be **highly absorptive** structures. For example, through the mucous membrane lining the digestive tract, nutrients are absorbed into the blood. Mucous membranes can also be **secretory.** The secretions produced may be of a rather watery consistency, with an abundance of **active enzymes,** as in serous cells, or more viscous where **lubrication** is the principal function, as in mucous cells. In the stomach and intestines, the **enzyme-rich digestive juices** of mucous membranes aid in the breakdown of food into simple nutrients available to the cells of the body. In the colon, the rather chemically inert, thicker mucous secretion serves as a necessary **lubricant** for the undigested material that moves down the tract. In the respiratory system, mucus **entraps foreign particles** from the inspired air and may also have bactericidal properties.

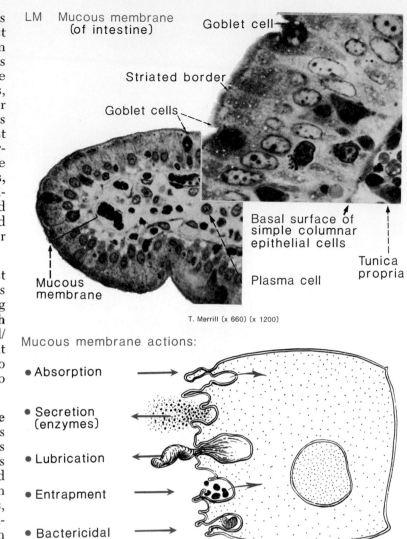

LM   Mucous membrane
        (of intestine)

Goblet cell

Striated border

Goblet cells

Basal surface of simple columnar epithelial cells

Plasma cell

Tunica propria

Mucous membrane

T. Merrill (x 660) (x 1200)

Mucous membrane actions:

- Absorption

- Secretion (enzymes)

- Lubrication

- Entrapment

- Bactericidal

For instance, recall that glands are masses of epithelial cells whose principal function is **secretion.** Their secretions either pass out of the cell into ducts, as in exocrine glands, or into the vascular system, as in endocrine glands.

In **exocrine glands** the secretory component may be a **single cell** interposed between epithelial cells, such as, goblet cells of the GI tract and respiratory system. All other exocrine glands are **multicellular** and usually drained by a system of ducts. They are classified by the morphology of their ducts, i.e., as simple (with one duct) or compound (with several ducts); or by their end-pieces, i.e., tubular (straight or coiled), acinar (grapelike), saccular (saclike), or alveolar (tublike).

The two principal types of secretions are produced by exocrine glands: (1) a thin, watery, **serous secretion,** rich in enzymes; or (2) a viscous, lubricating, **mucous secretion,** poor in enzymes. If the secretion is discharged from an intact cell, it is a merocrine gland. If the secretion contains ruptured cells detached from the gland, it is a holocrine type gland. If only a part of the cell breaks off into the secretion, it is an apocrine gland.

Endocrine glands are characterized by the **absence of ducts,** a **profuse blood supply,** and with cells arranged in cords, clusters, or follicles. Most of their secretions (hormones) are released into the bloodstream.

There are two types of epithelial membranes, serous and mucous. The **serous membrane** is a single layer of mesothelial cells and a thin sheet of connective tissue that line the pleural, pericardial, peritoneal, and joint cavities. The **mucous membrane** lines the open cavities of the digestive, respiratory, and urogenital systems. Typically, a mucous membrane consists of four layers: (1) a layer or layers of epithelium; (2) a thin basement membrane upon which these epithelial cells rest; (3) a layer of loose connective tissue, the tunica propria supporting this membrane; and (4) the deepest layer is a few smooth muscle fibers, the muscularis mucosa.

Table 5.1   *MORPHOLOGICAL CLASSIFICATION OF GLANDS*

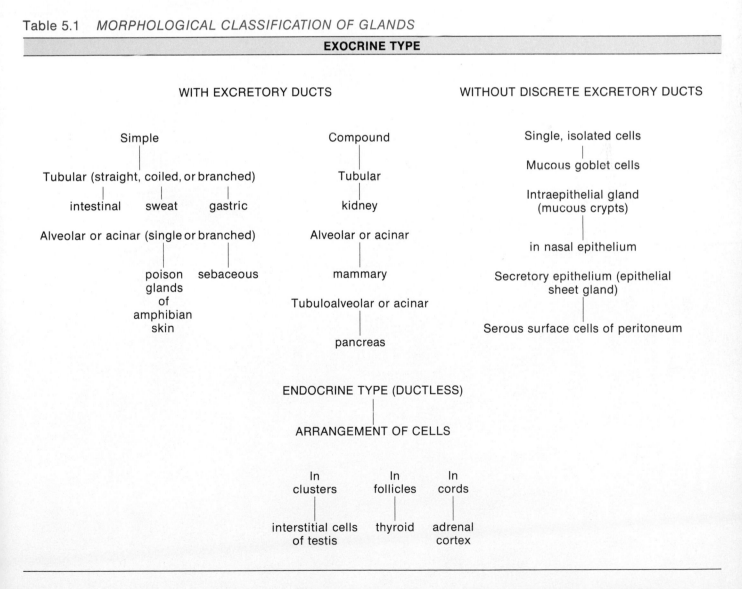

Chapter

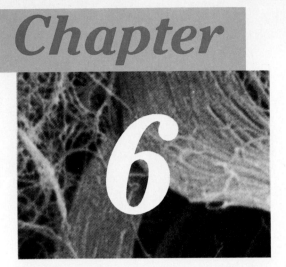

6

CONNECTIVE TISSUE

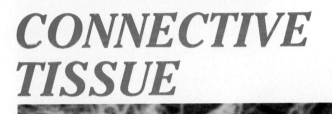

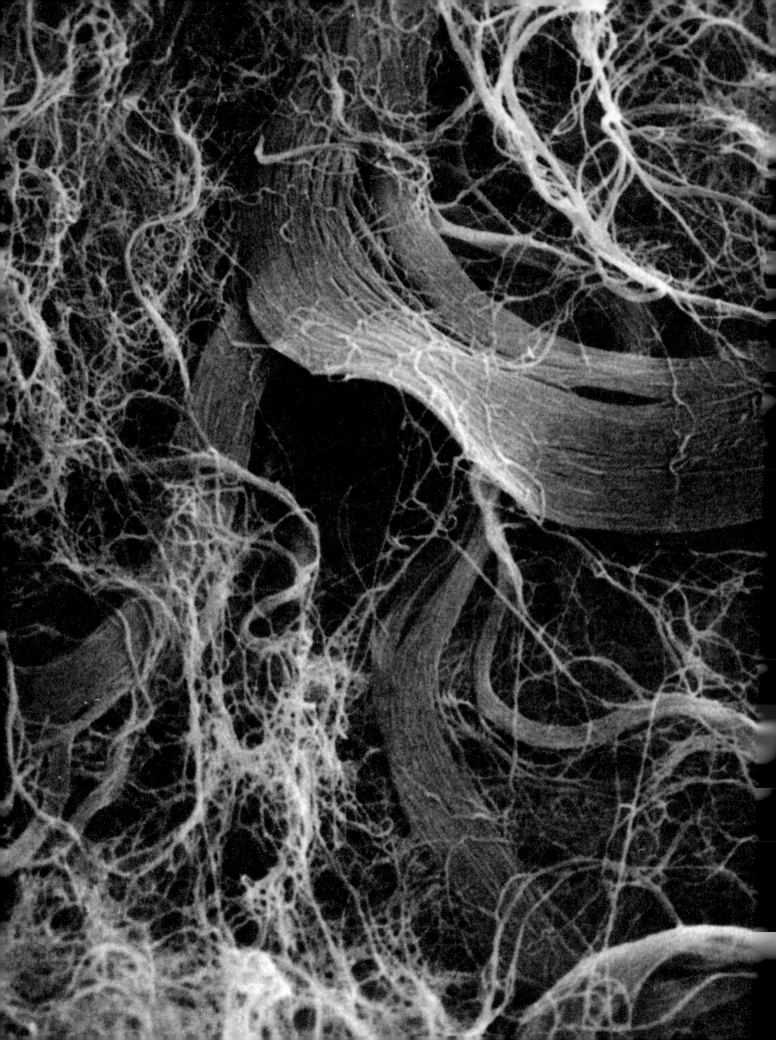

OBJECTIVES

THE SALIENT OBJECTIVES OF THIS CHAPTER ARE:

1. To be able to describe the morphology and to analyze functions of nine or more types of cells and three varieties of fibers, found in loose (areolar) connective tissue.

2. To compare accurately, histologically and functionally, fibroblasts vs. macrophages, plasma vs. mast cells, and collagenous vs. elastic fibers.

3. To formulate the sequential stages of collagen synthesis and factors that may limit its production.

4. To explain the origin and composition of the amorphous ground substance and explore how it influences the spread of infections and toxic substances in the body.

5. To contrast the locations and the structural and functional characteristics of dense and loose connective tissues.

6. To analyze the roles special types of connective tissues, e.g., mesenchyme, white and brown fat, and reticular tissue, play in the maintenance of health.

7. To evaluate the benefit of the macrophage system in the promotion of bodily defense mechanisms against infections.

In the traditional sense, connective tissues comprise all **supporting structures** of the body, including cartilage and bone. Less conventional is to include also fluid tissues, such as blood and lymph. Except for fluid tissues, these various structures serve many mechanical functions, such as binding, anchoring, and supporting the various parts of the body. With the exception of certain glial cells of the central nervous system and pigment cells, all connective tissues are **mesenchymal** in origin and contain three separate constituents: (1) **cells,** mostly fibroblasts; (2) extracellular **fibers,** i.e., reticular, collagenous, and/or elastic; and (3) a homogeneous **ground substance,** or matrix, which may be tissue fluid, an amorphous gellike material, or solid, as in cartilage and bone.

The relative amount and type of matrix, the type and arrangement of fibers, and the abundance and kinds of cells, are the criteria used for the **classification** of connective tissue. Because these elements vary greatly depending on the structural requirements of specific regions, classification is often imprecise, arbitrary, and difficult, and it should not be interpreted too rigidly. Nevertheless, these tissues are designated as being loose or dense, irregular or regular, elastic or collagenous, etc. Table 6.1 is a classification of these tissues.

LOOSE CONNECTIVE TISSUE

Loose or **areolar** (meaning small areas or spaces) connective tissue is a rather haphazard, loose arrangement of sheets of **unbound fibrous tissues.** It occurs throughout the body as a "filler" tissue between distinct regions within organs and between different organs and tissues. It is the poorly defined **subcutaneous tissue,** as well as the delicate network of fibers and cells beneath mucous membranes, called either the **tunica propria or submucosa.** It also surrounds peripheral nerves, blood and lymph vessels, excretory ducts, and forms the central core of mesenteries.

Within its rather viscid ground substance lie various cells and fibers. All connective tissue cells may be found here; however, most of them are **fibroblasts or macrophages. Collagenous fibers predominate** in the matrix with some elastic fibers but very few reticular fibers.

Cellular Components

Both fixed and wandering connective tissue cells arise from common embryonic stem cells, the **mesenchymal cells.** These primitive cells differentiate into various cell types to perform specific functions. However, certain cells retain some of their primitive plasticity and may differentiate into other connective tissue cells, such as macrophages, fibroblasts, chondroblasts, and osteoblasts.

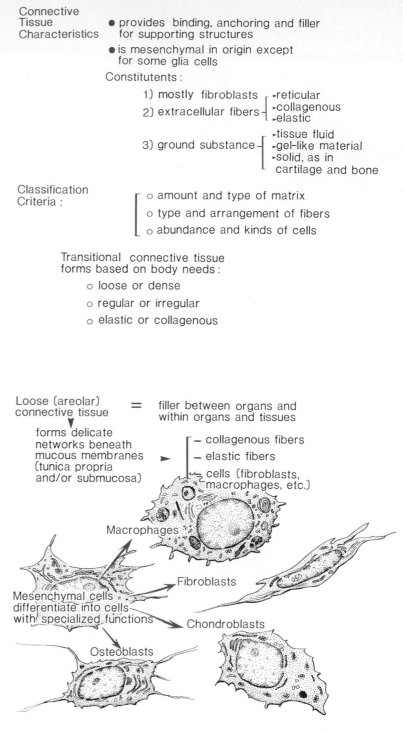

Connective Tissue Characteristics
- provides binding, anchoring and filler for supporting structures
- is mesenchymal in origin except for some glia cells

Constitutents:
1) mostly fibroblasts
2) extracellular fibers — reticular, collagenous, elastic
3) ground substance — tissue fluid, gel-like material, solid, as in cartilage and bone

Classification Criteria:
- amount and type of matrix
- type and arrangement of fibers
- abundance and kinds of cells

Transitional connective tissue forms based on body needs:
- loose or dense
- regular or irregular
- elastic or collagenous

Loose (areolar) connective tissue = filler between organs and within organs and tissues

forms delicate networks beneath mucous membranes (tunica propria and/or submucosa)
- collagenous fibers
- elastic fibers
- cells (fibroblasts, macrophages, etc.)

Macrophages
Fibroblasts
Mesenchymal cells differentiate into cells with specialized functions
Chondroblasts
Osteoblasts

Types of cells in loose areolar tissue

(1) Resident
- fibroblasts
- macrophages
- mesenchymal cells
- reticular cells

(2) Visitant
- fat cells
- plasma cells
- mast cells
- leukocytes
- pigment cells

LM   Fibroblast

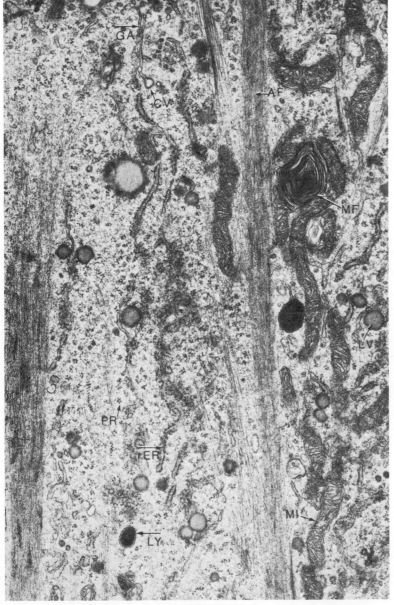

T. M. Crisp (x 30,000)

GA—Golgi apparatus   MF—Myelin figure   rER—Rough ER
AF—Actin filaments   LV—Lipid vesicle   LY—Lysosome
CV—Coated vesicle   PR—Polyribosome   MI—Mitochondrion

2368

Cells found in loose areolar tissue may be separated into two types: (1) **permanent residents,** i.e., fibroblasts, macrophages, and perhaps a few mesenchymal and reticular cells; and (2) **visitants or wandering cells** that may come and go depending on the functional needs of the body. These cells include fat cells, plasma cells, mast cells, various leukocytes, and pigment cells.

FIBROBLASTS Fibroblasts, a self-perpetuating group of cells, are the **most common.** As their name suggests, they are actively involved in **fiber formation, usually collagen,** and are also responsible for the elaboration of the amorphous matrix. Theodor Schwann, of the cell theory fame, reported in 1847 on the omnipresence of these cells in loose connective tissue and designated them as "fibre-cells of areolar tissue." Fibroblasts are involved in such diverse processes as the production of glue and leather, to the **healing of wounds.** In the latter function they have been dubbed "a ubiquitous ally for the surgeon," for in the absence of fibroblasts, wounds do not heal.

Under the light microscope **fibroblasts** are rather large, often flattened, ovoid or **stellate** cells, with long, tapering, **branching processes.** Each cell has a single prominent ovoid, light-staining nucleus with one or more distinct nucleoli; or as Schwann described the fibroblasts that he saw under his very simple microscope, ". . . they are represented as being spindle-shaped or longish corpuscles which are thickest in the middle and gradually elongated in both extremities into fine fibers."

Fibroblasts grow very well in tissue culture. When examined under dark-field illumination, they reveal **many mitochondria and fat droplets** in their cytoplasm. Electron microscopic studies show that when such cells are **metabolically active,** there is a marked **increase** in **free ribosomes,** granular endoplasmic reticulum, and an enlargement of the **Golgi complex.**

When fibroblasts pass into an **inactive stage,** as seen in tendons and ligaments, they are smaller, more flattened, and their **nuclei** are condensed, deeply stained, flattened **disks.** Some researchers prefer to call these inert cells **fibrocytes.**

MACROPHAGES Macrophages may be nearly as numerous in loose connective tissue as fibroblasts, which they closely resemble. As their name suggests they are **avidly phagocytic** (Gk. macro, big; phagein, to eat). They may be **fixed** or sessile in position and often are called **histiocytes.** Or they may be very mobile or **wandering** macrophages, i.e., the monocytes of the blood. The term macrophage is quite acceptable for both types of cells since any given cell may be fixed in position now but free to wander later.

How macrophages differ from fibroblasts is summarized in Table 6.2. **Macrophages,** as the major component of the macrophage (**reticuloendothelial**) **system,** are discussed in detail later in this chapter.

MESENCHYMAL CELLS Mesenchymal cells are **embryonic connective tissue cells** that may persist in the adult. They **resemble active fibroblasts** but are usually smaller. They tend to locate along blood capillaries where they are called **perivascular cells.** Unlike fibroblasts they are not closely associated with collagenous fibers. In a changing internal environment, they may be stimulated to differentiate into a variety of adult connective tissue cells.

RETICULAR CELLS Reticular cells are also a **primitive type of cell** similar to mesenchymal cells. They have long, cellular processes that extend over the intervening tissue spaces to form a three-dimensional network called a **cellular reticulum.** It is this fibrillar network or stroma that forms a **supportive framework** for bone marrow, lymph nodes and nodules, and spleen. In addition to support, the reticular cells **may be phagocytic** when stimulated. It is precisely this function that the famous German pathologist, Aschoff, recognized in 1924 when he coined the term reticuloendothelial system for all cells involved in phagocytosis. Reticular cells also may have a **hemopoietic** function by serving as possible precursors of the hemocytoblasts, the stem cells for all blood cells.

ADIPOSE CELLS Fat cells are a conspicuous and rather constant part of loose connective tissue. They may occur singly or in clusters, usually concentrated near blood vessels. Immature fat cells (**adipoblasts**) resemble fibroblasts containing a few **small vacuoles** of neutral fat. In the fetus, the fat droplets gradually increase in size, which greatly reduces the cytoplasm. Finally, the fat globules **coalesce** into a **single large globule** that essentially fills the cell, flattening the nucleus onto the plasmalemma. Thus, the **adult adipose cell** has a faint **ring of cytoplasm** on the edge of the fat droplet. With the **flat, discoid nucleus** a part of the cytoplasmic ring, the fat cell resembles a signet ring.

MAST CELLS Mast cells are large, oval cells about 15–20 μm in diameter. They are frequent **visitants** of loose connective tissue and are especially abundant along small blood vessels. They are called mast (Ger., to fatten) cells because of their fancied resemblance to cells that have been force-fed or fattened. Actually they are engorged with many **large, coarse granules,** so closely packed that they often obscure the small, pale nucleus.

These huge **secretory granules** are about 0.6–1 μm in diameter and are **metachromatic,** i.e., the color of granules is not the true color of the dye used to stain them.

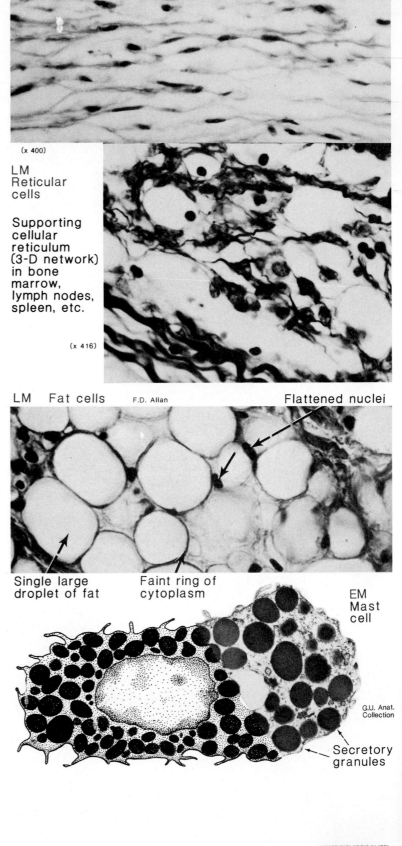

LM Mesenchymal cells

(x 400)

LM Reticular cells

Supporting cellular reticulum (3-D network) in bone marrow, lymph nodes, spleen, etc.

(x 416)

LM Fat cells   F.D. Allan   Flattened nuclei

Single large droplet of fat

Faint ring of cytoplasm

EM Mast cell

G.U. Anat. Collection

Secretory granules

4384

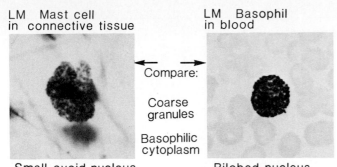

LM   Mast cell
in connective tissue

LM   Basophil
in blood

← Compare: →

Coarse
granules

Basophilic
cytoplasm

Small ovoid nucleus

Bilobed nucleus

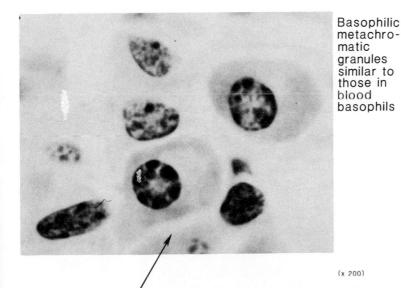

Basophilic
metachro-
matic
granules
similar to
those in
blood
basophils

(x 200)

LM   Plasma cells (thought to be postmitotic B- lymphocytes)

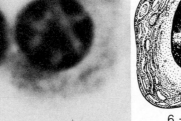

6 - 20μm

F.D. Allan

Round eccentric
nucleus with
prominent nucleolus

Translucent
area adjacent
to nucleus

Clock face or
spoke-like radial
arrangement
of chromatin

Abundant around blood vessels in inflammation
(synthesize and secrete antibodies)

Mast cells yield these metachromatic changes because of a high concentration of **heparin,** an effective anticoagulant. They also elaborate **histamine,** a vasodilator that increases the permeability of capillaries. Since both of these granules are water soluble, they are often washed out in most routine procedures and mast cells go undetected.

The **cell membrane** of mast cells is very fragile and often **ruptures,** allowing the granules to scatter. Often the first clue to the presence of mast cells in an area is the random dispersal of the granules in the region. Electron microscopic studies of mast cells reveal many small **villuslike projections** on the cell surface. Mitochondria are sparse and the endoplasmic reticulum scanty; however, the **Golgi apparatus** is well developed. The granules are membrane-bound and often their cytoplasm contains heterogeneous, lamellated whorls.

Mast cells resemble in many ways the **basophils** of the blood. In fact, they are often called **connective tissue basophils** because both cells have basophilic metachromatic granules that contain heparin and histamine. However, these are **two distinct cell types** arising from separate stem cells. Furthermore, the blood basophil has a bilobed nucleus while the single mast cell nucleus is smaller and spherical or ovoid.

PLASMA CELLS Plasma cells differentiate from a special population of cells, the **B-lymphocytes.** Their prime function is the **synthesis and secretion of antibodies,** i.e., the immune globulins of the blood, which primarily aid in the body's defenses against bacterial infections. They are oval or rounded cells varying in size from 6 to 20 μm. They have a marked resemblance to **lymphocytes.** The plasma cell has a homogenous, **basophilic cytoplasm,** suggestive of abundant rough endoplasmic reticulum. Closely adjacent to the nucleus is a clear, translucent area, the negative Golgi, unstained with H&E.

The plasma cell's most distinctive feature is its unusual **nucleus,** which is round, **eccentric** in position, and has a prominent nucleolus. Its **chromatin** is arranged in darkly staining clumps along the inner surface of the nuclear membrane. Such a unique, radial arrangement suggests the **spokes of a wheel, or a clock-face pattern.** This feature is used to identify a plasma cell.

Plasma cells are only occasionally found in the subcutaneous loose connective tissue, except **in infection,** when they are very **numerous,** especially around blood vessels. This is such a consistent phenomenon that "plasma cells are the hallmark of subacute and chronic inflammation." However, they are also quite **plentiful** in the highly cellular connective tissue of the **tunica propria,** especially beneath the lining epithelium of the digestive and respiratory systems.

Electron micrographs confirm that the deep basophilia of the cytoplasm of the plasma cell is due to an **extensive granular endoplasmic retic-**

ulum, studded by myriad ribosomes. These structures are suggestive of a cell actively involved in **protein production,** i.e., immunoglobulins. The **Golgi apparatus** is large and active, which would be expected by the extensive negative Golgi image seen under the light microscope. The **mitochondria** are large and spherical, few in number, and unremarkable in their internal fine structure.

The plasma cell is probably postmitotic, i.e., incapable of further division and differentiation. It is largely sessile, showing little of the mobility of the lymphocyte, its immediate ancestor.

LEUKOCYTES Leukocytes are frequent **emigrants** from the blood into loose connective tissue. By ameboid movement, these cells escape through the capillary walls into the surrounding tissue. Their numbers fluctuate greatly as they selectively collect in areas of **inflammation or infection.**

Many of these wandering cells are **monocytes,** which become **avid phagocytes** and are then indistinguishable from the resident macrophages in the area. **Neutrophils** are perhaps the next most common visitant. They leave the capillaries, especially in areas of **bacterial infection,** where they ingest the offending organisms. Because they have a distinct preference for bacteria, they are often referred to as **microphages.**

Eosinophils often leave the bloodstream to enter the connective tissue, especially in the breast, lung, and gastrointestinal tract. Here they are called **tissue eosinophils.** They increase in number in areas of parasitic infection, in asthma, and other allergic conditions. There is some evidence that they **phagocytize antigen-antibody complexes** and are attracted to areas where these complexes accumulate. This is an example of **positive tropism,** which is an innate tendency of cells (or organisms) to react to a stimulus by moving towards it. Movement away would be **negative tropism.** In this situation, the eosinophils move by ameboid motion towards the aggregates of antigen-antibody complexes.

PIGMENT CELLS Pigment cells or **melanocytes** occur in the connective tissue of the skin, iris, and choroid coat of the eye. Their shape is quite similar to fibroblasts, and their cell bodies and cytoplasmic processes contain **melanin granules.** With conventional histologic methods, melanocytes of the skin are difficult to visualize since they appear as small, clear, poorly stained cells. They are dispersed among the **basal cells of the epidermis** and, to a much lesser extent, among the collagenous fibers of the papillary layer of the dermis. They have the unusual capacity to transfer melanin through their protoplasmic processes to adjacent epithelial cells.

Melanocytes can be clearly identified only by a histochemical procedure, the **dopa reaction,** that blackens the cells. Briefly the dopa reaction

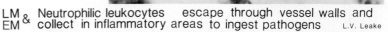
LM
Plasma cells

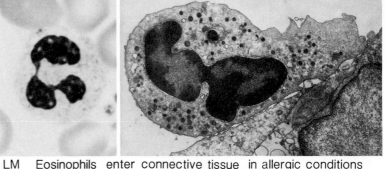
(x 200)

LM & EM Neutrophilic leukocytes escape through vessel walls and collect in inflammatory areas to ingest pathogens   L.V. Leake

LM   Eosinophils enter connective tissue in allergic conditions to phagocytize antigen-antibody complexes

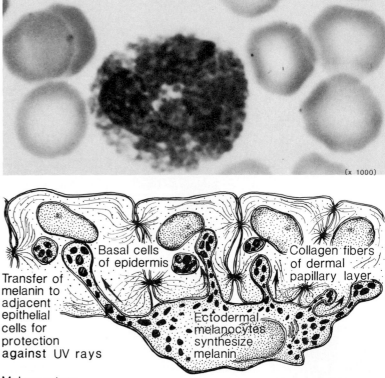
(x 1000)

Transfer of melanin to adjacent epithelial cells for protection against UV rays

Basal cells of epidermis

Collagen fibers of dermal papillary layer

Ectodermal melanocytes synthesize melanin

Melanocytes synthesize tyrosinase ⟩ oxidize into → tyrosine ⟶ dopa ⟶ dopaquinine ↓ Melanin

Support functions of extracellular fibers
1) fibrous capsules of organs
2) penetrating trabeculae of organs
3) dermis of skin
4) ligaments and tendons
5) bone and cartilage

Types of fibers
1) collagenous } Complex proteins of
2) reticular   } amino acids in
3) elastic   } polypeptide chains

EM   Collagen fibrils (in a fiber bundle)

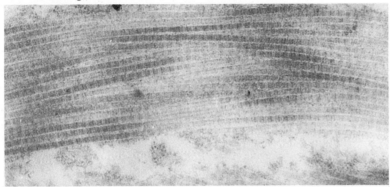

M.E. DeSantis (x 58,500)

Fibroblast – secretes
tropocollagen as rod
shaped macromolecules

Cross banding
of microfibrils
64nm intervals

Helix of three
polypeptides
held together by
hydrogen bonds

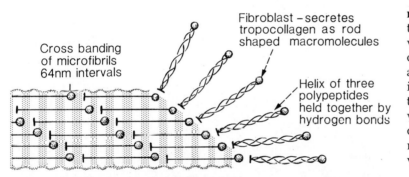

EM   Freeze-fracture replica of collagen

J.J. Anders (x 111,000)

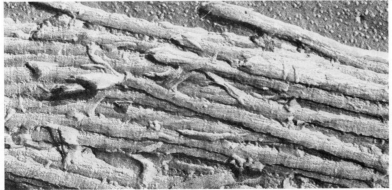

is as follows: **Melanocytes** synthesize the enzyme **tyrosinase**, which oxidizes **tyrosine**, an amino acid in melanocytes, first into dopa (3,4-dihydroxyphenylalanine) and then into dopaquinine. After several more oxidations and polymerizations, dopaquinine is transformed into the insoluble, dark brown or black pigment, **melanin.**

Unlike other connective tissue cells that arise from mesoderm, melanocytes are **ectodermal (neural crest) in origin.** They function to **absorb and disperse ultraviolet light** and thus prevent sunburn.

Fibrous Components

While the prime function of connective tissue is **support**, it is the **extracellular fibers** that are mainly involved. Evidence of their widespread, strengthening role is found: (1) in **fibrous capsules** that surround organs; (2) in the **trabeculae,** which penetrate glands for the support of tissues and cells; (3) in the **dermis** of the skin; (4) in the **ligaments and tendons** that help maintain the integrity of joints; and (5) in **cartilage** and **bone** that make up the skeleton which supports the muscles, viscera, and other soft tissues of the body.

Three connective tissue fibers, i.e., **collagenous, reticular,** and **elastic,** may occur singly or together and are unevenly scattered among the various types of connective tissue. They vary in concentration, arrangement, and relative amounts, as the function of a tissue or organ varies. All fibers contain long, parallel, complex protein molecules composed largely of **amino acids** with many **polypeptide chains.** They share the common chemical characteristic of **insolubility** in neutral solvents, which suggests why they survive in an often hostile internal environment.

COLLAGEN FIBERS Collagenous fibers are the **most numerous** of connective tissue fibers and have the **greatest tensile strength.** They are found in all types of connective tissue, except blood and lymph. Since collagen fibers are usually clustered together in **bundles,** these are the structures that are most obvious in histologic sections (L-A, plate 6). The bundles measure from 10 to 100 µm or more in width. The smallest collagen strand visible by the LM is the **fibril,** which is about 0.3–0.5 µm in diameter. Electron micrographs reveal that each fibril is composed of fine **microfibrils,** ranging from 45 to 100 nm in width, with repeating transverse **bands at 64-nm** intervals along its length.

Collagen fibers largely consist of the protein, **collagen,** the most abundant protein of the body. It is a **polymer** made up of fundamental units, or macromolecules of **tropocollagen** (Gk. tropos, turning, i.e., turning into collagen). These units are about 280 nm in length and 1.5 nm in diameter. They become polymerized to form the submicroscopic **microfibrils** of collagen.

Each **tropocollagen molecule** is composed of **three polypeptide chains** of equal length. As they twist around each other, the individual chains form a **helix**. The chains are held together by hydrogen bonds to form a single, elongated, rod-shaped macromolecule. These tropocollagen units are arranged end to end in parallel rows.

The principal **amino acids** in collagen are **glycine** (34%), **proline** (12%), and **hydroxyproline** (10%). The latter is a convenient marker for collagen since it is present in no other animal protein, except elastin, and then only in very small amounts. Thus, the **amount of collagen** in a tissue can be determined by measuring the **hydroxyproline level**. However, **ascorbic acid** is essential for the conversion of proline to hydroxyproline. In the absence of vitamin C, as in scurvy, this conversion does not occur and **wound healing** does not take place. **Scurvy** also develops other clinical symptoms, e.g., swollen, bleeding, malodorous gums; pain in the legs, especially the ankles; and the appearance of capillary hemorrhages usually related to trauma but often occurring spontaneously.

Most collagen is synthesized by **fibroblasts**; however, bone collagen is produced by osteoblasts and cartilage collagen by chondroblasts. There is also evidence that collagen associated with blood vessels, the uterus, and intestines may arise from smooth muscle cells.

Stages of Collagen Biosynthesis

1. Polypeptide chains are assembled on ribosomes which are bound to the rER. The chains are released into the cisternae where they form helical, tripeptide configurations, the **procollagen molecules**.

2. Procollagen molecules are transported to the **Golgi complex** by transport vesicles.

3. In the Golgi apparatus a carbohydrate component, **hexose**, is added. The procollagen is then packaged within **Golgi vesicles** and carried to the plasmalemma for release, by **exocytosis**, into the surrounding extracellular space. These triple-helical procollagen units are longer than the chains of mature collagen, due to extra peptides on both ends.

4. When the procollagen chains reach the extracellular space, the enzyme, **procollagen peptidase**, cleaves the extra lengths of peptides and procollagen is converted into **tropocollagen**. This is a stable form of collagen, assembled in a triple helix held together by hydrogen bonds between the three polypeptide chains.

5. In the extracellular matrix, the helical **tropocollagen units** are polymerized into linearly arranged, **rod-shaped molecules**. They overlap each other by one quarter of their length in a uniform, **staggered fashion**. Such extension creates a pattern of light and dark segments repeated

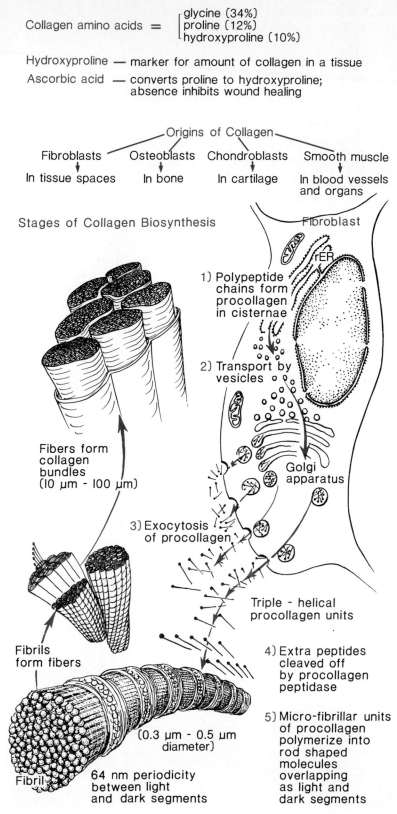

Collagen amino acids = glycine (34%)
proline (12%)
hydroxyproline (10%)

Hydroxyproline — marker for amount of collagen in a tissue
Ascorbic acid — converts proline to hydroxyproline; absence inhibits wound healing

Origins of Collagen
Fibroblasts — In tissue spaces
Osteoblasts — In bone
Chondroblasts — In cartilage
Smooth muscle — In blood vessels and organs

Stages of Collagen Biosynthesis

Fibroblast
rER
1) Polypeptide chains form procollagen in cisternae
2) Transport by vesicles
Golgi apparatus
3) Exocytosis of procollagen
Triple-helical procollagen units
4) Extra peptides cleaved off by procollagen peptidase
5) Micro-fibrillar units of procollagen polymerize into rod shaped molecules overlapping as light and dark segments

Fibers form collagen bundles (10 μm - 100 μm)

Fibrils form fibers

Fibril
(0.3 μm - 0.5 μm diameter)
64 nm periodicity between light and dark segments

LM   Collagen bundles

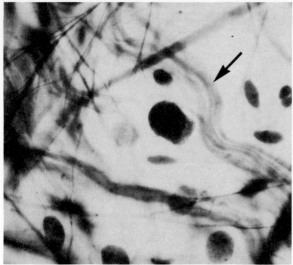

Hexose
cementing
substance
gives PAS
reaction
of
collagenous
fibers

(x 800)

Types of collagen
differing in tropocollagen
amino acid sequences:

I - tendon, bone, dentin, fibrous cartilage

II - fetal, hyaline & elastic cartilage

III - fetal skin, smooth muscle

IV - basal lamina of endothelium

V - placental basal lamina

LM
Reticular
fibers

Thin
collagenous
fibers in
stroma

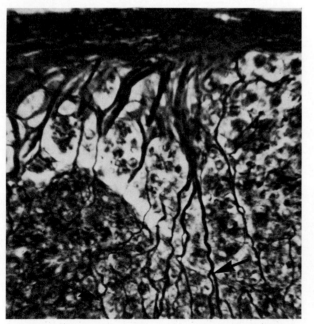

9756

along the length of the forming collagen fibril. This constant **periodicity of the 64-nm** intervals is a distinctive TEM characteristic of collagenous fibrils.

A cementing material binds the tropocollagen-containing microfibrillar units into **fibrils** (20–90 nm in diameter), which are bound together into **fibers,** visible by LM. The fibers are incorporated into collagen **bundles,** visible to the unaided eye. It is the presence of **hexose** in the cementing substance that gives the **PAS** reaction to collagenous fibers.

Types of Collagen Because the **amino acid sequences may differ** on the three-chain, coiled helix of the tropocollagen molecule, all collagen fibers in the body are not identical. Five different types have been identified.

Type I is the most common. It is found principally in loose connective tissue, tendon, bone, dentine, fibrous cartilage, and the sclerocorneal coat of the eye.

Type II is located in hyaline and elastic cartilage and in the vitreous body of the eye.

Type III is located in fetal skin, healing wounds, and smooth muscle, e.g., CVS.

Type IV is deposited mainly in basal laminae of epithelia, especially endothelium.

Type V is present in placental basal laminae, e.g., chorion and amnion, and tendon and muscle sheaths.

RETICULAR FIBERS Reticular fibers have a very **fine diameter** (100–500 nm) and are **branching,** anastomosing threads that tend to form a **network** (reticulum) instead of bundles. They stain very poorly with H&E, but are **argyrophilic,** i.e., they stain deeply with silver salts. They are **strongly PAS-positive,** indicating a substantial carbohydrate component. Because of these special staining reactions and the arrangement of fibers, it was formerly held that reticular fibers were distinctly separate and different from collagenous fibers. However, with the advent of the EM, it was discovered that reticular fibers consisted of **microfibrils** that presented a **64-nm periodicity** identical to collagen. It is now widely accepted that **reticular fibers** are actually **thin, collagenous fibers.**

The **staining differences** of reticular fibers are due to the **number and arrangement** of the collagen units, as well as the high content of **carbohydrates,** 6–12%, as hexoses, as compared to about 1% in adult collagen fibers. Furthermore, these two fiber types are often continuous, providing a gradual transition from one type to the other.

Reticular fibers are sparse in loose connective tissue but **plentiful** as the **stroma** of lymphoid and myeloid tissues, glandular structures, and in sheaths around blood vessels, muscles, and nerves. They are also the fibrous component of the **basal lamina** of epithelia, including endothelium.

ELASTIC FIBERS Elastic fibers (about 1 μm in width) have considerably **less tensile strength** than collagenous fibers but possess considerable **elasticity.** They can be stretched to over double their length and will return to their original dimensions without deformity. Because of this property, they are found in structures where frequent **stretching without breaking** is essential. Examples of these structures are **ligamenta flava** (between vertebrae), large arteries, and in cartilages where repetitive bending occurs, as in the **external ear** and epiglottis.

Elastic fibers are quite homogeneous and exhibit **no periodicity.** They remain essentially unstained with H&E but **stain selectively** with special dyes, e.g., resorcin fuchsin, aldehyde fuchsin, and orcein. In the **fresh state,** large concentrations of elastic fibers have a **yellow color,** hence they are often referred to as **yellow elastic,** while collagen fibers are called white fibrous connective tissue.

Electron micrographs reveal that elastic fibers have two components: (1) a **central amorphous zone** of the insoluble scleroprotein, **elastin;** and (2) an **enclosing sheath of microfibrils,** each 10 nm in diameter and collected into longitudinal bundles, which are embedded in the elastin core peripherally.

After considerable uncertainty about the genesis of elastic fibers, it is now accepted that they may arise from several different cells; for example, from **fibroblasts** in the tendons, ligaments, and dermis of the skin; from **smooth muscle cells** of the large blood vessels; and from undifferentiated **mesenchymal cells** in other areas of the body.

Ground Substance

The undistinguished name of **ground substance** belies the importance and complexity of this vital component of all connective tissues. It is variously described as an amorphous (shapeless), gellike substance with the capacity **to bind water** or as a **molecular sieve** screening out harmful microorganisms from entering the bloodstream. Optically, it is homogeneous and transparent and is seldom seen in routine histological sections.

Chemically, the ground substance is a complex mixture of water, mineral salts, glycoproteins, and various **mucopolysaccharides.** The very important latter group is divided into sulfated and nonsulfated types. The most common compound is the **nonsulfated hyaluronic acid** found in the skin, loose connective tissue, umbilical cord, vitreous body, and synovial fluid. It has the property to **bind water** and therefore influences the shifts of viscosity and permeability of the ground substance. These properties enable the ground substance to **control,** to an appreciable extent, the **spread of noxious substances** in localized infection sites.

LM Areolar connective tissue (x 200)

Wide bands of collagen fibers

Elastic fibers

LM Areolar connective tissue (x 400)

Collagen bundles

Elastic fibers

Fat cells

Plasma cells

Macrophage

Mast cells

Fiberblasts

Cross-section of elastic fiber (x 120,000)

Microfibrils

EM

Properties of "ground substance" (lies between cells and fibers)

➤ amorphous gel-like
➤ binds water
➤ acts as molecular sieve
➤ homogenous & transparent
➤ mixture of H_2O, minerals, glycoproteins & mucopolysaccharides
➤ altered by hyaluronidase

Composition of ground substance: --water--mineral salts--
  --glycoproteins--
  --mucopolysaccharides--

Nonsulfated group

➤ Hyaluronic acid
(in skin, loose conective tissue,
umbilical cord, vitreous body, &
synovial fluid) } breaks down
with hyaluronidase
"spreading factor"

➤ Chondroitin
(in cornea & embryonic cartilage)

Sulfated group

➤ Chondroitin-4-sulfate
(in cornea, skin, bone, & cartilage)

➤ Chondroitin-6-sulfate
(in tendons, cartilage, umbilical cord &
intervertebral disks)

➤ Dermatan sulfate
(in skin, tendons, ligaments & heart valves)

➤ Keratan sulfate
(in bone, cartilage, cornea & intervertebral disks)

--- Collectively termed "glycosaminoglycans"

Ground
substance
functions } ➤ controls passage of pathogens

➤ allows diffusion of O₂ & nutrients

SEM   Irregular dense connective tissue   G. U. Anat. Collection

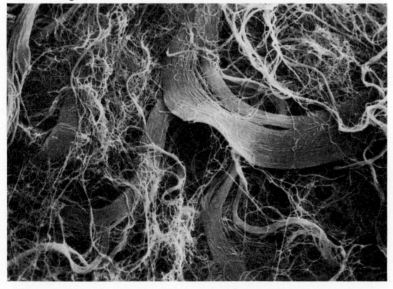

However, the presence of the enzyme **hyaluronidase** at the infection site causes the viscosity of the ground substance to be reduced and its permeability to increase, thus allowing the deleterious agents to spread into the surrounding tissues. This "**spreading factor**," as hyaluronidase is sometimes called, is present in snake and spider venoms, permitting them to be rapidly disseminated throughout the body of the poisoned victim, greatly enhancing their lethal potential. The other nonsulfated compound is **chondroitin,** found mostly in the cornea and embryonic cartilage. It is similar to hyaluronic acid, except it has galactosamine in place of glucosamine.

The **sulfated group** includes **chondroitin-4-**sulfate (in cornea, skin, bone, and cartilage), **chondroitin-6-**sulfate (in tendons, cartilage, umbilical cord, and intervertebral disks), **dermatan** sulfate (in skin, tendons, ligaments, and heart valves), and **keratan** sulfate (in bone, cartilage, cornea, and intervertebral disks). Recently, all of these mucopolysaccharides have been brought under the umbrella of the collective, descriptive term of **glycosaminoglycans (GAG)**, meaning polysaccharides that contain amino sugars.

Because of its relatively high concentration of GAG, the ground substance gives a positive **periodic acid-Schiff (PAS) reaction** and stains metachromatically with toluidine blue. Under the EM it appears as a poorly defined, medium dense, flaky substance.

Briefly, the functions of ground substance are:

1. As stated above, it **controls passage** of **pathogens** from connective tissues into the bloodstream.

2. Because of its high water content, it is a suitable medium for **nutrients** and O₂ to diffuse from capillaries into the often extensive intercellular space, and finally into the cells. By reverse action, **waste metabolites** are carried into the abundant lymph and blood capillaries for excretion. Thus ground substance is very important in **cellular nutrition** and waste removal.

3. Ground substance plays a vital role in **aging.** In the newborn, it is relatively abundant but gradually diminishes with age, especially in the skin, which becomes wrinkled and thinner, due, in part, to the gradual loss of the water-binding ground substance.

DENSE CONNECTIVE TISSUE

This tissue differs from loose connective tissue by a greater **abundance of collagenous fibers** arranged in heavy bundles. It also has fewer cells and less ground substance. Depending on the arrangement of the collagen bundles, two types of tissue are identified. If the bundles are irregularly woven into a feltlike fabric without a definite orientation, this is **irregular dense connective tissue.** If the bundles are constantly oriented in a uniform parallel pattern, it is **regular dense connective tissue.**

In **irregular dense connective tissue,** the randomly oriented collagen fibers are capable of responding to stress from all directions. Such a response is needed in the **dermis** of the skin; in **capsules** surrounding organs, e.g., lymph nodes and the spleen; and **sheaths** around tendons, large nerves, ganglia, and the periosteum.

In **regular dense connective tissue,** where the collagenous **fibers are arranged in parallel,** the fibers can respond to prolonged stress from a single direction. The **tendons and ligaments** are the best examples of this type of connective tissue. **Tendons** are virtually inextensible since they are made up almost entirely of collagenous fibers with only a few elastic fibers. However, **ligaments** are somewhat extensible since they have more elastic fibers. Both structures have a few flattened fibroblasts with limited, pale cytoplasm and flattened, dark-staining, discoid nuclei. Their fibers are separated by small amounts of amorphous ground substance.

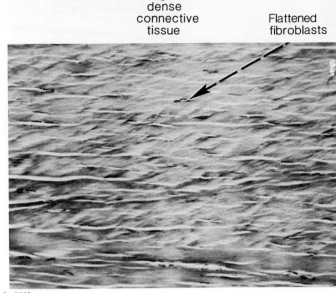

LM
Regular dense connective tissue

Flattened fibroblasts

(x 200)

SPECIAL TYPES OF CONNECTIVE TISSUE

Embryonic Connective Tissue

MESENCHYME Mesenchymal connective tissue (mesenchyme) is a meshwork of **stellate and fusiform cells** derived from **mesoderm.** They give rise to nearly all of the connective tissues in the body. These **multipotential cells** may persist in the adult to give rise to new generations of connective tissue cells, especially during periods of wound healing, bone repair, and tissue fibrosis.

Distinctive features of mesenchyme include: (1) the presence of scattered, mitotically active stellate cells with many branching processes that often attach to adjacent cells of gap junctions; (2) limited amorphous, viscid, ground substance; (3) contains only a few thin, mostly collagenous fibers; (4) an abundance of tissue fluid; and (5) in addition to giving rise to nearly all connective tissue cells, it is also the source, during embryonic development, for muscle fibers, blood and lymph vessels, including endothelium.

MUCOUS CONNECTIVE TISSUE This is a type of loose, embryonic connective tissue found primarily beneath the skin of the embryo and early fetus, and in the **umbilical cord,** as Wharton's jelly. It resembles mesenchyme except it has **very abundant,** jellylike amorphous **ground substance,** rich in glycosaminoglycans and glycogen, which gives a mucin staining reaction. In addition to the stellate-shaped fibroblastic cells, it also contains a few transient macrophages and lymphocytes.

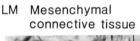

LM Mesenchymal connective tissue

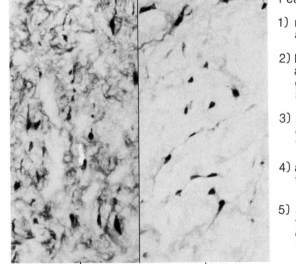

Meshwork of stellate and fusiform cells derived from mesoderm

Features:

1) mitotically active

2) limited amorphous ground substance

3) sparse collagenous fibers

4) abundant tissue fluid

5) source for other differentiated tissues

Wharton's jelly resembles mesenchyme but with abundant amorphous ground substance

Mesenchyme

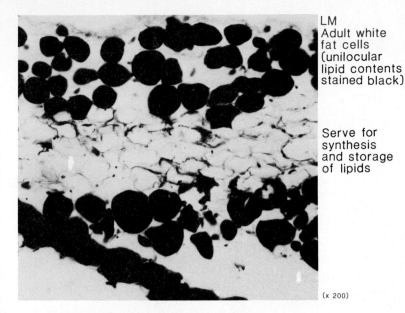

LM
Adult white
fat cells
(unilocular
lipid contents
stained black)

Serve for
synthesis
and storage
of lipids

(x 200)

Functions of fat:
- energy storage
- shock absorber
- viscera support
- heat loss insulator

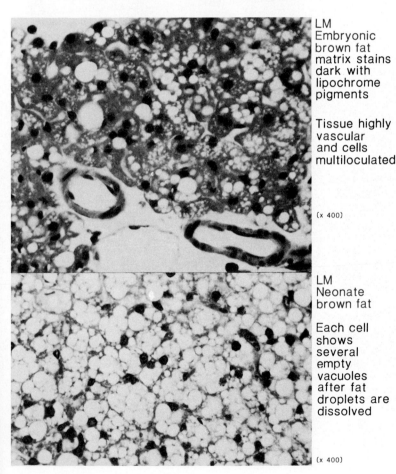

LM
Embryonic
brown fat
matrix stains
dark with
lipochrome
pigments

Tissue highly
vascular
and cells
multiloculated

(x 400)

LM
Neonate
brown fat

Each cell
shows
several
empty
vacuoles
after fat
droplets are
dissolved

(x 400)

Adipose Tissue

Fat cells are connective tissue cells specialized for the **synthesis and storage of lipids.** They probably arise from undifferentiated **mesenchymal cells** or from **modified fibroblasts** that develop an affinity for lipids. In either case, these cells enlarge, retract their cytoplasmic processes, and become typical, **spherical, adipose cells.** In fat tissue it is these many, rounded, clear cells that dominate the field and not the interstitial substance, which is largely a delicate reticular network and numerous capillaries.

Functionally and morphologically there are **two types of adipose tissue:** the abundant, **white or ordinary fat,** and the **brown or embryonic fat** that occurs in the embryo and fetus, and in limited amounts in certain locations in the adult.

WHITE ADIPOSE TISSUE In the **adult white fat cells,** the lipids, largely glycerides and fatty acids, are collected into a **single large droplet (unilocular)** or vacuole. It essentially fills the cell, crowding the cytoplasm and nucleus to the periphery. Thus the cell assumes a **signet-ring appearance** with a thin rim of cytoplasm as the circular part of the ring, while the flattened nucleus is the oval signet.

EM studies show that the usual **organelles** are **reduced** in size and amount, e.g., endoplasmic reticulum, Golgi complex, mitochondria, and a basement membrane complex that surrounds the entire cell. Delicate reticular fibers anchor the fat cells in position to the underlying structures. The plasmalemma has many pinocytotic vesicles.

Functions of white adipose tissue include (1) a **storage depot** of neutral fat that has a fairly rapid turnover. It is not a static deposit; it is mobilized in times of malnutrition and starvation. (2) It acts as **shock absorbing pads** between underlying tissues, such as soles of the feet and palms of the hands. (3) Fat **supports the viscera.** While the fat itself cannot suspend organs, it may act as a **padding** around them to prevent displacement by the tension of the surrounding muscles. For example, the kidney is held in position by its perirenal fat, which resists depletion even in inanition. (4) Fat is an excellent **insulator** against heat loss.

BROWN ADIPOSE TISSUE Brown fat cells are **multilocular,** i.e., the fat occurs in several droplets distributed throughout the cytoplasm. In the fresh state, it has a brownish color because of the presence of **lipochrome pigments,** many mitochondria, and its high vascularity. Brown fat is rather widespread in the **fetus and neonate,** but in the adult, it is confined to small areas in the **interscapular and inguinal regions.** It is especially abundant in hibernating animals as the **hibernating gland.**

SEM   Adipose cells

Area of
peripheral
nucleus

Rounded
clear
cells with
single
large fat
droplet

Capillary

Reticular
network

P.M. Motta

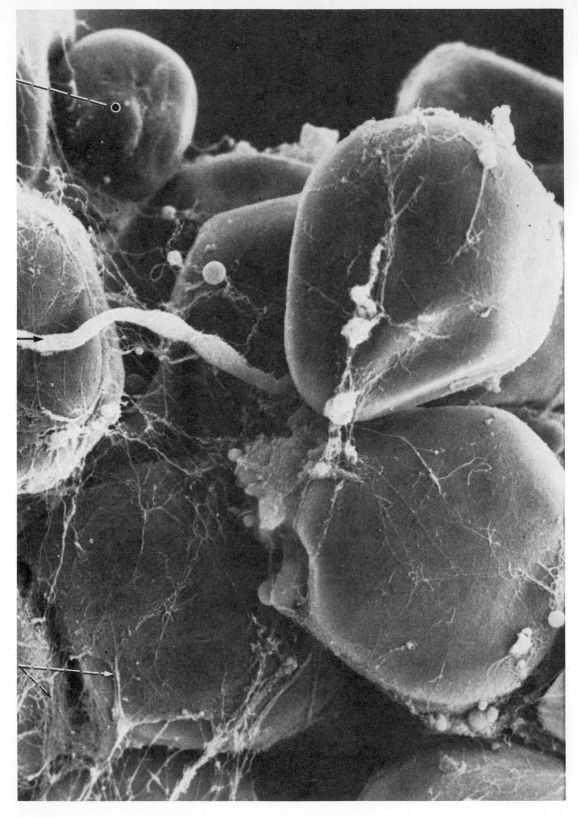

Observed by SEM, this group of typical mature adipose cells reveal their spherical or ovoid shape. They average about 100 μm in width which varies with the quantity of lipid in the cytoplasm. The peripheral nucleus of these cells can occasionally be seen bulging the plasmalemma. A delicate network of reticular fibers surround the cells. A possible capillary is seen crossing the field.

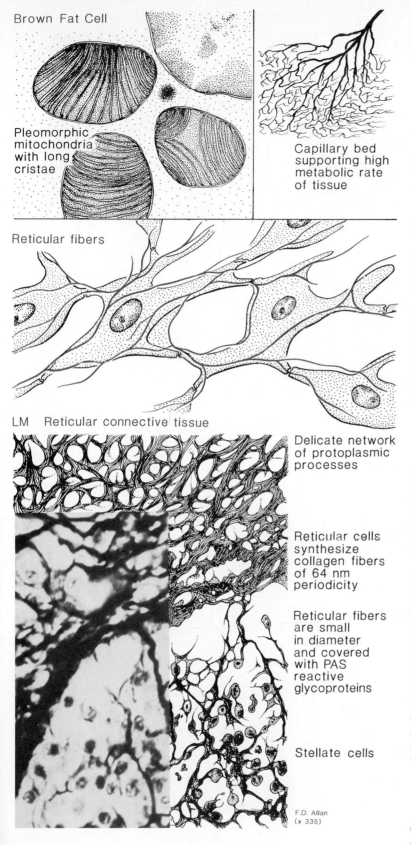

Brown Fat Cell

Pleomorphic mitochondria with long cristae

Capillary bed supporting high metabolic rate of tissue

Reticular fibers

LM   Reticular connective tissue

Delicate network of protoplasmic processes

Reticular cells synthesize collagen fibers of 64 nm periodicity

Reticular fibers are small in diameter and covered with PAS reactive glycoproteins

Stellate cells

F.D. Allan
(x 335)

Histologically, brown fat is distinctly **loculated** and **highly vascular.** Since these cells do not have a single, large, lipid droplet but several small fat vacuoles, the nucleus is not flattened but rounded and central in position. The cells are much smaller than the unilocular white adipose cell.

EM micrographs reveal only a few pinocytotic vesicles along the plasmalemma, a prominent Golgi apparatus, and the rER and sER are scanty. The abundant, large, pleomorphic **mitochondria** have long cristae that extend across the entire width of the organelle.

The function of brown fat is reflected in its abundance of mitochondria, rich capillary bed, and high metabolic rate. All of these features contribute to the main function of brown fat, namely, **heat production in the fetus and neonate** and in **hibernating animals.** At birth, the newborn is subjected to a relatively hostile, cold environment, which indirectly causes oxidation of brown fat to produce heat. The temperature of the blood passing through the brown fat deposits is markedly increased, resulting in a general increase in body temperature. Similar reactions occur during the arousal of animals from hibernation.

Reticular Tissue

Reticular connective tissue **resembles mesenchyme** with its many stellate cells which have large, pale nuclei surrounded by abundant, basophilic cytoplasm. Their long protoplasmic processes form an extensive, delicate **network (reticulum)** with adjacent cells. The interlocking meshwork supports free cells in such organs as lymph nodes, spleen, and bone marrow.

The **reticular cells,** similar to fibroblasts, **synthesize collagen,** the principal component of reticular fibers. It was earlier believed that the reticular fibers were composed of a protein called reticulin. However, when EM studies revealed that reticular fibers had the **same periodicity (64 nm) as collagen fibers,** it was concluded that the protein in reticular fibers was **collagen.** However, these fibers differed from collagen fibers in their **smaller diameter** and a covering of mucoprotein and glycoprotein, which gives a **strong PAS reaction.** Collagen fibers have only a faint reaction. Also, reticular fibers stain black with silver nitrate, while collagen remains unstained.

Blood and Lymph

Blood and lymph cells are unique connective tissue cells because they are free, i.e., they are not attached to other cells or fibers. These cells are discussed in Chapters 8 and 9.

14670

THE MACROPHAGE SYSTEM

The concept of grouping all phagocytic cells into a single system had its genesis in 1924 with the German pathologist, Aschoff. He coined the term **reticuloendothelial system (RES)** based on the **phagocytic function** of the **reticular cells** of the stroma of lymphoid tissue and the **endothelial cells** lining sinusoids of the liver, spleen, and bone marrow. Unfortunately, this term does not include the very abundant and important connective tissue macrophages, the **histiocytes.**

Recently, researchers have favored another term, the **mononuclear phagocyte system,** for a classification of all of the highly phagocytic, mononuclear cells. These authorities would exclude such faintly phagocytic cells as endothelial cells and fibroblasts. Perhaps the better term is simply the **macrophage system,** which identifies the principal function of the cells without attempting to limit the types of cells involved, i.e., reticular or endothelial, or limit phagocytes to the mononuclear variety.

As the term **macrophage** (Gk. makros, large; phagein, to eat) implies, these cells are "large eaters" or **scavenger cells** that ingest foreign material, e.g., carbon, heavy metals, cellular debris, senile fragmented RBCs, blood clot, and pathogenic bacteria. However, the term "system" is somewhat misleading for there is no single anatomical system involved. Instead, the macrophage system is a collective term connoting physiological and pathological relationships. Simply stated, the **macrophage system** is a **collection of highly phagocytic cells** widely distributed throughout the body. The phagocytic neutrophil, a white blood cell, is excluded from the system because of its small size. It is classified as a **microphage.**

For membership into this exclusive category, cells must meet the following criteria: (1) They must be **avidly phagocytic.** (2) They must have a **strong affinity for nontoxic dyes** and particulate matter, e.g., trypan blue and India ink. (3) The dye and particulate particles are isolated within the cell in discrete **storage vacuoles.** (4) In tissue culture, they **adhere firmly to glass** surfaces. (5) Their cell membranes possess **receptor sites** for antibodies (immunoglobulins).

Many of the cells that earlier comprised Aschoff's system do not meet the present criteria. For example, most **endothelial cells** are only slightly or not at all phagocytic and possess no antibody receptor sites. Likewise, **reticular cells** in lymphoid tissues are involved in reticular fiber production and not in phagocytosis. The highly phagocytic cells in the stroma of lymphatic organs associated with reticular cells are derived from monocytes and are not reticular cells.

Connective Tissue Macrophages (histiocytes)

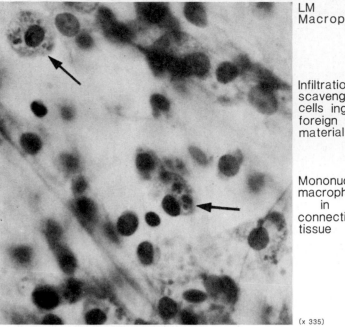

LM
Macrophages

Infiltration of scavenger cells ingesting foreign material

Mononuclear macrophages in connective tissue

(x 335)

Criteria for designating macrophages:

1) avidly phagocytic
2) strong affinity for dyes and particulates
3) store particulates in vacuoles
4) adhere to glass surfaces in culture
5) have antibody receptor sites on cell membranes

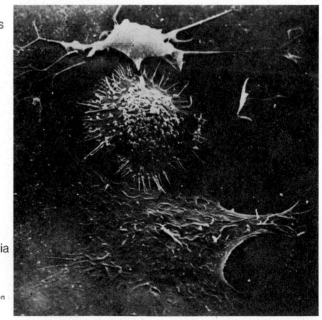

SEM
Phagocytes adhering to glass surface in tissue culture

Advancing pseudopodia

P.J. Edelson

EM Wandering
macrophage

Found in necrotic
tissue, resemble
fibroblasts

Short blunt
pseudopodia

Void of
nucleoli

Prominent
oval or
indented
nucleus with
dark staining
chromatin
granules

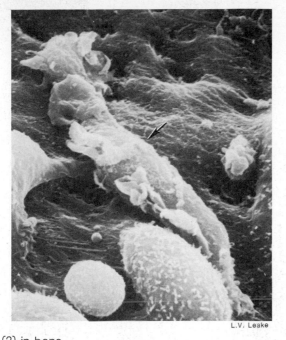

L.V. Leake

Macrophages arise (?) in bone
marrow from hemocytoblasts ──────→ monoblasts ─┐
                                                │
── monocytes ◄──── promonocytes ◄──────────────┘
│
▼
Escape into connective tissue as macrophages
│
▼
Return to bloodstream as monocytes

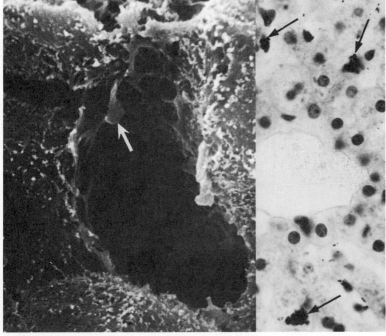

P.M. Motta   SEM   Kupffer cells in liver sinuses   LM

Normally macrophages are present in large numbers, either as **free (wandering) cells** or as **fixed (resident) cells,** in certain parts of the body, where they are given special names, e.g., alveolar macrophages of the lung and Kupffer cells of the liver (Table 6.3). However, they are in greatest concentration in areas of tissue necrosis.

Macrophages have few distinctive morphological features to distinguish them from other cells. They very closely **resemble fibroblasts,** as noted in Table 6.2. Nonetheless, a typical tissue macrophage is a large, ovoid or bean-shaped cell, with blunt, short **pseudopodia** that are contracted in fixed preparations. Its voluminous cytoplasm is pale staining and contains a prominent, **oval or indented nucleus** which is void of nucleoli but has coarse, dark-staining **chromatin granules.** If the cell is active, **phagocytosed material** is sequestered in discrete **vacuoles,** an excellent clue for identifying a phagocyte. EM micrographs reveal an abundance of **lysosomes,** especially if the cell has recently ingested materials.

While there is some question as to the common **origin of macrophages,** current consensus holds that perhaps these cells arise principally from precursor cells, probably **hemocytoblasts** in the bone marrow, although this has not been completely proven. They differentiate first into monoblasts, then into promonocytes, and finally into **monocytes.** When a monocyte escapes from a capillary into surrounding connective tissue, it is called a macrophage. If the cell returns to the bloodstream and resumes its spherical shape, it is recognized again as a monocyte.

In Table 6.3 the sinusoids of the **adrenal cortex** and the anterior lobe of the **hypophysis** were intentionally omitted, although earlier it was believed that the endothelium lining these blood sinusoids was phagocytic. From recent EM studies, it has been demonstrated that only certain **perivascular cells are phagocytic** and not the lining endothelial cells. Furthermore, the phagocytic property of cells lining the splenic venous sinuses is being questioned. Finally, it has been established that only the **Kupffer cells,** and not the endothelial cells lining liver sinuses, are highly phagocytic. From these various observations, virtually all of the endothelial elements of Aschoff's original reticuloendothelial system have been eliminated. Although this term is obsolete and should be discarded, it still lingers on in some textbooks.

Table 6.1 *CLASSIFICATION OF CONNECTIVE TISSUE*

	FIBERS	GROUND SUBSTANCE	TISSUE FLUID	CELLS	LOCATION(S)	FUNCTION(S)	COMMENTS
Embryonic • Mesenchyme	Primitive, thin collagenous fibers	Amorphous, jellylike	Abundant	Mesenchymal (early fibroblasts), branching, stellate with many processes	Embryo and early fetus	Precursor of nearly all connective tissues	Very active in mitosis
• Mucous	Delicate network of collagenous fibers	Abundant, amorphous, jellylike; gives mucin reaction with PAS; rich in mucopolysaccharides and glycogen	Abundant	Large, branching, stellate early fibroblasts; few macrophages and lymphocytes	Wharton's jelly in umbilical cord	Support around umbilical vessels	Also found in other parts of the fetus, e.g., beneath the skin
Adult • Connective tissue proper (loose-areolar)	Mostly collagenous, some elastic and a few reticular	Quite fluid, rich in mucopolysaccharides (GAG)	Abundant	Fibroblasts and macrophages; some visitants, e.g., mast and fat cells, leukocytes, etc.	Subcutaneous tissue, mesenteries, fasciae, etc.	Support and padding of tissues; lipid storage	Traversed by blood and lymph vessels, and nerves
• Dense—irregular	Nearly all collagenous fibers with a few elastic and reticular; arranged in disorganized sheets	Limited	Considerable	Flattened, elongated fibroblasts	Dermis, capsules of glands, periosteum	Support	Has considerable tensile strength
• Dense—regular	Parallel collagenous fibers; some elastic fibers in ligaments	Limited	Considerable	Flattened, elongated fibroblasts	Tendons and ligaments	Attachment of muscle to bone (tendons), bone to bone (ligaments)	Has great tensile strength; muscle or bone may be fractured by violent contraction, instead of tendon or ligament
Special • Adipose—white	Reticular fibers surround cells, some collagenous fibers between cells	Scanty	Negligible	Signet-ring-shaped fat cells with nucleus flattened on periphery of cell by large fat vacuole; few fibroblasts, leukocytes and mast cells	Subcutaneous layer, perirenal areas, and other fat depots	Energy (lipid) storage; insulation against temperature changes	Depleted during starvation and certain diseases; not a static tissue; has cycles of deposits and withdrawals; quite vascular
• Adipose—brown	Same as above	Scanty	Negligible	Fat cells smaller, nuclei spherical and centrally located; cytoplasm contains many small fat vacuoles	In man limited amounts in interscapular and inguinal regions; best developed as hibernating gland of certain animals	Source of heat production in newborn and animals in hibernation	More vascular; some pigment present; cells not easily depleted by nutritional deficits; many mitochondria
• Reticular	Reticular	Considerable	Abundant	Primitive reticular cells; often many lymphocytes and other blood cells	Stroma of glands and lymph nodes	Provide supporting framework for glands	Probably same as immature collagenous fibers

Table 6.1 *(continued)*

	FIBERS	GROUND SUBSTANCE	TISSUE FLUID	CELLS	LOCATION(S)	FUNCTION(S)	COMMENTS
Cartilage • Hyaline	Collagenous fibrils (submicroscopic); about 40% of dry weight is collagen	Dense, semisolid, rich in glycoaminoglycans and collagen	Abundant, is about 75% of wet weight of cartilage	Chondrocytes entrapped in lacunae, random distribution	Articular surfaces; fetal skeleton; tracheal rings	Support	Clear, glassy appearance; avascular, receives nutrients by diffusion; may calcify in old age
• Fibrous— white	Collagenous	Limited except in surrounding cells; heavily laced with entwined collagenous fibers	Limited except in nucleus pulposus of intervertebral disk	Same as above except cells usually arranged in parallel rows or in small clusters	Intervertebral disks; symphysis pubis	Support, especially where tough, tensile strength is needed	Lacks a perichondrium; is white in fresh state due to abundance of collagenous fibers
• Elastic— yellow	Mostly elastic with some collagenous in subperichondrial region	Limited, filled with branching network of elastic fibers	Limited	Similar to hyaline except cells more abundant and usually occur singly in lacunae	External ear; epiglottis	Support where flexibility and firmness are needed	Yellow color from elastic fibers; fracture healing is often uneven and incomplete, e.g., cauliflower ear
Bone • Cancellous	Collagenous fibrils (submicroscopic)	Rigid, calcified	Negligible	Osteocytes, osteoblasts, and osteoclasts	Centers of flat bones; ends of long bones	Support, also houses hemopoietic tissue	Also called spongy bone, forms a lattice work; osteons sparse
• Compact	Same as above	Same	Same	Same	Outer shell of bones	Provides most of support for skeleton	Also called cortical bone; has extensive osteons
Blood	Fibrin strands in clotting	Absent	Greatest amount (plasma)	Erythrocytes, leukocytes, and thrombocytes	Peripheral vascular system; red bone marrow	Erythrocytes for transportation of oxygen; leukocytes for body's main defense against infection	Also distributes heat; carries nutrients and waste products
Lymph	Same but fibrin forms more slowly		Same; however, composition less stable	Lymphocytes and a few granulocytes	Lymph vessels; lymphoid organs	Largely involved in immune reactions	In intestines, lymph (chyle) has a milky color due to large amount of fat droplets.

Table 6.2 *COMPARISON OF FIBROBLASTS AND MACROPHAGES*

	FIBROBLASTS	MACROPHAGES
Synonyms	Fibrocyte	Histiocyte, clasmatocyte, polyblast, wandering cell
Origin	Ordinarily from mesenchyme; also from macrophages, especially in wound healing	Mostly from monocytes, some from mesenchyme and fibroblasts
Functions	Synthesis of collagenous and reticular fibers, assist smooth muscle in synthesis of elastic fibers; produce mucopolysaccharides in ground substance	Important in defense against infections; are scavengers that rid the body of senile blood cells, cellular debris, bacteria and foreign bodies; contribute to the immune response of the body by engulfing, processing, and storing antigens; furnish receptor sites for antibodies; salvage and store iron from ingested RBCs for reuse in blood formation
Shape and size	Large, flattened, spindle-shaped cells with long branching processes	More rounded, often kidney-shaped; usually short, blunt processes
Nucleus	Large, pale, usually oval or indented, with finely granular chromatin and one or two prominent nucleoli	Smaller, oval or bean-shaped, coarser chromatin which stains darker; nucleoli absent or inconspicuous
Phagocytosis	Slight ability to engulf foreign particulate matter, e.g., trypan blue and carbon dust; do not ingest cellular fragments or bacteria	Highly active in ingesting foreign particulate material, cellular debris, and some bacteria
Motility	Move in a definite direction by slow streaming of protoplasm into processes	May be a rapid ameboid movement of entire surface involved; blunt pseudopodia or undulating (ruffled) membranes envelop foreign particles
Metaplasia	Into fat cells, some endothelial cells, macrophages, osteoblasts, and chondroblasts	Perhaps only into fibroblasts and monocytes

Table 6.3   *THE MACROPHAGE SYSTEM*

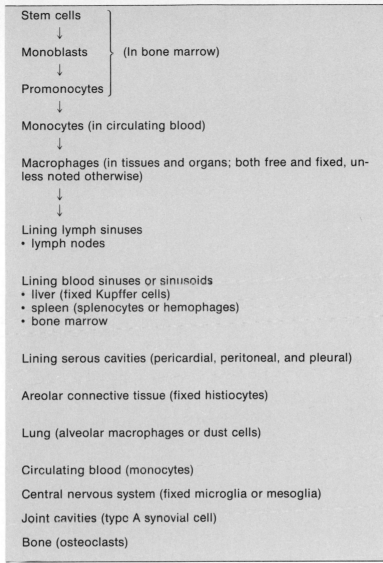

Stem cells
↓
Monoblasts   (In bone marrow)
↓
Promonocytes
↓
Monocytes (in circulating blood)
↓
Macrophages (in tissues and organs; both free and fixed, unless noted otherwise)
↓
↓
Lining lymph sinuses
• lymph nodes

Lining blood sinuses or sinusoids
• liver (fixed Kupffer cells)
• spleen (splenocytes or hemophages)
• bone marrow

Lining serous cavities (pericardial, peritoneal, and pleural)

Areolar connective tissue (fixed histiocytes)

Lung (alveolar macrophages or dust cells)

Circulating blood (monocytes)

Central nervous system (fixed microglia or mesoglia)

Joint cavities (type A synovial cell)

Bone (osteoclasts)

Chapter

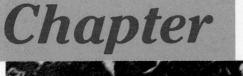

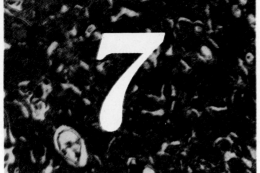

CARTILAGE, BONE, AND JOINTS

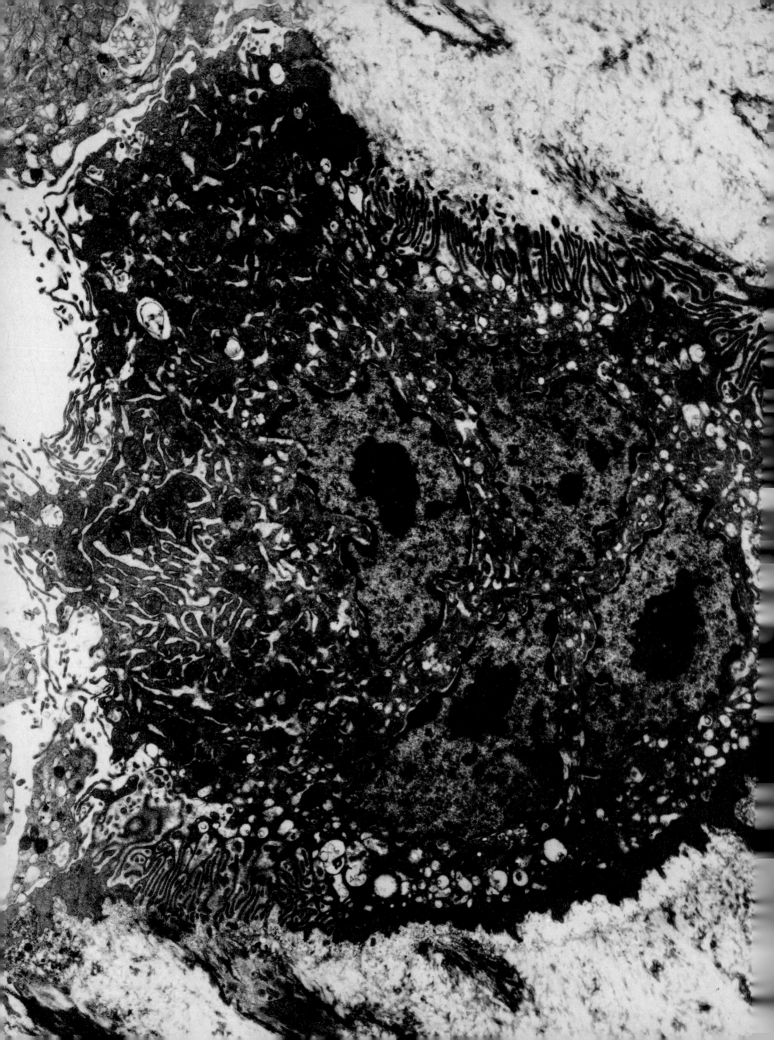

TO BE CONVERSANT ON THE FOLLOWING TOPICS:

1. The origin, location, and structure of hyaline, elastic, and fibrous cartilage and their growth and regeneration potentials.

2. The concept of bone as a tissue as contrasted to bone as an organ.

3. The comparison of intramembranous with endochondrial bone development, including the functions of osteoclasts, osteoblasts, and osteocytes in bone resorption and remodeling.

4. The correct chronological sequence of cellular events in bone repair.

5. The contrast of periosteum vs. perichondrium; bone growth in width vs. bone growth in length; interstitial vs. appositional growth; bone matrix vs. cartilage matrix; and fine structure of bone vs. cartilage ultrastructure.

6. The types of articulations and how arthritis and bursitis may affect them.

CARTILAGE

Cartilage and bone comprise the skeleton. Although **cartilage** plays a subordinate role to bone in support and protection of the body, it is a highly resilient tissue, capable of bearing considerable weight, having some rigidity, and yet giving remarkable flexibility to the body. Like all connective tissue, it consists of cells, fibers, and ground substance. Fibers, water, and ground substance constitute the **cartilage matrix.** It is the matrix, a hydrated amorphous gel embedded with collagenous and/or elastic fibers, that gives cartilage its resilience, firmness, elasticity, and tensile strength.

Development

In the human embryo, cartilage first appears during the fifth prenatal week. It originates from the everpresent, versatile **mesenchyme.** The stellate, mesenchymal cells differentiate into rounded, closely packed cells, the **chondroblasts,** which are interlaced with either collagenous or elastic fibers. Gradually these cells deposit layers of extracellular matrix until the cells become widely separated and securely imprisoned in lacunae (L. lacus, small lake or opening) in the matrix. The cells are then called **chondrocytes.**

Most cartilage that develops in the embryo is the **hyaline** type and serves as the **embryonic skeleton** until it degenerates and is replaced by bone. However, remnants of this chondroskeleton persist postnatally, such as the **epiphyseal growth centers** in long bones which enable

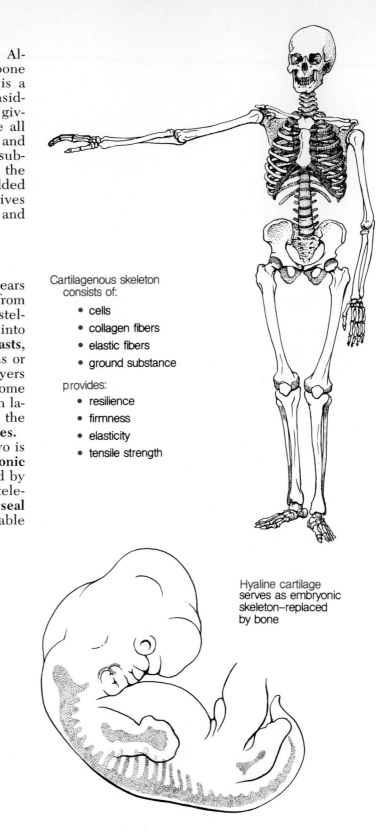

Cartilagenous skeleton consists of:

- cells
- collagen fibers
- elastic fibers
- ground substance

provides:

- resilience
- firmness
- elasticity
- tensile strength

Hyaline cartilage serves as embryonic skeleton–replaced by bone

Growth and Repair of Cartilage

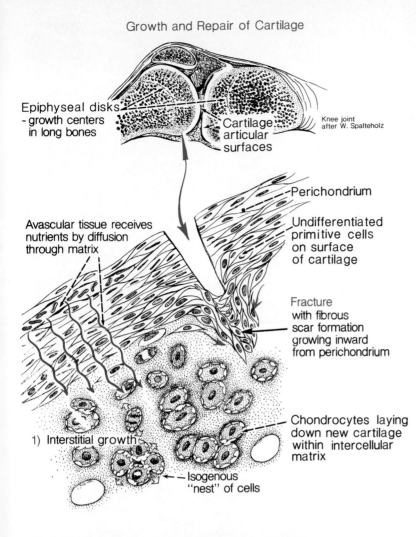

Epiphyseal disks - growth centers in long bones

Cartilage articular surfaces

Knee joint after W. Spalteholz

Perichondrium

Undifferentiated primitive cells on surface of cartilage

Avascular tissue receives nutrients by diffusion through matrix

Fracture with fibrous scar formation growing inward from perichondrium

Chondrocytes laying down new cartilage within intercellular matrix

1) Interstitial growth

Isogenous "nest" of cells

2) Appositional growth (surface deposition)   LM

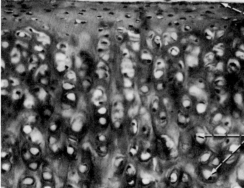

Undifferentiated primitive cells on surface of cartilage

Chondroblasts

(x 208)

Classification of Cartilage

1) Hyaline—no fibers visible under LM

2) Elastic—abundant elastic fibers

3) Fibro—dense collagenous fibers

13466

bones to grow in length. Other cartilages that persist in the adult body cover the **articular surfaces** of movable joints, the open or closed cartilage rings along the larger respiratory passageways and at the costosternal junctions between the ribs and sternum.

Growth and Repair

Cartilage is an **avascular** tissue that receives nutrients by diffusion through its matrix. Notwithstanding its poor nutrition, cartilage grows by two mechanisms:

1. By **interstitial** or **endogenous growth**; i.e., through mitosis the imprisoned chondrocyte multiplies to form a nest of cells, called **isogenous cells.** The surrounding matrix is sufficiently malleable to allow expansion of the lacunae housing the cells. The cells lay down more intercellular matrix, and interstitial growth occurs as they become separated by the new matrix.

2. **Appositional (exogenous) growth** occurs when a cartilage structure increases in size by new cartilage being **deposited on its surface.** This growth is dependent on the presence of **undifferentiated primitive cells** on the surface of the cartilage. These cells proliferate and differentiate into chondroblasts, which lay down new cartilage.

Interstitial growth **begins earlier** than appositional but **ceases early** in life because the rigid, maturing, intercellular matrix makes internal expansion very difficult. However, appositional growth may continue throughout life if diffusion gradients remain favorable.

Because cartilage has no blood supply, it has very **slight regenerative capacity.** If fractured, cartilage usually repairs itself by fibrous scar formation derived from the perichondrium (the fibrous investment around cartilage) and not by extensive new cartilage production.

Types of Cartilage

Classification of cartilage depends largely on the **character of the matrix** and the predominant type of **fibers** present. Using these two criteria, three varieties of cartilage can be identified under the light microscope, i.e., **hyaline** cartilage (no fibers visible), **elastic** cartilage (with an abundance of elastic fibers), and **fibrocartilage** (with dense collagenous fibers).

HYALINE CARTILAGE Hyaline cartilage is the most common type and is the **prototype** for all cartilage. The other types are simply variations on its generalized structure. It is called **hyaline** (Gk. hylos, glass) because in the fresh state it has a **glassy, translucent,** bluish white appearance. In the **embryo** it forms most of the **temporary skeleton** that is eventually replaced by bone.

In the **adult** it persists as the **articular** cartilage of movable joints; the **costal** cartilages; the cartilages of the nose, trachea, and bronchi; and most of the cartilages of the larynx.

As stated earlier, the **matrix components** are fibers, water, and ground substance. About 40–50% of the dry weight of hyaline cartilage consists of very fine **collagenous fibrils.** These fibrils are not visible under the LM because of their very small diameter (10–20 nm) and because they have about the same refractive index as the surrounding ground substance. The wet weight of the matrix is about 75% water, held in a gel structure. The remainder of the matrix, the **ground substance,** is largely composed of **glycosaminoglycans,** such as chondroitin sulfates, keratan sulfate, and hyaluronic acid. The basophilia of hyaline cartilage is due to the presence of the chondroitin sulfates. Also the positive periodic acid-Schiff (PAS) reaction of these sulfates indicates their carbohydrate nature.

The matrix immediately adjacent to the lacunae is poor in fibrils but rich in ground substance. Therefore, it has a deeper basophilia often associated with **metachromasia** (stains different colors with same dye) and a positive PAS reaction. These areas are called the **territorial** or **capsular matrix**—a distinctive characteristic of hyaline cartilage. There is also a direct correlation between the content of keratan sulfate and the hardness of the cartilage.

Cartilage cells, or **chondrocytes,** are rather evenly sprinkled throughout the matrix. They are entrapped, singly or in groups, **in lacunae.** On the periphery of the cartilage, these cells are flattened and lie parallel to the long axis of the cartilage. Those chondrocytes nearer to the center of the cartilage mass are rounded or ovoid. Each cell has a large, **spherical nucleus** with **one or more nucleoli.**

Under the LM, the **cytoplasm of chondrocytes** appears finely granular and is **basophilic** with H&E. This is due to the abundance of ribosomes, mitochondria, and rough endoplasmic reticulum **(rER).** Although chondrocytes fully occupy the lacunae during life, they shrink during histologic procedures, become irregular in shape, and separate from the wall of the lacunae.

Electron micrographs of an **active chondrocyte** reveal abundant free **ribosomes** and well-developed **rER** with dilated cisternae. The **Golgi complex** is large, with expanded saccules and vacuoles of various sizes. Mitochondria are limited. Some fat droplets are present as well as extensive clusters of **glycogen granules.**

Except for articular cartilage, all hyaline cartilage is invested in a dense connective tissue sheath, the **perichondrium,** which is essential for the growth of the cartilage. One can observe, in the junctional region where the perichondrium

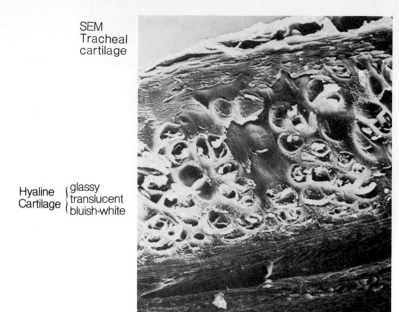

SEM
Tracheal
cartilage

Hyaline
Cartilage { glassy
translucent
bluish-white

M. J. Koering

Hyaline matrix components:
- 40–50% of dry weight
  fine collagenous fibrils (10–20 nm)
- 75% of H_2O in gel
- Ground substance consists
  of glycosaminoglycans,
  e.g. mucopolysaccarides { Chondroitin sulfates
Keratan sulfate
Hyaluronic acid

LM   Hyaline cartilage

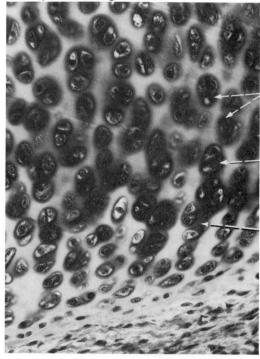

Metachromasia
(basophilia, positive PAS)

Basophilic
territorial matrix

Chondrocytes
trapped in lacunae

Spherical nucleus
1 or more nucleoli

Finely granular
basophilic cytoplasm
due to ribosomes,
mitochondria
and rER

Perichondrium

Transition from
fibroblasts to
chondroblasts

13487

Characteristics of Elastic Cartilage

1. Matrix impregnated with elastic fibers

4. Abundant packed cells

2. Bends without breaking

5. Does not ossify in old age

3. Fresh elastic fibers are opaque and yellow

6. Has little glycogen or lipid

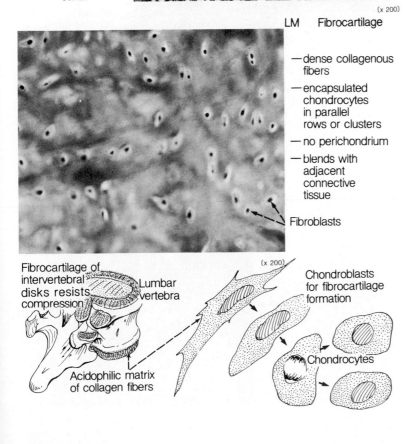

LM   Elastic cartilage

Perichondrium

Chondrocytes

Appositional growth area

Interstitial growth area

Found mostly in:
—external ear
—epiglottis
—auditory canal

(x 200)

LM   Fibrocartilage

—dense collagenous fibers

—encapsulated chondrocytes in parallel rows or clusters

—no perichondrium

—blends with adjacent connective tissue

Fibroblasts

(x 200)

Fibrocartilage of intervertebral disks resists compression

Lumbar vertebra

Acidophilic matrix of collagen fibers

Chondroblasts for fibrocartilage formation

Chondrocytes

meets the cartilage surface, a gradual transition from fibroblasts to chondroblasts. This is the inner, cellular, **chondrogenic layer** of the perichondrium; the outer layer is more fibrous and less cellular with essentially no chondrogenic potential.

ELASTIC CARTILAGE Elastic cartilage is quite similar to hyaline except that:

1. The matrix is impregnated with **elastic fibers,** which gives the tissue its accentuated resiliency and flexibility.
2. It is **yellow** in the fresh state due to the abundance of elastic fibers. Also it is more opaque than hyaline cartilage.
3. The **cells** resemble those of hyaline cartilage except that they are more **closely packed** and usually are found **singly** in lacunae; there are very few isogenic clusters of cells.
4. Normally it does not calcify or ossify in old age as does hyaline cartilage.
5. It shows less accumulation of glycogen and lipids.

Elastic cartilage is surrounded by a **perichondrium.** Growth occurs both **appositionally** from the perichondrium and **interstitially** by mitosis of chondrocytes internal to the perichondrium. Elastic cartilage is found only in a few isolated areas of the body where extra flexibility and support are needed, e.g., the **external ear,** certain laryngeal cartilages (especially the **epiglottis**), and the outer part of the external **auditory tube.**

FIBROCARTILAGE Fibrocartilage is an irregular, dense, fibrous tissue with thinly dispersed, **encapsulated cartilage cells** embedded within it. These **chondrocytes** are usually found in short parallel rows but may occur singly, in pairs, or occasionally in small clusters. Since it has **no perichondrium,** fibrocartilage never occurs alone. It blends with adjacent connective tissue structures, especially those associated with joints. For example, it blends with the articular (hyaline) cartilage of joints and with certain tendons where they insert into bone.

Fibrocartilage is best seen in the **intervertebral disks** and other articular disks associated with the knee, mandible, and sternoclavicular joints, where resistance to compression, durability, and tensile strength are needed. Its **matrix stains acidophilic** because of the concentration of **collagen fiber bundles.** Amorphous ground substance is scanty. It is best seen at the boundaries of the lacunae where it gives a positive PAS reaction and is slightly basophilic with H&E.

Fibrocartilage develops from dense fibrous tissue richly populated with fibroblasts which are separated by considerable matrix. When these fibroblasts differentiate into chondroblasts, fibrocartilage is formed (L-A, plate 2).

BONE

There are two somewhat divergent approaches to the study of bone, namely, (1) **bone as a tissue,** and (2) **bone as an organ,** that is, shaped out of bone tissue. Like other organs, bones are supplied with blood and lymph vessels, nerves, connective tissue investments and, unique to bones, their cavities are usually filled with **hemopoietic (blood-forming) tissue.** These two concepts complement each other, particularly when one considers how bones (as organs) develop, are remodeled, and repaired. These dynamic processes are best described on a cellular basis; however, the concept of bones as organs is the frame of reference.

Bone, as an **ossified tissue,** is the hardest tissue in the body, except dentine and enamel. It excels cartilage in its ability to **withstand compression, stress,** and **deformation.** Like other connective tissues, bone consists of cells, fibers, and ground substance. Although these elements are combined in a rigid, calcified matrix, **living bone** is a **dynamic, plastic tissue** capable of responding to life's stresses and strains by growth, remodeling, and reinforcement. Indeed, bone is one of the most plastic tissues in the body.

Bone As an Organ

With the unaided eye, one can distinguish two types of bone in a longitudinal section of a long bone. A shell of **compact** or dense bone makes up most of the **shaft (diaphysis),** while cancellous, or **spongy bone** occupies the center of the **ends (epiphyses)** of the bone. These two types are also called **cortical bone** and **medullary bone,** respectively. The small, irregular marrow spaces of the spongy bone in the epiphysis join with the large, hollow cavity of the diaphysis, called the **medullary cavity.** The spaces and cavity contain bone marrow. Two types of marrow are present in the adult: (1) **red marrow,** where active blood development (hemopoiesis), is occurring, and (2) **yellow marrow,** which has no active hemopoiesis but has a heavy concentration of adipose cells that gives the marrow its yellow color in the fresh state.

PERIOSTEUM Each bone is ensheathed by a tough, vascular, fibrous layer, **the periosteum.** It covers the bone except over the articular surfaces. Except where it is firmly attached to the articular margins, and at attachment sites of muscles, tendons, and ligaments, the fresh periosteum can be rather easily stripped free of the bone, especially its outer layer. Like the perichondrium, it has two layers. The **outer layer** is largely **collagenous fibers** with a small component of elastic fibers. The **inner layer** is highly vascular and cellular. This is the **osteogenic layer** that gives rise to concentric rings of new bone. The thin, poorly defined, cellular layer that lines the medullary cavity of the shaft and the spaces

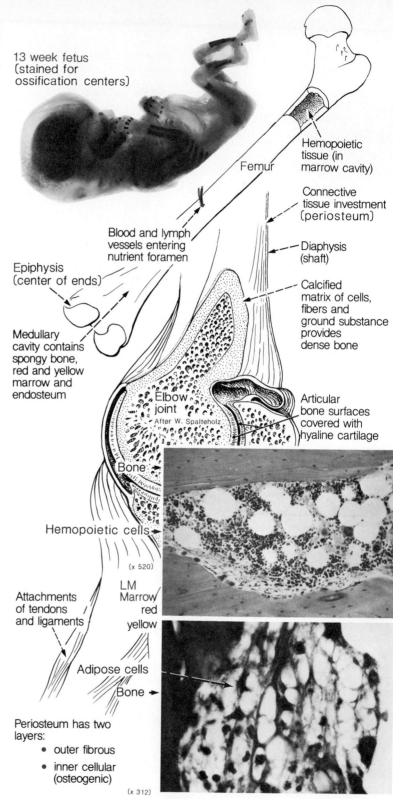

13 week fetus (stained for ossification centers)

Femur

Hemopoietic tissue (in marrow cavity)

Connective tissue investment (periosteum)

Diaphysis (shaft)

Blood and lymph vessels entering nutrient foramen

Epiphysis (center of ends)

Medullary cavity contains spongy bone, red and yellow marrow and endosteum

Calcified matrix of cells, fibers and ground substance provides dense bone

Elbow joint

After W. Spalteholz

Articular bone surfaces covered with hyaline cartilage

Bone

Hemopoietic cells

(x 520)

LM Marrow red yellow

Attachments of tendons and ligaments

Adipose cells

Bone

Periosteum has two layers:
- outer fibrous
- inner cellular (osteogenic)

(x 312)

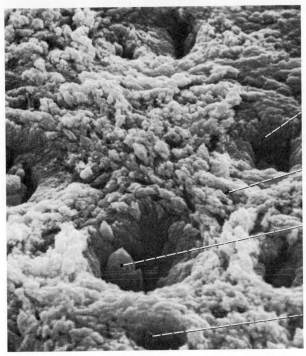

Blood vessels
enter
osteons
supplying
osteocytes

Calcified bone
matrix

Perforating
collagenous
fibers of
Sharpey

Small nerves
follow vessels
into osteons

T.E. Russell and
S.P. Kapur

Inorganic ←——— Intercellular matrix of bone
components
of bone:

- $Ca(PO_4)_2$ = 85%
- $CaCO_3$ = 10%
- other = 5%
  elements

$Ca(PO_4)_2$ forms
needle-like
hydroxyapatite
crystals (1.5nm–30nm)

Organic
components
of bone:

- collagen = 95%
- ground
  substance = 5%

Eosinophilic
stained collagen
(PAS positive)

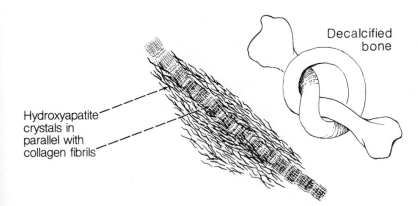

Hydroxyapatite
crystals in
parallel with
collagen fibrils

Decalcified
bone

of spongy bone, is the **endosteum.** It also has some osteogenic potential.

From the outer layer of the periosteum, fine bundles of collagenous fibers penetrate the underlying bone at regular intervals, especially at sites of attachment of tendons and ligaments. These are the **perforating fibers of Sharpey,** which effectively attach the periosteum to the bone as well as bind together the outer bone layers (lamellae).

BLOOD AND NERVE SUPPLY All bones are well supplied with blood vessels from several sources. For example, **periosteal vessels** penetrate the cortical bone of the diaphysis of long bones. The vessels divide into branches that enter the cylindrical **Haversian systems (osteons),** which are thin concentric layers of bone surrounding a tiny canal. These vessels supply the bone cells (**osteocytes**) embedded in the calcified matrix. Other larger vessels pierce the epiphysis to supply the spongy bone. Also a large artery traverses the **nutrient canal** near mid-shaft to supply the medullary cavity.

Small myelinated and nonmyelinated nerves follow the blood vessels into the Haversian canals. The periosteum is extremely sensitive to injury as evidenced by the acute pain elicited when one strikes a subcutaneous bone, such as the tibia (shin bone).

BONE MATRIX The **intercellular matrix** of bone tissue consists of organic and inorganic components. The **inorganic material** in compact bone is about 65% of the fat-free weight. It consists mainly of **calcium phosphate** (85%), about 10% **calcium carbonate,** and small quantities of magnesium, sodium, potassium, bicarbonate, fluoride, citrate, sulfate, and hydroxide. X-ray diffraction studies reveal that calcium and phosphorus form **hydroxyapatite crystals.** Electron micrographs show these crystals to be needlelike, about 1.5 × 30 nm in size. They are bound to the collagen fibrils in parallel rows, surrounded by ground substance.

The **organic component** is mostly **collagen** (95%). The amorphous **ground substance** contains **glycosaminoglycans** in combination with proteins (proteoglycans), most of which contain sulfates. The **matrix stains eosinophilic** because of its high collagen content and low concentration of sulfates. It gives a positive PAS reaction because of the presence of carbohydrates in the glycosaminoglycans.

The hardness and rigidity of bone are due to the intimate relationship between the hydroxyapatite crystals and the collagen fibrils that usually lie parallel to each other. Its slight flexibility is the property of the collagenous fibers.

Bone Development

Bone never develops alone. It always arises from a **preexisting tissue** which it eventually replaces. If the earlier tissue is a membrane, e.g., a sheet of mesenchyme or loose connective tissue, it is called **intramembranous** bone formation. If bone replaces cartilage which is largely resorbed before bone is formed, this is **endochondral** (intracartilaginous) bone development. In either case, the initial bone formed is **spongy**. Later, some or all of it is transformed into **compact bone** by a filling in of the spaces between the bony trabeculae or spicules.

In both processes, the early bone formed is of an **immature or primary** variety. This primary bone is temporary and is soon replaced by dense, **mature, lamellar bone.** Whether in early or late bone growth, there are often areas of immature, mature, and resorbing bone lying side by side. The production and removal of bone tissue is occurring continuously, beginning in the late embryo and continuing at a slower pace throughout adulthood. Thus, the structure of **bone is not static.** It is being changed constantly by a never-ending process of **bone resorption and remodeling.** In the elderly, bone resorption is often excessive, resulting in thin, porous, fragile bones.

INTRAMEMBRANOUS BONE DEVELOPMENT Intramembranous or membrane bone development usually begins near the center of well-vascularized connective tissue membranes, such as **mesenchyme.** Some of the mesenchymal cells differentiate into large, rounded, basophilic **osteoblasts.** Between these cells, **collagenous fibers** are found, largely masked by the dense ground substance. The matrix formed by osteoblasts is not initially calcified and is called **osteoid.** Later the matrix becomes calcified by an orderly deposition of hydroxyapatite crystals of calcium and phosphate.

Gradually the osteoid becomes fully calcified and small **spicules of bone** appear, surrounded by a layer of osteoblasts. By appositional growth, the spicule increases in size as layers of bone are laid down at the periphery of the spicules. During the process, **osteoblasts become entrapped** in lacunae in the bone. These cells are now called **osteocytes.** Gradually, the spicules coalesce and the definitive shape of the bone emerges, with osteoblasts lying on its surfaces. Through the osteogenic action of the periosteum, layers of compact (mature) bone surround the spongy (immature) bone. Most of the **flat bones** of the skull develop through **intramembraneous ossification.**

ENDOCHONDRAL (INTRACARTILAGINOUS) BONE DEVELOPMENT Endochondral bone formation begins in cartilage conforming to the shape of the future adult bone. This model serves as **a template** for most of the **developing skeleton.** The **cartilage** is subsequently **resorbed** and **replaced** by bone.

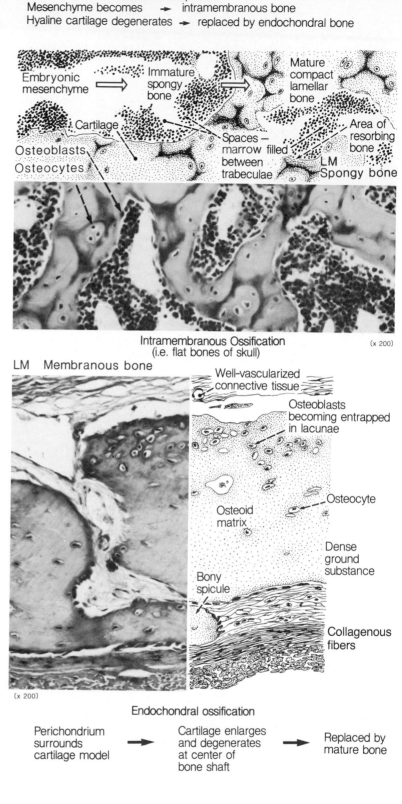

Bone Development
Mesenchyme becomes → intramembranous bone
Hyaline cartilage degenerates → replaced by endochondral bone

Intramembranous Ossification (x 200)
(i.e. flat bones of skull)

LM Membranous bone (x 200)

Endochondral ossification

Perichondrium surrounds cartilage model → Cartilage enlarges and degenerates at center of bone shaft → Replaced by mature bone

LM   Marrow formation in spaces of spongy bone

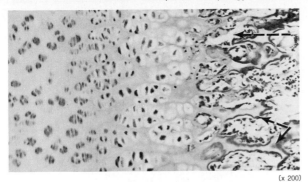

Cartilage cells
enlarge, creating
small cavities

Calcium
deposited on
cartilage spicules

(x 200)

LM   Endochondral bone

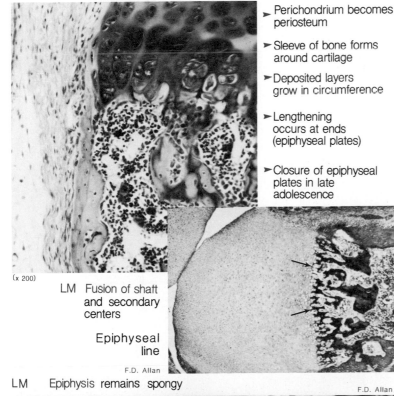

Compact Bone Formation

➤ Perichondrium becomes
   periosteum

➤ Sleeve of bone forms
   around cartilage

➤ Deposited layers
   grow in circumference

➤ Lengthening
   occurs at ends
   (epiphyseal plates)

➤ Closure of epiphyseal
   plates in late
   adolescence

(x 200)

LM   Fusion of shaft
      and secondary
      centers

      Epiphyseal
      line

F.D. Allan

F.D. Allan

LM   Epiphysis remains spongy

13739

Briefly, endochondral bone development in a typical **long bone** is as follows: The **perichondrium**, surrounding the cartilage model, is **invaded by capillaries**. Because of this vascular environment, the inner cells of the perichondrium differentiate into **osteoblasts.** These osteogenic cells (periosteum) lay down a thin **collar of bone** around the weakened midsection of the cartilage plate. Midway along the shaft of the cartilage model, changes begin to occur in the center of the cartilage, which later becomes the primary ossification center. The lacunae gradually enlarge, the **matrix** between them **calcifies**, the chondrocytes die, and small cavities form in the matrix.

While the calcified cartilage disintegrates, a collection or tuft of osteogenic cells (osteoblasts) and blood vessels, called the **periosteal bud,** penetrates the bony collar from the periosteum to reach the interior of the cartilage model. The osteoblasts surround the remnants of calcified cartilage and enclose them, first with osteoid (uncalcified bone) and then with calcified bone. Thus, the **cartilage spicules** are replaced by **bone spicules** that coalesce to form spongy bone. This general area becomes the **primary ossification center** of the long bone which expands toward both epiphyses as the **medullary cavity,** the site of hemopoiesis (blood formation).

While spongy bone is being laid down at the center of the cartilage model, bone of the same elements but different architecture, i.e., **compact bone,** is being formed at the periphery of the **shaft.** It arises from the **innermost cells** of the enveloping **perichondrium.** As these cells lay down a sleeve of bone around the center of the cartilage model, the **perichondrium becomes the periosteum.** As additional layers of bone are deposited, the **shaft grows in circumference.**

Simultaneously, the bone is being lengthened by proliferation of cartilage cells at the ends (epiphyses) of the shaft. Within the **epiphyses, secondary centers of ossification** form in which bone formation follows essentially the same pattern as in the shaft. The center of the epiphyseal cartilage gives way to spongy bone, and its diameter is increased by layers of compact bone. However, there are two differences: (1) the epiphyses are **mostly spongy bone without** a definitive **marrow cavity,** and (2) the cartilage on the **articular surface remains hyaline cartilage** rather than yielding to bone formation. The area between the shaft and epiphysis is the **epiphyseal plate.**

Long bones **grow in length** as a direct result of **interstitial growth** of the **epiphyseal cartilage.** As long as these disks contain mitotically active cells, the cartilage on either end of the shaft is constantly undergoing growth, ossification, and the shaft between the disks lengthens.

Histologic examination of an active epiphysis reveals an orderly series of **zones** that reflect the events of endochondrial bone formation. Beginning at the center of the disk and proceeding

Endochondral Bone Development
(Typical long bone)

After A.A. Maximow

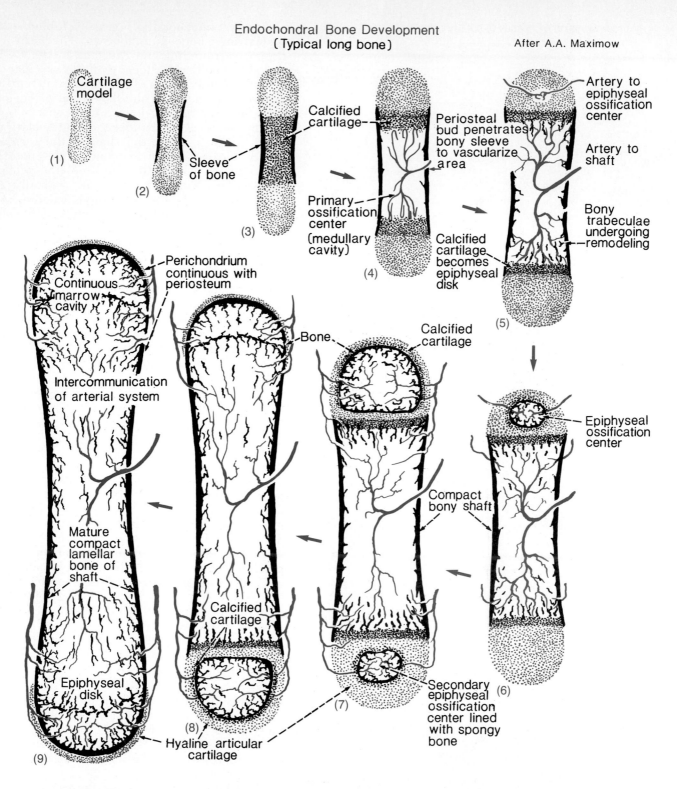

Sketches of successive stages of endochondral ossification in a typical long bone. These stages include: (1) an early hyaline cartilaginous model; (2) a periosteal sleeve (collar) of bone surrounds the midsection of the uncalcified cartilage; (3) the cartilage begins to calcify; (4) a periosteal bud of blood vessels carrying osteogenic mesenchymal cells penetrate the bony collar to vascularize the future medullary cavity (primary ossification center); (5) blood vessels with mesenchyme invade the upper epiphyseal cartilage; (6) it becomes calcified and is replaced by spongy bone, establishing a secondary ossification center; (7) a similar center is formed in the lower epiphyseal cartilage; (8) with closure of the epiphyseal disks, the bone ceases to grow in length; and (9) the marrow cavity becomes continuous throughout and the blood vessels of the various regions of the bone freely communicate.

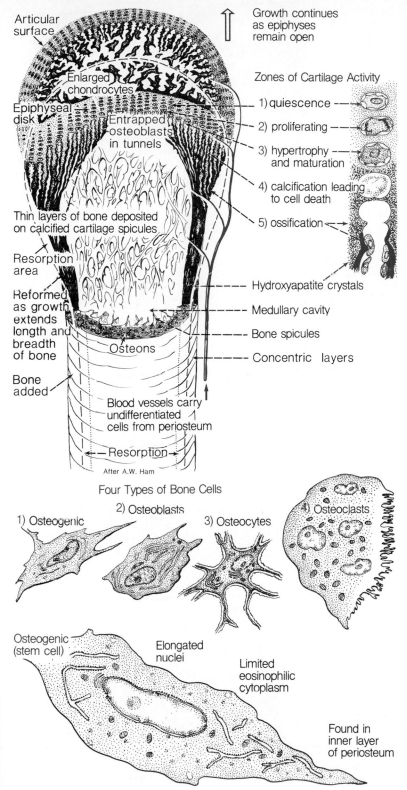

Epiphyses of Long Bones

Articular surface

Growth continues as epiphyses remain open

Enlarged chondrocytes

Epiphyseal disk

Entrapped osteoblasts in tunnels

Zones of Cartilage Activity

1) quiescence
2) proliferating
3) hypertrophy and maturation
4) calcification leading to cell death
5) ossification

Thin layers of bone deposited on calcified cartilage spicules

Resorption area

Reformed as growth extends length and breadth of bone

Bone added

Osteons

Blood vessels carry undifferentiated cells from periosteum

Resorption

Hydroxyapatite crystals

Medullary cavity

Bone spicules

Concentric layers

After A.W. Ham

Four Types of Bone Cells

1) Osteogenic
2) Osteoblasts
3) Osteocytes
4) Osteoclasts

Osteogenic (stem cell)

Elongated nuclei

Limited eosinophilic cytoplasm

Found in inner layer of periosteum

toward the diaphysis, the following zones are identified:

1. A zone of quiescence or **reserve cartilage** consists of typical hyaline cartilage cells.

2. A zone of **proliferating cartilage** shows active mitosis among chondrocytes which form parallel stacks of crowded, flattened cells. The stacks are aligned with the long axis of the bone.

3. A zone of **hypertrophy and maturation** is characterized by enlargement of chondrocytes which accumulate glycogen. No mitosis is occurring. The matrix is reduced to thin partitions (septa) between cartilage cells.

4. A zone of **calcification** signals the death of chondrocytes. The matrix between cells becomes impregnated with hydroxyapatite crystals of calcium and phosphorus and stains basophilic.

5. A zone of **ossification** shows thin layers of bone deposited on the surface of the spicules of calcified cartilage. **Blood vessels invade** the area carrying undifferentiated cells from the periosteum which give rise to osteoblasts. As the matrix calcifies, some osteoblasts are entrapped as osteocytes and **bone spicules** are formed. Coalescence of spicules creates spongy bone. Finally, resorption of spongy bone in the center of the diaphysis enlarges the medullary cavity.

Growth continues in this manner until early adulthood, when the epiphyseal plates close (ossify) and growth in length ceases. Simultaneously, the primary and secondary ossification centers fuse.

Growth in **diameter** keeps pace with growth in length by the addition of **concentric layers** of **bone** laid down by the **periosteum** on the external surface of the bony collar. Note that this new bone is **not endochondral** in origin **but periosteal,** i.e., it is derived from a membrane, the periosteum, and therefore is an example of intramembranous bone formation. At the same time, giant, multinucleate **osteoclasts** actively erode and remodel the internal surface of the long shaft. Thus, the marrow cavity increases in size, and the compact cortical bone remains a relatively thin, hollow cylinder. Without this osteoclastic activity, a long bone would become a solid cylinder with only a miniscule marrow cavity.

Bone As a Tissue

In both developing and adult bone, four types of bone cells are identified, namely, (1) osteogenic cells or osteoprogenitor cells, (2) osteoblasts, (3) osteocytes, and (4) osteoclasts.

OSTEOID CELLS As their name implies the **osteogenic cells** are primitive, pluripotential cells, similar to mesenchymal cells. They are found principally in the inner layer of the periosteum, the so-called **osteogenic layer.** They are also found, to a much more limited extent, in the cells lining the medullary cavity, the **endosteum,** and among the cells lining the nutrient canals of compact bone. They are **stem cells** capable of dividing and differentiating into any of the other bone cells.

OSTEOBLASTS Osteoblasts are involved in the **synthesis** of collagen, proteoglycans, and glycoproteins and are therefore responsible for the **formation and growth of new bone.** They are almost exclusively found on the surfaces of existing bone tissue or calcified cartilage where they initially deposit the new bone matrix (osteoid), which contains essentially no minerals. Later, mineralization occurs and the tissue is new bone. Because these cells usually line up side-by-side and are rather cuboidal in shape, they **resemble epithelium,** especially during the active synthesis of matrix. During this early active stage, the cytoplasm of the osteoblasts is **basophilic.** When activity declines, the cells tend to flatten out. During the active phase, there is marked alkaline phosphatase activity, which gives a positive PAS reaction in the cytoplasmic granules, indicating the presence of mucopolysaccharides.

During active bone synthesis, transmission electron micrographs reveal that **osteoblasts** contain well-developed **rER** and prominent **Golgi complexes,** which are typical of all protein-secreting cells. Secretory **vesicles** are also present which contain an amorphous substance, probably the precursor of the matrix. In the peripheral cytoplasm **microfilaments** are noted. These are about 5–10 nm in diameter and are especially numerous in the cytoplasmic processes projecting from the osteoblasts. These cells are **polarized,** that is, the secretion of the synthesized materials occurs on the cell surface next to the bone matrix, while the large, spherical nucleus, with its finely dispersed chromatin, is found on the cell surface opposite the bone matrix.

OSTEOCYTES Osteocytes are **bone cells** imprisoned in the **lacunae** of the surrounding **bone matrix.** They are poorly defined in most decalcified bone sections stained with H&E. However, under more favorable histological conditions, they appear as flat, elongated cells with numerous, small cytoplasmic processes which occupy the many minute canals, the **canaliculi,** that radiate in all directions from the lacunae. These intercommunicating canaliculi allow for the transfer of **nutrients.** This is essential to the survival of the incarcerated osteocytes since nutrients and oxygen cannot diffuse through the calcified bony matrix, as they do in the uncalcified matrix of cartilage.

Under the TEM, **osteocytes** resemble to some extent osteoblasts, their immediate ancestral cells. The rER and Golgi apparatus are less prominent, suggesting a **low level of cellular ac-**

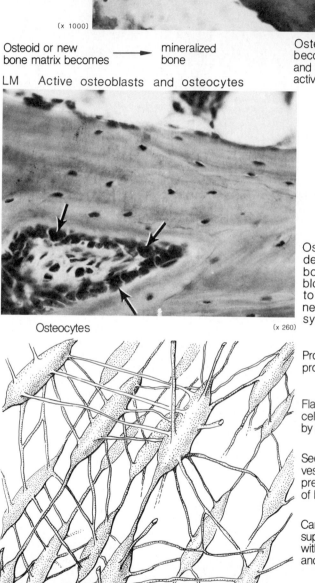

LM
Osteoblasts (synthesize collagen and glycoproteins in new bone)

Found on existing bone or calcified cartilage

(x 1000)

Osteoblasts become flattened and basophilic as activity declines

Osteoid or new bone matrix becomes ⟶ mineralized bone

LM   Active osteoblasts and osteocytes

Osteocytes   (x 260)

Osteoblasts depositing bone around blood vessel to begin new osteon system

Projecting processes

Flat elongated cells surrounded by bone matrix

Secretory vesicles contain precursor of bone matrix

Canaliculi supply cells with nutrients and oxygen

Osteocytes maintain bone that stores minerals

Osteocytes function in repair of fractures

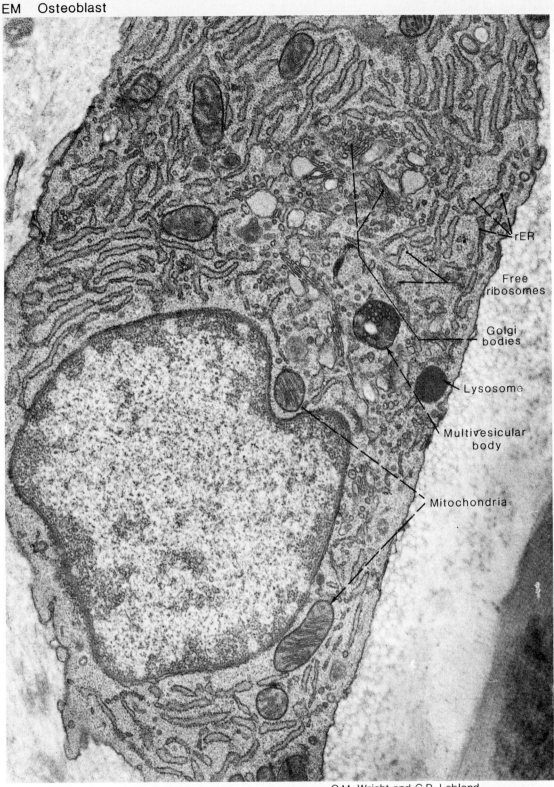

G.M. Wright and C.P. Leblond

Electron micrograph of an osteoblast from a rat tibia. Within the cytoplasm are an abundance of cellular organelles, characteristic of a cell involved in active protein synthesis, in this case, collagen. These structures include: (1) many profiles of rER (2) an abundance of free ribosomes (3) several Golgi bodies with stacks of saccules with pale, spherical or elongated distensions, and (4) frequent mitochondria. Also present are a few lysosomes and multivesicular bodies.

The osteoblast is surrounded by osteoid tissue that separates it from the mineralized, electron-dense bony matrix.

tivity. Yet, since these cells show some metabolic activity, they are not completely inert cells but aid in the **maintenance of bone tissue** and perhaps play some role in the storage of minerals in the tissue. Some osteocytes are released from bone during fractures and may round-up and **become active osteoblasts** again. This is one potential source of bone-forming cells that are urgently needed at fracture sites.

OSTEOCLASTS Osteoclasts are **giant, multinucleated cells** scattered along bone surfaces where resorption and remodeling of bone are occurring. They may have **40 or more nuclei** surrounded by eosinophilic, foamy cytoplasm. Typically they are nestled in shallow depressions on bone surfaces, called **Howship's lacunae.** Stained with H&E, the cytoplasm changes from basophilic in immature cells, to acidophilic in mature cells. Osteoclasts give a **positive acid phosphatase** reaction, probably due to the presence of numerous **lysosomes** in the cytoplasm. Under the electron microscope, these cells are characterized by the so-called **ruffled border** of the plasmalemma adjacent to the bone surface. In life, this border has a wavy, undulating appearance.

The function of osteoclasts is to **resorb bone** during bone remodeling. Although the mechanism is unclear, they secrete the enzyme **collagenase** with other proteinases, lactic acid and citrate, which, dissolve the bone matrix. The ruffled border increases the bone absorption area, making for a more effective removal of the bone, probably through enzymic action, or limited phagocytosis.

It was formerly held that the origin of osteoclasts was from the coalescence of osteoblasts. Recent investigations indicate that perhaps this is not correct and that **osteoclasts** may have their **origin** in the union of several phagocytic **monocytes** of the circulating blood.

Transmission electron micrographs show that **osteoclasts** have numerous mitochondria, considerable rER, and active Golgi complexes. Various-sized vacuoles are present, together with many lysosomes. There are two distinctive areas next to the plasmalemma. An **inner clear zone** is free of organelles except for considerable rER, and a **peripheral, ruffled border area** has numerous invaginations of the cell membrane, causing the ruffled appearance.

Microarchitecture of Bone

TYPES OF BONE As stated earlier, two types of bone are identified grossly: **spongy** and **compact.** Also, one recognizes two other varieties of bone microscopically: (1) **primary,** also referred to as woven, or immature; and (2) **secondary,** also called lamellar, or mature.

In **primary bone,** the collagenous **fibers** are arranged in a random, **interwoven** fashion. It has proportionally more cells and less mineral con-

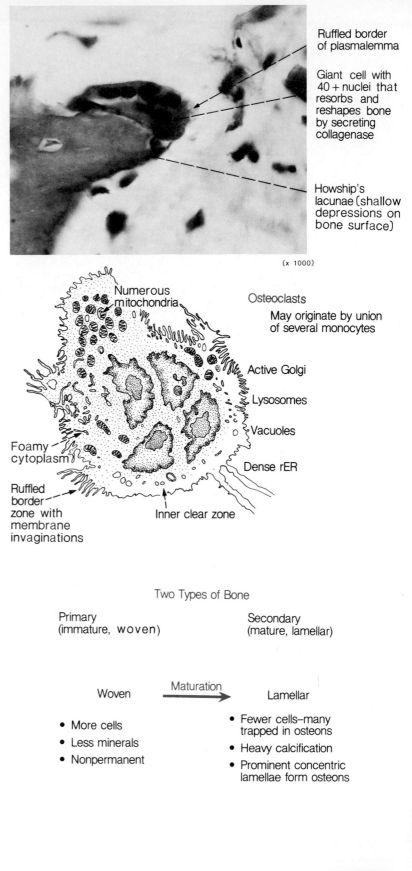

LM   Osteoclast

Ruffled border of plasmalemma

Giant cell with 40 + nuclei that resorbs and reshapes bone by secreting collagenase

Howship's lacunae (shallow depressions on bone surface)

(x 1000)

Numerous mitochondria

Osteoclasts

May originate by union of several monocytes

Active Golgi

Lysosomes

Vacuoles

Dense rER

Foamy cytoplasm

Ruffled border zone with membrane invaginations

Inner clear zone

Two Types of Bone

Primary (immature, woven)

Secondary (mature, lamellar)

Woven →Maturation→ Lamellar

- More cells
- Less minerals
- Nonpermanent

- Fewer cells–many trapped in osteons
- Heavy calcification
- Prominent concentric lamellae form osteons

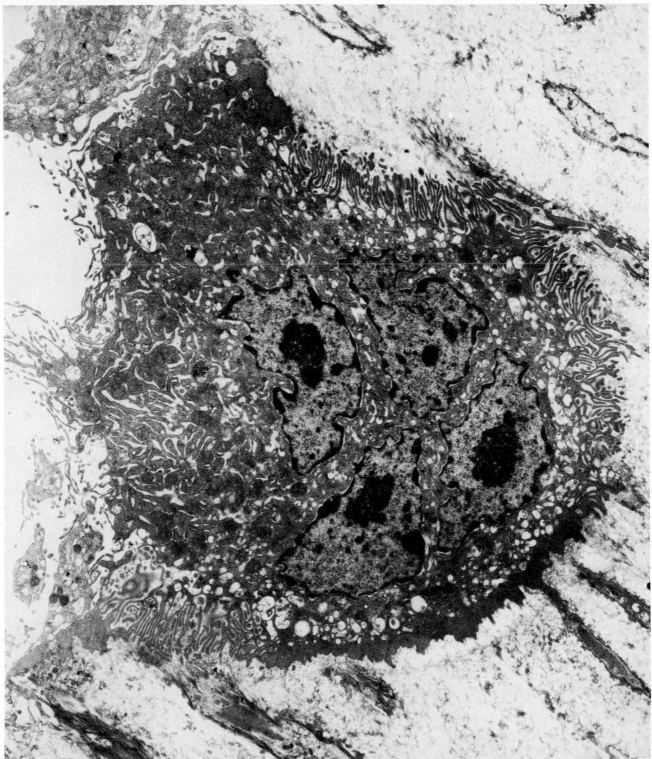

G. U. Anat. Collection   (x 8000)

This is an EM micrograph of a multinucleated osteoclast resting on the surface of a bone. The mineralized bone is the dark band at the lower right of the field. The remainder of the surrounding bone appears rather translucent. In these clear bony areas, elongated osteocytes can be seen. Surrounding most of the osteoclast, the plasmalemma is thrown into many, exaggerated infoldings, creating a ruffled border. Such a structure is indicative of a resorptive function and, in this case, bone is being resorbed. Criteria for the identification of osteoclasts should include: (1) multiple nuclei, (2) an extensive ruffled border, (3) abundant mitochondria, and (4) multiple vesicles.

13704

tent than mature bone. It is the first bone to appear in **development and repair** and is later replaced by mature bone.

Secondary bone is **mature**. It is also called **lamellar bone** because most of the calcium-impregnated, collagenous fibers are usually arranged in tight, **concentric layers or lamellae** enclosing small blood vessels. These concentric lamellae in long bones are about 4–12 μm thick and are laid down around small blood vessels during bone development to form **Haversian systems or osteons**.

OSTEONS OR HAVERSIAN SYSTEMS An **osteon** is the unit of structure of compact bone. It is a complex of 4–20 concentric, **bony lamellae** surrounding a central canal. The **canal** contains primarily blood vessels, with a few amyelinated nerve fibers, loose connective tissue, and flattened osteogenic cells that line the lumen of the canal. **Osteocytes** are sequestered in **lacunae** located within or between the lamellae. Osteons are found almost entirely in the **compact, cortical bone**. They are arranged as cylindrical tubes parallel to the longitudinal axis of the long bone.

A second arrangement of lamellae is found between the osteons, the **interstitial lamellae**. These are **remnants** of older, **partially resorbed Haversian systems,** disrupted during the remodeling of bone. Except that they are only a segment of a circle and the central canal has been lost, they are the same as the circular lamellae. A third arrangement is the **circumferential lamellae**, which are several rings of bone around the entire bone, immediately beneath the periosteum. These large, thick lamellae are not organized into osteons.

Radiating from the lacunae are many tiny channels, the **canaliculi**. Protoplasmic processes of the osteocytes enter these small canals and communicate with **adjacent osteocytes** and with the extravascular space within the Haversian canals. Here an exchange of O_2 and CO_2 occurs, nutrients are supplied to the cells, and metabolic wastes are eliminated. The Haversian canals have extensive communications with the marrow cavity, the periosteum, and with each other via the transverse **Volkmann's canals**, which run at right angles to the long axis of the bone. These latter canals are not surrounded by concentric lamellae but penetrate the lamellae to join the Haversian canals where anastomoses of their respective blood vessels occur.

There is great variation in the **diameter** of the Haversian canals. Since each system is formed by deposition of rings of calcified bone around a blood vessel beginning at the periphery, the younger systems have the wider canals.

In contrast to compact bone, spongy bone is not organized into osteons but is a **meshwork** of thin, irregular bars, or **trabeculae,** of bone. The many spaces within this bony latticework are filled with **bone marrow**. (Table 7.1.)

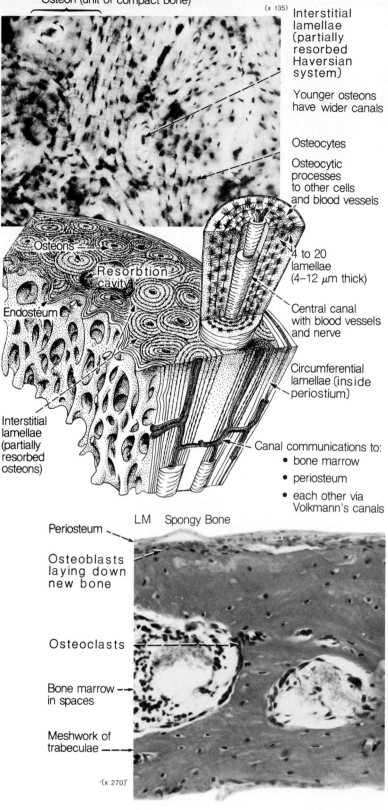

LM Secondary (mature) lamellar bone
Osteon (unit of compact bone)

(x 135)

Interstitial lamellae (partially resorbed Haversian system)

Younger osteons have wider canals

Osteocytes

Osteocytic processes to other cells and blood vessels

Osteons

Resorbtion cavity

Endosteum

Interstitial lamellae (partially resorbed osteons)

4 to 20 lamellae (4–12 μm thick)

Central canal with blood vessels and nerve

Circumferential lamellae (inside periostium)

Canal communications to:
• bone marrow
• periosteum
• each other via Volkmann's canals

LM   Spongy Bone

Periosteum

Osteoblasts laying down new bone

Osteoclasts

Bone marrow in spaces

Meshwork of trabeculae

(x 270)

13900

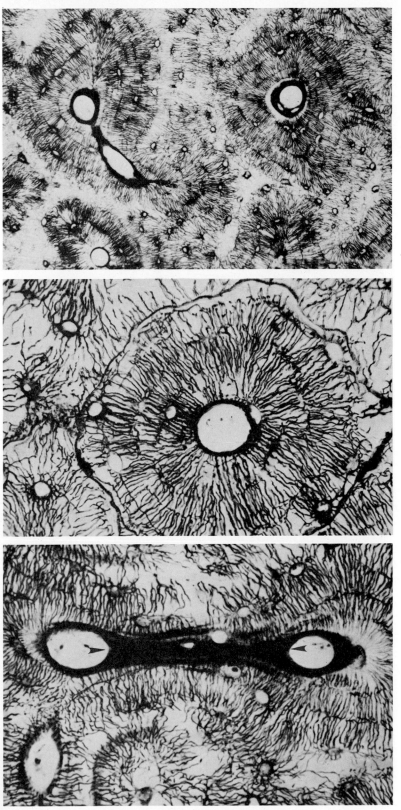

Volkmann canal

Upper. In this section of compact cortical bone, several osteons are sectioned transversely. Note that each Haversian canal is surrounded by several concentric bony lamellae. Interspersed along their margins are many lacunae, which in life are occupied by osteocytes. Delicate osteogenic processes occupy the tiny canaliculi that extend from the lacunae. They provide communicating links between osteocytes. Remnants of older degenerating osteons persist between the intact osteons, as interstitial lamellae. Left of center is an elongated Volkmann canal which joins an Haversian canal.

(x 200)

Middle. This is a higher magnification of an osteon with five to six concentric lamellae surrounding the central Haversian canal. Prominent lacunae are interspersed between or within the lamellae. The outer limit of the osteon is demarcated by a refractile line or lines, the cement line(s). In life, the canal is filled with small blood vessels, lymphatics, and nonmyelinated nerve fibers.

(x 400)

Lower. This is a view of a Volkmann canal connecting two osteons. Typically, Volkmann canals are conduits for blood vessels from the periosteum that supply the bone tissue, as well as vital communicating vascular channels between osteons. Observe that the Volkmann canal ends perpendicular on the much more abundant Haversian canals. The latter run parallel to the long axis of the bone. Unlike the Haversian canals, the Volkmann canals are not surrounded by concentric bony lamellae.

(x 400)

Bone Repair

The bare, dry, calcified bones of a cleaned skeleton disguise the true nature of living bone. Perhaps the most dramatic demonstration that bone is a **dynamic, living tissue** is in the repair of fractures.

When a **bone is broken,** the following cellular events immediately follow to **repair the damage.** They involve not only bone but also adjacent soft tissues.

1. Torn blood vessels in the area of fracture cause hemorrhage with the formation of a **blood clot** (hematoma).
2. Circulation to osteons in and near the fracture site is disrupted, causing death of osteocytes and **necrosis** (localized death) of the **bone fragments.**
3. Fibroblasts and new capillaries, largely from the periosteum, invade the clot to form the so-called **granulation tissue.**
4. As the granulation tissue becomes more fibrous, **temporary cartilage bars** are formed that are later replaced by bone. This newly formed fibrous connective tissue-cartilage bridge between the ends of the fractured bone is called the **callus.** It serves to temporarily stabilize and bind together the bone fragments.
5. As the callus is forming, the inner **osteogenic cells** of the periosteum become active and **lay down a sleeve of bone** around the callus, extending some distance beyond the fractured ends.
6. Gradually **periosteal buds** invade the callus and produce **spongy bone,** which replaces the temporary cartilage, a process similar to endochondral bone formation.
7. The newly formed spongy bone is transformed into **compact, lamellar bone.**
8. By absorption, the protruding surfaces and **excess bone are removed** and the broken bone is essentially returned to its normal contour and morphology.

It should be emphasized that it is the multipotentiality of **cells of the periosteum,** and to a much lesser extent of the endosteum, that affects bone repair. Perhaps another source of bone-forming cells are the osteocytes that are freed from the bone lacunae at the fracture site, which revert to active osteoblasts. Furthermore, an **ample blood supply** is required for bone repair. In the absence of adequate circulating blood, bone necrosis, and not bone growth, occurs at the fracture site.

In addition to an adequate blood supply, bone repair is also dependent on a **favorable metabolic environment.** Elements of such propitious surroundings include special nutrients, such as **calcium** and **vitamins C and D;** and proper blood levels of hormones.

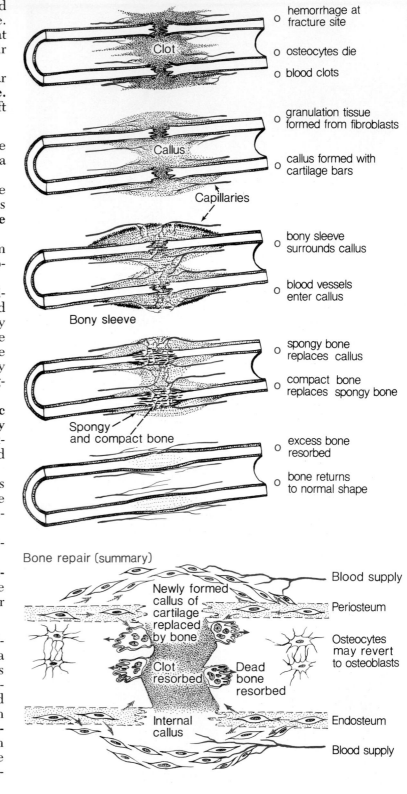

Sequence of Fracture Healing

Clot

o hemorrhage at fracture site

o osteocytes die

o blood clots

Callus

o granulation tissue formed from fibroblasts

o callus formed with cartilage bars

Capillaries

Bony sleeve

o bony sleeve surrounds callus

o blood vessels enter callus

Spongy and compact bone

o spongy bone replaces callus

o compact bone replaces spongy bone

o excess bone resorbed

o bone returns to normal shape

Bone repair (summary)

Blood supply

Newly formed callus of cartilage replaced by bone

Periosteum

Osteocytes may revert to osteoblasts

Clot resorbed

Dead bone resorbed

Internal callus

Endosteum

Blood supply

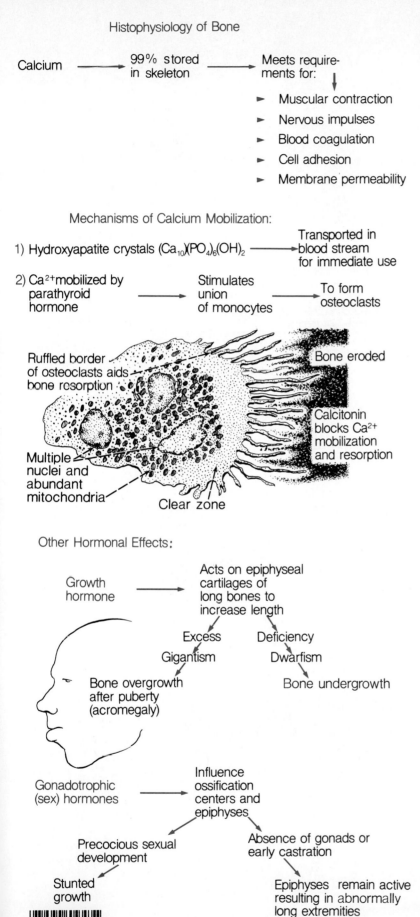

Histophysiology of Bone

Calcium → 99% stored in skeleton → Meets requirements for:

► Muscular contraction
► Nervous impulses
► Blood coagulation
► Cell adhesion
► Membrane permeability

Mechanisms of Calcium Mobilization:

1) Hydroxyapatite crystals $(Ca_{10}(PO_4)_6(OH)_2$ → Transported in blood stream for immediate use

2) Ca^{2+} mobilized by parathyroid hormone → Stimulates union of monocytes → To form osteoclasts

Ruffled border of osteoclasts aids bone resorption

Bone eroded

Calcitonin blocks Ca^{2+} mobilization and resorption

Multiple nuclei and abundant mitochondria

Clear zone

Other Hormonal Effects:

Growth hormone → Acts on epiphyseal cartilages of long bones to increase length

Excess — Gigantism

Deficiency — Dwarfism

Bone overgrowth after puberty (acromegaly)

Bone undergrowth

Gonadotrophic (sex) hormones → Influence ossification centers and epiphyses

Precocious sexual development

Stunted growth

Absence of gonads or early castration

Epiphyses remain active resulting in abnormally long extremities

13767

Histophysiology of Bone

CALCIUM STORAGE In addition to the supportive and protective functions provided by the skeleton, bone also serves as the **repository for calcium** in the body. About 99% of all body calcium is stored in the skeleton. It is from this reservoir that the body draws some of its daily calcium requirements. **Calcium is essential** for many diverse **biological processes,** such as muscular contraction, transmission of nervous impulses, coagulation of blood, the normal adhesion of cells, and the very essential control of cell membrane permeability.

To perform these functions **calcium is mobilized** from the bone by at least two different mechanisms: (1) Ions of **hydroxyapatite crystals** pass from bone matrix into the tissue fluid and then into the **blood stream** for immediate use. (2) Calcium is mobilized by the **action of parathormone,** a hormone of the parathyroid gland, on **osteoclasts.** The hormone stimulates the production of osteoclasts by active coalescence of mononuclear cells, i.e., monocytes. It also **stimulates bone resorption** by increasing the ruffled border of osteoclasts (the ultramicroscopic structure that assists the osteoclasts to resorb bone), thus releasing calcium into the blood. One of the thyroid hormones, **calcitonin,** has the opposite effect of parathormone, i.e., it inhibits bone resorption and calcium mobilization.

OTHER HORMONAL EFFECTS The skeletal system is affected by several other hormones. Perhaps the most important is **growth hormone** (somatotropin), which is synthesized by the pars distalis of the **hypophysis.** While it stimulates overall growth, it acts specifically on the **epiphyseal cartilage** that is responsible for growth in length of long bones and, therefore, for the ultimate height of an individual. Lack of this hormone before puberty causes **pituitary dwarfism;** excess of it, **gigantism.** However, after the epiphyses are closed at maturity, hypersomatotropism results in **acromegaly** (meaning large extremities), a disease that causes great thickening of the bones and overgrowth of the hands, feet, and face, especially the mandible. **Gonadotropic (sex) hormones** of both sexes have complex effects on bone development. They influence the **onset** and development of ossification centers, and the **closure** of epiphyses. Thus, in precocious sexual development, the epiphyseal cartilage is prematurely replaced by bone and body growth is stunted. Conversely with failure of gonads to develop (e.g., undescended testis) or in prepubertal castration, the epiphyses remain active and abnormally long extremities result, as seen in eunuchs.

Thyroxin, a hormone of the thyroid gland, influences cellular growth in general, and **bone growth** in particular, by acting synergistically with growth hormone. Removal of either the pituitary or thyroid produces **dwarfism** in the growing animal. When **hypothyroidism** occurs early in life the child develops into a **cretin,** with attendant physical and mental stunting. When it occurs after puberty, **myxedema** (mucus edema) results, characterized by marked edema (especially about the eyes), dry skin and hair, and loss of mental and physical vigor.

NUTRITIONAL FACTORS Normal growth and maintenance of bone are dependent upon adequate dietary levels of **vitamins A, C, and D,** and essential **amino acids.** Deficiencies of any of these dietary factors are often first detected in bone before becoming noticeable in soft tissues. There are two distinctly different processes involved here: (1) the **synthesis of organic materials,** such as collagen, and (2) the **calcification** of the intercellular matrix. While these processes occur independently, they are normally synchronized and act in harmony with each other.

Inadequate dietary protein results in a **deficiency of amino acids** that are essential for the synthesis of collagen by osteoblasts. **Vitamin C** is also involved in this process for in its absence, as in **scurvy,** collagen synthesis is blocked even though protein intake may be adequate. Thus, in these dietary deficiencies, growth is retarded, repair of fractures is hindered or even prevented, and wound healing is arrested.

In **vitamin D deficiency,** there is **poor absorption of calcium** from the small intestine creating a calcium deficiency which, in children, is called **rickets.** Their blood calcium may fall below the level required for calcification. Even though the epiphyseal cartilage continues to grow and its organic matrix is synthesized, there is little or no calcification of the thickened, irregular cartilage. Meanwhile, osteoblasts continue to lay down matrix, which remains essentially uncalcified osteoid tissue. These poorly ossified bones are easily bent by the weight they bear. Thus, rachitic children are usually **bowlegged** (genu varum; L. genu, knee; varum, bent).

Vitamin A is also necessary for normal bone growth. It is related to the distribution and level of activity of osteoblasts and osteoclasts. **Vitamin A** somehow helps to maintain a balance between the **synthesis** and the **remodeling** of bone. In its absence, the epiphyseal cartilage is rapidly replaced by bone or, in other words, the **epiphysis** is **prematurely closed** and body growth is stunted.

JOINTS

The site of union or junction of two or more bones is an **articulation or joint.** Some joints are **temporary,** i.e., they exist only during growth of the skeleton, such as the **epiphyseal disk** of long bones, which is the cartilaginous union of epiphysis and diaphysis. At maturity the two regions fuse and the joint disappears.

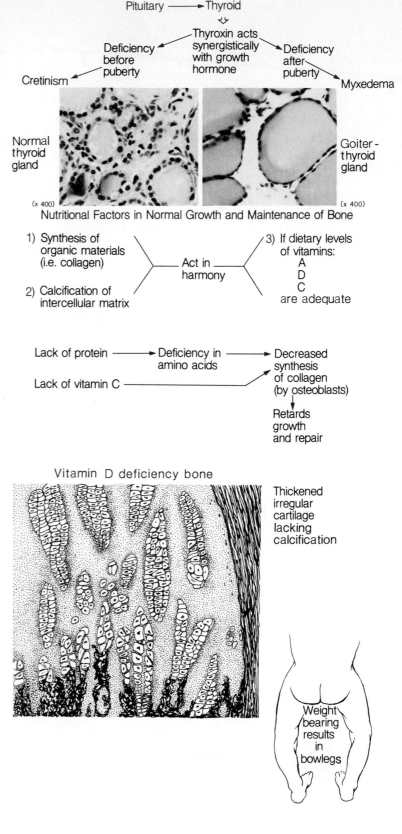

Nutritional Factors in Normal Growth and Maintenance of Bone

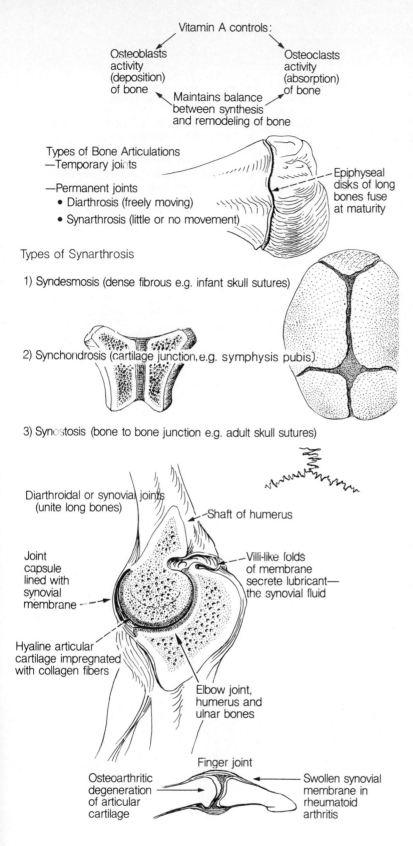

Vitamin A controls:

Osteoblasts activity (deposition) of bone

Osteoclasts activity (absorption) of bone

Maintains balance between synthesis and remodeling of bone

Epiphyseal disks of long bones fuse at maturity

Types of Bone Articulations
—Temporary joints

—Permanent joints
• Diarthrosis (freely moving)
• Synarthrosis (little or no movement)

Types of Synarthrosis

1) Syndesmosis (dense fibrous e.g. infant skull sutures)

2) Synchondrosis (cartilage junction, e.g. symphysis pubis)

3) Synostosis (bone to bone junction e.g. adult skull sutures)

Diarthroidal or synovial joints (unite long bones)

Shaft of humerus

Joint capsule lined with synovial membrane

Villi-like folds of membrane secrete lubricant— the synovial fluid

Hyaline articular cartilage impregnated with collagen fibers

Elbow joint, humerus and ulnar bones

Finger joint

Osteoarthritic degeneration of articular cartilage

Swollen synovial membrane in rheumatoid arthritis

Most articulations are **permanent** and may be classified either as **synarthroses** (Gk. syn, together; arthosis, articulation) with little or no movement or as **diarthroses** (Gk. dia, between), a freely moving joint.

There are three types of synarthroses: (1) **Syndesmosis** is the union of bones by dense fibrous connective tissue which permits **very limited movement,** such as in the cranial sutures of children, and the tibiofibular and radioulnar joints. (2) **Synchondrosis** is a junction by cartilage, either hyaline or fibrous. It is also called **amphiarthroidal** because it allows **limited movements,** as in the intervertebral joints and the symphysis pubis. (3) **Synostosis** is a joint united by bone where **no movement occurs,** as in sutures of the adult skull.

Diarthroidal or **synovial joints** usually unite long bones. They have **great freedom of movement.** They consist of an outer, robust, connective tissue capsule which encloses an articular or joint cavity. Except over the articular surfaces, the capsule is lined with a cellular, highly vascular, **synovial membrane,** which is thrown into folds or villi. It secretes a clear, viscous, lubricating, **synovial fluid.** The term synovial (Gk. syn + ovum) suggests egg white consistency.

Articular surfaces are **hyaline cartilage** impregnated with many **collagenous fibers** but have no perichondrium. Some of the larger joints communicate with extracapsular, blind-ended sacs, called **bursae,** which are also lined with synovial membrane. Inflammation of these bursae causes severe pain in or near the joints, a condition called **bursitis.**

Arthritis is a **joint disease** involving various connective tissues within the joint. For example, **rheumatoid arthritis** causes painful inflammation and swelling of the synovial membranes, especially of the fingers, causing digital deformities. Females are affected three times as often as males. Osteoarthritis or **degenerative arthritis** results in marked degeneration of the articular cartilage, usually a consequence of old age that at some time affects, to some degree, 70% of individuals over 50 years of age.

Table 7.1   *COMPARISON OF HYALINE CARTILAGE AND COMPACT BONE*

	HYALINE CARTILAGE	COMPACT BONE
Origin	Mesenchymal chondroblasts	Mesenchymal osteoblasts
Cells	Chondroblasts, chondrocytes	Osteoblasts, osteocytes, osteoclasts
Matrix	Submicroscopic collagenous fibrils randomly embedded in amorphous ground substance, composed mostly of chondroitin sulfates	Uniformly packed collagenous fibers embedded in rigid, calcified ground substance
Fibrils	Collagenous, about 10–20 nm in diameter, most do not have 64-nm cross-banding	Collagenous, about 50–70 nm in diameter with typical 64-nm cross-banding
Vascularity	None	Well developed in Haversian systems, and Volkmann and nutrient canals; derived largely from periosteal blood vessels
Nerves	None	Present, especially in periosteum and osteons
Lymphatics	None	Present in osteons
Nutrition	By diffusion	Between capillaries and osteocytes, via canaliculi
Growth	Interstitially and appositionally, very limited in adult	Appositionally only; increase in length and width until maturity; active throughout life in remodeling
Metabolism	Very limited	Active, bone being constantly remodeled and renewed; continuous mineral exchange, e.g., Ca, P, Na, Mg, F
Inorganic component	About 30–50%	About 60–75%, mostly Ca and P
Organic component	About 50–70%, mostly collagen	About 25–40%, mostly collagen
H$_2$O content	75% in fresh state	About 7% in fresh state
Regeneration	Very limited, fractures usually repaired by fibrous scar formation	Excellent, as in fracture healing
Fate of dead tissue	Resorbed or phagocytized as a foreign body	Same

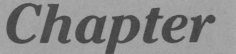

Chapter

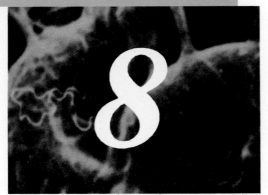

8

CIRCULATING BLOOD AND LYMPH

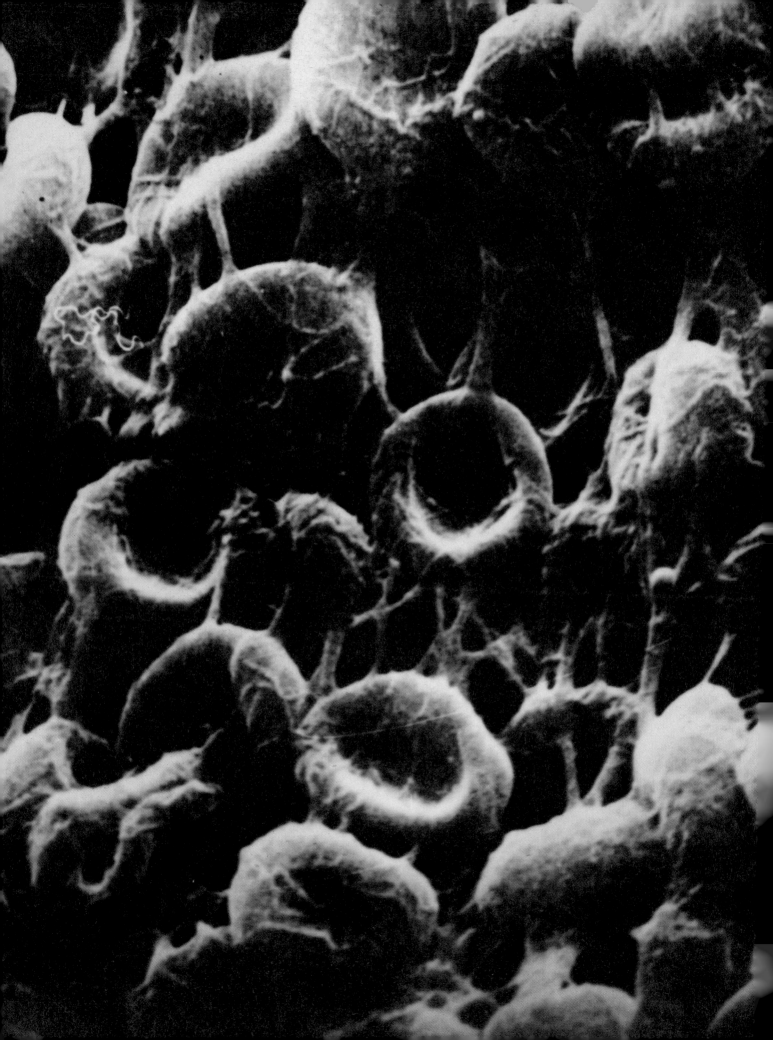

OBJECTIVES

CAREFUL STUDY OF THIS CHAPTER WILL ENABLE THE STUDENT TO:

1. Describe the life history of each blood cell, i.e., its origin, distribution, functions, life-span, and eventual fate.

2. Differentiate the various leukocytes by morphology, number in circulation, and staining reactions, especially of granules.

3. Describe how the erythrocyte is adapted for the transport of O_2 and CO_2.

4. Explain the clinical terms: hematocrit, anemia, polycythemia, sickle cell, crenation, leukocytosis, leukopenia, differential count, and polys.

5. Analyze the role of platelets in blood clotting and how clotting can be hastened or prevented.

6. Contrast B- and T-lymphocytes as to origin, locations, fine structure, and role in immunity.

7. Compare the lymph and blood circulatory systems as to their origins, cells, flow, and functions.

Blood is an atypical, specialized type of **connective tissue**. Its ground substance is a fluid, the **blood plasma**. Its fibers are strands of **fibrin**, which appear only in blood clot formation. And its cellular constituents are two populations of free cells, **erythrocytes** and **leukocytes**, suspended in the plasma. Other constituents of the blood include the noncellular blood **platelets** (thrombocytes), which are involved in blood coagulation, and small, lipid droplets called **chylomicrons**. Like most other connective tissue, blood is derived from **mesoderm**.

Because the blood circulates throughout the body, it influences the well-being of virtually every cell. It is the great **integrator** of body functions. As such, it is perhaps the most important **homeostatic force** acting to maintain each cell and tissue in a state of equilibrium with its environment. This is accomplished by its various **functions**, e.g., the exchange of respiratory gases (O_2 and CO_2), the transport of various nutrients to the cells, and the removal of metabolic waste. It is also involved in maintaining normal body levels of hormones, pH, osmotic pressure, and temperature.

When blood is allowed to stand exposed to air for a short time, it clots, entrapping cells in a jellylike mass. The clear, straw-colored fluid that remains is the **serum**, which differs from plasma by being free of fibrin. If the blood is prevented from clotting by the addition of an **anticoagulant**, e.g., heparin, and then centrifuged, three layers appear in the centrifuge tube. The top layer is **plasma**, comprising about 55% of the column. The thin, white, middle layer, the **buffy coat**, is composed of leukocytes and platelets, and is only about 1% of the column. The lowermost, red, **thick layer** consists of packed red blood cells, normally about 45% of the total blood volume. It is this percentage that is called the **hematocrit**—a very important clinical value. If the hematocrit drops below 30%, the patient may have **anemia**; if above 60%, the patient has **polycythemia**, which means too many red blood cells.

Formation of Circulating Blood

Mesoderm ⟶ Blood ⟨ Specialized connective tissue ⟩

In Plasma
- Erythrocytes
- Leukocytes
- Chylomicrons
- Thrombocytes

LM Normal blood smear

Blood, a homeostatic force that maintains:
- exchange of respiratory gases (O_2 and CO_2)
- transport of nutrients to cells
- removal of metabolic wastes
- functional levels of hormones, pH, osmotic pressures and temperature

Blood ⟶ Exposure to air ⟶ Clots with entrapped cells + Serum – free of fibrin

Anticoagulant added

Centrifuged layers:

1) about 55% plasma

2) 1% leukocytes and platelets (buffy coat)

3) about 45% packed RBC
= normal hematocrit

SEM RBC clot

L.S. Lessin

RBC levels (hematocrit)

Polycythemia above 60%

Normal

Anemia below 30%

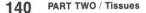

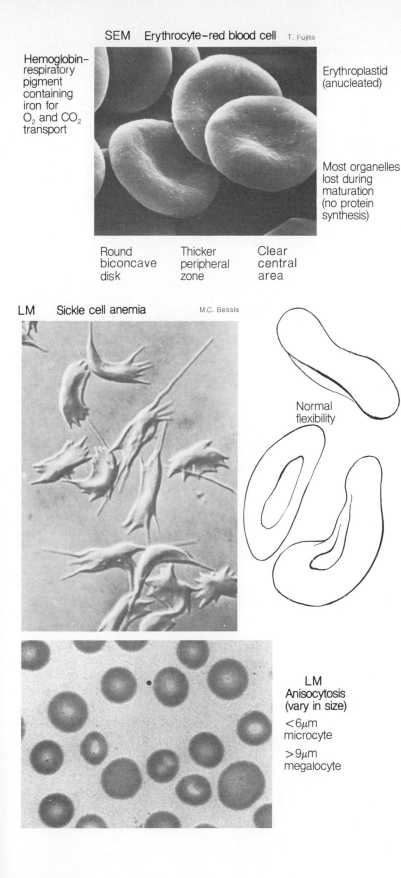

SEM Erythrocyte–red blood cell T. Fujita

Hemoglobin-respiratory pigment containing iron for O_2 and CO_2 transport

Erythroplastid (anucleated)

Most organelles lost during maturation (no protein synthesis)

Round biconcave disk

Thicker peripheral zone

Clear central area

LM Sickle cell anemia M.C. Bessis

Normal flexibility

LM Anisocytosis (vary in size)

<6μm microcyte

>9μm megalocyte

BLOOD CELLS (Table 8.1)

Erythrocytes

The mature **erythrocyte** or red blood cell (RBC) is a very specialized cell. It is a membranous sac of hemoglobin whose prime function is to **transport** O_2 from the lungs to the cells of the body and **return CO_2** to the lungs to be exhaled. It is uniquely qualified for these functions and its efficiency is enhanced by the **loss of the nucleus** as well as essentially all of its **organelles** during maturation. It has no capacity for protein synthesis but is filled with the iron-containing respiratory pigment, **hemoglobin**, whose molecules bind with the O_2 and to some extent CO_2 molecules for transport.

Since the cell is anucleate, the term erythrocyte is inappropriate and the name **erythroplastid** is more accurate. Yet this latter word has received little acceptance and the terms **erythrocyte,** red blood cell, and red blood corpuscle are most universally used.

The shape of the mature mammalian RBC is a round, **biconcave disk.** Since both surfaces are depressed, the center appears under the microscope as a clear area that blends into the thicker, darker periphery of the cell. In the fresh state each cell is about 8.5×2.5 μm in size. When fixed and stained, its size shrinks to about **7.5 × 2 μm.** Its discoid shape favors rapid diffusion of gases and increases its surface area exposed to the plasma by about 25%, as compared to a spherical cell. In the average human adult, the total surface area of RBCs is above 3800 m², or about 2000 times greater than the total body surface of an individual. The **cell membrane** of an erythrocyte is very **flexible,** which imparts plasticity to the cell and enables it to traverse capillaries smaller than its diameter, i.e., less than 8.5 μm.

Although the **shape of RBCs** is normally quite uniform, it may vary widely, especially in certain pathological conditions, such as **sickle cell anemia.** Here the cells assume many distorted, bizarre shapes, many resembling sickles. In other pathological states, and occasionally in normal individuals, the size of the erythrocyte may vary considerably, a condition known as **anisocytosis** (Gk. *anisos,* unequal). If cells are larger than 9 μm in diameter, they are termed megalocytes or **macrocytes;** if smaller than 6 μm, **microcytes.**

In expressing the number of RBCs in circulation, the number found in 1 mm³ of blood is used. In the adult human male, this value is **5–5½ million;** for the adult female, **4½–5 million.** Chronic exposure to high altitudes or to carbon monoxide will significantly increase the total blood volume, especially the number of erythrocytes, which may reach 9–10 million/mm³.

The life-span of RBCs averages **120 days** in the normal individual. Therefore, about 2,500,000 RBCs are lost per second and the same number of new cells must enter the bloodstream in the same period to maintain the normal hematocrit. Some of the **senile cells** are destroyed by phagocytosis in the liver and bone marrow, but most of them are **phagocytosed** in the spleen—the "graveyard" of the RBC. Here, the hemoglobin is degraded and the released **iron** is returned to the red bone marrow for reuse in the production of new hemoglobin. The recycled iron is incorporated into new RBCs. The nonferrous components of hemoglobin are converted in the liver into the bile pigment, **bilirubin**, which is excreted in the bile.

In fresh blood spreads, the cells often stick together in stacks or rolls resembling a stack of coins, called **rouleaux**. Also, when fresh cells are subjected to a hypertonic solution, they imbibe water, swell, and burst, i.e., they **hemolyze**. If placed in a hypotonic medium, they lose water and shrink, producing a prickly or notched appearance called **crenation** (L. crena, notch).

Since the mature RBC is void of a nucleus and organelles, it has an undistinguished EM appearance. Its **cytoplasm**, mostly hemoglobin, is quite impervious to the electron beam and, therefore, has a dense, amorphous appearance, which represents hemoglobin. Its **plasma membrane** is a typical trilaminar unit membrane, 7.0 nm thick. A good deal of the definitive data on the nature of the unit membrane has been obtained from research on the erythrocyte. Such research also suggests that a **polysaccharide layer** (glycocalyx) covers the external surface of the membrane, which contains blood group **antigens**, important in matching blood for transfusions, as well as an antigen for the **Rh blood factor**.

Reticulocytes

While nearly all RBCs stained with conventional blood dyes, e.g., Wright's or Giemsa's, have a clear pink or copper color, about 1–2% of the larger cells have a slight basophilic tint. These are immature RBCs, called **reticulocytes**, that have been recently released into the bloodstream from the red bone marrow. These cells can be more accurately identified if a drop of fresh blood is mixed with brilliant cresyl blue dye. Then, the cells reveal a deeply **basophilic**, threadlike **network** in their cytoplasm, hence the term reticulocytes, meaning cells with a small network. The basophilic network is the persistence of **ribosomes** in the cells. A **reticulocyte count** is of considerable clinical value in determining the rate of erythrocyte production. In anemic patients, an elevation of the count indicates that the RBC production is increasing and the patient is responding to treatment.

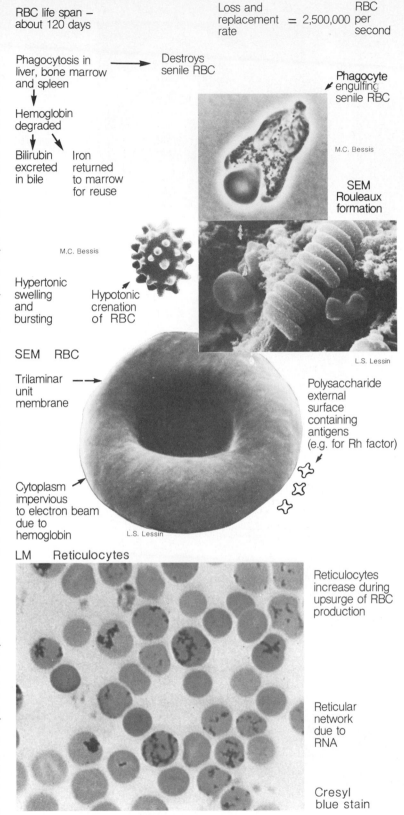

RBC life span – about 120 days

Loss and replacement rate = 2,500,000 RBC per second

Phagocytosis in liver, bone marrow and spleen → Destroys senile RBC

Hemoglobin degraded

Bilirubin excreted in bile

Iron returned to marrow for reuse

M.C. Bessis

Phagocyte engulfing senile RBC

M.C. Bessis

SEM Rouleaux formation

Hypertonic swelling and bursting

Hypotonic crenation of RBC

L.S. Lessin

SEM RBC

Trilaminar unit membrane

Cytoplasm impervious to electron beam due to hemoglobin

Polysaccharide external surface containing antigens (e.g. for Rh factor)

L.S. Lessin

LM Reticulocytes

Reticulocytes increase during upsurge of RBC production

Reticular network due to RNA

Cresyl blue stain

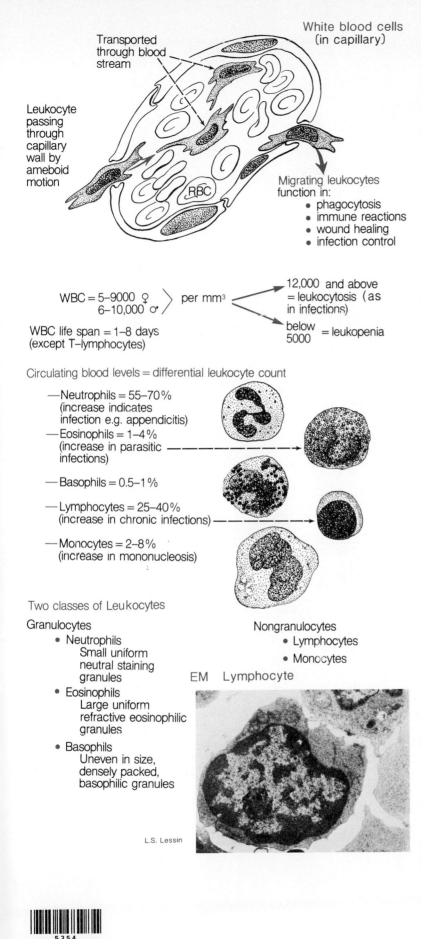

White blood cells (in capillary)

Transported through blood stream

Leukocyte passing through capillary wall by ameboid motion

RBC

Migrating leukocytes function in:
- phagocytosis
- immune reactions
- wound healing
- infection control

WBC = 5–9000 ♀
6–10,000 ♂ per mm³

12,000 and above = leukocytosis (as in infections)

below 5000 = leukopenia

WBC life span = 1–8 days (except T–lymphocytes)

Circulating blood levels = differential leukocyte count

—Neutrophils = 55–70% (increase indicates infection e.g. appendicitis)

—Eosinophils = 1–4% (increase in parasitic infections)

—Basophils = 0.5–1%

—Lymphocytes = 25–40% (increase in chronic infections)

—Monocytes = 2–8% (increase in mononucleosis)

Two classes of Leukocytes

Granulocytes
- Neutrophils
  Small uniform neutral staining granules
- Eosinophils
  Large uniform refractive eosinophilic granules
- Basophils
  Uneven in size, densely packed, basophilic granules

Nongranulocytes
- Lymphocytes
- Monocytes

EM   Lymphocyte

L.S. Lessin

Leukocytes

In contrast to RBCs, the **leukocytes** or white blood cells (WBCs) contain no pigment and are colorless in the fresh state. It is only when they aggregate together that they have a whitish appearance, as in the buffy coat after centrifugation. They are **true cells,** having a nucleus and cytoplasmic organelles, e.g., Golgi apparatus, centrioles, mitochondria, and lysosomes. They arise mostly in the **red bone marrow** and **lymphoid tissues,** and when mature, they enter the bloodstream. They use the bloodstream solely for transport to specific tissue areas. Here they pass through the capillary walls by ameboid movement into the **tissue spaces** to carry out their **functions,** e.g., phagocytosis, immune reactions, wound repair, and control of infections.

The WBCs are much less numerous than RBCs. The ratio is about 1:600, which comes out to about **5,000–9,000/mm³** of blood for adult females, and about **6,000–10,000** for adult males. The count rises rapidly in acute infections and when it reaches **over 12,000,** the condition is called **leukocytosis.** If the count is **below 5,000,** it is called **leukopenia.** Except for lymphocytes, all leukocytes have a short **life-span** of about **one to eight** days.

The percentage of the various leukocytes in the circulating blood of the normal adult is remarkably constant. Neutrophils are the most numerous, averaging 55–70%, eosinophils 1–4%, basophils 0.5–1%, lymphocytes 25–40%, and monocytes 2–8%. These relative proportions of the various types of circulating leukocytes are known as the **differential leukocyte count.** This is a valuable tool in the diagnosis of various diseases, since various disorders affect the number of each type of leukocyte differently. For example, in acute appendicitis, neutrophils may be 85% of all WBCs, while in certain parasitic infections, the eosinophils may reach 30–50% instead of the normal 1–4%.

Leukocytes are classified into two main classes on the basis of the type of cytoplasmic granules and the morphology of the nucleus, i.e., granular, with more than one lobe per nucleus (polymorphonuclear) and nongranular, with no lobulation of the nucleus (mononuclear) (see Table 8.1). The granular leukocytes or **granulocytes** are packed with specific granules. They are divided into three classes on the basis of the type of granules they contain. As demonstrated in conventional blood stains, **eosinophils** have large, uniform, refractive granules that stain strongly eosinophilic; **basophils** have less densely packed, uneven, basophilic granules; the granules of the **neutrophils** are very small, uniform in size, and stain poorly with all blood stains. They are essentially neutral in their staining reactions, giving a rather nondescript, stippled, grayish appearance.

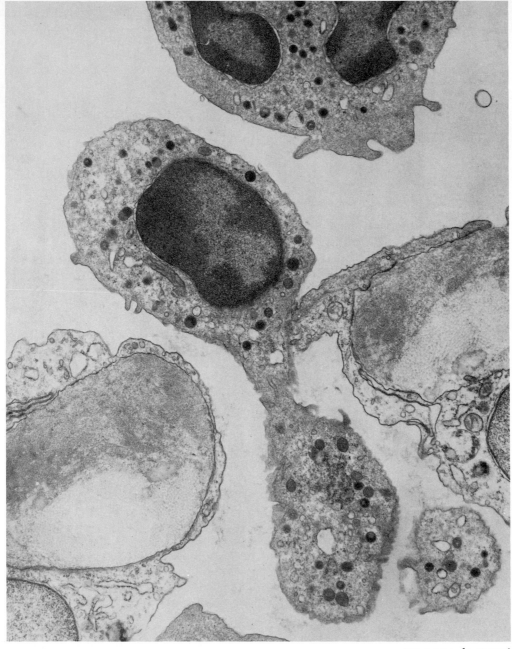

L.V. Leake (x 19,000)

In this EM micrograph of the inferior (peritoneal) surface of the diaphragm, a neutrophil is observed passing through a stoma (an opening between the mesothelial cells) to enter the lumen of a lymphatic vessel within the diaphragm. Such a view dramatically demonstrates the extreme plasticity of leukocytes, which enables them to traverse openings much smaller than their normal diameter. The movement of blood cells between endothelial lining cells of capillaries, called diapedesis, is probably very similar to the action of this neutrophil passing through a stoma.

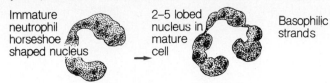

Polymorphonuclear (multilobed) nucleus of neutrophil

Immature neutrophil horseshoe shaped nucleus → 2–5 lobed nucleus in mature cell · Basophilic strands

Nuclei of nongranular lymphocytes and monocytes

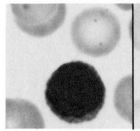 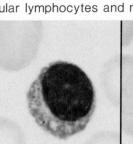

Spherical nucleus · Oval · Bean-shaped

Granulocytes

Neutrophils or "polys" = 55–70% of WBC = 3–6000 per mm³ or 15–20⁹ in circulation

Escape into tissue spaces to act as phagocytes

↓ Chemotaxis (ameboid)

Site of pathogenesis → Engulf bacteria and necrotic tissue → Destroyed by lysosomes ↓ Dead neutrophils (pus)

LM Mature neutrophils (diameter 10–12 μm)

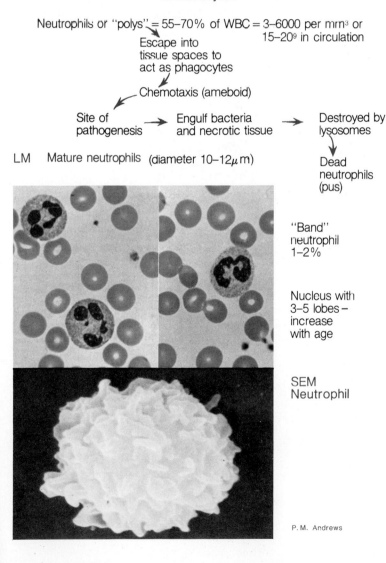

"Band" neutrophil 1–2%

Nucleus with 3–5 lobes – increase with age

SEM Neutrophil

P. M. Andrews

Adult granulocytes have an irregular, lobulated nucleus. In the immature cells, the nucleus has an elongated, banana shape. Later it becomes constricted at sites, dividing the nucleus into **two to five lobes,** which are joined together by strands of basophilic nuclear material. These cells do not have several nuclei, but only a **single, multilobed nucleus,** hence they are **polymorphonuclear** cells, not polynuclear.

The **nongranular cells** have **no specific granules** in their cytoplasm, although a few small, nonspecific azurophilic granules may be present. The cytoplasm varies from a clear, sky-blue color in **lymphocytes** to a bluish gray in **monocytes.** The nongranular cells have a single, large nucleus which may be spherical, oval, or bean-shaped. Although it may be curved or twisted, it is not lobulated.

GRANULOCYTES

Neutrophils The neutrophilic polymorphonuclear leukocytes, commonly called **"polys,"** are the most common WBC in the normal circulating blood, consisting of 55–70% of the total count. In absolute numbers, this amounts to about 3000–6000/mm³ of blood. Therefore, if the average person has five liters of blood in circulation, there are about **15–20 billion polys** in circulation. An approximately equal number adhere to the walls of blood vessels, forming the so-called **marginating pool** of neutrophils. There are also billions of additional neutrophils that have escaped from the capillaries into the tissue spaces or the internal cavities of the body. Here they are **avid phagocytes,** ingesting rather selectively bacteria, especially the pus-forming (pyrogenic) cocci variety. They are the first leukocytes to appear at an infection site and are the **first-line defense** against invading pathogenic organisms. They are attracted to the site of infection or inflammation by chemotaxis and move rapidly by ameboid movement to the infected area. However, most neutrophils are kamikaze cells, that is, in the process of killing, they are killed. They **engulf the bacteria** and release hydrolases which lyse surrounding cells. In the process, the neutrophils may die, contributing to the **formation of pus,** which consists of bacteria, necrotic cellular debris, but mostly of degranulated (dead) neutrophils.

Morphologically, the **mature neutrophil** is about 10–12 μm in diameter. It is characterized by a **multilobed nucleus** having three to five ovoid lobes connected by thin strands of chromatin. The number of lobes increases with age. A few immature neutrophils normally enter the bloodstream before lobulation of the nucleus has occurred, when the nucleus is elongated and assumes a horseshoe or S shape. These cells are called **band, or stab, neutrophils.** About 1–2% of the neutrophils are of this type. In massive infection, when the demand for polys is great, a higher percentage of band cells appears in the circulating blood.

In stained blood smears from women, the inactive female sex chromosome, or the **Barr body**, can be seen in about 3% of the neutrophils. It appears as a tiny, drumstick-shaped appendage attached to one of the lobes. It is probably present on all female neutrophils but is so closely adherent to the lobe that it is usually obscured. The frequent presence of the drumstick in a blood smear enables one to **determine the genetic sex** of an individual whose true sexuality may be in doubt. Such a question may arise in certain medicolegal situations and in patients desiring a sex-change operation.

The cytoplasm of neutrophils is filled with the small, uniform, **neutrophilic-specific granules**. They contain alkaline phosphatase and bactericidal proteins, called **phagocytins**, which destroy bacteria after they are ingested by the neutrophil. A much smaller population of larger, dense, nonspecific, **azurophilic granules** are interspaced throughout the cytoplasm. They are difficult to distinguish under the LM, but from EM micrographs and histochemical analyses, these granules have been determined to be **lysosomes**. They contain peroxidase, acid phosphatase, and possibly other enzymes.

These two types of **granules** act synergistically to **destroy bacteria** that have been ingested. The following sequence of events is thought to occur:

1. A specific (neutrophilic) granule fuses with the membranous sac containing the phagocytosed organism, e.g., *E. coli.*
2. The alkaline phosphatase and phagocytin within the granule are discharged into the sac.
3. A few minutes later azurophilic granules (lysosomes) fuse with the sac and empty their enzymes into it, and the bacteria undergo lysis.

TEM studies on the neutrophil reveal a cell with limited organelles. The nucleus has **heterochromatin** clustered along the inner surface of the nuclear envelope, which has only a few pores. In general, the cytoplasmic organelles are inconspicuous, represented usually by an inactive, small Golgi apparatus and a few scattered mitochondria. The most prominent feature is the large, granular component consisting principally of the densely packed, small, **specific neutrophilic granules** that essentially fill the cell. The larger, much less numerous nonspecific **azurophilic granules** (lysosomes) are ovoid or spherical in shape and are very electron dense.

LM   Neutrophil with Barr body

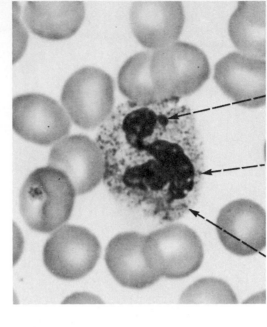

Barr body seen in about 3% of ♀ neutrophils

Neutrophilic specific granules containing alkaline phosphatase and phagocytins

Nonspecific azurophilic granules are lysosomes containing peroxidase, acid phosphatase and other enzymes

Steps in Destruction of Bacteria

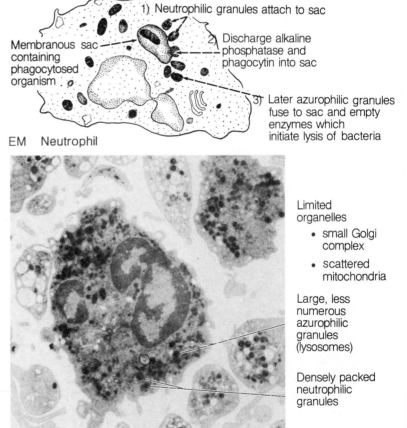

Membranous sac containing phagocytosed organism

1) Neutrophilic granules attach to sac

2) Discharge alkaline phosphatase and phagocytin into sac

3) Later azurophilic granules fuse to sac and empty enzymes which initiate lysis of bacteria

EM   Neutrophil

Limited organelles
- small Golgi complex
- scattered mitochondria

Large, less numerous azurophilic granules (lysosomes)

Densely packed neutrophilic granules

L.C. Lessin

5291

LM   Eosinophil

Lysosomal
orange-red
granules
(0.5–1.5μm)

Bilobed
nucleus

Granules
contain:
- peroxidase
- histamine
- hydrolytic
  enzymes

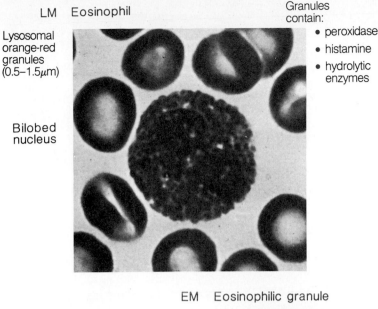

EM   Eosinophilic granule

Properties of
eosinophils
- 11–14μm diameter
- 2–4% of circulating leukocytes
- show diurnal rhythm
- increase in allergies
- sluggish ameboid movement
- accumulate in tissue spaces
- limited activity against bacteria
- phagocytize antigen-antibody complexes
- corticosteroids decrease
  circulating eosinophils

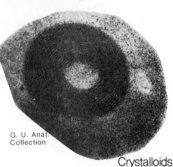

G. U. Anat.
Collection

Crystalloids
in granules

EM   Eosinophil

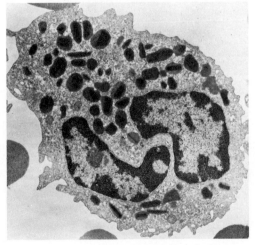

D. Zucker-Franklin
(x 25,000)

Eosinophils When stained with conventional blood dyes, **eosinophils** are characterized by an abundance of **orange-red, refractile granules,** each about 1.0 μm in diameter. They essentially fill the cell and may partially obscure the **bilobed nucleus.** The granules are considered to be **lysosomes** since they contain large quantities of peroxidase, histamine, some hydrolytic enzymes, and possibly other enzymes similar to those found in the azurophilic granules of neutrophils.

Frequently, in TEM micrographs the eosinophilic-specific granules contain an electron-dense, rectangular, **central crystal** that may occupy half the area of the granule. These crystalloids are stable structures that resist osmotic lysis and mechanical disruption. Their function is unknown.

Eosinophils are slightly larger than neutrophils (11–14 μm) and normally comprise about 2–4% of circulating leukocytes. They show a modest diurnal rhythm in normal individuals, having a slightly higher count at night than during the day. They may increase dramatically in heavy **parasitic infestations,** e.g., in trichinosis, where they may exceed 50% of the total WBC count. Also, they increase in number in chronic infections and in most **allergic reactions,** especially those affecting the digestive and respiratory tracts.

Unlike neutrophils, eosinophils exhibit only sluggish ameboid movement, yet they move freely through the capillary walls into the tissue spaces where they may accumulate in large numbers, especially in the intestinal mucosa. They show very **limited phagocytic activity** against bacteria, but actively phagocytize antigen-antibody complexes, as demonstrated by fluorescence studies.

Clinically, it has been demonstrated that the administration of corticosteroids causes a dramatic decrease in circulating eosinophils. However, these chemicals have no effect on the number of eosinophils in the red bone marrow. It appears, therefore, that these hormones somehow interfere with the release of eosinophils from the bone marrow into the bloodstream.

5277

Basophils Basophils are difficult to locate in normal blood smears since they number only about **0.5–1%** of the circulating WBCs. They are usually smaller than the other granulocytes, with a diameter ranging from 8–10 μm. However, they are readily identified by the presence of many round, deeply **basophilic granules** of various sizes (0.2–0.5 μm). These granules are scattered over the large **bilobed nucleus**, obscuring its outline. TEM studies show these granules are membrane-bound and contain delicate, electron-dense particles. They contain **serotonin, histamine, and heparin.**

The precise functions of basophils are unclear. They are **slightly phagocytic** and collect at infection sites. They produce about 50% of the **histamine** in the blood and appear to play some role in allergy control. They increase in chronic granulocytic leukemia and in chicken pox.

Basophils are not to be confused with connective tissue **mast cells.** Yet, they have similarities, e.g., both have basophilic, water-soluble granules that react metachromatically to certain stains, and both cells produce heparin and histamine. However, their dissimilarities are many, such as:

1. The ultrastructure of the **mast cell** granules includes **lamellar structures;** granules of basophils have fine particles of varying size.
2. The round mast cell **granules** are larger, more uniform in size, and more densely packed in the cell.
3. The mast cell nucleus is larger and **nonlobulated.**
4. Mast cells originate in loose connective tissue, while basophils are derived from cells in the red bone marrow.
5. Mast cells are not phagocytic, while basophils have a limited phagocytic capability.

NONGRANULAR LEUKOCYTES

Lymphocytes These are the most numerous of the agranular leukocytes. Normally, about **20–30%** of circulating WBCs are **lymphocytes.** They vary considerably in size, ranging from 6–14 μm in diameter. For convenience, they are arbitrarily divided into small cells (6–8 μm), medium-sized cells (8–10 μm), and large cells (10–14 μm) in diameter.

They are spherical cells with a large, round, **dark-staining nucleus** surrounded by a **halo of sky-blue cytoplasm.** The larger the cell, the more cytoplasm is visible. A few, small, azurophilic (lysosomal) granules may be present. The most prominent cell organelles are the ribosomes. Because of their abundance, they impart a strong **basophilia** to the cytoplasm. Most of the ribosomes are free, but some are aggregated into polyribosomes. Only a few adhere to the scanty rER. Limited spherical mitochondria are present, and the Golgi body is small and inactive. A pair of centrioles is often seen.

EM   Basophil

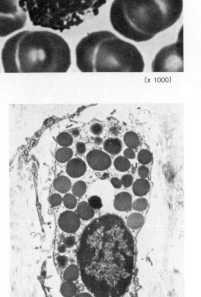

(x 1000)

Properties of basophils:

- 0.5–1% of circulating WBC
- smallest of granulocytes (8–10μ diameter)
- contain basophilic membrane-bound granules (0.2–0.5μm)
- obscured bilobed nucleus
- produce about 50% of histamine in blood
- increase in granulocytic leukemia and chicken pox

EM Mast cell

Mast cells differ from basophils by:

- larger granules with fine structure differences
- larger nucleus
- arise from connective tissue cells
- slightly phagocytic

G. U. Anat. Collection

EM   Lymphocyte (large)

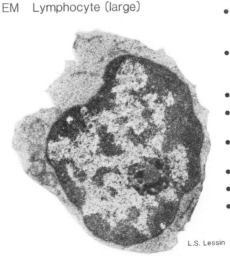

L.S. Lessin

Properties of lymphocytes:

- most numerous agranular leukocytes (20–30% of circulating WBC)
- vary in size —small 6–8μm —large 10–14μm
- spherical
- dark staining nucleus occupies most of cell
- numerous basophilic free ribosomes
- limited mitochondria
- inactive Golgi
- centrioles often present in pairs

Small lymphocyte
(in blood stream)

- large round basophilic
  nucleus filling cell
- thin rim of blue
  cytoplasm
- oldest of
  lymphocytes
- some recirculate
  into lymphoid
  organs transforming
  into large lymphocytes capable of mitosis

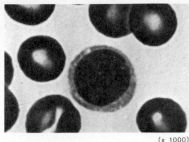

(x 1000)

Two Populations of Lymphocytes—T and B Types

1) T–lymphocytes

Undifferentiated ⟶ migrate to ⟶ Thymus and
hemocytoblasts   differentiate into
                                  ↓

T–lymphocytes which move
via blood and lymph to be

sequestered in lymph
organs to initiate
immune reactions

2) B–lymphocytes

Bone marrow ⟶ migrate to ⟶ Lymphoid tissues
hemocytoblasts   and differentiate into
                                  ↓

B–lymphocytes
stored for antibody
production

SEM
T and B lymphocytes

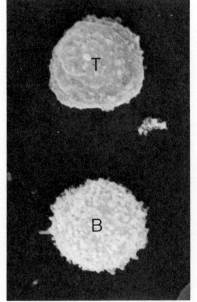

P.M. Andrews

Recycled B–lymphocytes have
"memory" for foreign
antigens (primary immune response)

Subjected to
familiar antigen

► Undergo mitosis
► Give rise to plasma cells that
► Synthesize antibodies
► Destroy foreign antigens

Repeated for secondary
immune response

► Rapid antibody synthesis
► Lifetime protection
  to specific diseases

The **small lymphocyte** is the **principal type** of lymphocyte in the bloodstream. It is characterized by a deeply basophilic nucleus that nearly fills the cell, leaving visible only a thin rim of purplish blue cytoplasm. Many of these cells circulate through the spleen, thymus, lymph nodes, and diffuse lymphoid tissue. Here, in the presence of various antigens, the small lymphocyte **undergoes transformation** and becomes a **large lymphocyte** capable of mitosis. Thus, new generations of lymphocytes are produced.

ROLE OF LYMPHOCYTES IN IMMUNE RESPONSES

There are **two populations** of small lymphocytes. One type arises from undifferentiated cells in the bone marrow and the embryonic liver. They migrate to the **thymus,** where they multiply and differentiate into thymus-dependent **T-lymphocytes.** After a period of maturation in the thymus, they enter the bloodstream or lymph to be sequestered or "seeded" in the various lymphoid organs until their services are needed to initiate immune reactions against invading antigens.

The other class, the bursa or bone marrow-dependent **B-lymphocyte,** is derived in birds from the bursa of Fabricius, a lymphoid organ in the cloaca; or in man, probably from stem cells in the bone marrow. They also take up residence in the lymphoid tissues until needed to set in motion **antibody production** by differentiating into **plasma cells** (see Table 8.2).

In the thymus and bone marrow, each lymphocyte is programmed to respond to a **specific antigen,** such as a virus, a bacterium, or a foreign protein. When an antigen makes its first appearance in the body, it elicits a reaction, called a **primary immune response.** That is, the small lymphocytes that **recognize the antigen** transform into large lymphocytes in the lymphoid tissues. Here they undergo mitoses to **produce clone cells** that recognize the antigen. The transformed **B-lymphocytes** produce cells that differentiate into **plasma cells** capable of synthesizing antibodies specific to the antigen.

The mitosis of T-lymphocytes produces several types of cells, including: (1) **T-helper cells,** which release a factor that, when it contacts **B-lymphocytes,** causes these cells to be transformed into **plasma cells,** capable of manufacturing antibodies; (2) **suppressor T-cells** that depress the production of antibodies by suppressing the conversion of B-cells into plasma cells; (3) **cytotoxic or killer T-cells** capable of destroying cells that are carrying an antigen that the T-cell recognizes as foreign; and (4) **memory T-cells,** to be discussed later. In order to destroy the cell, direct contact must be established between the target cell, carrying the antigen, and the killer cell. This is called **cell-mediated immunity,** in contrast to **humoral (antibody) mediated immunity,** where no cell contact is required.

There is some evidence that the cytotoxic

T-cells release cytotoxic or cytolytic substances directly into the target cell. This causes swelling, lysis, and death of the target cell. Body **rejection of organ transplants** and tissue (skin) grafts are excellent examples of cell-mediated immune responses.

Another subgroup of lymphocytes produced in a primary immune response is **memory cells.** These are primarily **long-lived T-cells,** and some B-cells, with a life-span of many months or even years. They are programmed to "remember" an earlier exposure to a foreign antigen, such as a virus. Such a recognition explains why, upon second exposure to the same antigen, the response, **called secondary immune response,** is faster and more efficient than the initial primary response. This is the mechanism **responsible for immunity** to a previously experienced disease.

FINE STRUCTURE OF LYMPHOCYTES

Although the T- and B-lymphocytes have different origins and functions, they cannot be distinguished under the LM. However, when viewed with the scanning EM, the outer surface of the **B-lymphocyte** may be covered with many projecting, **long microvilli,** giving the cell an irregular, roughened appearance. The **T-cell** has a relatively smooth outer surface with only a few **short microvilli.**

Under the transmission EM, the resting (unstimulated) B- and T-cells are very similar. Electron micrographs of such interphase lymphocytes reveal the following common features. The large nucleus has a small nucleolus, and most of the nucleoplasm is electron opaque heterochromatin, *not* involved in DNA synthesis. In the cytoplasm only a few rER profiles are found scattered among many free ribosomes. Clusters of intermediate filaments, microtubules, several mitochondria, a few azurophilic granules, and a poorly developed Golgi apparatus complete the list of organelles.

When activated by antigen to proliferate and differentiate, the T- and B-cells are distinguishable by alterations in their fine structure. For example, the cytoplasm of an **activated B-lymphocyte** has a **large Golgi complex** and is filled with **rER cisternae** distended with antibody molecules, with only a few free ribosomes, similar to a plasma cell. Recall that plasma cells are derived from B-lymphocytes. In contrast, the **activated T-lymphocyte** has an **abundance of free ribosomes,** a paucity of rER profiles, a small Golgi body, a few lysosomes, and no evidence of antibody production.

Other important differences in these cells are the subtle variations in their plasma membrane proteins, which serve as distinguishing markers. For example, the **B-cells possess surface immunoglobin,** which is readily revealed by immunofluorescence. T-cells do not give this response. Another marker, the **Thy-1 glycoprotein,** is found in T-lymphocytes but not on B-cells.

T–lymphocytes react to specific antigen from previous exposure in blood or lymph

↓

Enlarge, undergo mitoses and differentiate into subgroups with special functions, e.g.:

1) T–memory cells

2) T–helper cells—aid to transform B-lymphocytes into plasma cells that produce antibodies

3) T–killer cells—cytotoxic to cells carrying antigens

Organ tissue graft rejection

Mobile T–killer cells

↓

Target cells carrying foreign antigens

↓

Lysis of graft cells → K⁺ leakage

EM
T-lymphocyte

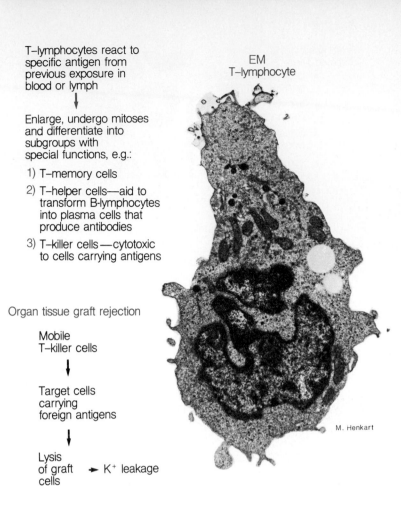

M. Henkart

LM   Monocyte

Monocyte—the macrophage of peripheral blood

- largest WBC (12–20µm)
- no specific granules
- some azurophilic granules
- large bean-shaped, eccentric nucleus
- loose chromatin network
- 2–3 nucleoli

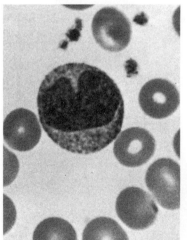

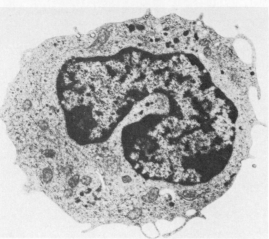

EM   Monocyte

- prominent nucleoli
- heterochromatin along inner surface of nuclear membrane
- numerous rER profiles
- few ribosomes
- many small mitochondria
- active Golgi

M.C. Bessis

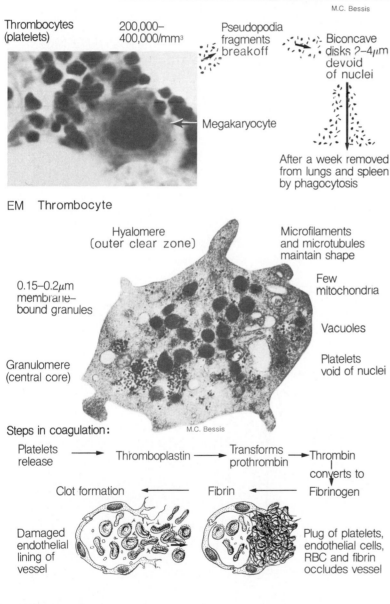

Thrombocytes (platelets)   200,000–400,000/mm³

Pseudopodia fragments breakoff

Biconcave disks 2–4μm devoid of nuclei

Megakaryocyte

After a week removed from lungs and spleen by phagocytosis

EM   Thrombocyte

Hyalomere (outer clear zone)

Microfilaments and microtubules maintain shape

0.15–0.2μm membrane-bound granules

Few mitochondria

Vacuoles

Granulomere (central core)

Platelets void of nuclei

M.C. Bessis

Steps in coagulation:

Platelets release → Thromboplastin → Transforms prothrombin → Thrombin converts to → Fibrinogen

Clot formation ← Fibrin ←

Damaged endothelial lining of vessel

Plug of platelets, endothelial cells, RBC and fibrin occludes vessel

Monocytes Monocytes are the **macrophages** of the bloodstream. Upon passing through the capillary wall, they enter the connective tissue where they are called **tissue macrophages** or histiocytes. Here they belong to the macrophage (reticuloendothelial) system.

Monocytes are spherical, **large agranulocytes** about **12–20 μm** in diameter and constitute 2–6% of the circulating WBCs. Perhaps their most distinctive feature is a large, **bean-shaped,** usually **eccentric nucleus.** The nuclear chromatin network is looser and less dense than in a lymphocyte and, therefore, stains a lighter blue. Often two to three nucleoli are present. The ample cytoplasm is a bluish gray color and usually contains a few, fine **azurophilic granules.** Their positive peroxidase reaction suggests that they are lysosomes.

TEM studies of **monocytes** reveal prominent nucleoli and heterochromatin clustered along the inner surface of the nuclear membrane. Considerably more **rER profiles,** and **fewer free ribosomes** and polyribosomes are present than in lymphocytes. Many small, elongated **mitochondria** are observed, as well as an **active Golgi apparatus.** Numerous microfilaments and microtubules are present, especially in the indentation of the nucleus.

Monocytes are often confused with large lymphocytes. Under the LM the monocytes can be distinguished by (1) their usually larger size; (2) deeply indented, lighter-staining, flocculent nucleus; (3) more abundant cytoplasm which stains a grayish blue color; and (4) more azurophilic granules. (L-A, plate 3)

Platelets

Thrombocytes or platelets are fragments of cytoplasm from the **pseudopodia of megakaryocytes** (giant cells in red bone marrow). Platelets are **void of nuclei** and are roughly biconvex disks about 2–4 μm in diameter. Their concentration in human blood varies greatly, ranging from 200,000 to 400,000/mm³. They remain in the peripheral blood about a week before they are removed in the lungs and spleen by phagocytosis. Each thrombocyte has a **central core (granulomere)** containing small, uneven, basophilic granules, and a clearer, light blue **peripheral zone, the hyalomere.**

TEM micrographs show electron-dense, round, membrane-bound granules (0.15–0.2 μm), a few mitochondria, and occasional vacuoles within the granulomere. The hyalomere contains numerous microfilaments and microtubules, which probably help to maintain the shape of the platelet. The external surface of the plasma membrane is covered with a fuzzy coat consisting of glycoproteins that enable the platelets to adhere to each other, the first event in **clot formation.**

Briefly the **steps in coagulation** are as follows:

A few minutes after a blood vessel is cut or ruptured, **platelets begin to adhere** and aggregate along the damaged endothelial lining of the vessel near the site of injury. Platelets liberate the enzyme **thromboplastin,** which transforms **prothrombin into thrombin.** The latter, in turn, is converted into **fibrinogen** and finally into **fibrin.** The structureless mass of platelets, damaged endothelial cells, and fibrin **forms a clot** that partially or totally blocks the lumen of the vessel. While the clot is forming, RBCs become entrapped in the mass, giving the blood clot its red color. As the clusters of platelets and fibrin increase in size, the damaged vessel is occluded and the bleeding stops.

In a deficiency of platelets (**thrombocytopenia**), small, spontaneous, hemorrhages occur, especially beneath the skin and mucous membranes. The absence or malfunction of any of the various clotting factors can cause excessive and sometimes uncontrollable bleeding, a condition called **hemophilia.** It is an inherited deficiency. The gene transmitted is a sex-linked recessive trait. Although the female is the carrier, she is asymptomatic and the disease is manifested only in her affected sons. Hemophilia occurs once in 10,000 individuals of the general population.

LYMPH

Lymph consists of **intercellular fluid** in which is suspended many **small lymphocytes** (about 14,000/mm³), occasionally a few neutrophils and monocytes, and usually, after heavy meals, abundant fat droplets called **chylomicrons.** Lymph capillaries transport the lymph from connective tissue to lymph nodes where lymphocytes are added. Efferent lymph vessels of the lymph nodes, especially in the abdomen, drain the lymph into a large saclike reservoir, the **cisterna chyli.** Its continuation, the **thoracic duct,** ascends into the lower neck region to join the beginning of the left brachiocephalic vein. The short, **right lymphatic duct** drains the upper right quadrant of the body, to empty into the right subclavian vein. Thus, the lymph flow is unidirectional, beginning in blind capillaries and ending where it joins the bloodstream in the neck.

Considerable variation in the content of the lymph is found in various regions of the body. Lymph from the small intestine, called **chyle,** is milky in appearance because of the high **fat** content, especially after a fatty meal. Lymph from the **liver** is rich in **protein,** while lymph from the extremities is poor both in fat and proteins. Like blood, lymph coagulates, but much more slowly, and the clot is soft and colorless.

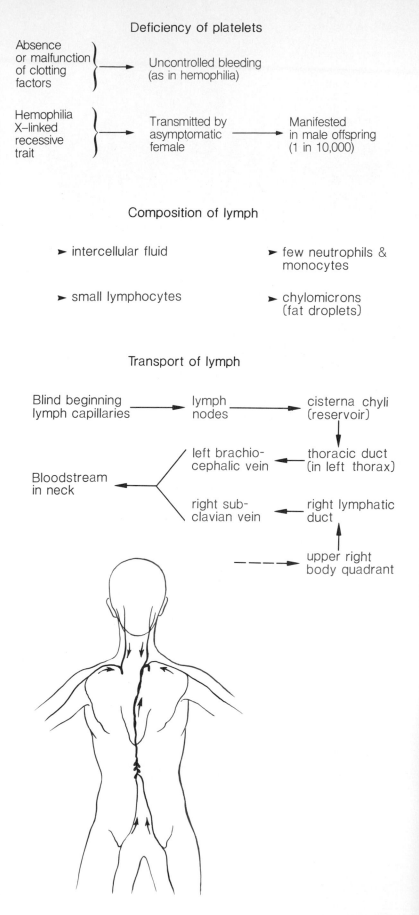

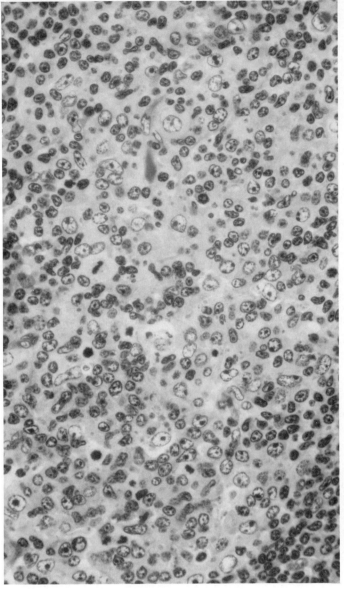

(x 400)

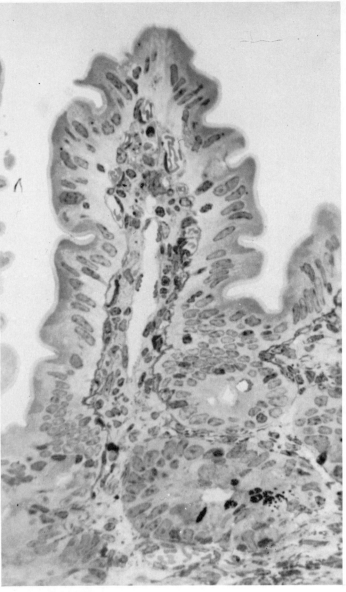

T. G. Merrill (x 440)

Left LM photograph. A lymph nodule with a pale germinal center that occupies most of the field. It is largely populated by light-staining, large lymphocytes, many in mitosis. Other cells include macrophages and large, clear reticular cells. Beyond the germinal center, postmitotic, dark-staining, small lymphocytes dominate the right margin of the field.

Right LM photograph. A view of an intestinal villus whose central core is largely occupied by an empty lymph capillary, called a lacteal. Such a structure, lined with endothelium, is the beginning of the intestinal lymphatic system.

Table 8.1　*COMPARISON OF CIRCULATING BLOOD CELLS*

TYPE	DIAMETER (μm)	NUMBER/mm³	MORPHOLOGY	PHAGOCYTOSIS	INCREASE IN DISEASE	FUNCTIONS
Erythrocytes (RBC)	8.5 (fresh) 7.5 (stained)	5–5.5 million♂ 4.5–5 million♀	Anucleate, bi-concave disks; pliable	None	Polycythemia	Aided by hemo-globin, they transport O_2 and CO_2; responsible for about 70% of buffering action of blood
Leukocytes (WBC)	6–20	5000–9000	Variable	From very active to none	Leukemias	Include phago-cytosis, detoxifi-cation, immune response, etc.
Neutrophils	10–14	3000–6000 (60–75% of WBC)	3- to 5-lobed nu-cleus; many small uniform, faintly staining, neutrophic granules	Very active, es-pecially of bac-teria	Acute pus-form-ing infections and myelogen-ous leukemia	Active phagocy-tosis of bacteria and cellular de-bris in inflam-matory condi-tions; promote wound healing
Eosinophils	11–14	100–400 (2–4% of WBC)	Large bilobed nucleus; cell filled with large, coarse, uniform, refractive eosin-ophic granules	Slight	Parasitic infec-tions and aller-gies; also in var-ious autoimmune re-actions	May act in de-toxification of foreign proteins and neutralizing of certain anti-gen-antibody complexes
Basophils	8–10	25–50 (0.5–1% of WBC)	Bilobed nucleus obscured by ir-regular, coarse, basophilic gran-ules	Slight	Chicken pox Chronic granulo-cytic leukemia	Release hista-mine, heparin, and seratonin; involved in in-flammatory re-actions, some of allergic origin
Lymphocytes	6–8 (small) 8–10 (medium) 10–14 (large)	1000–3000 (20–30% of WBC)	Spherical dark-staining nucleus nearly fills cell; nongranular, sky-blue cyto-plasm; occa-sionally a few azurophilic granules	Active	Chronic infec-tions, mononu-cleosis, whoop-ing cough, and lymphatic leuke-mia	Active in hu-moral and cell-mediated im-mune responses
Monocytes	12–20	100–600 (2–6% of WBC)	Single, kidney-shaped, lighter-staining nu-cleus; consider-able, grayish blue cytoplasm with few azuro-philic granules	Very active, es-pecially ingest-ing cellular de-bris and particulate mat-ter	Tuberculosis and protozoal infections	Phagocytosis; upon escape from blood-stream into tis-sue spaces they become tissue macrophages (histiocytes)
Platelets (thrombo-cytes)	2–4	200,000–400,000	Anucleate, bi-convex disks, basophilic cen-tral area (chro-momere) with granules, and light-staining peripheral zone (hyalomere)	None	Thrombocy-themia may be associated with polycythemia, chronic myelog-enous leuke-mia, severe hem-orrhage and splenectomy	Clotting of blood

Table 8.2 *ANATOMICAL LOCATIONS OF T- AND B-LYMPHOCYTES*

	B LYMPHOCYTES	T LYMPHOCYTES
Thymus	Rare	+ + + +
Bone marrow	+ + + + (as precursors)	+
Circulating blood	+	+ + +
Lymph node	+ + (germinal centers	+ + + (deep thymus-dependent cortex)
Spleen	+ + (germinal centers)	+ + + (periarterial lymphatic sheaths)
Thoracic duct	+	+ + +

Modified from H. N. Claman's *Cellular Immunology,* in *Immunology,* 1981, p. 52, The Upjohn Co., Kalamazoo, Michigan.

Chapter

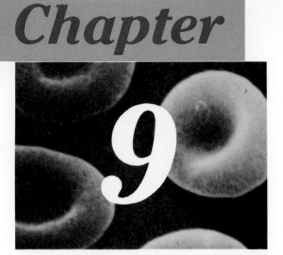

9

HEMOPOIESIS

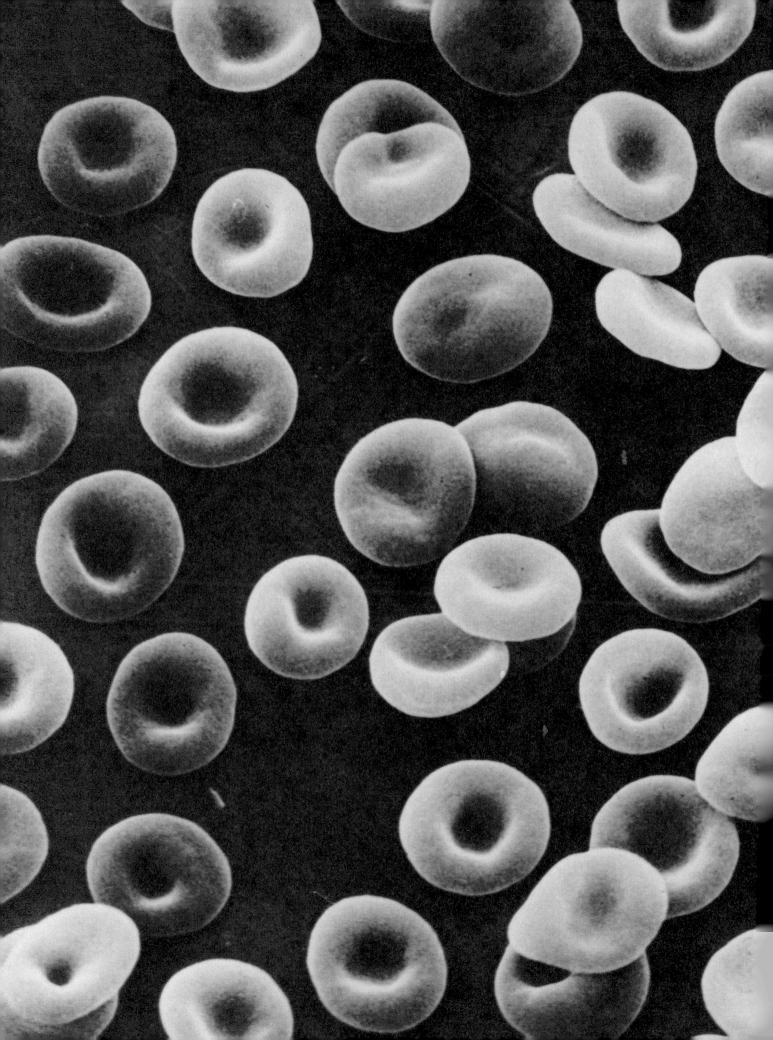

FROM THIS CHAPTER, ONE SHOULD BE ABLE TO:

1. Evaluate the need for various temporary sites of blood development in the human embryo and fetus.

2. Formulate the sequences of changes in size, color, and chromatin pattern common to all maturing blood cells.

3. Differentiate between the erythrocytic, agranulocytic, and granulocytic precursor cells in red bone marrow.

4. Explore the clinical implications of the appearance of immature blood cells in circulating blood.

5. Prepare a schema showing the origin, storage, pathway, distribution, and fate of iron in the bloodstream.

6. Analyze the phagocytic elements of the blood as to their origins, sites of phagocytosis, and roles in health and disease.

Hemopoiesis (Table 9.1) means "to make blood" (Gk. hemo, blood; poiein, to make); however, the term is generally used in a more restricted sense to refer to the **production of blood cells.** It does not include the formation of blood plasma or the other noncellular components, such as lipid droplets (chylomicrons) and blood dust (hemoconia).

Although blood cells are constantly being formed and destroyed and are always entering and leaving the bloodstream, the number of formed elements in the circulating blood remains remarkably constant. A sensitive **feedback mechanism,** as yet poorly understood, carefully monitors minor variations in blood cell populations and sends the information to blood stem cells in the red bone marrow and lymphoid organs. These parent cells respond appropriately by either accelerating or decelerating the production of each type of blood cell. Thus, a delicate balance of the number and type of cells in the bloodstream is maintained.

PRENATAL HEMOPOIESIS

At about the end of the second week of life of the human embryo, the **first blood cells** appear in **blood islands** that form in the mesenchyme of the yolk sac. These nests of cells are composed largely of **erythroblasts,** the early red blood cells (RBCs). Their appearance heralds the beginning of the **mesoblastic stage** in embryonic blood development. In about the sixth week, this stage is followed by the **hepatic phase,** a shift of hemopoiesis to the liver. Somewhat later, during the tenth to twelfth week, RBC and WBC formation begins on a limited scale in the spleen. The **splenic phase** ends in the fifth month when the hepatic stage is also phased out. At this time, the **red bone marrow** replaces the liver and spleen as the major site for fetal and postnatal hemopoiesis.

MATURATION SEQUENCES IN HEMOPOIESIS

For a clearer understanding of the flow of events that give rise to the various adult blood cells, the following **sequence of maturation** stages, developed by Dr. L. W. Diggs and associates, will be helpful. Such a conceptual approach to the study of hemopoiesis brings some order and logic to this rather difficult and complicated subject.

Since all blood cells initially arise from undifferentiated **mesenchymal cells,** the earliest and most primitive cells of each cell line closely **resemble each other.** When they cannot be differentiated by morphology alone, other techniques are needed, e.g., immunological and histochemical markers. However, as these primitive cells mature, a series of changes occurs in the nucleus, cytoplasm, and cell size which are distinctive for each cell line.

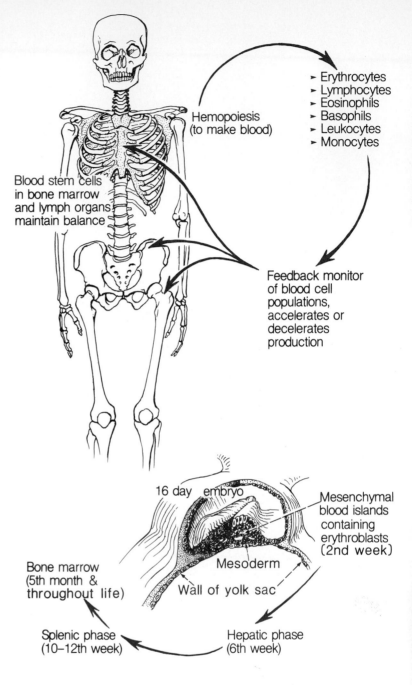

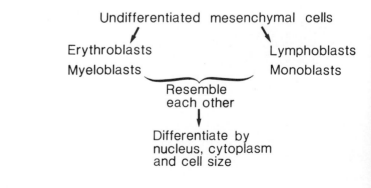

Maturation sequences:

Undifferentiated mesenchymal cells

Erythroblasts   Lymphoblasts

Myeloblasts   Monoblasts

Resemble each other

Differentiate by nucleus, cytoplasm and cell size

Origin of blood cells

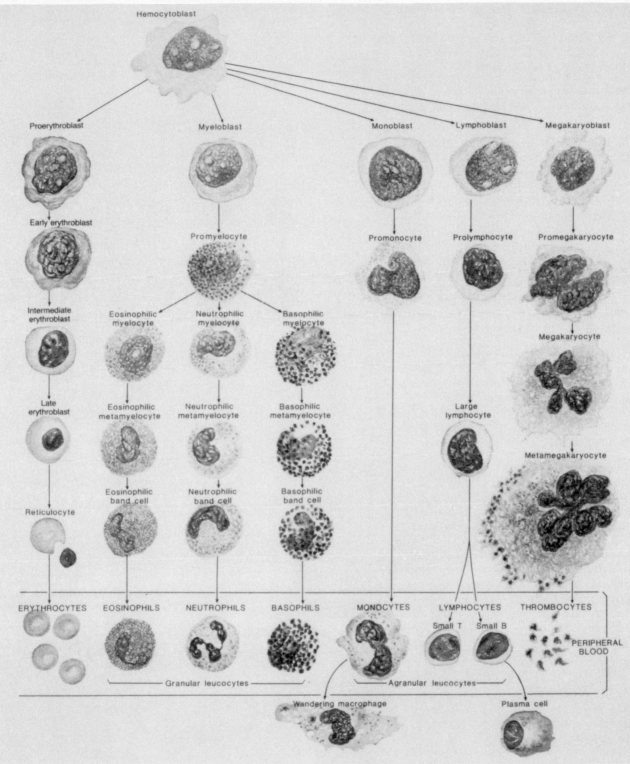

G. J. Tortora/N.P. Anagnostakos

This schema shows blood cell lineages arising from pluripotential stem cells in the red bone marrow. Also shown are the interrelationships and morphological changes that occur during the maturation of the erythrocytic, granulocytic, and lymphatic series. These structural variations, e.g., shape, size, staining reactions, and shift of nuclear and cytoplasmic ratios, change constantly during development. To keep these changes in proper perspective, all cells were sketched at essentially the same magnification.

These maturation changes follow a definite sequence common to all cells. Examples of these sequential changes, principally during development of the **red blood cells,** are shown in the accompanying illustrations. As observed in **conventional blood stains,** they include:

1. The **most immature** blood cells are usually the **largest** of a given cell line and become gradually smaller as the cell matures.

2. The nucleus of **primitive blood cells** is relatively large, occupying about 70–80% of the entire cell area. The nuclear chromatin strands usually stain uniformly and are light in color. As the **cell becomes older,** the absolute and relative **size of the nucleus decreases** and the chromatin becomes a pattern of dark-staining ropes or clumps (heterochromatin). In the **adult stage** the nucleus is a small, round, or lobulated, dark purple body which, in the erythrocytic series, is expelled.

3. One or more **nucleoli** appear in the metabolically active **early cells.** As the cell ages, its metabolism slows and the nucleoli disappear.

4. The **cytoplasm** of immature blood cells is a deep blue color due to the presence of abundant ribosomes. With the synthesis of various secretory products, such as hemoglobin and lysosomes, the cytoplasm shifts from blue to the color of the adult cell, e.g., in the RBC to a reddish copper color.

In granulocyte development, the immature stem cells are essentially free of specific granules; however, in early granulocytes these granules gradually appear. As the cell matures the granules become more numerous and selectively stain as eosinophilic, neutrophilic, or basophilic granules. Finally, in the reproductive sequence, the primitive cells increase in size during mitosis and then decrease during maturation.

Such a sequence of maturation stages emphasizes the concept that hemopoiesis is a dynamic continuum of constant change. Hence, the classical stages of development are rather dogmatic, idealized phases of development, which may not correspond to most of the cells observed in red bone marrow sections.

FORMATION OF ERYTHROCYTES (ERYTHROPOIESIS)

In RBC production (**erythropoiesis**), the multipotential, undifferentiated stem cell, the **hemocytoblast** in the bone marrow, undergoes a series of morphological and physiological changes to develop into a **mature erythrocyte.** Depending on their state of maturation, these cells are classified as proerythroblasts, basophilic erythroblasts, polychromatophilic erythroblasts, normoblasts, reticulocytes, or erythrocytes.

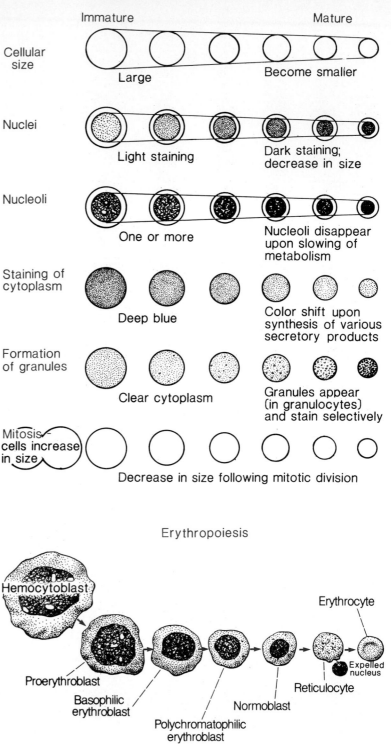

Maturation Sequences of Blood Cells After L.W. Diggs

Erythropoiesis

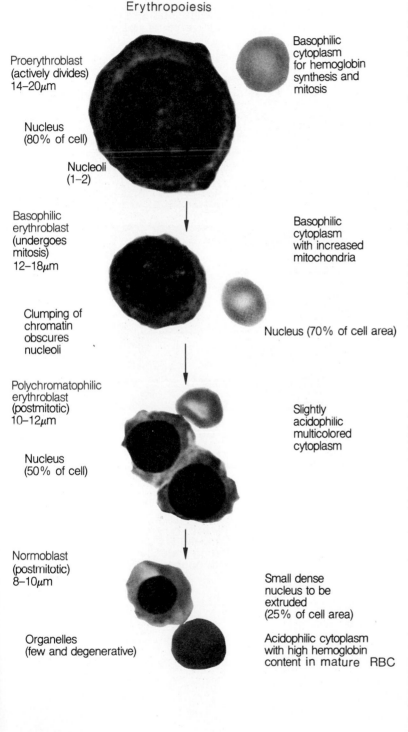

Purposes served in maturing of RBCs

1) to develop cells producing hemoglobin
(uniting with O_2 forming oxyhemoglobin for transport)

2) to fashion smallest cells with greatest surface areas for gas exchange

Erythropoiesis

Proerythroblast
(actively divides)
14–20μm

Nucleus
(80% of cell)

Nucleoli
(1–2)

Basophilic
cytoplasm
for hemoglobin
synthesis and
mitosis

Basophilic
erythroblast
(undergoes
mitosis)
12–18μm

Clumping of
chromatin
obscures
nucleoli

Basophilic
cytoplasm
with increased
mitochondria

Nucleus (70% of cell area)

Polychromatophilic
erythroblast
(postmitotic)
10–12μm

Nucleus
(50% of cell)

Slightly
acidophilic
multicolored
cytoplasm

Normoblast
(postmitotic)
8–10μm

Organelles
(few and degenerative)

Small dense
nucleus to be
extruded
(25% of cell area)

Acidophilic cytoplasm
with high hemoglobin
content in mature RBC

Proerythroblasts

The proerythroblast is the initial cell in this series to be differentiated. It is a large (14–20 μm) actively **dividing cell,** with a spherical, **central nucleus** occupying about 80% of the cell area. There are one to two **nucleoli** that stain pale blue with blood stains and are sometimes difficult to identify under the LM. The scanty **basophilic cytoplasm** contains the ingredients for active **protein (hemoglobin) synthesis** and **mitosis,** e.g., numerous free ribosomes, polyribosomes, mitochondria, an active Golgi apparatus, a pair of centrioles, and some rER. Although the amount of hemoglobin synthesized here is too small to be identified histologically, it can be detected spectroscopically.

Basophilic Erythroblasts

The proerythroblast becomes reduced in size (12–18 μm) as it divides to form the **basophilic erythroblast.** Clumping of the chromatin obscures the nucleoli, giving the nucleus a rather compact, dark appearance. The **nucleus** dominates about 70% of the cell. The **cytoplasm** is deeply **basophilic** and devoid of granules. Its fine structure resembles that of the proerythroblast; however, **ribosomes and polyribosomes** are more numerous and are responsible for the intense **basophilia** of the cytoplasm. Also, mitochondria increase in number and size. These cells also undergo **mitosis.**

Polychromatophilic Erythroblasts

In the mitotically active **polychromatophilic erythroblast,** the **hemoglobin** is synthesized in quantities sufficient to be detected in stained preparations. Thus, the basophilia of the cytoplasm is reduced and replaced by a **slight acidophilia.** Polychromatophilic means "many colored." The cell is truly multicolored, since its cytoplasm may have various shades of blues and pinks, or a mixture which gives a gray color. The **smaller nucleus** has coarser clumps of chromatin, with no observable nucleoli, and occupies about one half the cell area. The cell is reduced in size to about 10–12 μm.

Normoblasts

The normoblast has a very distinctive appearance. It is a **small cell** (8–10 μm), with a small, dense (**pyknotic**) **nucleus,** with no chromatin pattern. The nucleus occupies about 25% of the cell area. The **pink cytoplasm,** reflecting a high **hemoglobin** content, has only a trace of the blue-gray color. The cell organelles are scarce and degenerative. Normoblasts are **postmitotic cells.** Their final act of maturation in the red bone marrow is the **extrusion of the nucleus,** which is ingested by macrophages.

Reticulocytes

The reticulocyte is a normoblast that has lost its nucleus. As an **immature erythrocyte**, it has only about 80% of the normal amount of hemoglobin of mature RBC.

Under normal conditions, 48–72 hours are required to complete the maturation process from the hemocytoblast to the expulsion of the nucleus resulting in the formation of the **reticulocyte**. During this period, the early cells undergo many mitotic divisions. Also during this interval the machinery for **hemoglobin synthesis** is developed, i.e., polyribosomes, a Golgi apparatus, mitochondria, and ferritin (iron-protein complex) bodies. By the end of the synthesis period, the reticulocyte has largely rid itself of these same organelles. They are now no longer needed by the final cellular product, the erythrocyte.

In the **reticulocyte**, a few ribosomes are present and continue to **synthesize hemoglobin** for about 48 hours until the cell has its full adult complement. When reticulocytes are stained with brilliant cresyl blue dye, their remaining ribosomes stain a deep blue and are arranged in delicate strands or a **small network**. Hence their name, reticulocytes, which means "cells with a net." About 1% of RBCs in the circulating blood are reticulocytes.

Erythrocytes

The mature RBC, with its **full complement** of **hemoglobin,** has a deep pink, salmon, or **eosinophilic color** when exposed to conventional blood stains. It has a uniform **size (7–8 μm)** and is shaped like a biconcave disk. Erythrocytes remain in circulation for about **120 days** before they become rather rigid and fragile. These **senile cells** are largely sequestered in the sinusoids of the **spleen and liver** where they are engulfed by macrophages and degraded by lysosomes. In the process, their hemoglobin is broken down into **bilirubin and iron.** The latter is eventually joined with protein to form **ferritin.** The ferritin is phagocytized and stored within the macrophage. It is later released for transport by carrier proteins in the blood to the red bone marrow where it is **reincorporated** into erythroblasts by a process resembling pinocytosis.

Factors Affecting Erythropoiesis

Perhaps the most fundamental stimulus to RBC production is a deficiency of cellular oxygen, i.e., hypoxia. **Hypoxia** may occur following severe hemorrhage, in anemias, and in exposure to high altitudes. In all of these situations, the oxygen supply to cells and tissues is inadequate. It has been demonstrated experimentally that hypoxic cells release into the blood a factor (hormone) called **erythropoietin.** It stimulates the production of more RBCs for transmitting the

48-72 hour cycle

Hemocytoblast → Reticulocyte → Erythrocyte

| Contains many organelles; undergoes frequent mitoses | Contains organelles for final hemoglobin synthesis | Loses organelles no longer needed for hemoglobin production |

LM Reticulocytes = Normoblasts after loss of nuclei
(cells with a net)　　(immature erythrocytes - 1% of total)

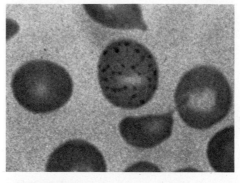

Contain 80% of hemoglobin of adult RBCs

3–5% indicates increase in RBC production

Remnants of ribosomes (stain with brilliant cresyl blue)

SEM Mature RBCs

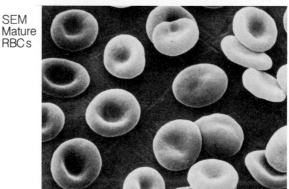

Stain salmon color

Shaped as a biconcave disk (7–8μm)

L.S. Lessin

Circulate ± 120 days then engulfed by macrophages, e.g. in spleen → Hemoglobin degraded to bilirubin and iron; latter recycled into ferritin for future use by erythroblasts

Hypoxia → Stimulates RBC production through release of erthropoietin

↑

Hemorrhage
Anemia
High altitude

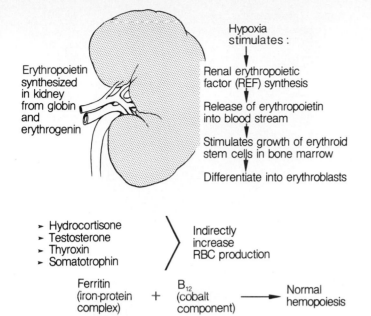

Erythropoietin synthesized in kidney from globin and erythrogenin

Hypoxia stimulates:

Renal erythropoietic factor (REF) synthesis

Release of erythropoietin into blood stream

Stimulates growth of erythroid stem cells in bone marrow

Differentiate into erythroblasts

► Hydrocortisone
► Testosterone
► Thyroxin
► Somatotrophin

Indirectly increase RBC production

Ferritin (iron-protein complex) + B_{12} (cobalt component) → Normal hemopoiesis

Granulopoiesis

Myeloblasts
Promyelocytes
Myelocytes
Metamyelocytes
Mature granulocytes (neutrophils, eosinophils, basophils)

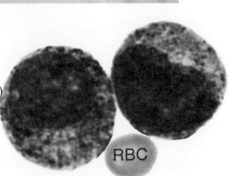

LM
Myeloblast (12–18μm)
- resemble proerythroblasts, monoblasts & lymphoblasts

Nucleus (75% of cell area)

1 to 3 nucleoli

Basophilic cytoplasm

LM
Promyelocytes (15–25μm)

Large nucleus (60% of cell area)

Basophilic cytoplasm with azurophilic granules

RBC

needed oxygen to the hypoxic cells.

Erythropoietin is a glycoprotein formed by the interaction of precursor compounds, mainly **erythrogenin** and the hemoglobin protein, **globin.** Since most of the erythrogenin is produced in the kidney, it is called **renal erythropoietic factor (REF).** Hypoxia stimulates REF synthesis, which results in an increased release of the hormone erythropoietin into the bloodstream.

Other **hormones,** e.g., hydrocortisone, testosterone, thyroxin, and somatotrophin (growth hormone), acting indirectly, also contribute to increased RBC production. Another factor needed for normal hemopoiesis is an adequate, usable supply of iron in the form of the iron-protein complex, **ferritin.** However, ferritin cannot be utilized by the erythroblasts except in the presence of vitamin B_{12}, the **antipernicious anemia factor.** A critical part of the vitamin B_{12} molecule is **cobalt,** which is a limiting factor in the synthesis of the vitamin. The absence or deficiency of cobalt in the diet may result in anemia.

DEVELOPMENT OF GRANULOCYTES (GRANULOPOIESIS)

All **granulocytes** arise in the red bone marrow. The **myeloblast,** the most primitive cell of the granulocyte series, gives rise to three types of granulocytes. The other stages in the development of the granulocytes, in order of their immaturity, are, promyelocytes, myelocytes, metamyelocytes, band forms, and mature granulocytes, i.e., neutrophils, eosinophils, and basophils.

Myeloblasts

The myeloblast (Gk. myelos, marrow) is a large, spherical cell, 12–18 μm in diameter. Its large, **round nucleus** occupies about 75% of the cell area. It has delicate, netlike chromatin and one to three coarse nucleoli. The **basophilic cytoplasm** is scanty, with **no granules** visible under the LM. However, the EM reveals an abundance of **free ribosomes,** a few profiles of rER, and numerous small, spherical mitochondria. In LM studies, the morphology of the myeloblast resembles several other immature blood cells, e.g., proerythroblasts, monoblasts, and lymphoblasts.

Promyelocytes

Promyelocytes are larger than myeloblasts, ranging from 15–25 μm. The large round or oval **nucleus** occupies less cell area, about 60%. Early **clumping of the chromatin** is present, and the nucleoli are less visible. The **cytoplasm** is more **basophilic** and contains nonspecific **azurophilic** (reddish purple) **granules,** *the* diagnostic feature that distinguishes the cell from a myeloblast. When specific granules appear, the promyelocyte is called a myelocyte.

Myelocytes

The myelocyte varies greatly in size. The early forms may be as large as the promyelocyte (15–25 μm) but the late myelocyte is smaller, 12–18 μm. The **nucleus**, with dark clumps of chromatin, is smaller, **slightly indented,** and occupies about 50% of the cell area. The distinctive features of the myelocyte are: (1) the appearance of **specific granules,** and (2) the presence of a **perinuclear clear zone** occupied by the **unstained Golgi** apparatus. As the cell matures, the specific granules become more abundant and **stain selectively.** Now one can recognize neutrophilic, eosinophilic, and basophilic myelocytes. All cells are mitotically active.

Metamyelocytes

The metamyelocyte, as the name implies (Gk. meta, beyond), is the **intermediate stage** between the myelocyte and the adult granular leukocyte. It has a full complement of **specific granules** and an oval, **indented (bean-shaped) nucleus.** Nucleoli are absent. This is perhaps the most abundant, nucleated cell in bone marrow, comprising about 22–30% of all cells present. It is a **postmitotic cell.**

Band Cells

The stage beyond metamyelocyte is called a **band or stab cell.** These are also called **juvenile granulocytes** because the nucleus is not yet lobulated but is in the form of a band, a horseshoe, or a slightly coiled rod. It is a smaller cell (10–15 μm), and its cytoplasm is filled with **specific granules of only one type.** In common usage the term band cell is used almost exclusively to identify **neutrophilic juvenile cells.** A few band cells escape from the bone marrow and enter the bloodstream. One to two percent of all circulating granulocytes may be band forms. If a significant **increase (3–5%)** of band cells reach the bloodstream, it is called a "shift to the left" and may suggest some clinical abnormality, such as **granulocytic leukemia.**

Mature Granulocytes

The various mature granulocytes are distinguished by the staining characteristics of their specific granules. Specifically, acidic **eosin** selectively stains granules of the **eosinophil; basic methylene blue** reacts to granules in the **basophil,** while granules of the neutrophil have little or no affinity for either stain but take on a greyish tint.

Also occurring simultaneously are morphological changes in the band-shaped nucleus of the juvenile cell. The **mature neutrophil** develops **two** to **five lobes,** while the eosinophil and basophil are **bilobed.**

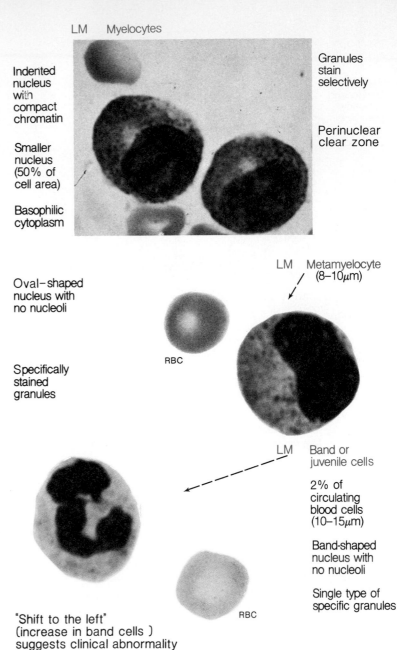

LM   Myelocytes

Indented nucleus with compact chromatin

Smaller nucleus (50% of cell area)

Basophilic cytoplasm

Granules stain selectively

Perinuclear clear zone

Oval-shaped nucleus with no nucleoli

Specifically stained granules

RBC

LM   Metamyelocyte (8–10μm)

LM   Band or juvenile cells

2% of circulating blood cells (10–15μm)

Band-shaped nucleus with no nucleoli

Single type of specific granules

RBC

"Shift to the left" (increase in band cells) suggests clinical abnormality

Granular cell staining characteristics

Stain	Granulocyte
Acidic eosin	Eosinophil
Basic methylene blue	Basophil
No affinity	Neutrophil

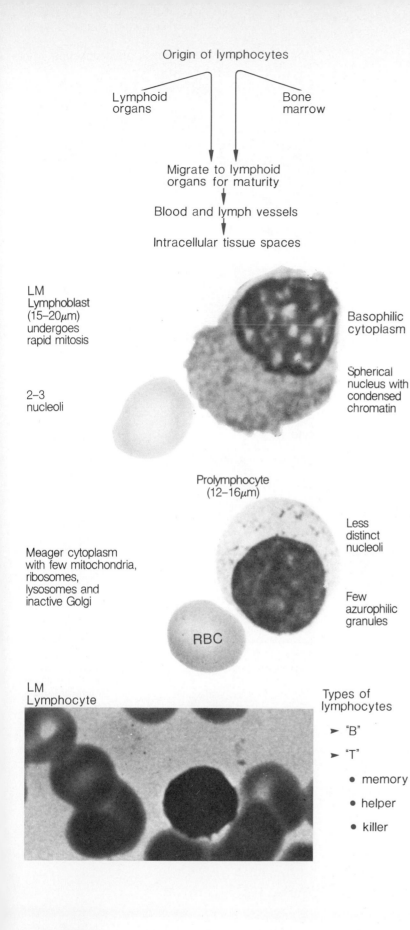

Origin of lymphocytes

Lymphoid organs

Bone marrow

Migrate to lymphoid organs for maturity

Blood and lymph vessels

Intracellular tissue spaces

LM
Lymphoblast
(15–20μm)
undergoes
rapid mitosis

2–3
nucleoli

Basophilic
cytoplasm

Spherical
nucleus with
condensed
chromatin

Prolymphocyte
(12–16μm)

Meager cytoplasm
with few mitochondria,
ribosomes,
lysosomes and
inactive Golgi

Less
distinct
nucleoli

Few
azurophilic
granules

RBC

LM
Lymphocyte

Types of
lymphocytes

➤ "B"

➤ "T"

• memory

• helper

• killer

AGRANULOCYTE DEVELOPMENT (AGRANULOPOIESIS)

Lymphocyte Production (Lymphopoiesis)

There is no clear consensus on the origin of the lymphocyte; however, **three distinct lineages** are suggested. (1) An older view held that the lymphocytes developed only in **lymphoid organs.** (2) Radioautographic studies have found this view to be untenable for, clearly, many lymphocytes **arise in the red bone marrow** and later migrate to, and mature in, the various lymphoid organs. (3) Another current opinion would have **all lymphocytes** and their precursors **originate in the bone marrow.** In our discussion we shall hold to the dual-origin concept, i.e., that lymphocytes develop both in lymphoid organs and bone marrow (see Table 9.1).

LYMPHOBLASTS The first definitive cell in the lymphocyte genealogy, beyond the undifferentiated stem cell (hemocytoblast), is the **lymphoblast,** which closely resembles the myeloblast. It is the largest cell of the lymphocyte series, being about 15–20 μm in diameter. Its basophilic cytoplasm is **devoid of azurophilic granules.** Its large, spherical nucleus has an abundance of **condensed chromatin,** a portent of the deeply staining bluish purple nucleus of the mature cell. The nucleus also has two to three nucleoli. These cells undergo rapid **mitosis,** especially in the thymus, bone marrow, and secondary lymphoid organs.

PROLYMPHOCYTES The prolymphocyte shows signs of maturity, e.g., the cell is **smaller** than the lymphoblast, the nuclear **chromatin is condensed,** and the nucleoli are less distinct or invisible under the LM. A few **azurophilic granules** may appear in the cytoplasm. The prolymphocyte transforms into the circulating large lymphocyte, then the medium lymphocyte, and finally into the small lymphocyte.

LYMPHOCYTES It should be noted that the mature, **small (7–9 μm) lymphocytes** are actually a **family of cells.** In LM studies, they are **morphologically indistinguishable** spherical cells, with a dense nucleus filling most of the cell and a narrow rim of blue cytoplasm. However, **functionally** there are **many types,** e.g., B-lymphocytes and T-lymphocytes; the latter divide further into memory cells, helper cells, killer cells, etc. (discussed on page 280). Although these cells engage in rather complicated and diverse activities, their ultrastructure is quite simple. The meager cytoplasm contains only a few small mitochondria and ribosomes; a small, inactive Golgi apparatus; and a few lysosomes (azurophilic granules).

Monocyte Production (Monopoiesis)

Earlier it was widely held that **monocytes** developed in lymphoid tissue and were simply a variation of the large lymphocyte, their "lookalike" cell. Recently, through EM studies, and radioautography and chromosome marker techniques, the origin of monocytes has been determined. They arise from **precursors in the bone marrow,** probably **hemocytoblasts** that may differentiate into **monoblasts.** In support of this theory, monocytes show a kinship with neutrophils in that the metabolism involved in the destruction of phagocytosed bacteria is similar in both cells. Since it is now generally held that the precursor of the neutrophil, the myeloblast, and the monoblast are perhaps morphologically indistinguishable, they probably share a **common ancestor** of all blood cells, the **hemocytoblast.**

MONOBLASTS Monoblasts resemble **myeloblasts** in their rounded shape, size (about 10 μm), and fine structure. Both cells have free ribosomes, polyribosomes, a few rER profiles, and a limited number of small, spherical mitochondria. **Monoblasts** can be identified only when they begin to show the two morphological features that will be predominate in the promonocyte, namely, (1) the **indentation of the nucleus,** and (2) the appearance of **azurophilic granules** in the cytoplasm.

PROMONOCYTES In the promonocyte the above-mentioned diagnostic features of the monoblast gain prominence. In addition, the cell is uneven in size, ranging from 8–15 μm, and its cytoplasm is lighter staining. Its **indented nucleus** is also lighter staining, due to the fine network of **heterochromatin** and the abundance of **euchromatin.** Two or three **nucleoli** are present. Promonocytes are **mitotically active** in the bone marrow. As the cell gradually matures, the nucleus decreases in size, and ribosomes are less numerous; however, **azurophilic granules increase** in number and size.

MONOCYTES Monocytes are released from the bone marrow into the bloodstream shortly after their immediate precursors (promonocytes) have completed the last mitotic division. They **circulate in the blood** for perhaps **one to two days** before they pass, by diapedesis, through the capillary wall into the surrounding connective tissue or body cavities. Here they mature into free or fixed **macrophages.** The structure and functions of these tissue macrophages are discussed in Chapter 6.

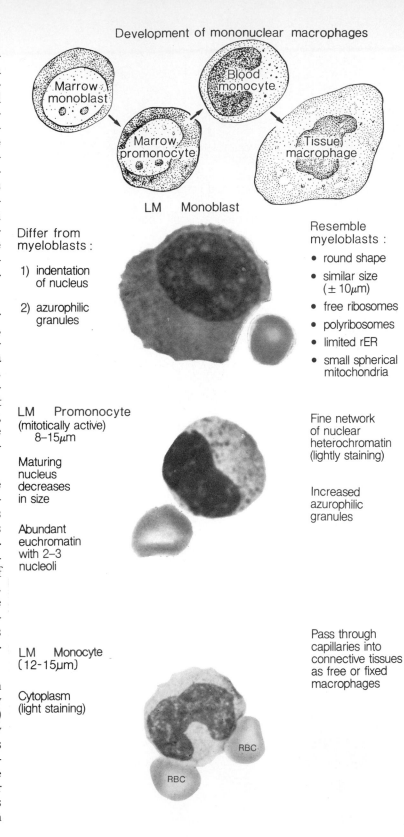

Development of mononuclear macrophages

Marrow monoblast

Marrow promonocyte

Blood monocyte

Tissue macrophage

LM   Monoblast

Differ from myeloblasts:

1) indentation of nucleus

2) azurophilic granules

Resemble myeloblasts:
- round shape
- similar size (± 10μm)
- free ribosomes
- polyribosomes
- limited rER
- small spherical mitochondria

LM   Promonocyte (mitotically active) 8–15μm

Maturing nucleus decreases in size

Abundant euchromatin with 2–3 nucleoli

Fine network of nuclear heterochromatin (lightly staining)

Increased azurophilic granules

LM   Monocyte (12-15μm)

Cytoplasm (light staining)

RBC

RBC

Pass through capillaries into connective tissues as free or fixed macrophages

Development of platelets

Stem cells in
red bone marrow ——→
give rise to:

LM
Megakaryoblasts
(25–50μm)

Oval indented
nucleus with
multiple nucleoli
(nucleus largest of
hemopoietic cells)

Homogenous
basophilic
cytoplasm

(x 400)

LM
Early
megakaryocytes
(40–100μm)

Twisted multilobulated
polypoid nucleus

Incomplete
mitosis
lacking
division
of nuclei
or cytoplasm

Extensive
rER

Increase in
azurophilic
granules

Pinching off
of cytoplasm
as platelets
(life span
8–10 days)

Few:
□ mitochondria
□ ribosomes
□ granules
□ vacuoles

(x 800)

LM   Late megakaryocyte

EM
Platelet

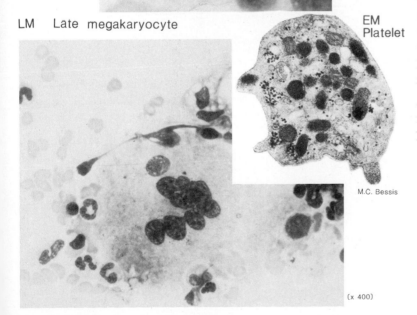

M.C. Bessis

(x 400)

PLATELET DEVELOPMENT (THROMBOPOIESIS)

Megakaryoblasts

In their development, **platelets**, like other formed elements of the blood, develop from stem cells in the red bone marrow. The first differentiated cell is the early **megakaryoblast**. It is distinguished from its precursor, the hemocytoblast, by its **larger size (25–50 μm)** and a large, oval, **indented nucleus** with multiple nucleoli. Its nucleus is the largest of the early hemopoietic cells. Its cytoplasm is homogeneous and quite basophilic due to the abundance of **ribosomes**. The cell contains other organelles, e.g., many small, round mitochondria, a prominent Golgi apparatus, and a few membrane-bound granules, i.e., the azurophilic granules, as seen under the LM.

Megakaryocytes

Gradually the late megakaryoblast differentiates into a **megakaryocyte**. The transformation is made by a series of unusual **incomplete mitoses** where neither the daughter nuclei nor the cytoplasm separate. These aberrant cell divisions result in a **giant cell (40–100 μm)**, with an abundance of slightly basophilic cytoplasm surrounding a very large, twisted, **multilobulated, polyploid nucleus**. The azurophilic granules are greatly increased. TEM studies reveal the same organelles as in the megakaryoblast but they are greatly increased in number.

When differentiation is complete, a pinching off of bits of cytoplasm occurs. These cytoplasmic fragments are the **platelets (thrombocytes)**. The segments of cytoplasm usually contain a few small mitochondria, ribosomes, considerable sER, limited rER, and some granules and vacuoles. From isotope studies the **life-span** of platelets in the bloodstream has been determined to be about **eight to ten days**. The megakaryocyte, deprived of its cytoplasm, degenerates and is removed by phagocytosis. The adult functional platelet is discussed on page 151.

Table 9.1   *LINEAGES OF BLOOD CELLS*

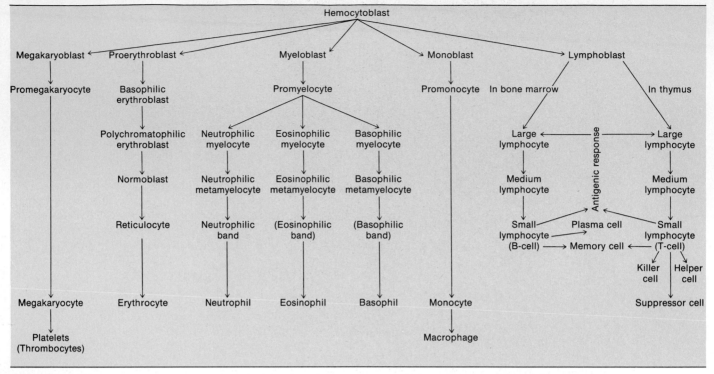

Chapter

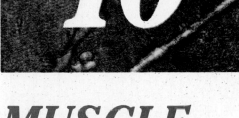

10

MUSCLE TISSUE

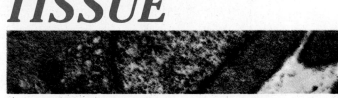

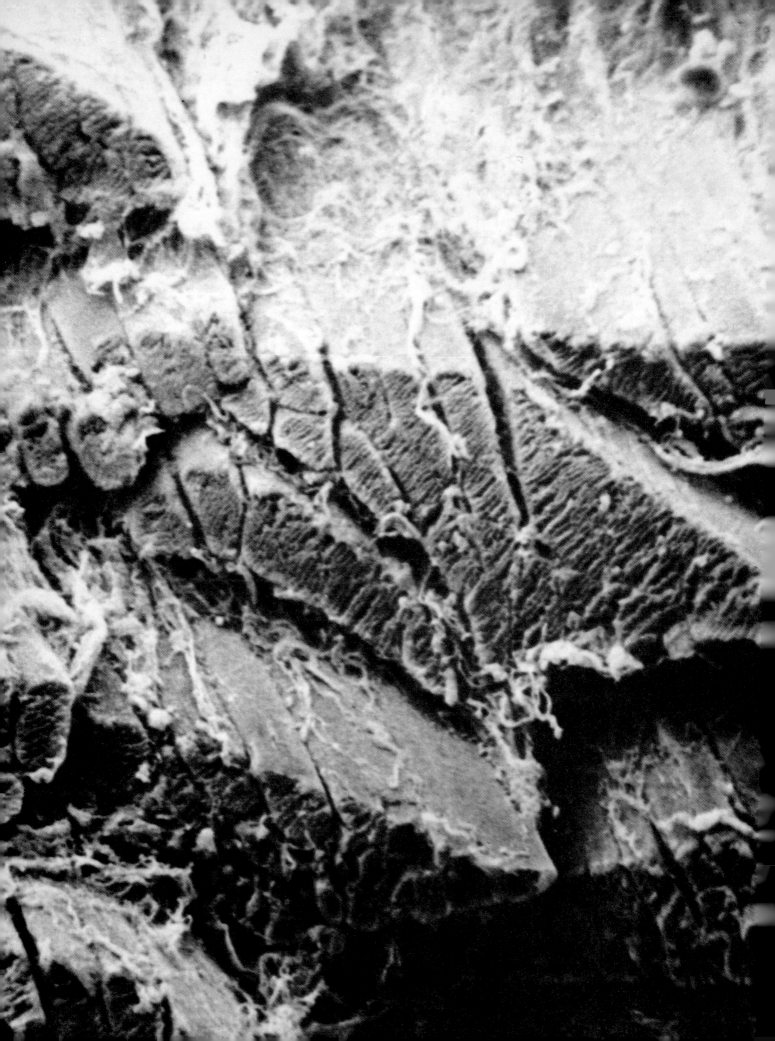

OBJECTIVES

THOUGHTFUL STUDY OF THIS CHAPTER WILL ENABLE THE STUDENT TO CONCEPTUALIZE:

1. The morphological and functional differences and similarities between smooth, skeletal, cardiac, and Purkinje muscle types.

2. The structural and size relationships of an entire skeletal muscle, fascicles, fibers, myofibrils, and myofilaments.

3. How the arrangement of the actin and myosin filaments create cross striations in cardiac and skeletal muscle.

4. The sliding filament concept of contraction and how it applies to the various muscle types.

5. Why skelctal muscles have the potential for partial regeneration, while cardiac fibers do not.

Motility is a prime attribute of living animals. "If it moves, it's alive" is an axiom we learned as children. From hydra to man, muscular tissue endows the animal kingdom with movement. Such muscle action is not limited to obvious gross body movements but includes, for example, the rhythmic contraction of the heart or the sluggish, peristaltic action of the intestines.

In vertebrates, muscles develop from **mesoderm** except some intrinsic muscles of the eye, which are ectodermal in origin. Three types of muscle fibers are present in the body. (1) **Smooth muscle fibers** are the predominant tissue in the walls of blood vessels, ducts, and hollow viscera (except the heart) and are usually arranged in sheetlike layers. Their contraction propels the contents of viscera along their course. (2) **Cardiac muscle fibers** are found only in the heart and in the origins of the large vessels issuing from it. The walls of the heart contract to pump the blood throughout the body. (3) **Skeletal muscle fibers** make up the various named muscles that usually attach to the skeleton to move the body or its parts.

LIGHT MICROSCOPY OF MUSCLE

Smooth Muscle

Smooth muscle, also called **involuntary** or **visceral** muscle, is structurally the simplest of the muscle types. It is called smooth because it has no visible cross striations, involuntary because it is not under conscious control, and visceral because it is predominantly found in organs. The individual fibers are elongated, tapered, **spindle-shaped cells** with great range in length (20–200 μm). Their length depends on the organ. For example, in the pregnant uterus the length may be increased to 600 μm. The diameter of the smooth muscle cell may vary from 3–9 μm.

A **cigar-shaped nucleus** lies near the center of each fiber. If the fibers are contracted at fixation, the nuclei have a corkscrew appearance. The cytoplasm, which in muscle cells is called **sarcoplasm,** appears rather homogeneous even though it is filled with very fine contractile elements, the **myofilaments.** The delicate cell membrane cannot be seen with the light microscope.

The involuntary smooth muscle fibers are innervated by the **autonomic nervous system.** All nerve fibers are postganglionic and unmyelinated. Not every fiber receives a nerve terminal; the stimulus passes from one fiber to another by **gap junctions** (nexuses). Smooth muscle has only a moderate blood supply. Capillaries course in the connective tissue that invests the muscle bundles but do not directly supply individual fibers (L-A, plate 5).

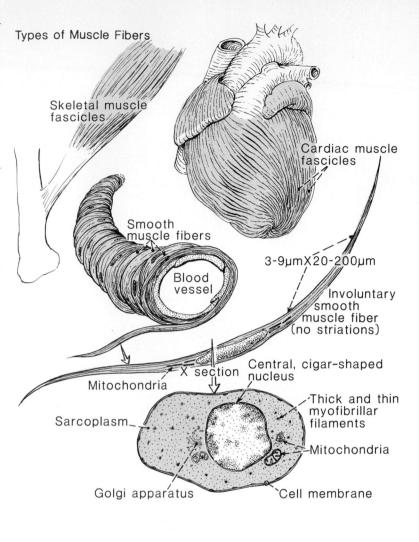

Types of Muscle Fibers

Skeletal muscle fascicles

Cardiac muscle fascicles

Smooth muscle fibers

Blood vessel

3-9μmX20-200μm

Involuntary smooth muscle fiber (no striations)

Mitochondria

X section

Central, cigar-shaped nucleus

Sarcoplasm

Thick and thin myofibrillar filaments

Mitochondria

Golgi apparatus

Cell membrane

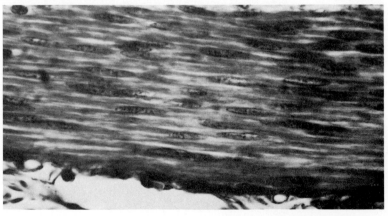

LM   Smooth muscle

P. M. Andrews

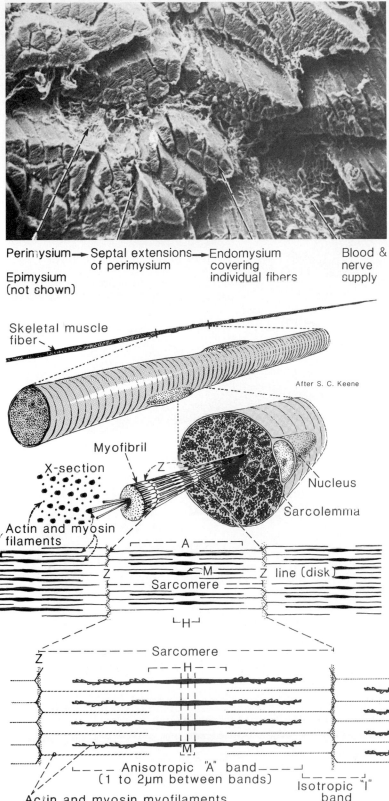

Perimysium ⟶ Septal extensions ⟶ Endomysium   Blood &
                of perimysium   covering   nerve
Epimysium   individual fibers   supply
(not shown)

Skeletal muscle
fiber

After S. C. Keene

Myofibril

X-section

Nucleus

Sarcolemma

Actin and myosin
filaments

A

Z   M   Z line (disk)
Sarcomere

H

Sarcomere
Z
H

M

Anisotropic "A" band
(1 to 2μm between bands)   Isotropic "I"
                                         band
Actin and myosin myofilaments

Skeletal Muscle

Skeletal muscle, also called **voluntary or striated muscle,** forms the muscles of the body that respond to conscious control. Neither skeletal, voluntary, nor striated are entirely appropriate descriptive terms. Some skeletal muscles do not attach to the skeleton, others are not always under the control of the will, and all striated muscles, i.e., cardiac, are not skeletal muscle.

Externally, a dense connective tissue sheath, the **epimysium,** encloses an entire muscle. In gross anatomy this tough investment is called the deep fascia. Each **fascicle** (bundle) of muscle fibers within the epimysium is invested with a thinner covering, the **perimysium.** It is derived from septal extensions of the epimysium, which carries with it a rich blood and nerve supply to the individual muscle fibers. (The nerve terminals, i.e., sensory endings of muscle spindles and motor end plates, are discussed in Chapter 11.) A delicate layer of reticular fibers, the **endomysium,** surrounds and separates individual muscle fibers within a fascicle.

The typical fiber of skeletal muscle is a giant, multinucleated, **cylindrical cell,** enclosed in a distinct cell membrane, the **sarcolemma.** The fibers may attain relatively great differences in lengths (1–40 mm), and the diameter varies from 10–100 μm. Many flattened, **elongated nuclei** are located at the **periphery** of the cell just internal to the sarcolemma. The fiber is filled with **myofibrils** that are prominently **cross striated** with light and dark bands.

The **dark and light bands** of one fibril are accurately **aligned in register** with the dark and light bands of other fibrils in the same muscle fiber. Hence, the entire fiber appears cross-banded. It should be noted that these bands are actually three-dimensional cylinders and not simply surface markings. The dark band is called the **anisotropic, or A,** band because it is doubly refractive (anisotropic) to polarized light and appears dark in the fresh state. The light, or **isotropic I, band** is singly refractive to polarized light and is pale in the living fiber.

Since the myofibril is about 1–2 μm in diameter, it can be seen with the LM. In cross section the **myofibrils** appear as dots of variable sizes, separated by a limited amount of clear sarcoplasm. Only in longitudinal and some oblique sections can the banding be seen. Careful examinations of the light and dark bands reveals additional structures. Each **light I band** is bisected by a dark, transverse partition, the **Z line.** The segment of a myofibril between two Z lines is a **sarcomere,** the smallest subunit of contraction along a myofibril. Likewise, the **dark A band** is divided by a thin, light-staining band or disk, called the **H band.** The significance of these structures is discussed later.

RED AND WHITE MUSCLES In fresh skeletal muscles, one can distinguish **red and white fibers.** The red color is due to an abundance of the muscle pigment, **myoglobin;** an increase in mitochondria, and a richer vascularity in the smaller red, muscle fibers. The larger, pale, **white fibers** have fewer mitochondria, less pigment, and a poorer blood supply. These variations are not conspicuous in routine staining procedures. However, they become so with special histochemical methods for identifying enzymatic activity. For example, staining for the enzyme, **succinic dehydrogenase,** gives a clear, positive test in the red muscle fibers because of the abundance of **mitochondria.**

Functionally, red and white muscles are also different. The **red muscles** contract more slowly than the white and are therefore also called **slow muscles** as contrasted to the **fast acting, white muscles.** Red muscles, as in **postural muscles,** do not fatigue easily; while the fast, white muscles fatigue rather quickly, as in muscles used in running. An intermediate type of fiber also exists with some characteristics of both the red and white muscles (see Table 10.1).

The duration of isometric contractions differs sharply in red and white muscles. For example, the gastrocnemius muscle of the leg (largely white fibers) has a duration of contraction of about ⅟30 second, while the adjacent soleus muscle, with mostly red fibers, has a contraction time of ⅟10 second. Thus, the gastrocnemius muscle can contract rapidly and forcefully, providing great velocity for leaping and running. In contrast, the soleus, a postural muscle, is involved principally in giving constant, sustained support to the body against gravity.

Other examples of slow and fast muscles are found in the **neuromuscular spindle,** discussed in Chapter 11, where the longer, thicker "bag" fibers are slow fibers that act in a tonic fashion, similar to other slow (red) muscles. The more numerous, thinner, "chain" fibers act in phasic contractions, a common feature of fast (white) muscles.

Other physiological data support the concept that the differentiation of muscle fibers into white and red types is dependent on the innervation. If red and white fibers are cross innervated, that is, their neurons are severed, crossed-over, and allowed to regenerate, then the muscle fibers change their structure and function to match the new innervation.

In man, essentially all muscles are composed of both types, with one dominant type. However, lower animals, such as chickens and rabbits, have some all red and all white muscles (light and dark meat), but many of their muscles are also mixed.

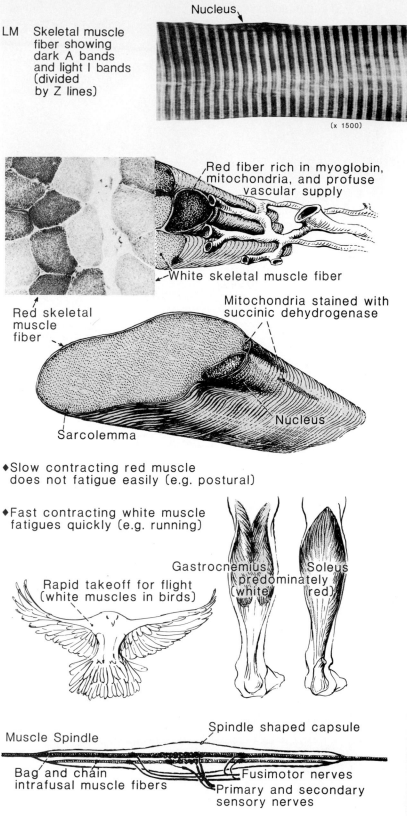

LM Skeletal muscle fiber showing dark A bands and light I bands (divided by Z lines)

Nucleus

(x 1500)

Red fiber rich in myoglobin, mitochondria, and profuse vascular supply

White skeletal muscle fiber

Red skeletal muscle fiber

Mitochondria stained with succinic dehydrogenase

Nucleus

Sarcolemma

♦Slow contracting red muscle does not fatigue easily (e.g. postural)

♦Fast contracting white muscle fatigues quickly (e.g. running)

Rapid takeoff for flight (white muscles in birds)

Gastrocnemius predominately (white)

Soleus (red)

Muscle Spindle

Spindle shaped capsule

Bag and chain intrafusal muscle fibers

Fusimotor nerves

Primary and secondary sensory nerves

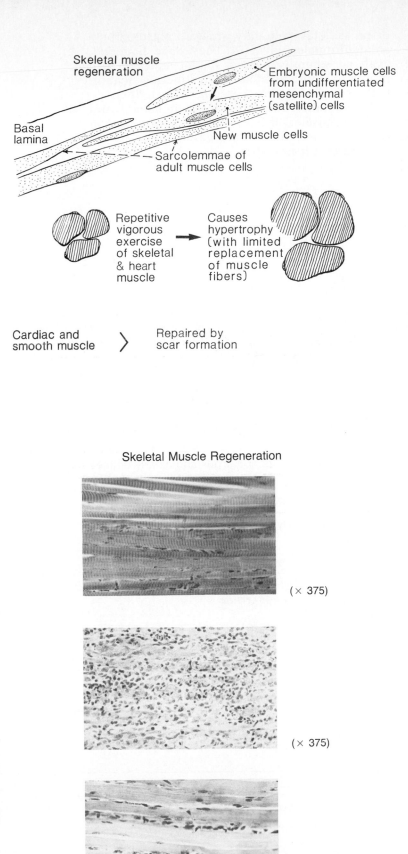

Skeletal muscle regeneration

Embryonic muscle cells from undifferentiated mesenchymal (satellite) cells

Basal lamina

New muscle cells

Sarcolemmae of adult muscle cells

Repetitive vigorous exercise of skeletal & heart muscle → Causes hypertrophy (with limited replacement of muscle fibers)

Cardiac and smooth muscle ⟩ Repaired by scar formation

Skeletal Muscle Regeneration

(× 375)

(× 375)

(× 375)

Normal (upper photo), degenerated (middle photo), and regenerated muscle (lower photo) in rat nutritional muscular dystrophy.

Consequently **regeneration** of damaged muscular tissue is very **limited**. Repair is usually accomplished by fibrous scar formation laid down by fibroblasts. Nonetheless, muscle types respond somewhat differently to fiber loss and, under special conditions, limited regeneration may occur.

In skeletal muscle shortly after injury, a few new **myoblasts** appear, which fuse together to form new muscle fibers. This phenomenon is especially prominent in some of the various **muscular dystrophies**. The principal source of these embryonic muscle cells are small, **satellite cells** that are enclosed within the basal lamina next to the sarcolemma of adult muscle cells. These are probably undifferentiated **mesenchymal cells** left over from earlier embryonic stages. However, in severe muscle trauma, their contribution is minimal and the tissue deficit is replaced by scar tissue.

Vigorous repetitive muscular exercise will cause normal muscle fibers to increase in diameter, i.e., they **hypertrophy**, but the number of fibers probably do not increase. Conversely, muscles that are not exercised **atrophy** by decrease of fiber diameter.

There is essentially **no regeneration of cardiac fibers** after injury since they do not possess satellite cells and the damaged fibers rapidly degenerate and are replaced by fibrous scars. However, after sustained, severe strain on the heart, the cardiac fibers increase in size but with no increase in number. In other words, the heart, like skeletal muscle, may undergo **hypertrophy but not hyperplasia.**

During pregnancy the **smooth muscle cells** of the uterus increase in number, by mitosis (**hyperplasia**), as well as size (**hypertrophy**). However, the smooth muscle of the uterus should be considered an exception, for elsewhere in the body smooth muscle fibers do not undergo mitosis and, when damaged, the wound is usually healed by fibroblastic activity.

To recapitulate briefly, smooth (nonstriated, involuntary) muscle consists of sheets of spindle-shaped fibers, each enclosed by a very thin plasma membrane. Each cell contains a central, cigar-shaped nucleus. Branching cardiac (involuntary, striated) muscle fibers have faint cross striations with central, ovoid nuclei. Each fiber is enclosed by a sarcolemma and is divided into several cardiac cells by intercalated disks. Cylindrical skeletal (voluntary, striated) muscle fibers are multinucleated cells. They have flattened, oval, peripherally located nuclei adjacent to a prominent sarcolemma. A distinctive feature is the prominent cross banding of each fiber.

Regeneration is very moderate in smooth and skeletal muscles; it is essentially nonexistent in cardiac fibers. Muscle damage may be repaired by fibrous scar formation.

Table 10.1 *TYPES OF SKELETAL MUSCLE FIBERS*

DISTINGUISHING CHARACTERISTICS	TYPE I (red or slow)	TYPE II (white or fast)
Fresh gross appearance	Dark red color due to rich blood supply, large amount of myoglobin, and abundant large mitochondria	Whitish grey color due to less blood, less myoglobin, and fewer mitochondria
Location	Perhaps in all muscles but predominates in slow-fatiguing, postural (antigravity) muscles, e.g., soleus m.	In all muscles; however, concentrated in easily fatigued, fast-acting muscles, e.g., gastrocnemius m.
Blood supply	Greater	Lesser
Average diameter	Smaller (27 μm rat diaphragm)	Larger (44 μm rat diaphragm)
Neuromuscular junctions	Smaller with shallow functional folds	Larger with deep functional folds
Myofibrils	Less numerous and poorly defined, cross striations less regular	More numerous and clearly defined, cross striations regular and prominent
Z lines	Thicker	Narrower (about half as wide)
Nuclei	Maybe scattered throughout fiber, not always hypolemmal in position	Hypolemmal in position
Sarcoplasm	Granular, large amount	Less granular, lesser amount
Mitochondria	Larger size and numbers, concentrated on periphery of fiber and between myofibrils; have closely packed, abundant cristae	Smaller, sparse; no pattern of accumulation; fewer cristae
Sarcoplasmic reticulum	Complex especially near H band	Simpler
Myoglobin	Abundant	Less abundant
Glycogen	Lesser amount	Greater amount
Oxidative enzymes	Abundant	Less abundant
Myofibrillar ATPase activity	Low	High
Maturation	Less mature	More mature
Respiratory activity	High	Low

Table 10.2 *COMPARISON OF MUSCLE FIBERS*

	SMOOTH	SKELETAL	CARDIAC	PURKINJE
Location	GI, GU, respiratory, and vascular systems	Usually attached to skeleton	Myocardium	Myocardium adjacent to endocardium
Shape	Long, tapering, fusiform cells	Cylindrical or prismatic fibers	Cylindrical, short, branching fibers	Similar to cardiac but greater diameter and shorter
Arrangement of cells	As individual cells usually in sheets or layers	Very long, multinucleated giant cells arranged in bundles	Joined at intercalated disks to form short fibers	Form rows of thick, short cells
Size	Variable, from 12 × 600 μm (gravid uterus) to 2 × 10–15 μm (small arteriole)	Extremely variable, 3–4 mm to 10–15 cm: long; diameter 10–100 μm	Length variable, diameter 9–20 μm	About 50 × 100 μm
Sarcolemma (plasmalemma)	Delicate	Prominent	Less prominent	Poorly developed
Nuclei	Single, central, cigarshaped	Multiple, peripheral, ovoid	1–2 central, ovoid to spherical shape	2–3 central, round
Myofibrils	Nonstriated, fill cell, evenly distributed	Cross striated, often arranged in clusters as Cohnheim's fields, nearly fill cell	Cross striated, may be in groups, fill cell except near nucleus	Cross striated, sparse and confined to periphery of cell
Intercalated disks	Absent	Absent	Present	Present but seldom seen
Sarcoplasm	Scanty	Scanty	Large amount especially surrounding nuclei	Largest amount, fills most of cell
Glycogen	Least amount	Considerable amount	Greater amount	Greatest amount
Mitochondria	Few, clustered near nuclei	Abundant near nuclei and surrounding myofibrils	Most abundant, largest, form in rows along myofibrils	Abundant, random distribution
Golgi complex	Small, single, near nucleus	Small, multiple, near nuclei	Single, small, near nucleus	Same as cardiac
Junctional complexes	Mostly nexuses (gap)	Absent	Desmosomes at intercalated disks, nexuses at lateral borders	Same as cardiac
Sarcoplasmic reticulum	Poorly developed	Network of cisternae and tubules. Triads at A-I junctions	Similar to skeletal except diads at Z line, no triads	Same as cardiac, except no T-tubules
Blood supply	Moderate	Rich	Twice that of skeletal but anastomoses are poor	Similar to cardiac
Nerve supply	Autonomic, sparse, simple nerve endings	Cerebrospinal, multiple specialized endings (motor end plates)	Autonomic, sparse, simple nerve endings	Same as cardiac
Contraction	Involuntary, sluggish, maybe rhythmic	Voluntary, rapid	Involuntary, vigorous, rhythmic	Involuntary, very limited

Chapter

11

NERVOUS TISSUE

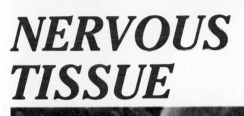

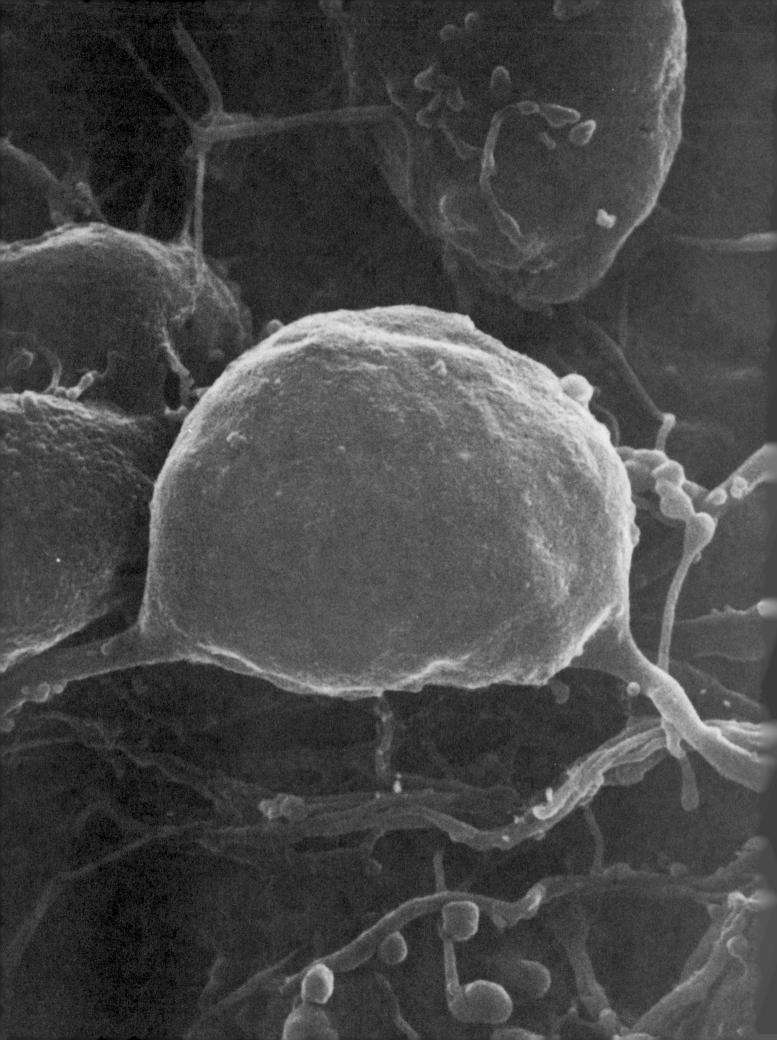

OBJECTIVES

AFTER CAREFUL PERUSAL OF THIS CHAPTER, ONE SHOULD BE ABLE TO:

1. Discriminate between axons and dendrites; glial cells and neurons; myelinated and nonmyelinated nerves.

2. Evaluate the present status of the neuron doctrine.

3. Contrast the central nervous system (CNS), peripheral nervous system (PNS), and autonomic nervous system (ANS) as to component parts, functions, and coverings.

4. Discuss the morphology and functions of reflexes and synapses.

5. Recognize the differences of the structural components and functions of receptor and effector nerve endings.

6. Describe the process of myelination and the clinical picture of demyelination.

7. Make an appraisal of the regeneration potential of the PNS and CNS.

This discussion of nervous tissue will introduce the basic elements and organization of the nervous system. With very few exceptions, nervous tissue is found in all tissues and organs of the body. Over 10 billion nerve cells (neurons) and innumerable nerve fibers are required to accomplish the tremendous task of initiating and transmitting impulses throughout the body. These signals cause movements of muscles, secretion of glands, and maintain, with the endocrine system, the homeostasis of the body by sensing changes in the external and internal environments. This information allows the body to adjust to these environmental factors and thus maintain an equilibrium among its various organ systems.

DIVISIONS

Anatomically the nervous system is divided into three main divisions. (1) The central nervous system (**CNS**) consists of the brain and spinal cord enclosed in bone, i.e., the skull and vertebral column (discussed in Chapter 12); (2) the peripheral nervous system (**PNS**); and (3) the autonomic nervous system (**ANS**), a subdivision of the PNS.

PERIPHERAL NERVOUS SYSTEM

The peripheral nervous system lies outside the CNS and consists of nerves and their special endings, and ganglia. **Nerves** are collections of processes (**axons**) whose nerve cell bodies are usually within the CNS. Nerves leave the CNS in pairs, one nerve for each side of the body. Emerging from the brain are the 12 pairs of **cranial nerves.** Those arising from the spinal cord are the 31 pairs of **spinal nerves.**

In addition to nerve fibers, the PNS contains clusters of neurons, the **ganglia**, which are surrounded by connective tissue capsules. These are two types: (1) the **spinal or sensory ganglion,** a fusiform swelling on each dorsal (sensory) root of spinal nerves; and (2) the **autonomic ganglia,** contained either in two parallel chains of connective tissue, the **sympathetic chain ganglia,** extending along the anterior surface of the vertebrae, or as small, poorly **encapsulated parasympathetic ganglia** near or within various organs.

Afferent and Efferent Fibers

Functionally the PNS is divided into two types of fibers, **sensory or afferent fibers** (meaning, to carry toward the CNS) and **motor or efferent fibers** (meaning to carry away from the CNS). The **afferent division** consists of nerve fibers that convey information (impulses) from **receptors,** e.g., in skin, organs, and special senses, to the CNS. Those sensory fibers, distributed to the body wall and limbs, e.g., skin, muscles, and bone, are called **somatic** (Gk. soma, body) **afferents.** Those innervating the viscera, e.g., organs and glands, are called **visceral afferents.**

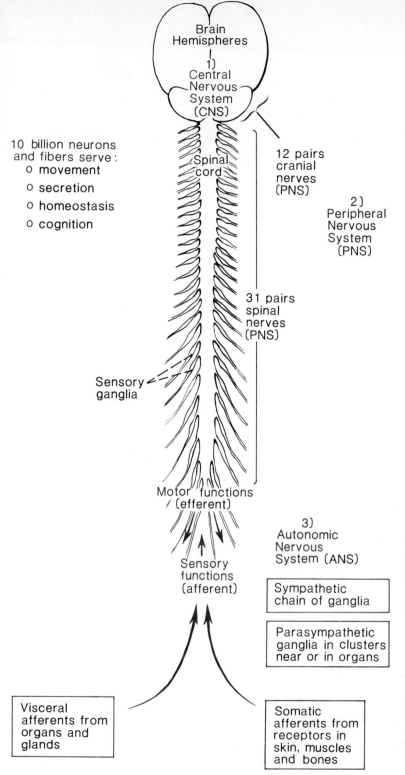

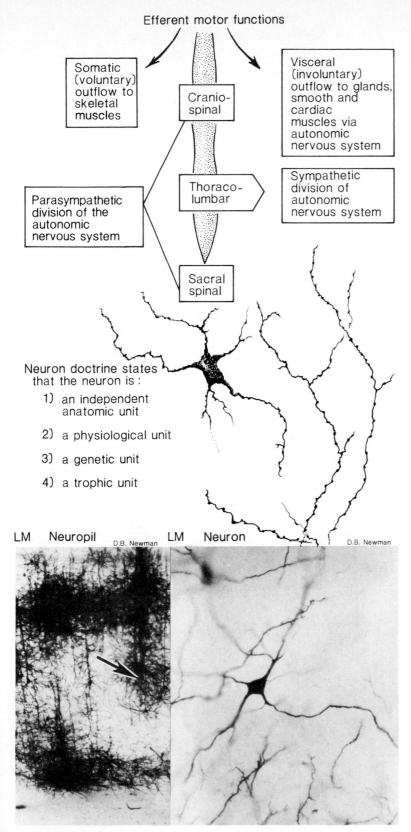

Efferent motor functions

Somatic (voluntary) outflow to skeletal muscles

Cranio-spinal

Visceral (involuntary) outflow to glands, smooth and cardiac muscles via autonomic nervous system

Thoraco-lumbar

Sympathetic division of autonomic nervous system

Parasympathetic division of the autonomic nervous system

Sacral spinal

Neuron doctrine states that the neuron is:

1) an independent anatomic unit

2) a physiological unit

3) a genetic unit

4) a trophic unit

LM   Neuropil   D.B. Newman   LM   Neuron   D.B. Newman

The **efferent parts** of the PNS are **motor** in function, i.e., they cause muscles to contract and glands to secrete. **Somatic (voluntary) efferent** fibers arise in the spinal cord and end on skeletal muscles. **Visceral (involuntary) efferents** comprise most of the autonomic nervous system (ANS). They convey impulses from the CNS to smooth and cardiac muscles, causing them to contract, and to glands, stimulating them to secrete. If their cells of origin are in the thoracic and upper lumbar levels of the spinal cord, they belong to the **thoracolumbar division** of the ANS, or better known as the **sympathetic division.** Those arising from certain cranial nerves and the sacral spinal nerves are the **craniospinal** or **parasympathetic division.**

Most organs are innervated by both divisions, which usually are antagonistic to each other. For example, parasympathetic (vagus) impulses to the heart cause reduction in the heart rate, while sympathetic stimulation accelerates the heart beat.

THE NEURON DOCTRINE

In 1891 the then known facts of the anatomy and physiology of neurons were incorporated into a theory by Waldeyer, a German anatomist, and verified by Cajal, a Spanish neurologist. This theory became known as the **Neuron Theory or Doctrine.** It was essentially an extension of the earlier cell theory of Schleiden and Schwann as it applied to nervous tissue.

Briefly, the present version of the theory states: (1) Each nerve cell with its axon and dendrite(s) is an **independent anatomic unit** of the nervous system. It has contiguity by synapses with other neurons but no physical continuity. (2) The neuron also is a **physiological unit.** Only through neurons is an impulse detected and transmitted by chains of such units. Other nervous tissue cells, i.e., neuroglia, can neither receive nor transmit a nervous signal. (3) The neuron is a **genetic** (developmental) **unit.** A neuroblast gives rise to a single nerve cell and its processes. (4) The nerve cell is a **trophic** (meaning, to nourish) **unit.** When an axon is severed from the cell body, the distal portion degenerates while the proximal part survives and regenerates because it still is attached to and nourished by the cell body. These tenets have been proven correct so often that Waldeyer's theory is no longer simply a working hypothesis—it is now accepted as a fact, a law. Therefore it is quite appropriate to call it the **Neuron Doctrine.**

THE NEURON

The neuron is a unique cell capable of receiving a variety of signals about its external and internal milieu. It then conducts and transmits this information as an impulse to an effector organ for an appropriate response. To accomplish this complex task, the nerve cell consists of (1) usually many short, branching processes, the **dendrites**; (2) a single, often very long, **axon** with few branches; and (3) a large cell body or **perikaryon** (Gk. peri, around; karyon, nucleus). Dendrites conduct impulses **toward** the cell body, while the axon transmits signals **away from** the perikaryon towards the effector region or organ.

Morphological Classification

The number of cell processes provides a method of classifying neurons. A cell with a single process attached to the cell body is a **unipolar neuron.** Yet during development these neurons are bipolar, with a process growing from each pole of the cell body. Later the two processes join and a single T-shaped extension projects from the cell surface. One end is directed toward the periphery and the other toward the central nervous system. These cells may also be considered to be **pseudounipolar** because initially they had a dendrite and an axon that later fused and then separated a short distance from the cell body as a peripheral extension and a proximal process. In other words, there were always two processes—they simply became united in the later stages of development. Such neurons are found in the **sensory (spinal) ganglia** of the spinal cord and in most of the cranial ganglia.

Bipolar neurons consist of two processes, a dendrite and an axon. **Neuroblasts** are mostly bipolar as are the adult neurons of the **special senses,** e.g., retina, cochlear (hearing) and vestibular (equilibrium) ganglia, and the olfactory epithelium.

Most neurons are **multipolar,** i.e., they have a single axon but more than one dendrite. Most neurons of the **brain and spinal cord** are multipolar with many short dendrites.

Perikaryon

The perikaryon or **nerve cell body** varies in size from 4 μm of the granule cells of the cerebellum, to over 135 μm of the motor neurons of the spinal cord. Its relatively large, **light-staining nucleus** (2–8 μm) has a prominent dark-staining **nucleolus.** Under the LM the most distinctive features are the many dark-staining **Nissl bodies** which, under the EM, are identified as aggregates of **rER**—sites for protein synthesis. Otherwise the contents of the cell body consist of the usual **cell organelles,** such as a well-developed Golgi apparatus, many elongated mitochondria, numerous lysosomes, a considerable number of microtubules and microfilaments, and lipofuscin

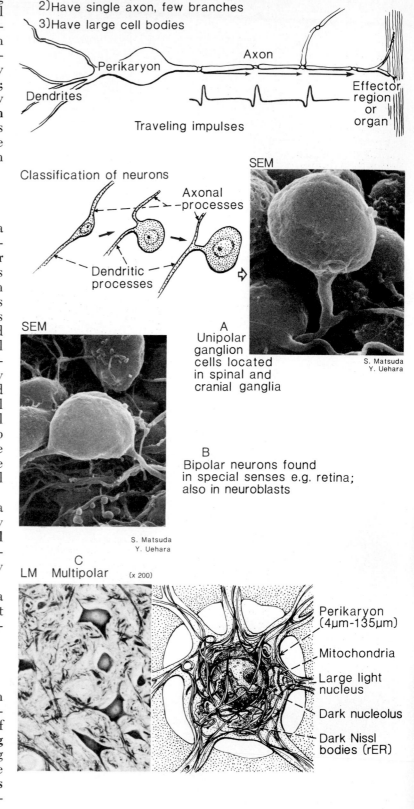

Characteristics of neurons:
1) Have dendrites with many short branches
2) Have single axon, few branches
3) Have large cell bodies

Perikaryon

Axon

Dendrites

Effector region or organ

Traveling impulses

Classification of neurons

Axonal processes

Dendritic processes

SEM

A
Unipolar ganglion cells located in spinal and cranial ganglia

S. Matsuda
Y. Uehara

SEM

B
Bipolar neurons found in special senses e.g. retina; also in neuroblasts

S. Matsuda
Y. Uehara

C
LM Multipolar (x 200)

Perikaryon (4μm-135μm)

Mitochondria

Large light nucleus

Dark nucleolus

Dark Nissl bodies (rER)

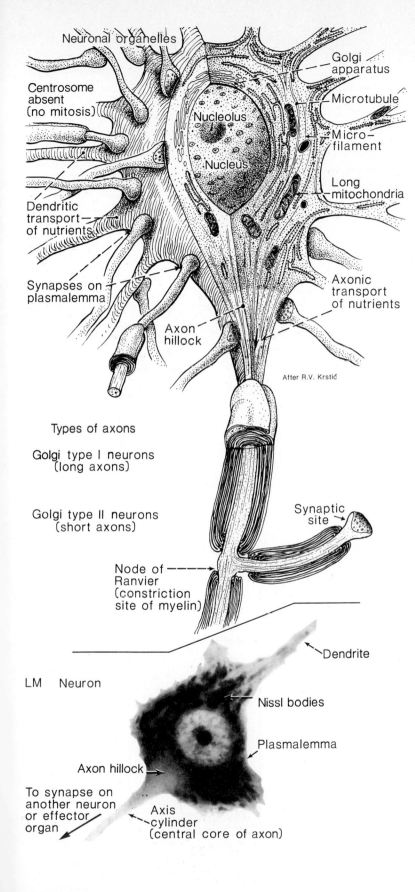

Neuronal organelles

Golgi apparatus

Centrosome absent (no mitosis)

Microtubule

Nucleolus

Micro-filament

Nucleus

Long mitochondria

Dendritic transport of nutrients

Axonic transport of nutrients

Synapses on plasmalemma

After R.V. Krstić

Axon hillock

Types of axons

Golgi type I neurons (long axons)

Golgi type II neurons (short axons)

Synaptic site

Node of Ranvier (constriction site of myelin)

LM   Neuron

Dendrite

Nissl bodies

Plasmalemma

Axon hillock

To synapse on another neuron or effector organ

Axis cylinder (central core of axon)

pigment. The latter is especially prominent in the nerve cells of the elderly. Absent are the centrosomes, which reflects the fact that neurons are incapable of mitosis and therefore **cannot reproduce.** Once a nerve cell dies, it is not replaced. Furthermore, at birth or shortly thereafter, the total inventory of neurons is established, which then gradually diminishes throughout life.

As a receptor center, the **plasmalemma** of the cell body participates in a great number of **synapses** which transmit inhibitory and excitatory signals generated by other neurons. As the **trophic center,** the cell body **nourishes** the processes by axonic and dendritic transport of nutrients and oxygen. Table 11.1 tabulates other distinctive features.

Cell Processes

All neurons have cytoplasmic processes with varying degrees of branchings, extending from the perikaryon for various distances. The **single, usually long branch** that carries impulses **away** from the cell body is the **axon.** The relatively **short dendrites** with **many branches** convey impulses **toward** the cell body.

AXON The single **axon** arises from an elevated cone of the perikaryon, the **axon hillock.** The axon gives off a few branches, which arise as right angle collaterals at constriction sites (**nodes of Ranvier**) of the fatty **myelin sheath** that surrounds the axon in myelinated neurons. The branches end synaptically on neurons in the immediate vicinity. These collateral branches are about the same diameter as the axon itself.

The axon proper may extend highly variable distances from the cell body, ranging from a few millimeters to a meter or more. It may pass through a **fiber tract** in the brain or spinal cord, or through a **peripheral nerve** to end in a **synapse** on another neuron, or on an effector organ, such as a muscle or gland. Neurons with these long axons are termed **Golgi type I cells.** If the axons are short, terminating on nearby neurons, they are designated as **Golgi type II neurons.**

Under the LM the **axon hillock** is a relatively unstained, **clear area** because of the **absence** of the deeply basophilic **Nissl bodies.** Particularly in larger neurons, it appears as if a barrier may exist between the axon hillock and the cytoplasm of the neuron which screens out the relatively large, dark-staining Nissl bodies.

The plasmalemma of the perikaryon continues as a covering over the axon, which is now called the **axolemma.** It encloses the thin layer of protoplasm of the axon, the **axoplasm,** and the central core of the axon, the **axis cylinder.** The axon may or may not be covered by a myelin sheath. The axon terminates by an extensive arborization, the **telodendron,** on effector organs or regions. Because of this extensive branching, a single axon may innervate many muscle fibers or secretory cells of glands.

From EM micrographs the following observations about **axons** are of special interest. The **abundant microtubules** of the cell body change their orientation and flow into the axon hillock and form bundles as they enter the initial segment of the axon. Their numbers gradually decrease distally. The axon has **no ribosomes or rER** but considerable **sER. Neurofilaments** are numerous, especially in the larger axons. For some unknown reason they appear to increase after trauma to the axon. The long, thin **mitochondria** are dispersed along the axoplasm but are concentrated in the **axonal terminal.**

DENDRITES As their name implies, **dendrites** resemble branches of a tree. They are tapered processes with many tiny, rough projections or spines called **gemmules,** which are often sites of axodendritic synapses. Their extensive and profuse arborizations **terminate near the perikaryon** and never extend any great distance, as do axons. Hence, dendrites of neurons of the CNS are not found in the PNS, as are axons. Typically, dendrites are **nonmyelinated;** however, the larger processes may be finely myelinated.

The ultramicroscopic features of dendrites are summarized in Table 11.1. Since **dendrites** are direct protoplasmic continuations of the perikaryon, they contain most of the **inclusions and organelles** found in the cell body. Exceptions include fewer neurofilaments and lysosomes, a poorly developed Golgi apparatus, more sER, and an increase in free ribosomes.

COMPARISON OF AXONS AND DENDRITES Structural differences between axons and dendrites are tabulated in Table 11.1. Perhaps the most striking features are: In **axons**

1. **Nissl bodies** (rER + free ribosomes) do not extend into the axon hillock or axon proper; however, they extend throughout **dendrites.**
2. **Myelin** usually surrounds them; in dendrites it is absent.
3. A **constant diameter** is maintained throughout their length; dendrites are tapered.
4. Branching occurs only at terminals and at some nodes; **dendrites branch profusely** throughout their length.
5. Their surfaces are smooth, while dendrites have roughened surfaces due to **spines** (gemmules).
6. Many **presynaptic vesicles** are present; dendrites have none.

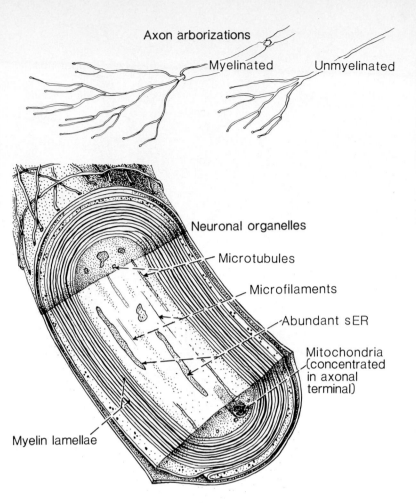

Axon arborizations — Myelinated — Unmyelinated

Neuronal organelles
— Microtubules
— Microfilaments
— Abundant sER
— Mitochondria (concentrated in axonal terminal)

Myelin lamellae

	Comparison	
	Axons	Dendrites
1) Nissl bodies	absent	present
2) Microtubules	proximal segment only	present throughout
3) Microfilaments	abundant e.g. in hillock	few
4) Myelin	present	absent
5) Shape	large, uniform diameter	small, tapering in diameter
6) Branching	limited to nodes and terminal	profuse throughout
7) Organelles	few	more
8) Gemmules (spines)	absent	many
9) Presynaptic vesicles	present	absent

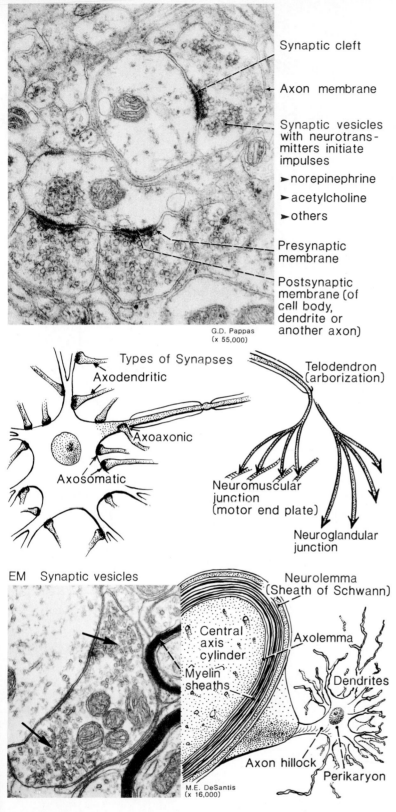

Synaptic cleft

Axon membrane

Synaptic vesicles with neurotransmitters initiate impulses

➤norepinephrine

➤acetylcholine

➤others

Presynaptic membrane

Postsynaptic membrane (of cell body, dendrite or another axon)

G.D. Pappas
(x 55,000)

Types of Synapses

Axodendritic

Axoaxonic

Axosomatic

Telodendron (arborization)

Neuromuscular junction (motor end plate)

Neuroglandular junction

EM Synaptic vesicles

Neurolemma (Sheath of Schwann)

Central axis cylinder

Axolemma

Myelin sheaths

Dendrites

Axon hillock

Perikaryon

M.E. DeSantis
(x 16,000)

Synapses

A **synapse** is a junction or site of stimulus transfer of one neuron with another. Functionally, it is the location for **chemical transmission,** i.e., where an impulse from the axon of one neuron creates a chemical signal in the dendrite, axon, or cell body of a second neuron. There is **no protoplasmic continuity** between these neurons. A **synaptic cleft,** about 20 nm wide, separates the two cell membranes.

A **neurotransmitter** is released from the preceding cell into this cleft, which initiates the impulse. Such chemical synapses are found in nerves of the PNS, CNS, and ANS. These chemical neurotransmitters, e.g., **norepinephrine, acetylcholine,** and others, diffuse across the cleft, **depolarizing the cell membrane.** This ionic shift generates a nerve impulse that will be propagated along the second neuron. Under the EM this neurotransmitter is seen located in small **synaptic vesicles,** a characteristic of the terminal **boutons** (Fr., buttons) of the axon. Its membrane is called presynaptic membrane, while the membrane of the dendrite or perikaryon is the postsynaptic membrane.

Synapses have a variety of shapes, ranging from simple contacts of an axon with a dendrite, to complexes of synaptic end bulbs with many morphological variations. While synapses are most common between an axon and a dendrite, called **axodendritic synapses,** they are also found between the axon and the cell body, called **axosomatic synapses.** In a few cases synapses exist between two axons and are **axoaxonic.**

A single dendrite and cell body of a given neuron may receive as many as 15,000 synapses. A single **axon** may terminate on many synapses since it has an extensive arborization at its terminal, the **telodendron.** If the termination of a motor fiber is on a skeletal muscle fiber, it is called a **motor end-plate or a neuromuscular junction.** If the motor axon ends on a gland, it is called a **neuroglandular junction.** Both are basically similar to synapses between neurons. They will be discussed in later chapters.

Peripheral Nerves

Each **nerve fiber** is composed of a central **axis cylinder** covered by a delicate plasma membrane, the **axolemma,** and surrounded by one or more sheaths. All of the individual fibers have an outer, thin cellular **neurolemma, or sheath of Schwann,** which invests the axon beyond the axon hillock. The larger peripheral nerve fibers are also enclosed by a fatty covering called the **myelin sheath,** which lies within the neurolemma. The axons of smallest diameter may be either finely myelinated or the myelin sheath may be entirely lacking, i.e., they are unmyelinated.

11898

INVESTMENTS In gross anatomy one identifies peripheral nerves by their rather glistening, tough, connective tissue investment. This is the **epineurium** composed of collagenous fibers containing small blood vessels. Under the LM nerve fibers can be seen arranged in bundles called **fascicles.** These bundles are also surrounded by a connective membrane much thinner than the epineurium, the **perineurium.** Further LM examination of the fascicles reveals that each individual nerve fiber is surrounded by a delicate reticular tissue investment, the **endoneurium.**

Peripheral nerves have a rich blood supply. Frequent anastomosing capillary plexuses can be seen entering the epineurium to supply the underlying nervous elements.

NODES OF RANVIER Under the LM, the myelin sheath can be seen to be constricted at intervals by the overlying neurolemma, like a string of link sausages. These indentations are called the **nodes of Ranvier.** While these nodes are equidistant for a given fiber, their distance varies greatly depending on the width of the fiber, i.e., the thicker the fiber, the longer the internodal spaces. These nodes are important because they represent the **sites of depolarizations** and the origin of the right angle branches. Also, mitochondria collect in the area, suggesting a higher level of metabolic activity at the node, which in large, myelinated nerves is where depolarization occurs. In such nerves the impulse jumps from node to node. This is **saltatory** (L. saltare, to jump) conduction, which is much faster than continuous conduction. Therefore large, heavily myelinated nerves have the highest velocity of nerve impulse transmission, i.e., 120 m/s, as compared to 0.5 m/s for very small unmyelinated fibers.

SENSORY NERVE ENDINGS (RECEPTORS) Decision making by the brain is possible because of the information it is constantly receiving from **sensory receptors** about our internal and external environments. There are a variety of these information gatherers scattered throughout the epithelia, connective tissues, muscles, and joints. They mediate **somesthetic sensations,** that is, stimuli from the body. Another group of receptors occurs in specialized areas of the head and are associated with the **special senses,** i.e., hearing, equilibrium, sight, smell, and taste. These are discussed in Chapter 26.

SOMESTHETIC RECEPTORS The **somesthetic receptors** may be subdivided: (1) **Exteroceptors,** which receive sensations near or in the skin, such as pain, heat, cold, pressure, and touch. (2) **Interoceptors** receive stimuli from within the body, arising from the viscera and blood vessels. These sensations include pain, pressure or fullness, and thermal changes. (3) Last, the **proprioceptors** relay information to the

LM   Fascicles of nerve fibers

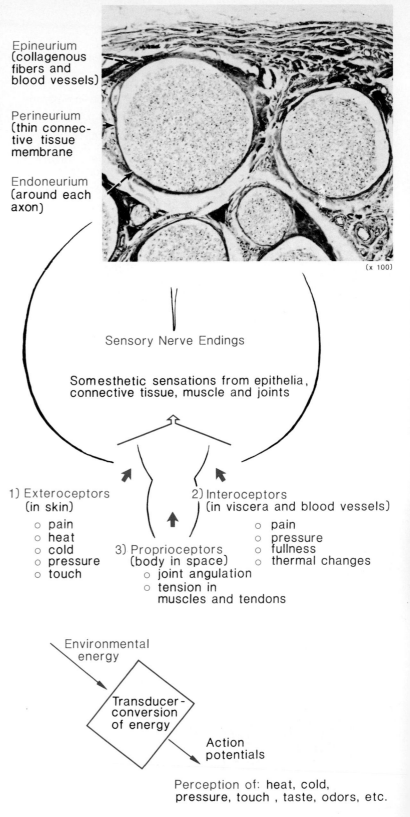

Epineurium (collagenous fibers and blood vessels)

Perineurium (thin connective tissue membrane

Endoneurium (around each axon)

(x 100)

Sensory Nerve Endings

Somesthetic sensations from epithelia, connective tissue, muscle and joints

1) Exteroceptors (in skin)
- pain
- heat
- cold
- pressure
- touch

2) Interoceptors (in viscera and blood vessels)
- pain
- pressure
- fullness
- thermal changes

3) Proprioceptors (body in space)
- joint angulation
- tension in muscles and tendons

Environmental energy

Transducer - conversion of energy

Action potentials

Perception of: heat, cold, pressure, touch, taste, odors, etc.

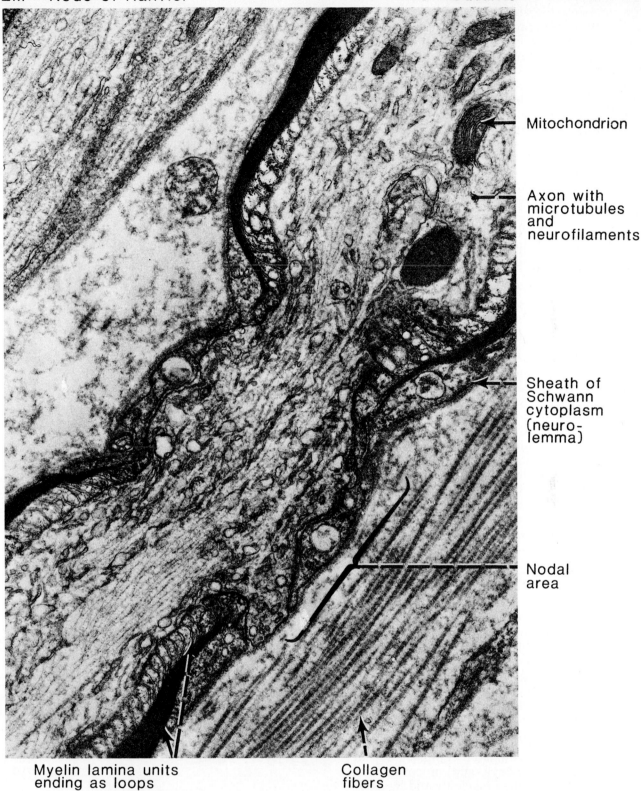

Mitochondrion

Axon with microtubules and neurofilaments

Sheath of Schwann cytoplasm (neuro-lemma)

Nodal area

Myelin lamina units ending as loops

Collagen fibers

As viewed transversely in this TEM micrograph, a node of Ranvier reveals electron-dense laminae of the myelin sheath gradually reduced in number and in size, by a peeling-off of the individual laminae as spiral loops. These spiral processes are covered with cytoplasm from Schwann cells. Gradually the myelin is entirely lost at the edge of the nodal area with only a thin layer of Schwann cell cytoplasm to bridge the node and cover the naked axon. The exposed axonal exoplasm contains many cell organelles, such as mitochondria, sER, microtubules, and neurofilaments. Abundant collagenous fibrils are seen in the lower right region.

11499

brain concerning the relation of the body or its parts in space, the angulation of joints, and the tension of muscles and tendons.

All receptors perform like **transducers,** i.e., they convert one form of energy in the environment into action potentials in neurons. For example, changes in **thermal energy** are interpreted as heat or cold; **mechanical energy** may be perceived by the brain as pressure or touch and **chemical energy** as taste or odor.

Traditionally each receptor has been assigned a particular sensation, e.g., touch, pain, heat, cold, etc. While this concept of **receptor specificity** is valid for many receptors, especially the special senses, it does not necessarily hold for cutaneous receptors. We are all aware that we can discriminate a stimulus being either cold or hot but when the thermal receptors are excessively stimulated, the brain interprets the stimulus as pain.

In addition to classifications of receptors on the basis of their sensory modalities or their location in the body, they are also grouped as **free (naked)** or **encapsulated nerve endings.**

FREE NERVE ENDINGS Free nerve endings are nothing more than **filamentous terminations** of afferent nerve fibers stripped of their neurolemmal and myelin sheaths and are therefore called **naked or unsheathed axons.** Most of them **mediate pain** sensations and terminate among the cells of the **stratum germinativium** of the epidermis, or around the base of hairs, as peritrichal fibers. Other free receptors end as small, **expanded disks (of Merkel)** that lie adjacent to epidermal cells or hair follicles. Some bare nerve endings terminate as pain or touch receptors on the cornea, mucous membranes, joint surfaces, and the periosteum.

ENCAPSULATED SENSORY NERVE ENDINGS Encapsulated nerve endings have a special connective tissue **capsule** of varying thickness **surrounding a naked axon or axons.** The capsule is usually characterized by its **lamellated structure** but is extremely variable in its degree of encapsulation. For example, it varies from a few thin, loose connective tissue layers around an **end bulb of Krause,** to the many concentric, robust connective tissue lamellae of the **Pacinian corpuscle.**

Krause's End Bulb Krause's end bulb is the simplest of the encapsulated receptors. They are found in the conjunctiva and mucous membranes, especially of the oral cavity and lips, dermis, glans penis, and clitoris. It is a small (about 50 μm), oval or spherical **bulb** with a thin, **loose lamellated capsule** of collagenous fibers. A small, myelinated, afferent nerve fiber loses its myelin sheath as it enters the capsule. The bare axon usually terminates in a number of branches that intertwine into a loose ball-like mass called a **glomerulus.**

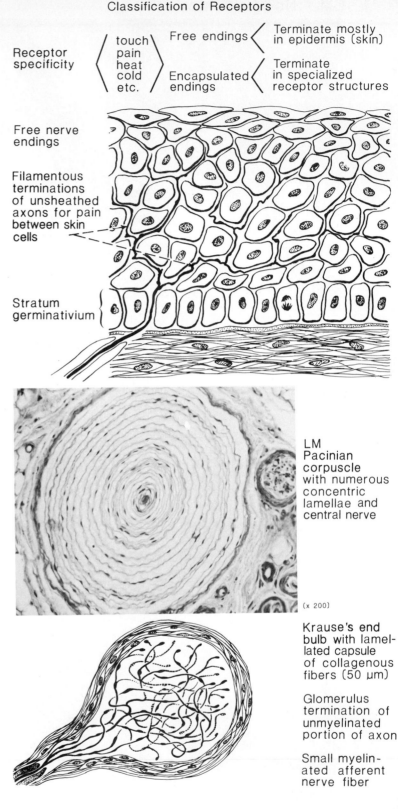

Classification of Receptors

Receptor specificity { touch pain heat cold etc. } Free endings < Terminate mostly in epidermis (skin) Encapsulated endings < Terminate in specialized receptor structures

Free nerve endings

Filamentous terminations of unsheathed axons for pain between skin cells

Stratum germinativium

LM Pacinian corpuscle with numerous concentric lamellae and central nerve

(x 200)

Krause's end bulb with lamellated capsule of collagenous fibers (50 μm)

Glomerulus termination of unmyelinated portion of axon

Small myelinated afferent nerve fiber

Encapsulated Nerve Endings:

Krause's end bulb	— general touch & pressure
Meissner's corpuscle	— touch discrimination
Pacinian corpuscle	— vibration & deep pressure
Ruffini ending	— position & motion
Golgi tendon organ	— muscle tension
Muscle spindle	— muscle control

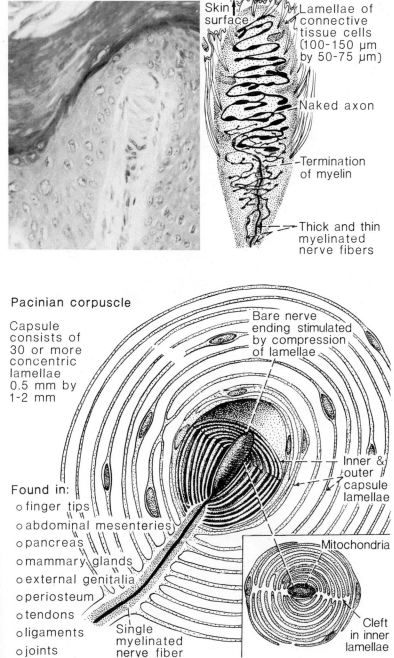

LM
Meissner's corpuscle – tactile receptor in dermal papillae

Skin surface

Lamellae of connective tissue cells (100-150 μm by 50-75 μm)

Naked axon

Termination of myelin

Thick and thin myelinated nerve fibers

Pacinian corpuscle

Capsule consists of 30 or more concentric lamellae 0.5 mm by 1-2 mm

Bare nerve ending stimulated by compression of lamellae

Inner & outer capsule lamellae

Mitochondria

Cleft in inner lamellae

Single myelinated nerve fiber

Found in:
- finger tips
- abdominal mesenteries
- pancreas
- mammary glands
- external genitalia
- periosteum
- tendons
- ligaments
- joints

Although historically these end bulbs have been accepted as receptors of cold, this is now seriously questioned since many areas of skin are devoid of the end bulbs yet cold is detected here. Many authorities now believe these structures are primarily **mechanoreceptors**, i.e., they detect touch and pressure sensations.

Meissner's Corpuscle Meissner's tactile **corpuscle** is a more complex encapsulated nerve ending. It is an oval, cylindrical structure about 100–150 μm long and 50–75 μm wide. It consists of loose **stacks of lamellae** of flattened connective tissue cells (perhaps Schwann cells) surrounding one or two naked axons, which follow a tortuous course among the connective tissue cells and fibers. Most of the axons are from myelinated fibers which shed their myelin sheaths as they enter the corpuscle. Other axons are unmyelinated fibers.

Meissner's corpuscles are sensitive, **tactile receptors.** They are concentrated in the **dermal papillae** of the **finger and toe tips,** palms of the hands, and soles of the feet. They serve as a **discriminative touch organ** enabling one to accurately distinguish very slight differences in roughness, sharpness, size, shape, and texture of an object by passing it over the epidermal ridges, especially of the finger tips. These tactile corpuscles may be drastically reduced in number with age.

Pacinian Corpuscle The **Pacinian corpuscle** is the largest of the encapsulated nerve endings, often reaching a length of 1–2 mm and about 0.5 mm in diameter; therefore they are visible to the unaided eye. The prominent capsule is formed by **30 or more concentric rings** of connective tissue fibers with an abundance of tissue fluid between the layers. In a transverse section these lamellae resemble a cut onion. Each corpuscle is supplied by a single myelinated fiber which loses its myelin as it enters the corpuscle. The bare axon extends through the center of the structure to terminate in a spray of delicate, knoblike branches.

These corpuscles are best seen beneath the **dermis** of the fingers, in abdominal **mesenteries,** pancreas, mammary glands, external genitalia, periosteum, tendons, ligaments, and joints. They **respond to vibrations** and **to deep pressure.** They are especially sensitive to limb or body displacement, thus signaling mechanical deformations, an important **proprioceptive function.**

Ruffini Endings **Ruffini endings** are less lamellated than Pacinian or Meissner's corpuscles. They are **spindle-shaped** structures about 1 mm long and 0.1 mm wide. They are surrounded by a loose connective tissue capsule that is continuous with the endoneural sheath of afferent fibers. As the myelinated sensory fibers enter the capsule they lose their myelin sheaths. The axons immediately break up into a spray of branches with terminal knobs that intermesh with the collagenous fibers and fibroblasts that form the connective tissue core of the nerve endings.

When Ruffini described these nerve endings in 1894, he simply indicated that they were loosely encapsulated nerve endings, intermediate in size between the Krause's end bulbs and the Pacinian corpuscles. He assigned to them a **tactile function,** intermediate between Meissner's (light touch) corpuscle and Pacinian (deep pressure) corpuscles. Later, on questionable evidence, these endings were thought to be specific receptors of heat, a misconception that still persists. Present thinking favors the idea that "these endings are now regarded as one of the commonest forms of slowly adapting **mechanical receptors.**" In other words, they are **joint proprioreceptors** that respond to mechanical distortions of limbs or the body, as well as reacting to changes in position and motion, a very important **proprioceptive** function.

Golgi Tendon Organs **Golgi tendon organs** resemble Ruffini endings. They are small (about 1 mm long) fusiform bodies enveloped in a thin capsule of loose collagenous fibers and cells. The single afferent nerve fiber that enters the end organ immediately loses its myelin and then breaks up into sprays of naked branches with club-shaped endings that become entwined with the connective tissue cells and fibers. They are found in **tendons** near musculotendonous junctions and in **aponeuroses** of muscles.

These tendonous endings are **stimulated reflexly** by tension arising within the muscle. Their response is to inhibit excessive contractions. For example, upon vigorous muscular contraction, the tendon organ is reflexly stimulated. The reflex causes appropriate motor neurons in the spinal cord to be inhibited and further muscular contraction is prevented, thus **avoiding muscle damage** from over exertion.

MUSCLE SPINDLES Muscle spindles are found in nearly all skeletal muscles. They are especially numerous in muscles involved in fine, delicate movements, e.g., intrinsic muscles of the hand and muscles of the eye. They respond to dynamic changes in muscles during contractions, acting as **mechanoreceptors** (stretch receptors) similar to miniature strain and pressure gauges. When spindles are stimulated, their **afferent (sensory) output,** from annulospiral and flower-spray endings, travels to the spinal cord and syn-

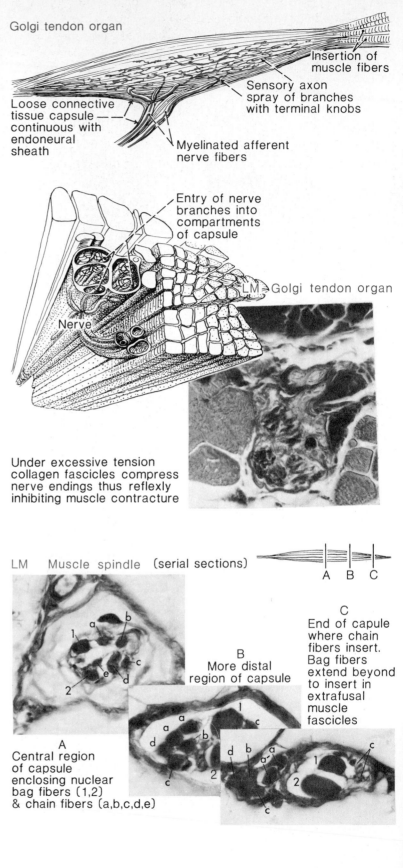

Golgi tendon organ

Insertion of muscle fibers

Sensory axon spray of branches with terminal knobs

Loose connective tissue capsule — continuous with endoneural sheath

Myelinated afferent nerve fibers

Entry of nerve branches into compartments of capsule

LM Golgi tendon organ

Nerve

Under excessive tension collagen fascicles compress nerve endings thus reflexly inhibiting muscle contracture

LM   Muscle spindle   (serial sections)

A B C

C
End of capule where chain fibers insert. Bag fibers extend beyond to insert in extrafusal muscle fascicles

B
More distal region of capsule

A
Central region of capsule enclosing nuclear bag fibers (1,2) & chain fibers (a,b,c,d,e)

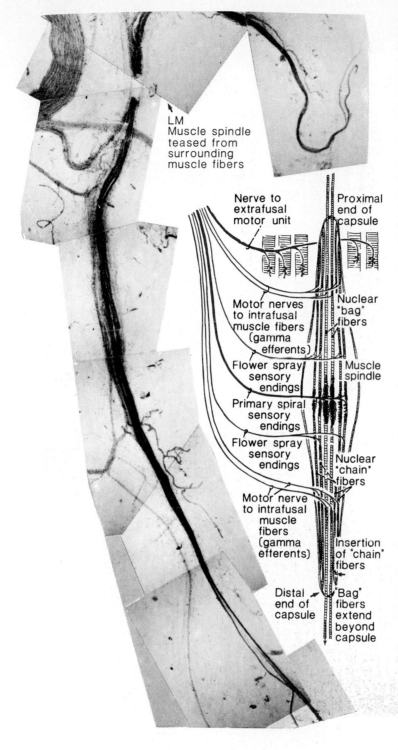

LM
Muscle spindle teased from surrounding muscle fibers

Nerve to extrafusal motor unit

Proximal end of capsule

Motor nerves to intrafusal muscle fibers (gamma efferents)

Nuclear "bag" fibers

Muscle spindle

Flower spray sensory endings

Primary spiral sensory endings

Flower spray sensory endings

Nuclear "chain" fibers

Motor nerve to intrafusal muscle fibers (gamma efferents)

Insertion of "chain" fibers

Distal end of capsule

"Bag" fibers extend beyond capsule

apses with the motor neurons supplying corresponding motor units in a muscle (motor units are discussed on page 204). The efferent (motor) fibers transport impulses back to **muscle motor units** causing them to contract. Thus muscle motor units are coordinated for **on-and-off contractile tension** upon muscle tendons, perhaps protecting the muscle from damage due to excessive stretching.

In their simplest action, muscle spindles act in **stretch reflexes,** as in the **knee jerk.** When the taut patellar tendon is struck sharply, the quadriceps femoris muscle is slightly stretched causing reflex contraction of the muscle to move the leg. Thus the muscle reflexly shortens. Hence, muscle spindles monitor the contractility of motor units and **control the length and tonus** of skeletal muscles.

Each muscle spindle is about 2 mm in length and 0.5 mm wide and is composed of several miniature, specialized skeletal muscle fibers enclosed in a fusiform, loose connective tissue capsule. These are called **intrafusal** fibers because they lie within the spindle (L. fusus, spindle). Each muscle's population of spindles is located near the center of the muscle's fascicular mass and is oriented parallel to the regular muscle fibers, the **extrafusal fibers.** Microscopically, two populations of intrafusal fibers are recognized. The large diameter **"bag"** fibers have an expanded noncontractile central region, called the bag, where nuclei aggregate. There are about one to four bag fibers within each spindle. They extend beyond both ends of spindle capsules to **insert in parallel** with **extrafusal muscle fascicles.** The other fiber type is more numerous (two to ten). They are smaller in diameter and extend the length of spindle capsules to **insert at the ends.** They have no bag area, and their elongated nuclei are arranged in linear fashion along the length of the fibers. Hence their name, **nuclear chain fibers.**

Acting together, muscle spindles, neurotendinous Golgi organs, joint receptors (Ruffini endings), Pacinian corpuscles, and some free nerve endings comprise a **group of proprioceptors.** Except for the free endings, they all exhibit a similar, encapsulated design, suggesting perhaps a common developmental origin. Each responds to specific physical stimuli serving to **measure** the **magnitude of physical forces** or other events impinging upon or within the body. These endings initiate impulses that are coded to carry specific sensory information to the CNS.

Finally, the chemoreceptors for taste and olfaction are discussed with the oral or nasal cavities, respectively. (Receptors are summarized in Table 11.2.)

MOTOR NERVE ENDINGS (EFFECTORS)

Motor Unit As a large motor axon approaches the skeletal muscle it innervates, it terminates by branching into many small endings. Each branch will supply a single muscle fiber. Such a motor neuron and the cluster of muscle fibers it innervates constitutes a **motor unit.** The muscle fibers of motor units interdigitate with those of neighboring motor units, thus providing a smooth, **even tension on tendons.**

Motor End-plate The specialized site where the motor axon terminates on the sarcolemma of a muscle fiber is the **motor end-plate** or **neuromuscular junction.** As the axon converges on the muscle fiber, it loses its myelin sheath but retains its neurolemmal investment.

Typically, a motor end-plate consists of (1) the expanded, **bulbous terminal part of the axon;** (2) the delicate neurolemma covering the end of the axon; (3) a shallow trough (**primary synaptic cleft**) about 50 nm deep that separates the membranes of the axon and the muscle fiber and is filled with basal laminae of the muscle fibers, and (4) numerous deep folds in the sarcolemma (the **secondary synaptic cleft**) called the **junctional folds.**

TEM micrographs reveal that the expanded synaptic ends of axons are filled with many clear vacuoles, the presynaptic vesicles, each about 40 nm in diameter. In cholinergic neurons, they contain the chemical neurotransmitter, **acetylcholine.** Structures in the postsynaptic motor end-plate include many muscle nuclei (called **sole plate nuclei**), abundant mitochondria, ribosomes, and glycogen particles.

Muscle contraction begins when the motor neuron fires, causing a **release of acetylcholine** from the vesicles. This transmitter substance diffuses through the primary synaptic cleft to **bind to receptor sites** in the junctional folds (secondary synaptic cleft) of the sarcolemma. By this action the sarcolemma is made more permeable to sodium and is **depolarized.** The resulting electrical impulse is carried throughout the muscle cell by the extensive T-tubule system, causing the muscle fiber to contract.

The enzyme **acetylcholinesterase,** sequestered in the junctional folds, hydrolyzes the liberated acetylcholine. As a result, the nervous impulse is terminated, calcium is transported back to the cisternae of the sarcoplasmic reticulum, the muscle membrane is again **polarized,** and the **muscle relaxes.** The motor end-plate is now primed to transmit nerve impulses again.

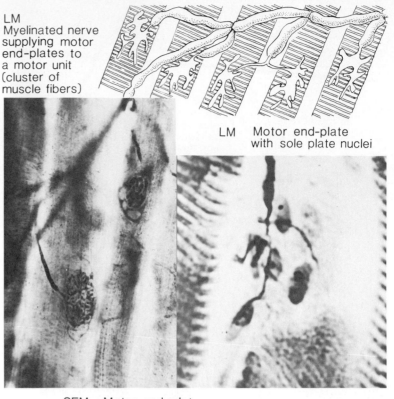

LM Myelinated nerve supplying motor end-plates to a motor unit (cluster of muscle fibers)

LM Motor end-plate with sole plate nuclei

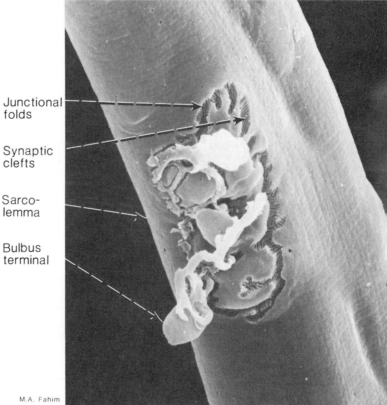

SEM Motor end-plate

Junctional folds

Synaptic clefts

Sarcolemma

Bulbus terminal

M.A. Fahim

Myelination Process

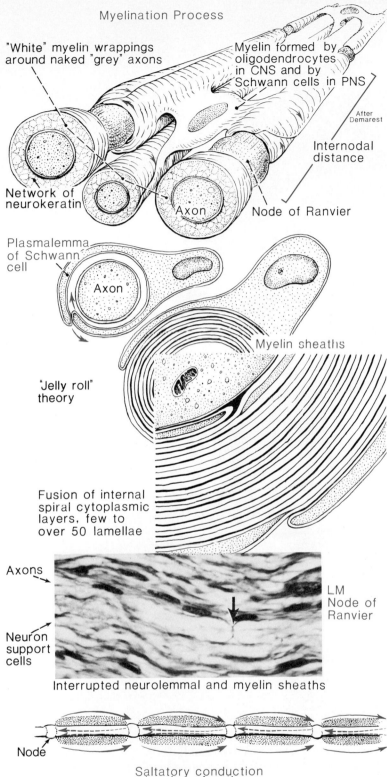

"White" myelin wrappings around naked "grey" axons

Myelin formed by oligodendrocytes in CNS and by Schwann cells in PNS

After Demarest

Internodal distance

Network of neurokeratin

Axon

Node of Ranvier

Plasmalemma of Schwann cell

Axon

Myelin sheaths

"Jelly roll" theory

Fusion of internal spiral cytoplasmic layers, few to over 50 lamellae

Axons

Neuron support cells

LM Node of Ranvier

Interrupted neurolemmal and myelin sheaths

Node

Saltatory conduction – leaping of action potentials from node to node speeds up nervous conduction

Myelination

In the fresh state, most nerves have a white, glistening appearance, while others are lackluster and grey in color. Under the LM, the white fibers reveal an **outer fatty covering** of varying thickness, the **myelin sheath**, hence their name, **myelinated fibers**. The grey fibers lack myelin and are, therefore, called **unmyelinated** or nonmedullated nerves.

Myelination is the process whereby an insulating layer of myelin is wrapped around a naked axon. **Myelin is elaborated** by the neurolemmal (**Schwann**) **cells** in the PNS and by **oligodendrocytes** in the CNS. Since myelin is a lipoprotein complex, the lipid component is removed in routine histological procedures. However, the protein component is preserved as a fine, lacy network around the axon, called **neurokeratin**. Certain fat stains, e.g., osmium tetroxide, preserve (fix) the myelin and stain it black.

During the fourth month of fetal life, myelination in peripheral nerves begins by a **naked axon** coming in contact with the **plasmalemma of a Schwann cell**. As the axon sinks into the cell membrane, a groove is formed whose edges come together over the axon. As the axon is further buried into the cell, the edges fuse to form a **double membrane**, which increases in length as it wraps around the axon.

The dynamics of myelination involve the **rotation of the Schwann cell** and its sheetlike protoplasmic processes **around the axon**, not the reverse. Furthermore, in some axonal nodal segments, the spirals are clockwise, others counterclockwise. The mechanism of spiraling is unknown. However, this wrapping of the sheath around the axon in a "jelly-roll" fashion continues until a certain amount of **myelin is laid down**. It may be a few **lamellae** or over 50, depending on the diameter and length of axon. Only one Schwann cell is involved in myelin synthesis for each internode.

The myelin sheath is not continuous but is **interrupted** at regular intervals by constrictions, the **nodes of Ranvier**, where a minute portion of the **axolemma is exposed** since both the neurolemmal and myelin sheaths are absent. These nodes are not merely anatomical curiosities but have an important function. The exposure of the axon at the node enables an **action potential to leap from node to node** instead of traveling along the entire length of the axolemma, thus greatly **increasing the velocity** of the impulse. Such a transmission of a nerve impulse along a myelinated nerve is called **saltatory conduction**, previously discussed on page 198.

11541

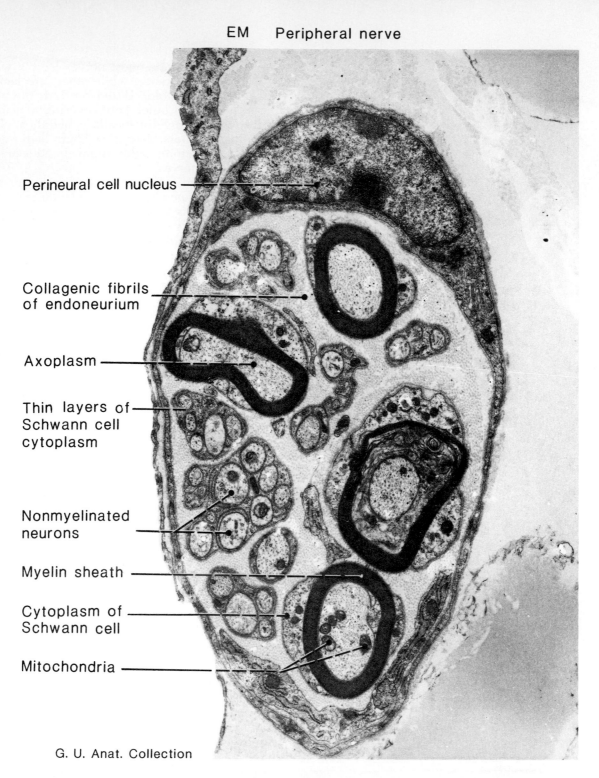

Perineural cell nucleus

Collagenic fibrils
of endoneurium

Axoplasm

Thin layers of
Schwann cell
cytoplasm

Nonmyelinated
neurons

Myelin sheath

Cytoplasm of
Schwann cell

Mitochondria

G. U. Anat. Collection

   Transmission electron micrograph of a cross-section of a nerve fascicle (bundle) showing four axons enclosed in myelin sheaths. The myelin consists of a variable number of regular, parallel, electron-dense, concentric lamellae. The sheath completely surrounds the axoplasm which contains several spherical mitochondria. Externally the meylin is incompletely covered by Schwann cell cytoplasm. The larger axons develop myelin sheaths, while the smaller ones usually do not. Between the myelinated axons are clusters of unmyelinated nerves. Except for their smaller diameter and absence of myelin, they are structurally similar to myelinated fibers.

   Located in the upper part of the micrograph is a large perineurial cell (fibroblast) with a prominent oval nucleus. Its cytoplasmic processes completely surround the nerve fascicle and thus contribute to the blood-nerve barrier which protects nerve fibers from noxious agents.

11485

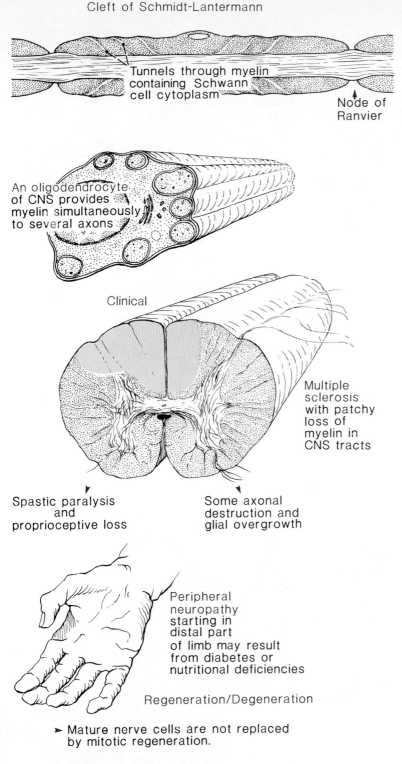

Cleft of Schmidt-Lantermann

Tunnels through myelin containing Schwann cell cytoplasm

Node of Ranvier

An oligodendrocyte of CNS provides myelin simultaneously to several axons

Clinical

Multiple sclerosis with patchy loss of myelin in CNS tracts

Spastic paralysis and proprioceptive loss

Some axonal destruction and glial overgrowth

Peripheral neuropathy starting in distal part of limb may result from diabetes or nutritional deficiencies

Regeneration/Degeneration

► Mature nerve cells are not replaced by mitotic regeneration.

► Peripheral nerves with intact perikaryon regenerate.

Another interruption of a myelin sheath is the **Schmidt-Lantermann clefts.** These are a series of staggered breaks or **funnel-shaped tunnels** in the sheath, connecting the outside and inside of the sheath. From EM micrographs they appear as widened areas between the myelin lamellae where the Schwann cell cytoplasm persists due to incomplete compaction. Their function is uncertain.

In the CNS a glial cell, the **oligodendrocyte,** is responsible for **myelin formation.** Unlike a Schwann cell, which provides myelin to a single internode, an oligodendrocyte may form myelin around **several axons.** This is accomplished by multiple axons becoming embedded in the expansive cytoplasm of an oligodendrocyte. The "jellyroll" process of myelinization then proceeds as in peripheral nerves.

CLINICAL OBSERVATIONS Loss of myelin sheaths is a defect in certain disorders of the CNS, such as **multiple sclerosis (MS).** Its etiology is unknown, and its cure still eludes us. It attacks primarily individuals between the second and fifth decades of life. It is a chronic, remitting disease that often leads to total disability. It **may affect any myelinated tract** causing, for example, partial or complete blindness, mild to severe sensory or motor disorders of limbs, cerebellar incoordination, etc. Its prime pathological lesion is simply a **loss of myelin,** which is **selective and patchy** in its occurrence, hence the term multiple sclerosis, meaning many degenerative lesions. In addition to demyelinization, there will also be **axonal destruction** as well as **overgrowth of glial tissue.** The most frequent symptom of MS is **spastic paralysis** of both legs with some impairment of proprioception and vibratory sense.

Peripheral neuropathy, i.e., any noninflammatory disease of peripheral nerves, and **neuritis,** an inflammatory disorder, are common **degenerative changes in peripheral nerves** that may result in sensory loss, motor weakness, or both. Usually the symptoms appear in the distal part of the limb, such as in the hands or feet, and then proceed proximally. Various nutritional deficiencies, such as **vitamin B deficiency** or **diabetes,** may precipitate such attacks.

Reflex Arc

The anatomical unit of the nervous system is the neuron, while its **basic functional unit,** at lower levels, is the **reflex arc.** The simplest path an impulse follows from its origin, e.g., in a skin receptor, to its termination, perhaps on a skeletal muscle, is a reflex arc. The most basic of these pathways contains only **two neurons.** The first component is an **afferent (sensory) neuron,** which propagates an impulse from the periphery towards the CNS. The second part is an **efferent (motor) neuron** that ends on a muscle or gland.

However, the **three-neuronal reflex arc** is more common. The **first sensory neuron** ends in the **gray matter** as it enters the spinal cord. Here it synapses on a short, **interconnecting neuron**, which in turn conveys the impulse to the third neuron, the out-going **efferent neuron**. This is the usual pattern of the simple reflex arc.

Most actions involve these reflex arcs. An example is the common knee jerk (**stretch reflex**), which is used clinically to test the integrity of the nervous system. When one taps the patellar tendon just below the knee, the limb swings forward. Such a movement is also carried out in the act of kicking. But the **first movement** is **reflex** (a two-neuronal arc) and the **second** is **voluntary**, under the control of the will. Specifically, a reflex is an **involuntary response to a stimulus**. It is an automatic act. The person may be aware of the movement and may even be able to inhibit it under some conditions, but when activity results, it occurs involuntarily, without conscious assistance.

Under normal conditions **reflexes** are immediate responses to changes in our internal and external environment; in other words, they help to **maintain homeostasis**. The reflexes that cause contraction of the skeletal muscle are called **somatic reflexes**. Those that cause secretion of glands or contraction of cardiac and smooth muscle fibers are **visceral (autonomic) reflexes**.

Ganglia

By definition a **ganglion** (Gk., a knot) is a cluster of neuronal cell bodies **outside the CNS**. (Similar aggregations within the brain and spinal cord are called nuclei.) There are two principal types: (1) the **craniospinal (sensory)** ganglia attached to some cranial nerves, and to all spinal nerves, such as the dorsal root ganglia; and (2) the **autonomic ganglia**, which are **motor (visceral)** in function and associated with the autonomic nervous system (L-A, plate 7).

A minor class of visceral ganglia are the small intramural ganglia. They are clusters of a few ganglionic cells located near or within the walls of organs, especially of the alimentary tract. They belong to the parasympathetic division of the ANS. Most of the cells are multipolar and stellate in shape, although a few bipolar and pseudounipolar cells may be present. The dendrites are often coiled to form a ball-like structure, a glomerulus (L., small ball). Typical examples of intramural ganglia are the myenteric (Auerbach's) plexus between the muscle layers of the gut wall and the submucosal (Meissner's) plexus beneath the epithelial lining of the lumen of the intestines. (The more prominent sympathetic ganglia are discussed on page 211.)

Two neuron reflex arc

Sensory to motor synapse

Spinal cord level

Population of spindles with afferent sensory endings

① Tap on patellar ligament stretches spindles in muscle initiating knee jerk

② Efferent endings are stimulated to contract motor units within muscle resulting in knee jerk

Components of a somatic reflex

1) receptor nerve endings
2) afferent neuron to CNS
3) synapse with intermediate neuron
4) synapse with efferent neuron
5) efferent fiber terminates on an effector (e.g. motor end-plate)

Reflex arcs maintain homeostasis

➤ Spinal reflexes   ----solely in spinal cord

➤ Somatic reflexes   ----skeletal muscle contractions

➤ Visceral reflexes
- ----glandular secretions
- ----heart contractions
- ----smooth muscle contraction

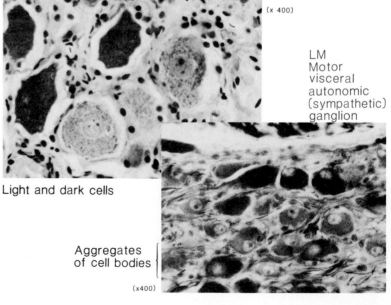

LM   Craniospinal (sensory) ganglia

(x 400)

LM Motor visceral autonomic (sympathetic) ganglion

Light and dark cells

Aggregates of cell bodies

(x400)

Spinal cord sections reveal the scatter pattern of demyelination (de) in multiple sclerosis

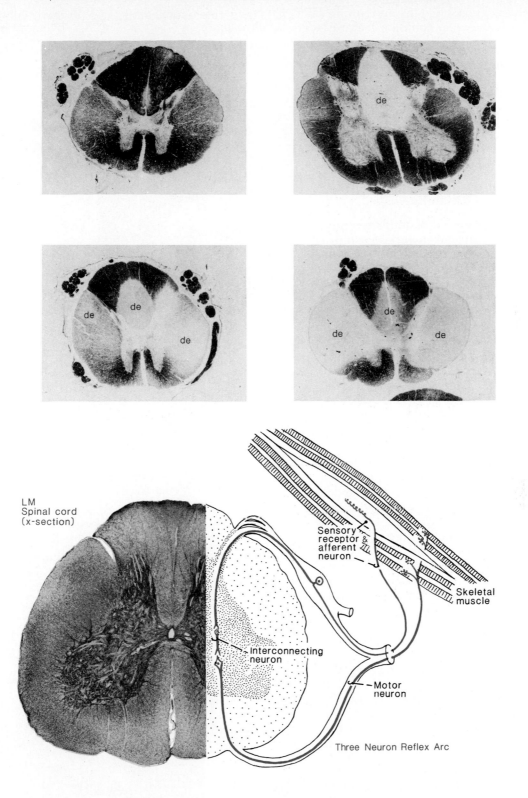

LM
Spinal cord
(x-section)

Sensory
receptor &
afferent
neuron

Skeletal
muscle

Interconnecting
neuron

Motor
neuron

Three Neuron Reflex Arc

The simple reflex arc consists of two elements: (1) a sensory receptor, e.g., skin, with its afferent neuron; and (2) an efferent (motor) neuron, which carries the impulse to an effector organ, e.g., muscle. However, the most common reflex involves three neurons. Here the sensory neuron synapses with a short interconnecting (internuncial) neuron in the grey matter of the spinal cord. This intermediate neuron conveys the impulse to the efferent neuron, completing the three neuronal reflex arc.

Although the principal types of ganglia (sensory and motor) vary greatly in size and number of neurons, they have several common features.

1. They are surrounded by a connective tissue **capsule** which, in larger ganglia, is quite robust. The capsule consists of collagenous and reticular fibers blending with the epineurium and perineurium of nerves.

2. Each ganglion cell is surrounded by a layer of small, flattened, or cuboidal cells called **satellite cells,** similar to Schwann cells.

3. A thin layer of connective tissue invests each ganglion cell with its satellite cells.

4. Blood vessels, axons, and dendrites traverse the connective tissue **meshwork** that binds the ganglion cells together into a discrete knot or body.

5. **Nissl bodies** are present in the cell bodies, especially noticeable in the larger ganglionic cells.

CRANIOSPINAL GANGLIA On the dorsal (posterior) root of each spinal nerve is a fusiform swelling, the **spinal ganglion.** Along the course of some cranial nerves a similar enlargement is noted, the **cranial ganglion.** Except for their location, they are essentially identical structures. Therefore, the term **craniospinal** is used for both ganglia.

The neurons of these ganglia are **pseudounipolar cells,** i.e., they have a single myelinated process, but it functions as both an axon and a dendrite. A short distance from the cell, the **single axonal process becomes T-shaped,** sending a larger well-myelinated branch to the periphery as the **dendrite** to innervate a receptor organ or region. The smaller, less myelinated branch is the **axon,** which proceeds centrally into the spinal cord to **synapse** with other sensory neurons. As the axon of the larger cell leaves the perikaryon, it may form several loops or convolutions to fashion an intracapsular glomerulus or net.

Here is a very curious anomaly, namely, the **dendrite is not an extension of the cell body** but of the axon. Furthermore, the impulse in sensory ganglia appears to proceed directly from the periphery, such as the skin, to the spinal cord **without entering the ganglionic cell body.** Since there are **no synapses** on the perikaryon, it cannot receive any impulses and, therefore, the role of the cell body is exclusively **trophic,** i.e., it serves only to nourish and maintain the integrity of its single axon and subsequent branches.

The rather spherical, **spinal ganglion cells** are roughly divided into two groups: (1) **small, dark-staining cells** about 15–25 μm in diameter, whose processes are unmyelinated or finely myelinated; and (2) a population of **larger, lighter-staining cells** that may reach 120 μm in diameter.

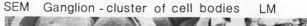

Similarities between craniospinal and autonomic ganglia:

1) extensive outer connective tissue capsule
2) cell bodies surrounded by satellite cells
3) thin CT investment over cell bodies
4) blood vessels, axons & dendrites traverse CT network
5) Nissl bodies present

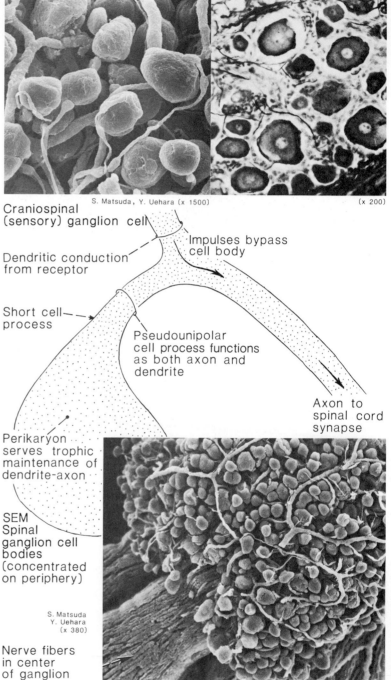

SEM   Ganglion - cluster of cell bodies   LM

S. Matsuda, Y. Uehara (x 1500)   (x 200)

Craniospinal (sensory) ganglion cell

Impulses bypass cell body

Dendritic conduction from receptor

Short cell process

Pseudounipolar cell process functions as both axon and dendrite

Axon to spinal cord synapse

Perikaryon serves trophic maintenance of dendrite-axon

SEM Spinal ganglion cell bodies (concentrated on periphery)

S. Matsuda Y. Uehara (x 380)

Nerve fibers in center of ganglion

Two Groups of Spinal Ganglion Cells

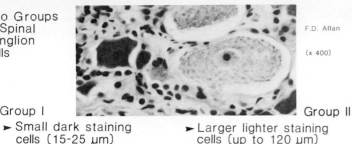

F.D. Allan

(x 400)

Group I
- ► Small dark staining cells (15-25 µm)
- ► Unmyelinated or finely myelinated axons

Group II
- ► Larger lighter staining cells (up to 120 µm)
- ► Well-myelinated axons

Distinctive Features of Autonomic Ganglia

Sympathetic ganglion cells   LM

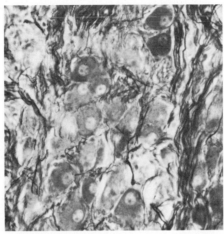

1) Located in two parallel chains along vertebral column
2) Mostly multipolar stellate (15-45 um) cells evenly distributed
3) Round, vesicular, eccentric nuclei
4) Lipofuscin present
5) Axodendritic and axosomatic synapses between two visceral motor neurons
6) Few satellite cells

(x 400)

Parasympathetic ganglion cells   LM

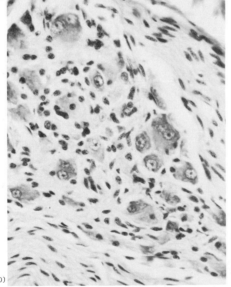

1) Located near or in wall of innervated viscus (terminal)
2) Consist of small clusters of cells
3) Devoid of connective tissue capsules

Autonomic Nervous System regulates:
- ► smooth muscle activity
- ► cardiac rhythm
- ► secretion of glands

(x 400)

AUTONOMIC GANGLIA Sympathetic and parasympathetic ganglia are the ganglia of the autonomic nervous system. Although anatomically the **sympathetic ganglia** resemble sensory ganglia, they have several significant differences: (1) Sympathetic ganglia are located in the **two, parallel, connective tissue chains** that run along the anterolateral surface of the vertebral column. Lateral ramifications of the chains, called **intermediate ganglia**, are near the viscera they innervate. (2) Nearly all of the sympathetic ganglionic cells are **multipolar**, stellate in shape, smaller, and more even in size. They do not cluster on the periphery of the ganglion body but are rather evenly distributed throughout. (3) The round, vesicular **nucleus** is typically **eccentric** in position. (4) **Lipofuscin** (wear-and-tear pigment) is usually prominent and accumulates with age within the cells. (5) Satellite cells are less prominent. (6) Axons usually are unmyelinated and do not form bundles.

The **parasympathetic ganglia** are found directly **on, or within, the wall of the viscus** they innervate. They closely resemble sympathetic cells, except that they do not form discrete structures but rather **small clusters** of ganglion cells, or even a single cell. They are devoid of connective tissue capsules but are loosely held together by the stroma of the organ they supply. These are also called **terminal or intramural ganglia** discussed on page 214).

NERVE DEGENERATION AND REGENERATION

Peripheral Nervous System Response

Since mature **nerve cells do not undergo mitosis**, they cannot be replaced. We are literally losing neurons from the day of our birth until we die. Yet there may be **regeneration of damaged peripheral nerves**, providing their axons are still attached to the cell bodies.

When a peripheral **nerve fiber is cut or severely damaged**, certain pathological changes occur on either side of the site of injury. The **proximal segment of the axon**, still attached to the cell body, has the **potential to regenerate**, while the **distal segment**, separated from the trophic center, the cell body, undergoes complete **disintegration**, called Wallerian or secondary degeneration. Eventually, it is phagocytosed by tissue macrophages. However, the **neurolemmal sheaths** of these degenerating axons **remain intact** and play a vital role in reinnervation, which will be discussed later.

The **proximal nerve segment** undergoes less severe **degeneration**, which usually **extends for only a few nodes**. These changes are called **primary or retrograde degeneration** because they are moving proximally against the axonal flow of material along the axon from the cell body.

The nerve cell body does not escape damage following axonal injury, especially if the injury occurs close to the cell body. The **changes** occurring **in the perikaryon** include: (1) **chromatolysis**, i.e., dispersal and reduction of Nissl bodies; (2) **increase of cytoplasm**, which causes the cell to swell; and (3) **displacement of the nucleus** to the periphery of the cell.

Later, when the cell returns to normal, the **proximal damaged stump** proceeds to form outgrowths called **sprouts** or **filaments**. They extend beyond the injury site and are "attracted" toward the cords or columns of **neurolemmal (Schwann) cells** that have continued to proliferate in the degenerating distal stump. Under the stimulation of the degenerative processes at the site of injury, the Schwann cells have laid down several layers of basement membranes of neurolemmal sheaths which provide effective **conduits** for the newly regenerated axons to reach their **original areas of innervation.**

Obviously only those axons that enter these neurolemmal sheaths will reach the denervated area. The other axons will become lost in a skein-like ball of nerve and neurolemmal fibers called a **neuroma.** Also if only sensory axons should enter a sheath that terminates on a muscle, no motor functions would follow.

Nerve Grafts

Extensive proliferation of Schwann cells makes several **surgical procedures** possible. They include the **suturing** of the regenerating end of a cut nerve to its degenerating segment. Thus, it is possible to have axons grow into the same locale that they formerly innervated. A surgeon may also **cross-suture** an intact functioning nerve to a degenerating segment of a different nerve. Consequently, the intact nerve will grow into an area foreign to it and innervate muscles or skin that were originally innervated by the damaged nerve.

Nerve transplants are also used to repair extensive nerve damage, such as when a portion of a peripheral nerve is destroyed, as by a gunshot wound. The surgeon will remove a section of an intact sensory nerve to the skin and splice it between the proximal and distal fragments of the damaged nerve. The regenerating axons of the proximal segment of the severed nerve will grow into the neurolemmal sheaths of the nerve graft and continue on into the sheaths of the degenerating distal fragment. Eventually, the regenerating axons will enter the denervated area and function is restored.

Regeneration/Degeneration

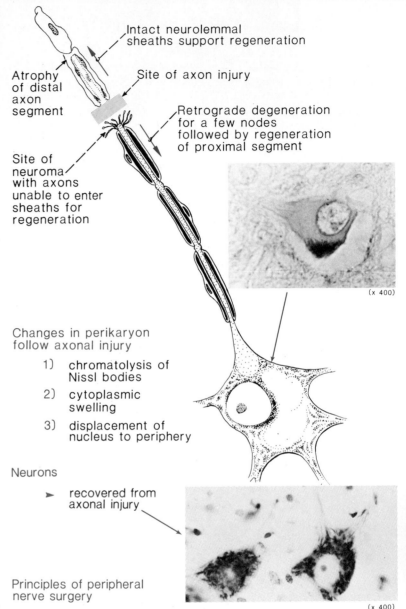

Intact neurolemmal sheaths support regeneration

Atrophy of distal axon segment

Site of axon injury

Retrograde degeneration for a few nodes followed by regeneration of proximal segment

Site of neuroma with axons unable to enter sheaths for regeneration

(x 400)

Changes in perikaryon follow axonal injury

1) chromatolysis of Nissl bodies

2) cytoplasmic swelling

3) displacement of nucleus to periphery

Neurons

➤ recovered from axonal injury

(x 400)

Principles of peripheral nerve surgery

1) suture matching cut segments

2) may cross suture to different nerve, replacing damaged nerve innervation

3) may transplant intact sensory nerve segment to replace destroyed portion

Nerve grafts

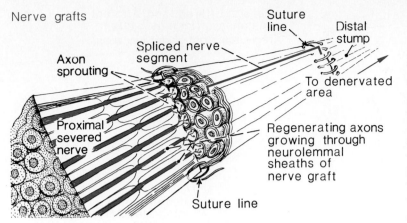

CNS regeneration failure due to:

1) lack of endoneurial and neurolemmal tubes for axon guidance

2) deficiency in nerve growth factor

3) lack of glial properties favoring axonal growth (e.g. glia scar formation at injury site forms mechanical barrier)

Role of
Autonomic Nervous System (ANS)

Controls at subconscious level:

➤ smooth muscle activity

➤ cardiac rhythm   } homeostasis

➤ secretion of glands

Serves vital role in:

➤ visceral reflexes

➤ alerting to organ malfunctions

Central Nervous System Response

Permanent **regeneration** of axons **does not occur** to any appreciable extent in the mammalian **brain or spinal cord.** Failure of the severed axons to reestablish their original site of innervation is not necessarily the fault of the damaged neurons. If the cell bodies are still intact, **regenerating axons** will grow into the lesion site for a short distance, where they lose their "sense" of direction and **become lost in a tangled ball** of nerve filaments and glial processes. Possible reasons why the regenerating axons become lost are: (1) **the absence,** in the injury site, of **endoneurial** and **neurolemmal tubes** for guidance, (2) the deficiency of a **nerve growth factor,** and (3) the neurolemmal cells of peripheral nerves may have unique properties favoring axonal regeneration not shared by their counterparts in the CNS, the oligodendrocytes. Furthermore, it is precisely the reaction of glial cells to nerve injury that produces a **glial scar,** which is an effective mechanical barrier to nerve regeneration in the CNS.

AUTONOMIC NERVOUS SYSTEM

Although anatomically the **autonomic nervous system (ANS)** is a part of the peripheral nervous system, it primarily is a discrete **functional unit** concerned with **regulating bodily functions.** In other words, it controls smooth muscle activity, variations in cardiac rhythm, and the secretion of glands. These activities are all involved in maintaining a constant internal environment of the body, i.e., a state of **homeostasis.**

As the system was defined by Langley in 1921, it included only **visceral efferent (motor) fibers.** Unfortunately, this narrow definition is still current even though the visceral **afferent (sensory) fibers** play a vital role in visceral reflexes and in alerting us with visceral pain or discomfort about **organ malfunctions.** These **sensory fibers,** originating in the various organs and tissues, **accompany the motor fibers** of the autonomic system and should be considered part of it.

Although the ANS functions are at the **subconscious level,** the term autonomic may be misleading for it suggests that the system operates automatically, i.e., independently of the CNS. This is not the case, for most, if not all, of its functions are being constantly monitored and **influenced by conscious (CNS) activity,** especially our emotional responses to our surroundings. In fact, it is the hypothalamus that integrates the activities of the ANS with the other nervous elements.

Traditionally, the anatomical components of the ANS are **two motor neurons.** The primary or **preganglionic neuron** has its cell body located either in the **gray matter** of the spinal cord or in the brain stem. The secondary or **postganglionic neuron** is housed in an **autonomic ganglion** outside the CNS. The axons of these latter cells innervate organs and tissues.

Sympathetic Division

The **two divisions of the ANS** are identified by the location of their neurons in the spinal cord or brain and by their functions. The **sympathetic division** consists of preganglionic neurons whose cell bodies lie in the lateral gray column of the **12 thoracic nerves** and the first through the third **lumbar segments** of the spinal cord. For this reason, their outflow fibers are also called the **thoracolumbar** division of the ANS. These myelinated **preganglionic fibers leave the spinal cord** via the ventral (motor) roots of spinal nerves but soon terminate either in **synapses** in the **sympathetic chain ganglia** or the prevertebral ganglia. The unmyelinated postganglionic fibers arising from these ganglion cells have relatively long axons extending from the chain or prevertebral ganglia to smooth muscle in viscera often a considerable distance away. They also terminate on blood vessels, sweat and oil glands, and arrector pili muscles.

Depending on their location, the ganglia of the sympathetic division are designated as (1) paravertebral, (2) prevertebral, or (3) terminal. Two parallel chains (trunks), containing the **paravertebral ganglia,** extend on each side of the vertebral column. In each chain, in the neck region, are three swellings, the superior, middle, and inferior **cervical ganglia.** Ten or eleven ganglia are evenly spaced in the thoracic region, while the lumbar and sacral regions each have four ganglia.

The **prevertebral ganglia,** in front of the vertebral column, form plexuses near to the abdominal organs they innervate, i.e., celiac (solar), superior mesenteric, and inferior mesenteric plexuses. **Terminal ganglia** are located more peripherally, e.g., very close to the viscera they supply.

Some of the specific **reactions** that result from **sympathetic stimulation** are: (1) blood pressure is elevated, (2) heart rate is increased, (3) the pupils are dilated, (4) the external sphincters are tightly closed, (5) salivary and other digestive secretions are inhibited, and (6) cells of the adrenal medulla release epinephrine into the bloodstream. Opposing actions result from activity of the parasympathetic division.

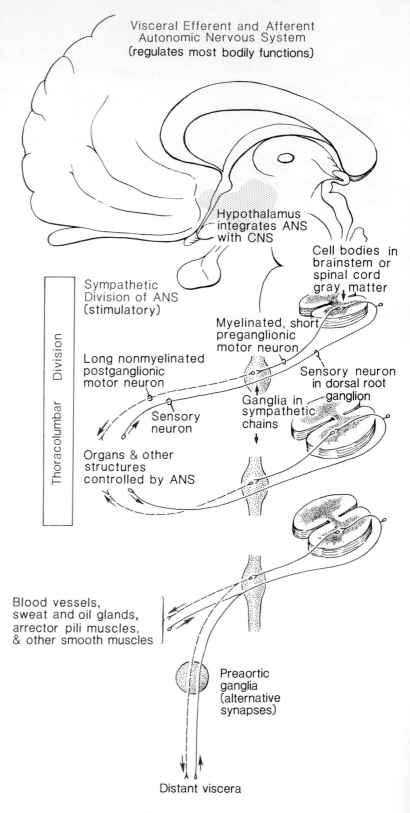

Visceral Efferent and Afferent Autonomic Nervous System (regulates most bodily functions)

Hypothalamus integrates ANS with CNS

Cell bodies in brainstem or spinal cord gray matter

Sympathetic Division of ANS (stimulatory)

Myelinated, short preganglionic motor neuron

Thoracolumbar Division

Long nonmyelinated postganglionic motor neuron

Sensory neuron in dorsal root ganglion

Sensory neuron

Ganglia in sympathetic chains

Organs & other structures controlled by ANS

Blood vessels, sweat and oil glands, arrector pili muscles, & other smooth muscles

Preaortic ganglia (alternative synapses)

Distant viscera

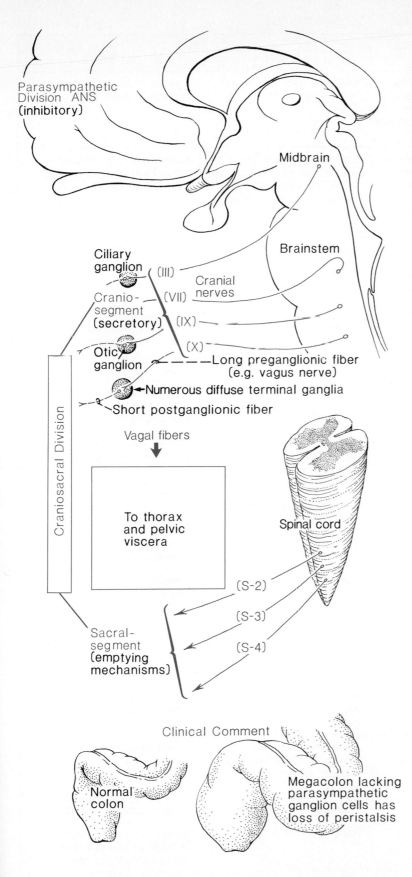

Parasympathetic
Division ANS
(inhibitory)

Midbrain

Brainstem

Ciliary
ganglion
(III)

Cranio-
segment
(secretory)
(VII)

Cranial
nerves

(IX)

Otic
ganglion
(X)

Long preganglionic fiber
(e.g. vagus nerve)

Numerous diffuse terminal ganglia

Short postganglionic fiber

Vagal fibers

To thorax
and pelvic
viscera

Spinal cord

Craniosacral Division

(S-2)

(S-3)

(S-4)

Sacral-
segment
(emptying
mechanisms)

Clinical Comment

Normal
colon

Megacolon lacking
parasympathetic
ganglion cells has
loss of peristalsis

Parasympathetic Division

The **parasympathetic division** of the ANS **differs** from the sympathetic division in several aspects. (1) The outflow of the preganglionic fibers is found in cranial nerves III, VII, IX, and X emerging from the midbrain and brain stem, and from the 2nd, 3rd, and 4th sacral nerves. Therefore, it is also called the **craniosacral division.** (2) The **preganglionic neuron has a long course,** extending from the brain or sacral spinal cord to synapse on terminal ganglia located within or near the viscera they innervate. Hence, the **postganglionic fibers are very short.** (3) Parasympathetic ganglia are not arranged in chains but as small, **diffuse clusters of cells** scattered within the capsule or between tissues of an organ. Parasympathetic cells are also located in the head region as tiny, discrete, thinly **encapsulated ganglia** associated with certain **cranial nerves.**

Preganglionic fibers arising from nuclei of cranial nerves are largely **secretory in function.** They supply the lacrimal and salivary glands and the mucous membranes of nose and mouth. **Preganglionic vagal fibers** (cranial nerve X), the largest component of the parasympathetic division, end synaptically on ganglion cells, which supply postganglionic fibers to all **thoracic and abdominal viscera.** Likewise, the **sacral outflow** fibers supply **pelvic viscera,** e.g., colon, rectum, and the reproductive and urinary systems. They are primarily concerned with **emptying mechanisms,** i.e., urination, defecation, and parturition.

Most organs are innervated by both sympathetic and parasympathetic fibers. These innervations frequently have **opposing effects.** Generally speaking, if an organ is stimulated by sympathetic impulses, it is inhibited by parasympathetic action. For example, sympathetic stimulation of smooth muscle of the iris dilates the pupil, whereas parasympathetic stimulation constricts the pupil.

Table 11.1   *COMPARISON OF PERIKARYON, AXON, AND DENDRITES*

	PERIKARYON (CELL BODY)	AXON	DENDRITE
Size	From 4 μm diameter of smaller neurons of cerebral cortex, to 135 μm larger motor cells of spinal cord	Diameter 1–3 μm; length <1 mm to >1 m	Length indeterminate, diameter about 1 μm
Plasmalemma	Typical unit membrane averages 7–8 nm in diameter; modified at synaptic and junctional areas by electron-dense material; very permeable	Continues over axon as the axolemma; often protected by myelin sheath; perhaps less permeable	Continues over dendrites; more exposed; no myelin; highly permeable
Nucleus	Large (2–8 μm), spherical, pale staining except for dispersed clumps heterochromatin, and prominent, basophilic nucleolus (RNA)	Not applicable	Not applicable
Nissl bodies	Abundant, especially in larger neurons; widely distributed as rER, site of protein synthesis	Absent	Abundant, especially in proximal segment of larger cells; may be absent in smaller neurons
Rough endoplasmic reticulum (rER)	Especially plentiful in larger cells; widely distributed as Nissl bodies as seen in LM	Absent	Considerable amount with flattened saccules in proximal segment
Free ribosomes	Few	Few in initial segment; absent beyond beginning of myelin sheath	Numerous in proximal part
Smooth endoplasmic reticulum (sER)	Largely absent	Limited amount; vesicular and tubular types	Considerable, mostly saccular variety
Golgi apparatus	Very well developed	Absent	Maybe present, especially in proximal segment
Mitochondria	Thin, elongated; average diameter 0.1 μm; quite abundant	Slender, long, widely dispersed; concentrated in terminals	Plentiful; increase in number in distal segment
Lysosomes	Many of primary type; secondary type (residual bodies or lipofuscin) increase with age	Limited	Limited
Microtubules (neurotubules)	Numerous, scattered singly or in fascicles. About 20–30 nm in diameter	Abundant, mostly in proximal segments linked together in bundles	Very abundant, arranged in parallel fascicles. A distinctive feature
Microfilaments (neurofilaments)	Abundant; average diameter about 7–10 nm. May act as support in cytoskeleton	Abundant, especially in larger axons. Increase in number after injury	Fewer in number
Glycogen		Scanty	Considerable
Pigment	Considerable lipofuscin, especially in old age	Rare	As lipofuscin accumulates in large amounts within nerve cells of the elderly

Table 11.1 *(continued)*

	PERIKARYON (CELL BODY)	AXON	DENDRITE
Processes (branches)	Single axon; dendrites may be single, as in bipolar cells, or multiple, as in multipolar cells	Few branches largely limited to the terminal ramification, the telodendria. Some right angle processes occur at nodes. All branches about same diameter of axon, which is uniform in diameter throughout course. No spines	Many, short, diffuse, tapering, acute-angled branches with rough, spiny appearance. All ramify close to cell body. Diameter decreases distally
Synaptic contacts	Very numerous; both axosomatic and dendrosomatic types	Plentiful, mostly axodendritic and axosomatic varieties	Scanty; axodendritic and dendrodendritic types
Spines	Absent	Absent	Very plentiful; most axodendritic synapses occur here
Synaptic vesicles	Absent	Abundant in endings, presynaptic variety. An important diagnostic feature	Absent
Transport potential	Highly efficient system to move synthesized proteins, fats, etc. into processes	Extensive movement of nutrients and waste products via axon transport system. Great variations in velocity of flow	Less movement but similar to axons
Relative volume	Least	Greater	Greatest
Myelinization	Absent	Usually present; unmyelinated axons relatively scarce. Presence of myelin sheath usually diagnostic of axon	Usually absent. Myelinated dendrites relatively rare
Function(s)	1. Reception center of synapses which convey excitatory and inhibitory stimuli generated by other neurons. 2. Trophic (nourishing) center for synthesis of proteins for maintenance of axon and dendrites	Primarily concerned with conduction and transmission of impulses	Primarily involved with synapses

Table 11.2 *SENSORY NERVE ENDINGS (RECEPTORS)*

TYPE	NAME	STIMULUS	LOCATION	MODALITY	EXTEROCEPTORS (E), INTEROCEPTORS (I), PROPRIOCEPTORS (P), SPECIAL SENSES (SS)
Free	Naked nerve fibers	Excessive stimulation of exteroceptors, especially if tissue damage results	Skin, cornea, mucous membranes, connective tissues	Pain	E
		Gentle stroking	Cornea	Touch	E
	Basket or peritrichal fibers	Hair movement	Around base of hairs	Movement	E
	Merkel's disks	Light touch	On outermost sheath of hair base; on spinous and basal cells of skin	Touch	E
Encapsulated	Meissner's corpuscles	Light pressure and touch	In dermal papillae of skin, especially fingers, palms, nipples, lips, genitalia	Light touch	E
	Pacinian corpuscles	Pressure and vibration	In dermis, mesenteries, periosteum, joints, tendons, etc.	Deep touch Pressure and vibration	E P
	Krause's end bulbs	Thermal change	In dermis, lips, oral mucosa, conjunctiva, and genitalia	Cold(?)	E
	Ruffini corpuscles	Thermal change (?); position shift	In dermis, subcutaneous tissue of sole of foot and joint capsules	Heat(?), Touch(?) Position sense	E P
	Golgi tendon organs	Changes in tension	Musculotendon junctions; aponeuroses	Tension	P
	Muscle spindles	Stretching	Skeletal muscles	Stretch reflex	P
Chemoreceptors	Taste buds	Substances in solution	Mostly in circumvallate, few in fungiform papillae of tongue	Acid, bitter, sweet, and salty tastes	SS
	Olfactory epithelium	Any odoriferous substance	Mucous membrane in roof of nasal cavity	Smell	SS

Table 11.2   *(continued)*

TYPE	NAME	STIMULUS	LOCATION	MODALITY	EXTEROCEPTORS (E), INTEROCEPTORS (I), PROPRIOCEPTORS (P), SPECIAL SENSES (SS)
	Carotid and aortic bodies	Changes in CO_2 and O_2 concentrations in blood	Bifurcation of common carotids; adjacent to subclavian arteries near aortic arch	Monitor O_2 and CO_2 levels in blood	I
Baroreceptors	Pressure receptors	Changes in arterial pressure	Walls of carotid sinus and aortic arch	Monitor blood pressure	I
Photoreceptors	Rods and cones cells	Light	Retina	Sight	SS
Audioreceptors	Auditory hair cells	Sound vibrations	Internal ear (organ of Corti)	Hearing	SS
Vestibulo-receptors	Vestibular hair cells	Movement of endolymph	Saccule, utricle and semicircular canals of internal ear	Equilibrium	SS P

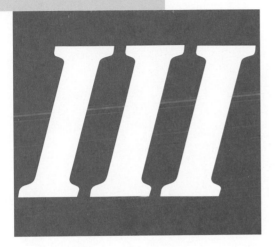

Part

III

ORGAN SYSTEMS

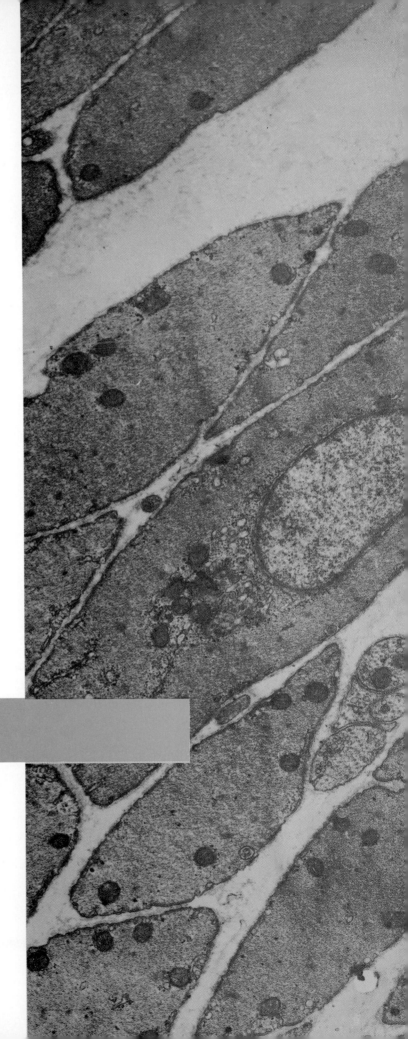

Chapter

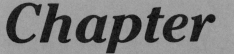

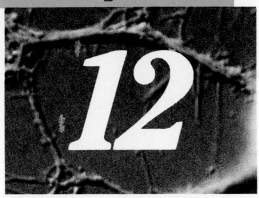

12

CENTRAL NERVOUS SYSTEM

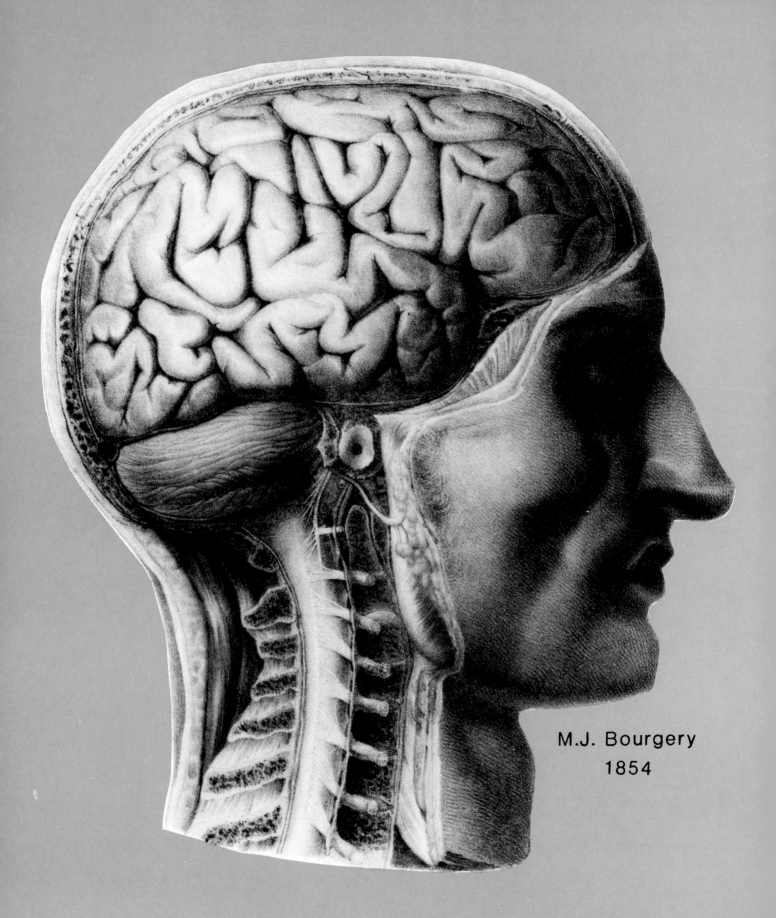

M.J. Bourgery
1854

OBJECTIVES

ALTHOUGH THE CENTRAL NERVOUS SYSTEM (CNS) IS THE DOMAIN OF NEUROANATOMY, THIS CHAPTER WILL ENABLE THE READER TO ORGANIZE AND DISCUSS BASIC INFORMATION ABOUT THE BRAIN AND SPINAL CORD, SUCH AS:

1. Their anatomical subdivisions and coverings (meninges).

2. The histological composition and distribution of the gray and white matter.

3. The concept of ascending and descending tracts, and motor (efferent) and sensory (afferent) pathways.

4. The microarchitectural patterns of the cerebral and cerebellar cortices, interspersed with many supportive neuroglial cells.

5. The cerebral spinal fluid (CSF) surrounding the brain and spinal cord acts as a protective fluid cushion or buffer.

The brain and spinal cord constitute the **central nervous system (CNS).** Its functions are to receive and integrate incoming information (stimuli) concerning our internal and external environment received from **sensory receptors. Motor impulses** are then generated and discharged to effector organs (muscles and glands) for appropriate action, or the information may be stored as memory for future reference.

In the fresh condition, the spinal cord and especially the brain are very soft, almost jellylike in consistency. If it were not for the blood vessels and investing membranes (meninges), the brain would be almost formless since it **lacks** collagenous and other **connective tissue fibers** to give it firmness. Only after thorough fixation is the form and shape of the brain stabilized.

HISTOLOGICAL STRUCTURES

The histological elements of the CNS consist of: (1) **Neurons** in the spinal cord are located in a longitudinal, **H-shaped column** in the center of the cord; while in the brain they are either in clusters **(nuclei)** deep in the brain, or in layers **(laminae)** in the superficial cortex. (2) **Glia** are nonneuronal cells that are the supportive or insulating elements throughout the CNS. (3) **Nerve fibers** are mostly long axons which may be myelinated or nonmyelinated. They traverse and connect various regions of the brain and spinal cord. Most of the fibers are in definite bundles called **tracts.** (4) Accessory structures that support and nourish the nervous elements are the investing **meninges,** abundant **blood vessels,** and the **cerebral spinal fluid** in spaces, or reservoirs, called cisternae and ventricles.

The study of the intricacies of the organization of neurons into centers, groups, and layers, and their axons into tracts is the province of **neuroanatomy.** However, the **architecture** of the brain and spinal cord and the types of cells and fibers encountered in the various regions, will be briefly described.

GRAY AND WHITE MATTER

The brain and spinal cord are each divided into gray and white matter. In **gray matter** nerve **cell bodies** and **unmyelinated fibers** predominate and, in fresh tissue, have a dull, gray color. The cell bodies are separated by a **dense fibrous network** consisting of dendrites, axons, and glial processes, all permeated by a diffuse capillary bed. These areas of entangled elements, where most synapses occur, constitute the **neuropil** (Gk. pilos, feltlike). EM micrographs of neuropils reveal a space of 20–25 nm between nerve cell bodies and glial processes, creating an important **extracellular compartment** in the gray matter. This space is about 20–30% of the total tissue volume.

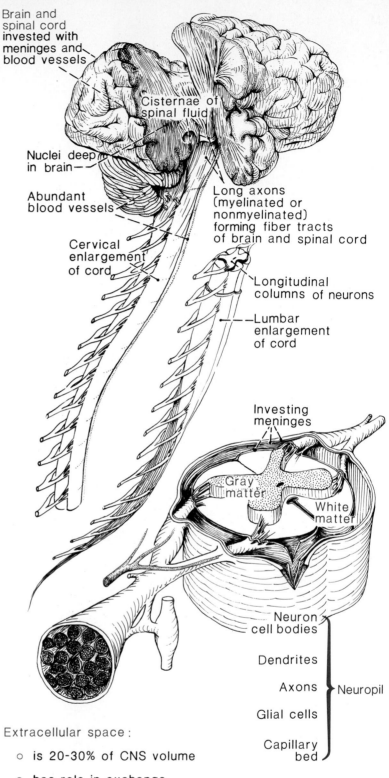

Brain and spinal cord invested with meninges and blood vessels

Cisternae of spinal fluid

Nuclei deep in brain

Abundant blood vessels

Cervical enlargement of cord

Long axons (myelinated or nonmyelinated) forming fiber tracts of brain and spinal cord

Longitudinal columns of neurons

Lumbar enlargement of cord

Investing meninges

Gray matter

White matter

Neuron cell bodies

Dendrites

Axons

Glial cells

Capillary bed

} Neuropil

Extracellular space:

○ is 20-30% of CNS volume

○ has role in exchange of gases and nutrients

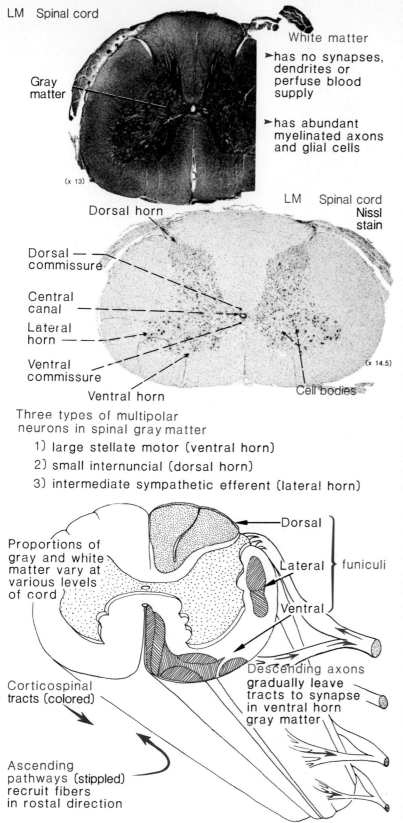

LM Spinal cord

Gray matter

White matter

→ has no synapses, dendrites or perfuse blood supply

→ has abundant myelinated axons and glial cells

(x 13)

LM Spinal cord
Nissl stain

Dorsal horn

Dorsal commissure

Central canal

Lateral horn

Ventral commissure

Ventral horn

Cell bodies

(x 14.5)

Three types of multipolar neurons in spinal gray matter
1) large stellate motor (ventral horn)
2) small internuncial (dorsal horn)
3) intermediate sympathetic efferent (lateral horn)

Proportions of gray and white matter vary at various levels of cord

Dorsal
Lateral } funiculi
Ventral

Descending axons gradually leave tracts to synapse in ventral horn gray matter

Corticospinal tracts (colored)

Ascending pathways (stippled) recruit fibers in rostal direction

In **white matter,** parallel fascicles (L., small bundles) of **myelinated axons dominate** and exhibit a white, glistening appearance in the fresh condition. There are relatively few capillaries and very little extracellular space. Since the function of white matter is largely **conductive,** it has considerably less metabolic activity. It differs greatly from gray matter by having **no synapses, no dendrites,** and a **limited blood supply.**

Various glial cells are found in both areas. Their distribution and functions are discussed on page 232.

SPINAL CORD

A typical cross section of the spinal cord is demarcated into an **outer** thick zone of **white matter** and an **inner** butterfly or H-shaped zone of **gray matter.** Near the center of the crossbar of the H is the small **central canal** lined with **ependymal cells,** a type of glial cell. On each side of the cord, the gray matter extends caudally and rostrally as **two vertical columns** called the **dorsal** (posterior) and **ventral** (anterior) **horns.** A small **lateral horn** is also seen in the thoracic and upper lumbar regions.

There are three types of **multipolar neurons** in spinal gray matter: (1) the large, stellate **motor cells** in the ventral horns: (2) the small and medium-size **sympathetic efferent neurons** in the lateral horns; and (3) the medium-size, **sensory neurons** in the dorsal horns. All of these cells are confined to layers called **laminae.**

The **white matter** of the spinal cord consists of **bundles of axons** having specific functions, either motor or sensory, e.g., pain, touch, proprioception. There are three of these large **fiber columns or funiculi** (L., cords), named from their position, i.e., dorsal, lateral, and ventral. Each funiculus is subdivided into smaller nerve bundles, the **fasciculi, or tracts.** From the name of the tract, one can tell the location of the cells of origin and the termination of the fibers. For example, in the corticospinal tract, the cell bodies are in the cerebral cortex and their axons end synaptically on neurons in the spinal cord.

While the pattern of gray and white matter is constant, their relative proportions vary at various levels. The greatest amount of **gray matter** is found in the **cervical and lumbar enlargements** of the cord because of the marked increase of neurons that are needed to serve the upper and lower limbs. The **white matter increases** in a **caudal to rostral direction** because the ascending pathways, connecting the spinal cord with the brain, are constantly **recruiting fibers** as they approach the brain. Furthermore, the axons of the descending tract gradually **leave the tract** to terminate in **synapses** on the motor cells of the gray matter (ventral horn) of the cord. Recall that, unlike the gray matter, white matter contains only axons and glial cells.

BRAIN

The brain is subdivided into the large **cerebrum**, the much smaller **cerebellum** (meaning small brain), and the inferiorly situated, funnel-shaped **brain stem.** The latter is composed of nerve tracts entering and leaving the brain, as well as nuclei subserving various reflex functions.

Cerebrum

The **cerebrum** is divided into two equal **hemispheres** by a deep, longitudinal fissure that contains the **falx cerebri,** a vertical extension of the dura mater. The **cortex** (gray matter) is highly convoluted, i.e., thrown into deep folds which greatly increase its surface area. The convolutions are called **gyri** (Gk., circles; singular, gyrus) and the intervening depressions are **sulci** (L., furrows; singular, sulcus).

Histologically the **cerebral cortex** shows **six, ill-defined layers** or zones that vary in their cytoarchitecture from area to area of the brain. Three morphologically different cell types make up most of the neurons, i.e., stellate or granular, fusiform, and pyramidal. By far the most conspicuous are the various sized **pyramidal cells.** The largest cortical neurons are the large pyramidal cells in layer five. They are identifying landmarks of this layer and are involved in executing motor commands.

All pyramidal cells have an **apical dendrite** that projects towards the outer surface of the cortex. Its **axon,** emerging from the base of the pyramid, penetrates the deeper layers of the cortex to eventually form the efferent pathways of the brain in the white matter of the cortex.

The layers of the cerebral cortex are summarized as follows:

I. The Molecular or Plexiform layer. This is the **outermost layer** of the cortex. It is called molecular because in cross section the delicate, fine fibers stain as tiny dots, giving it a molecular or punctate appearance. It is also plexiform in appearance because many dendrites and axons are sectioned longitudinally and appear as a network or plexus. Only a **few neurons** are present which are mostly the horizontal cells (of Cajal). It is an important **synaptic area.**

II. The Outer Granular layer. Such a term is a misnomer since most of the cells are **small, pyramidal cells.** The remaining cells are small, **stellate cells** which, when stained, appear as granules. Dendrites of both types of cells terminate in this layer or ascend into layer I. Their axons may descend into lower layers or continue deeper into the white matter.

III. The Outer Pyramidal layer. Most cells are **medium-sized, pyramidal cells** whose apical dendrites extend into the molecular layer. Their axons descend into the deeper layers or enter the white matter.

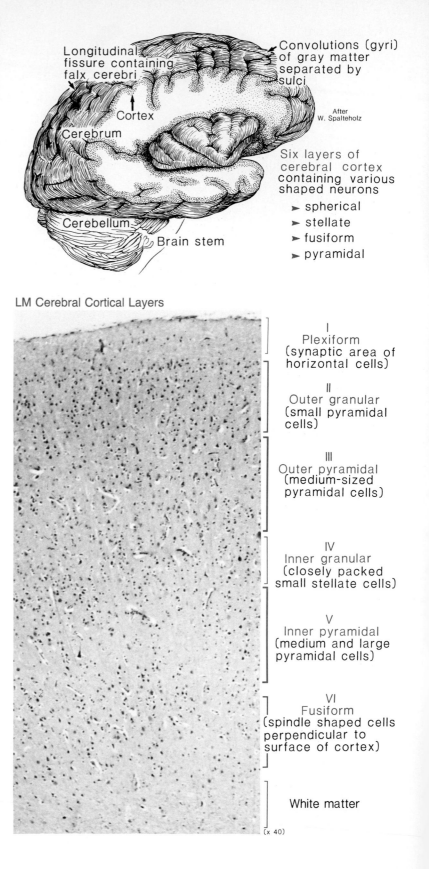

Longitudinal fissure containing falx cerebri

Convolutions (gyri) of gray matter separated by sulci

Cortex

Cerebrum

After W. Spalteholz

Cerebellum

Brain stem

Six layers of cerebral cortex containing various shaped neurons

► spherical
► stellate
► fusiform
► pyramidal

LM Cerebral Cortical Layers

I
Plexiform (synaptic area of horizontal cells)

II
Outer granular (small pyramidal cells)

III
Outer pyramidal (medium-sized pyramidal cells)

IV
Inner granular (closely packed small stellate cells)

V
Inner pyramidal (medium and large pyramidal cells)

VI
Fusiform (spindle shaped cells perpendicular to surface of cortex)

White matter

(x 40)

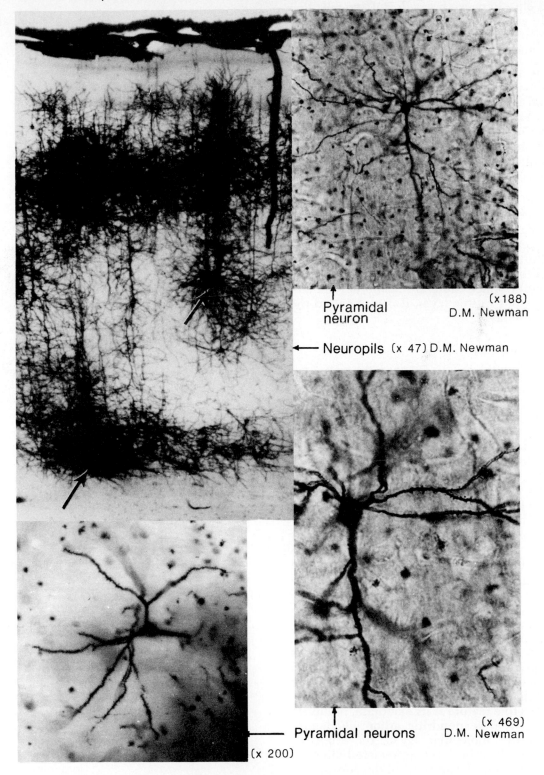

Pyramidal
neuron   (x188)
                          D.M. Newman

← Neuropils (x 47) D.M. Newman

Pyramidal neurons   (x 469)
                           D.M. Newman

(x 200)

LM photomicrographs of silver impregnated, pyramidal neurons of the cerebral cortex.
   Upper left. Many of these neurons have prominent apical dendrites projecting into the
upper light-staining layers, while their axons extend into the lower levels. Arrows
indicate rather solid masses of entangled axons, dendrites, and glial processes,
collectively called neuropils because of their matted, feltlike texture (Gk., pilos, felt).
   Other pyramidal cortical neurons show extensive branching of dendrites studded with
fine projections or spines, termed gemmules, which are sites for synapses.

IV. The Inner Granular layer. The principal cells are closely packed, **small, stellate cells** that resemble **granules.** Many of their axons are short and remain within the layer; others pass into layers V and VI.

V. The Inner Pyramidal or Ganglionic layer. The predominant cells are the **medium and large pyramidal cells.** In the motor cortex, the **giant pyramidal cells (of Betz)** are landmarks. The apical dendrites of the large pyramidal cells may penetrate into layer I; dendrites of the smaller cells terminate in layer IV. **Axons of all cells enter the white matter.**

VI. The Fusiform or Multiform layer. Here the main cell type is the **fusiform or spindle cell** whose long axis lies perpendicular to the surface of the cortex. Apical dendrites of the smaller cells end within the layer; those of the larger cells extend into layers IV and V. All **axons enter the white matter.** Since there are also other cells of various shapes in this layer, it is also called the **polymorphic layer.**

Cerebellum

Like the cerebrum, the **cerebellum** is divided into **right and left hemispheres,** which are separated by a wormlike, segmented band of gray matter called the **vermis** (L., worm). The surface of the hemispheres is thrown into many thin, parallel folds or leaflets called **folia** (L., leaves; singular, folium). A thin cortex of gray matter covers the folia. Collections of neurons are buried in the underlying white matter, comprising the **cerebellar nuclei.**

A section through the cerebellar cortex reveals a **trilaminar structure.** It has an **outer molecular layer** consisting of a few, small, basket- and stellate-type neurons; myriad parallel fibers derived from granule cells; and a massive dendritic arborization largely arising from the deeper Purkinje cells. The **intermediate layer** is the **Purkinje layer,** consisting of a single layer of very large Purkinje cells whose cell bodies rest on the innermost granular layer. The **Purkinje cell** has a large, prominent, **flask-shaped cell** body with a clear vesicular nucleus. Many Nissl granules are scattered throughout the cytoplasm. However, its most **distinctive feature** is its elaborate, profusely branching, **treelike dendritic arbor** which projects into the molecular layer. Its extensive branches can best be fully appreciated after silver staining of sagittal sections of the cortex. The thin, myelinated axons of Purkinje cells project deep into the cerebellar nuclei.

The **innermost granular layer** is the most conspicuous layer of the cerebellar cortex because it consists of a large population of closely packed, **small granular cells** whose nuclei essentially fill the cell. Under low-power, they resemble lymphocytes.

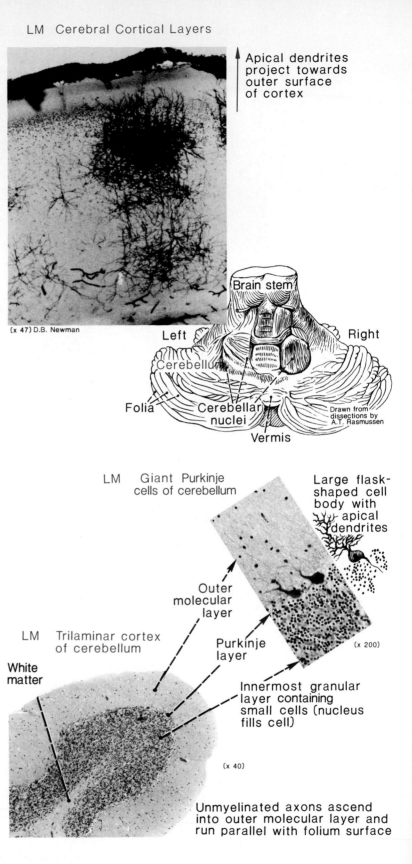

LM Cerebral Cortical Layers

Apical dendrites project towards outer surface of cortex

(x 47) D.B. Newman

Brain stem

Left   Right

Cerebellum

Folia   Cerebellar nuclei

Vermis

Drawn from dissections by A.T. Rasmussen

LM   Giant Purkinje cells of cerebellum

Large flask-shaped cell body with apical dendrites

Outer molecular layer

LM   Trilaminar cortex of cerebellum

White matter

Purkinje layer

(x 200)

Innermost granular layer containing small cells (nucleus fills cell)

(x 40)

Unmyelinated axons ascend into outer molecular layer and run parallel with folium surface

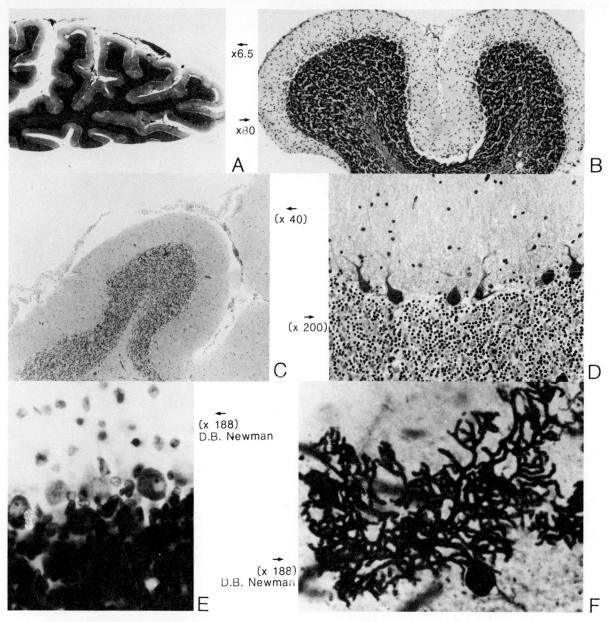

Various stains reveal different histological features. These LM micrographs of the cerebellar cortex show the reactions of several common stains that are utilized in the study of the cytoarchitecture of the nervous system.

A. Section of cerebellar folia stained with the Weigert-Weil stain (ferric ammonium sulfate and hemotoxylin) reveals selective black staining of the central white matter (myelinated fibers) and the lightly stained cortical gray matter (nerve cell bodies and nonmyelinated fibers).

B. Section of the cerebellar cortex stained with a Nissl stain (thionin), specific for nerve cell bodies containing Nissl substance (rER). Note the three cellular layers: (1) the outer molecular (pale) layer; (2) the inner granular (dark) layer; and (3) the narrow intermediate layer of a single row of large Purkinje cells, poorly seen at this magnification.

C. Cerebellar cortex stained with conventional hemotoxylin and eosin (H&E). The three layers are less well-defined than in B.

D. Higher magnification of B. showing large Purkinje cells in the middle layer.

E. Cresyl violet, a Nissl stain, reveals: (1) few cells in outer, light-staining molecular layer; (2) row of large Purkinje cells in middle layer; and (3) the highly cellular inner granular layer.

F. The single axon and extensive dendritic arborization of a Purkinje cell have been impregnated with silver nitrate, a Golgi-type staining procedure.

Brain Stem

The **brain stem** houses the **main sensory and motor tracts** of the brain. They are collected and concentrated into this cylindrical mass of white matter, which tapers caudally to form the **spinal cord.** The cerebellum rests astride the central portion of the brain stem, called the **pons** (L., bridge). Other parts are the **medulla oblongata,** located between the spinal cord and the pons, and the midbrain, situated rostral to the pons. The diencephalon, extending rostrally from the midbrain, is also included in the brain stem by some authors.

Histologically the **brain stem** exhibits a variety of neuronal structures. It is the **funnel** through which all the **nerve pathways** between the cerebrum and spinal cord must pass. Practically all of the tracts are composed of **heavily myelinated fibers.** It is in the brain stem that most of the **cranial nerves** arise or terminate. Therefore in the gray matter, where these events take place, neurons will be sequestered in clusters (**nuclei**). For additional information consult neuroanatomy textbooks.

NEUROGLIA

About 70–80% of all cells of the CNS are nonnervous, i.e., they are mostly **supportive cells,** not neurons. Collectively they are called **glial cells or neuroglia.** This is a very appropriate term since it means "nerve glue." Certainly these cells "glue" together the various cells and parts of the CNS. As reinforcing cells, they **function similar to connective tissue cells** in other parts of the body. But unlike the mesodermal connective tissue cells, glial cells, except microglia, are **ectodermal** in origin.

Neuroglia include **astrocytes** (protoplasmic and fibrous), **oligodendroglia, microglia,** and **ependyma.** With conventional stains, only the nuclei of glial cells stain. For accurate identification, special silver stains are used to delineate the characteristic morphology of each cell type (Table 12.2).

Astrocytes

Star-shaped **astrocytes** (Gk. astron, star) are of two types: (1) **protoplasmic or mossy,** and (2) **fibrous or spiderlike.** They are probably the same cell type, merely representing functional differences as reflected in their structural variations. They serve as **support** of neuronal and vascular structures of the gray and white matter of the brain and spinal cord. Astrocytes are about 8–10 μm in diameter.

Protoplasmic astrocytes are found chiefly in the **gray matter.** They have a rather large, round, **light-staining nucleus** surrounded by abundant **granular cytoplasm.** Many cytoplasmic processes

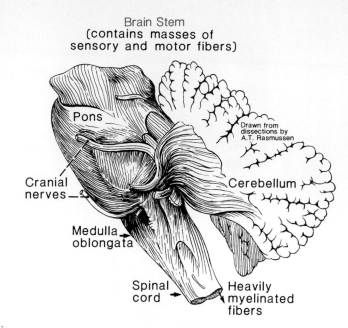

Brain Stem (contains masses of sensory and motor fibers)

Pons

Drawn from dissections by A.T. Rasmussen

Cranial nerves

Cerebellum

Medulla oblongata

Spinal cord

Heavily myelinated fibers

Neuroglia

70-80% of CNS cells are nonnervous glia providing support for neurons

Glia cells are ectoderm in origin (except microglia) and include:
- astrocytes
- oligodendroglia
- microglia
- ependyma

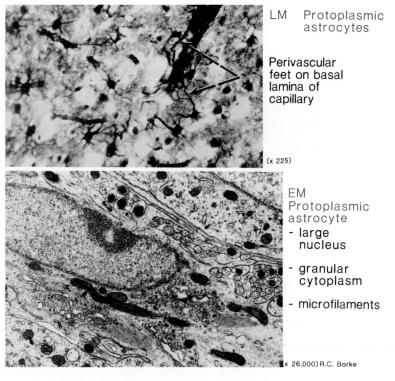

LM Protoplasmic astrocytes

Perivascular feet on basal lamina of capillary

(x 225)

EM Protoplasmic astrocyte
- large nucleus
- granular cytoplasm
- microfilaments

(x 26,000) R.C. Borke

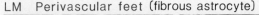

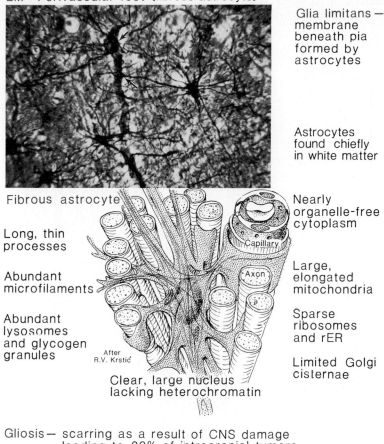

Glia limitans —
membrane
beneath pia
formed by
astrocytes

Astrocytes
found chiefly
in white matter

Fibrous astrocyte

Nearly
organelle-free
cytoplasm

Long, thin
processes

Abundant
microfilaments

Capillary

Axon

Large,
elongated
mitochondria

Abundant
lysosomes
and glycogen
granules

Sparse
ribosomes
and rER

After
R.V. Krstić

Limited Golgi
cisternae

Clear, large nucleus
lacking heterochromatin

Gliosis — scarring as a result of CNS damage
leading to 20% of intracranial tumors
(astrocytomas)

EM Oligodendrocyte — most common support cells for CNS

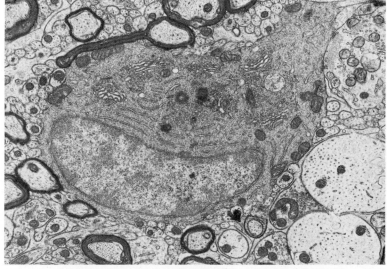

R.C. Borke
(x 18,200)

Two types of oligodendroglia, perivascular cells rest
on capillaries and satellite cells collect around neurons

terminate as expanded endings, called **perivascular feet,** which attach to the basal lamina of capillaries. These expansions may cover most of the blood vessels, thereby contributing to the **blood-brain barrier** of the CNS. The barrier restricts the passage of substances of a certain molecular size from entering the brain or spinal cord from the bloodstream. These processes also form most of the packing material between neurons. Some of the processes extend to the **surface of the brain and spinal cord** where they form a thin, superficial, glial sheath beneath the pia mater, the **glia limitans.**

Fibrous astrocytes (spider cells) are found mainly in the **white matter.** As their name implies, they have long, thin, **sparsely branching, processes** that extend considerable distances from the cell body. Otherwise, they are similar to protoplasmic astrocytes.

Both types of astrocytes have essentially the same ultramicroscopic features. Their most distinguishing feature is the presence of many **microfilaments** scattered throughout the cytoplasm. These extend as parallel bundles into the glial processes. Many large, elongated **mitochondria** are oriented parallel to the microfilaments. Another EM characteristic is the **large, electron-lucent nucleus,** largely devoid of heterochromatin.

In damage to the CNS, astrocytes may increase in number and size to form a **glial scar.** This process is called **gliosis.** Furthermore, a common brain tumor, **astrocytoma,** is derived from astrocytes. About 20% of all intracranial tumors are of this type.

Oligodendroglia

The **oligodendrocyte** is the **most common** of the supporting elements of the CNS. It has a **smaller cell body** than astrocytes (measuring 6–8 μm in diameter) and contains a small, often eccentric, **dark nucleus** with abundant heterochromatin. As its name implies, it has **only a few** (Gk. oligo, few) **processes.** It has considerably less cytoplasm and is more granular in appearance than the astrocyte. The oligodendrocytes do not have perivascular feet, yet their bodies may rest upon capillaries. Such cells are classified as **perivascular oligodendrocytes,** while the more abundant cells that cluster around neurons are called **satellite cells.** It is not unusual to see rows of these cells along neurons with their glial processes anastomosing with nerve processes.

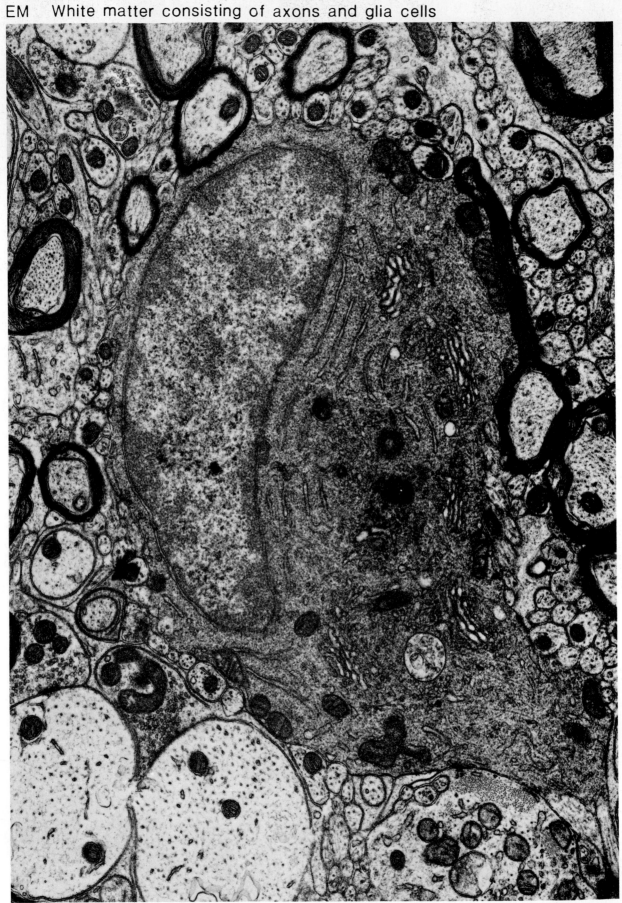

R.C. Borke (x 18,200)

Oligodendrocyte among myelinated and nonmyelinated axons

LM Oligodendroglia

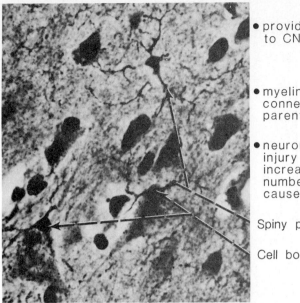

- provide myelin to CNS axons

- myelin remains connected to parent cell

- neuronal injury causes increase in number and may cause tumors

Spiny processes

Cell bodies

At the ultrastructural level, the most characteristic feature of an oligodendrocyte is its **electron-dense cytoplasm,** which is filled with **abundant rER** and free ribosomes. Other diagnostic EM features are the prominence of numerous **microtubules,** the absence of neurofilaments, and a well-developed Golgi apparatus.

Oligodendrocytes are responsible for **myelination** of axons in the CNS. Thus, they are analogous to the neurolemmal (Schwann) cells of the peripheral nervous system. In myelination, a single oligodendrocyte may provide myelin for a number of adjacent axons. The **cytoplasmic connection** between the myelin sheath and these glial cells is **permanent** and therefore provides a method or route through which **nutrients** may pass from the oligodendrocytes to the myelin sheath to maintain its integrity. Thus, myelin sheaths are functionally and anatomically connected to their parent cell, much as an axon is related to the perikaryon from which it is derived.

In some neuronal injuries, the oligodendrocytes proliferate, which may result in a tumor, a **glioma,** or more specifically, an oligodendroglioma. These are not nearly as frequent (5–10%) as astrocytomas.

Microglia or Mesoglia

Microglia are the only glial cells derived from **mesoderm** and are therefore also called **mesoglia.** They are the **smallest** of the glial cells, about 5–7 μm in diameter. Their **nuclei** are small, irregular in shape, and stain deeply. The cells have very **limited, granular cytoplasm** and only a **few stubby, twisted processes.** They make up about 4–5% of the total population of glial cells in the white matter but about 18% in the gray matter of the cerebral cortex. Their salient ultrastructural characteristics include the many, **dense inclusion bodies, lysosomes,** and lipofuscin granules, which are suggestive of the cell's **phagocytic activity.** Also the rER has long, attenuated cisternae, as contrasted to the short cisternae of oligodendrocytes.

Microglia are **phagocytic cells,** a part of the macrophage (reticuloendothelial) system. When engorged with cellular debris, principally degenerating myelin, they are called **gitter** (Ger., lattice) **cells.** Their numbers greatly increase following damage to the central nervous system. They may be brought to the site of injury by the general circulation or by migration from other areas of the CNS by ameboid movement (L-A, plate 9). (See Table 12.2.)

EM Microglia
(smallest glial cells 5-7 μm)

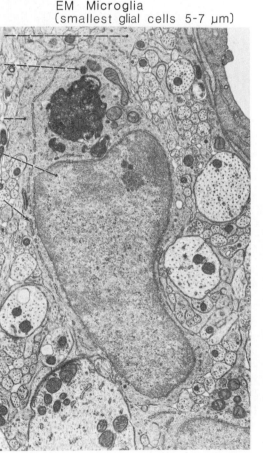

Few stubby processes

Many dense inclusion bodies

Limited granular cytoplasm

Small nuclei, irregular shape, deep staining

RER long cisternae

Few microtubules, no glycogen or neurofilaments

Less prominent Golgi

➤ phagocytic activity (gitter cells)

➤ 4-5% of total glial cells in white matter, 18% in gray

➤ microglia increase during and following damage to CNS

R.C. Borke
(x 18,200)

B. Kachar   T. Behar
M. Dubois-Daleq

(x 1,800)

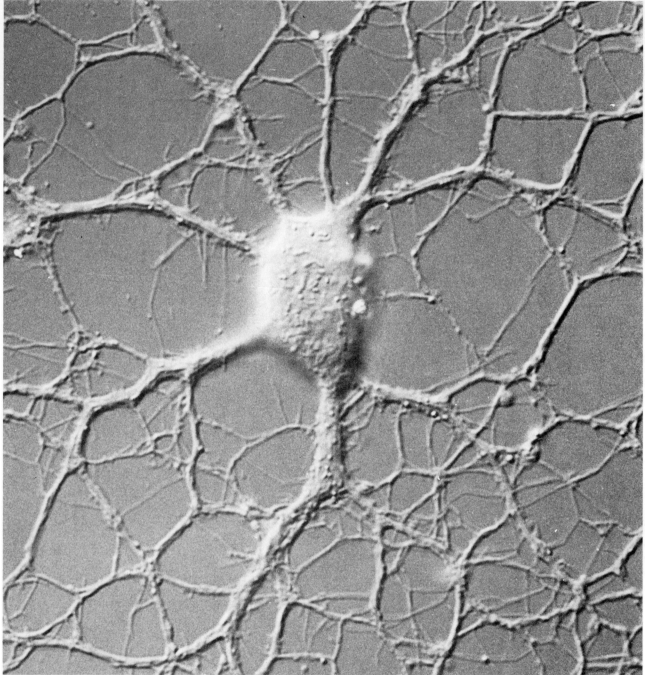

An oligodendrocyte characterized by an oval or round cell body with several long beaded cytoplasmic projections. With differential interference contrast microscopy, eight main processes and many smaller lateral branches are revealed. Each process may be associated with the formation of a myelin internode along a nerve fiber of the central nervous system.

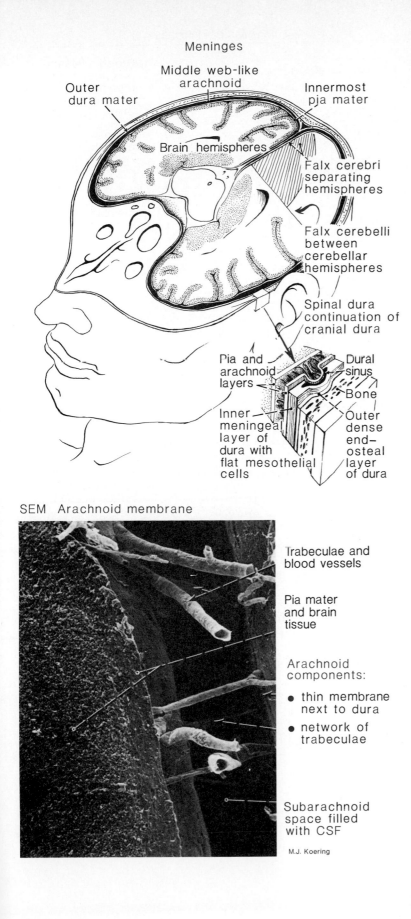

Meninges

Outer dura mater

Middle web-like arachnoid

Innermost pia mater

Brain hemispheres

Falx cerebri separating hemispheres

Falx cerebelli between cerebellar hemispheres

Spinal dura continuation of cranial dura

Pia and arachnoid layers

Dural sinus

Bone

Inner meningeal layer of dura with flat mesothelial cells

Outer dense endosteal layer of dura

SEM Arachnoid membrane

Trabeculae and blood vessels

Pia mater and brain tissue

Arachnoid components:
- thin membrane next to dura
- network of trabeculae

Subarachnoid space filled with CSF

M.J. Koering

MENINGES

The central nervous system is protected from external trauma by bony encasements (the skull and vertebral column), as well as by three membranous investments, the **meninges.** These fibrous coverings are the outermost, robust **dura mater,** the middle, spider-web-like **arachnoid,** and the innermost, delicate, vascular **pia mater.** The three layers enclose the brain and spinal cord. They also sheathe the cranial nerves as they leave the cranium and the spinal nerves as they exit the vertebral canal.

Dura Mater

The **cranial dura** is a tough, relatively thick collagenous sheath consisting of two layers: (1) An outer, dense connective tissue, the **endosteal layer,** adheres to the inner surface of the bones of the skull. It is well supplied with blood vessels and nerves. (2) An **inner meningeal layer** consists of a thinner fibrous tissue membrane which is covered on its inner surface by a single layer of flat, **mesothelial** cells. These two layers separate from each other at certain locations to form the extensive **venous (dural) sinuses.**

The dura also sends out extensions that form partitions for the brain. The largest of these is the sickle-shaped **falx cerebri,** which extends along the superior longitudinal fissure and partially separates the left and right cerebral hemispheres. An extension of the dura over the cerebellum is the **falx cerebelli,** a thick septum between the cerebellar hemispheres. Separating the cerebellum and cerebrum is another extension of the dura, the tentlike **tentorium cerebelli.** At its anterior aspect is an oval gap, the **tentorial notch,** which allows the brain stem to pass from the undersurface of the cerebrum into the posterior cranial fossa.

The **spinal dura** is a continuation of the inner layer of the cranial dura. From its attachment to the margins of the foramen magnum of the skull, it descends as a closed tube to **surround the spinal** cord. It terminates as the coccygeal ligament that invests the **filium terminale,** the filamentous ending of the spinal cord.

Arachnoid

The arachnoid is a delicate, nonvascular membrane immediately beneath the dura. It has two components: (1) a thin, **connective tissue component** in contact with the dura, and (2) a network of delicate **trabeculae,** which are covered with flat or low cuboidal epithelium. The trabeculae expand into the rather large space between the connective tissue and the underlying pia mater. This cavity is the very important **subarachnoid space** which is filled with **cerebrospinal fluid (CSF).**

In some areas adjacent to the venous dural sinuses, the arachnoid perforates the dura mater to open into the venous sinuses. These protrusions, carrying a central core of trabeculae, are the **arachnoid villi**, which function to transfer the CSF back into the bloodstream.

Pia Mater

The pia mater is the **innermost layer** of the meninges. It is a thin, highly **vascular sheath** that adheres closely to the brain and spinal cord. It follows all of their surface irregularities. Therefore, unlike the dura and arachnoid, the pia closely **covers the convolutions (gyri)** of the brain and extends into the **depths of the sulci.** As blood vessels penetrate the brain and spinal cord, they carry the pia with them for a short distance, creating a **perivascular space.**

The pia mater consists of two, poorly defined layers. The **inner, thinner layer** of reticular and elastic fibers is firmly attached to the underlying nervous tissue. The more **superficial layer** receives fibrous attachments (**trabeculae**) **from the arachnoid.** Its external surface is a single layer of squamous cells of mesodermal origin. This cellular covering is continuous with cells covering the arachnoid. Since both the pia and arachnoid are so closely related, they are often described as a single structure, the **pia-arachnoid membrane,** or leptomeninx (Gk., slender membrane).

CEREBROSPINAL FLUID

Most of the **cerebrospinal fluid (CSF)** is produced in **choroid plexuses** (folds of pia mater), located in the ventricles of the brain. The remainder of the fluid, perhaps as much as 40%, is formed at other sites, e.g., at the blood vessels of the subarachnoid space, cerebral vessels, and the ependymal lining cells of the ventricles and spinal canal.

Ependymal Cells

In embryonic development, the brain and spinal cord develop as a hollow tube. Lining this neural tube are **primitive neuroepithelial cells** that later persist as **ependymal cells,** a type of neuroglia. They line the four ventricles of the brain and the central canal of the spinal cord and cover the choroid plexuses. They are simple cuboidal or low columnar cells.

Many of these cells have an abundance of **microvilli** and one or two cilia on their luminal surfaces. The presence of cilia is not unexpected since all of the cells had cilia during some stage in their development. The basal ends of these ependymal lining cells do not rest on a basement membrane, instead, the **base is tapered to form a single, branched process** that extends into the underlying nervous tissue. In thin regions of the

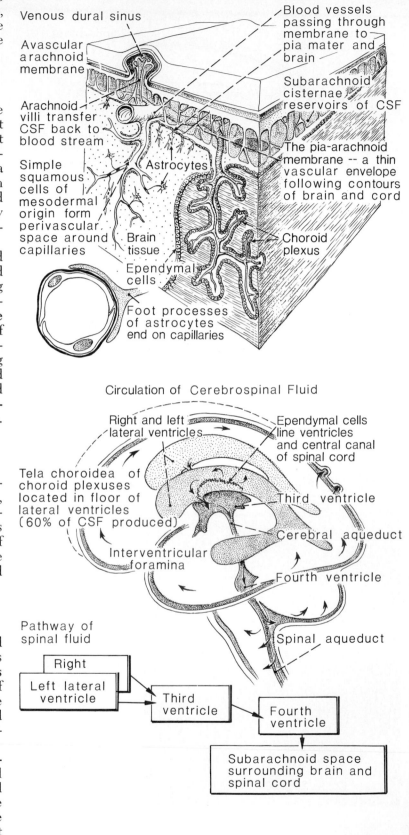

Relationships of Meninges

Venous dural sinus

Avascular arachnoid membrane

Arachnoid villi transfer CSF back to blood stream

Simple squamous cells of mesodermal origin form perivascular space around capillaries

Astrocytes

Brain tissue

Ependymal cells

Foot processes of astrocytes end on capillaries

Blood vessels passing through membrane to pia mater and brain

Subarachnoid cisternae, reservoirs of CSF

The pia-arachnoid membrane -- a thin vascular envelope following contours of brain and cord

Choroid plexus

Circulation of Cerebrospinal Fluid

Right and left lateral ventricles

Tela choroidea of choroid plexuses located in floor of lateral ventricles (60% of CSF produced)

Interventricular foramina

Ependymal cells line ventricles and central canal of spinal cord

Third ventricle

Cerebral aqueduct

Fourth ventricle

Spinal aqueduct

Pathway of spinal fluid

Right

Left lateral ventricle → Third ventricle → Fourth ventricle → Subarachnoid space surrounding brain and spinal cord

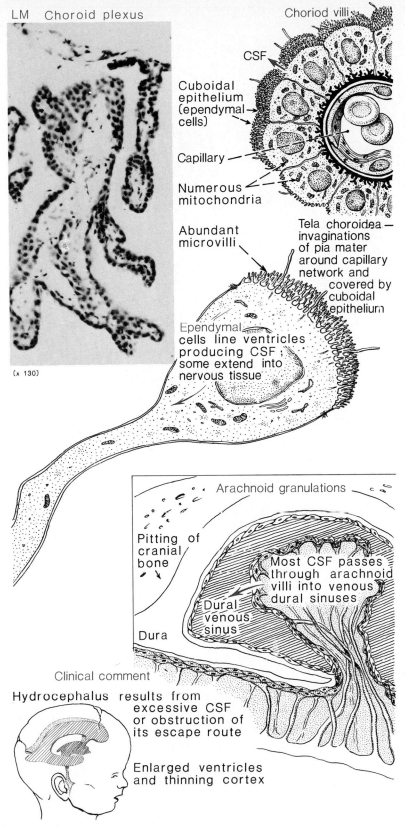

LM Choroid plexus

Choriod villi

CSF

Cuboidal epithelium (ependymal cells)

Capillary

Numerous mitochondria

Abundant microvilli

Tela choroidea — invaginations of pia mater around capillary network and covered by cuboidal epithelium

Ependymal cells line ventricles producing CSF; some extend into nervous tissue

(x 130)

Arachnoid granulations

Pitting of cranial bone

Most CSF passes through arachnoid villi into venous dural sinuses

Dural venous sinus

Dura

Clinical comment

Hydrocephalus results from excessive CSF or obstruction of its escape route

Enlarged ventricles and thinning cortex

brain, some of these processes may extend to the external surface of the brain. Along with other glial cell processes, they contribute to the formation of the **glia limitans,** discussed on page 233.

TEM micrographs of the lining ependymal cells reveal large accumulations of **mitochondria** in the apices of the cells. The other cell organelles are similar to the astrocyte, e.g., limited rER and ribosomes, small Golgi complexes, and many bundles of **microfilaments;** each filament is about 6–10 nm in diameter.

In certain regions of the ventricles of the brain, the lining ependymal cells cover tufts of capillaries, called **choroid plexuses.** This special layer of ependyma is the choroid plexus epithelium, which is involved in the production of the **cerebrospinal fluid (CSF).**

Choroid Plexuses

The choroid plexuses are delicate **capillary networks** formed by invaginations of the pia mater called **tela chorioidea.** As the plexuses invaginate into the ventricles, they are covered by a layer of cuboidal epithelium, **the ependymal cells** that line the ventricles. This epithelium shows evidence of high metabolic activity, involving the expenditure of energy in the **production of CSF.** Such cytological characteristics of the epithelium include numerous mitochondria; abundant cytoplasm; and a large, clear, vesicular nucleus. Also the plasma membrane of the free surface of these cells has irregular microvilli, suggesting an absorptive function.

Eventually, the CSF leaves the interior of the brain by way of three foramina to enter the **subarachnoid space** surrounding the brain. The fluid then flows down the subarachnoid space surrounding the spinal cord. Thus, the CSF serves as an effective **fluid buffer** or cushion for the CNS, protecting it against sudden movements of the head and body.

As the fluid diffuses over the brain, it escapes from the subarachnoid space by passing through villi that perforate the dura into the **dural venous sinuses** of the brain. These arachnoid villi become hypertrophied with age and are then called Pacchionian bodies or **arachnoid granulations.** They may be of sufficient size to produce a pitting of the cranial bones, which can be seen in the dried skull.

Hydrocephalus

If there is an excess of CSF in the ventricles, a pathological condition results called **hydrocephalus,** which means "water in the head." It may result from an **obstruction to the flow of CSF** out of the ventricles via the cerebral aqueduct. Since the CSF cannot escape from the lateral ventricles, the fluid causes pressure, which greatly **enlarges the ventricles** resulting in a **thinning** out of the **cerebral cortex** as it is pressed

11919

against the bony cranium. If this condition is congenital, the baby develops a very large head since the cranial sutures are still open (not ossified) which allows the cranial bones to be forced apart. The child is usually mentally retarded.

Hydrocephalus can be cured, or at least relieved, by a **subcutaneous bypass operation.** This consists of taking a section of a peripheral vein and anastomosing it with the lateral ventricles and to one of the large veins of the neck. Such a procedure allows the excess CSF to drain into the general blood circulation and relieves the pressure in the lateral ventricles. However, if the cause of the pressure is overproduction of CSF, then periodic aspirations of the fluid, or surgical removal of some of the choroid plexuses, may be adequate therapy.

Blood-brain Barrier

When certain drugs, pigments, or dyes are administered intravenously to animals, these substances do not enter the tissues of the brain or spinal cord, yet they penetrate most other tissues of the body. Such absorptions suggest the presence of a barrier between the capillaries of the CNS and the surrounding nervous tissue, i.e., a **blood-brain barrier.**

However, it was not until EM studies were available that the **elements of the barrier** were identified. They include the presence of: (1) many **tight junctions** between adjacent endothelial cells that line the continuous-type capillaries of the CNS, (2) a well-developed **basal lamina** surrounding these capillaries, and (3) the extensive covering of the external surface of the capillaries by myriad **end-feet processes** from astrocytes. Such a physiohistologic barrier normally allows only O_2, CO_2, and small nutrient molecules to pass which sustain the easily damaged neurons and less delicate glial cells.

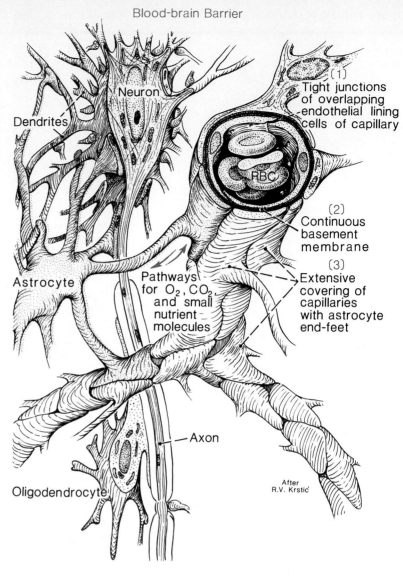

Blood-brain Barrier

Neuron

Dendrites

Astrocyte

(1) Tight junctions of overlapping endothelial lining cells of capillary

RBC

(2) Continuous basement membrane

(3) Extensive covering of capillaries with astrocyte end-feet

Pathways for O_2, CO_2, and small nutrient molecules

Axon

Oligodendrocyte

After R.V. Krstić

Table 12.1   COMPARISON OF LAYERS IN CENTRAL NERVOUS SYSTEM

LAYER NUMBER	NAME	NERVE CELL BODIES	PROCESSES AND SYNAPSES
Cerebrum I	Molecular or plexiform	Only few cells, mostly horizontal cells (of Cajal) and a few Golgi type II cells	Terminal dendrites of fusiform and pyramidal cells from deeper layers; also axonal synapses with neurons possessing ascending axons, i.e., Martinotti cells
II	Outer granular	Many small pyramidal and stellate cells which appear as granules	Dendrites of both cell types terminate here, while their axons descend to deeper layers; axons of deep Martinotti cells synapse here
III	Outer pyramidal	Most cells are medium-sized pyramidal cells; others are small pyramidal and Martinotti cells	Apical dendrites extend into molecular layer; axons descend to synapse in deeper layers
IV	Inner granular	Chiefly small, stellate cells that resemble granules under low magnification	Axons of smaller cells largely remain in layer; axons of larger cells descend to synapse in deeper layers
V	Inner pyramidal or ganglionic	Principally large and medium-sized pyramidal cells; in motor cortex giant cells of Betz are prominent	Axons pass into white matter while apical dendrites ascend into molecular layer or may arborize within layer
VI	Fusiform or multiform	Fusiform (spindle) cells dominate; their long axes are perpendicular to cortical surface	Apical dendrites of smaller spindle cells arborize within layer; others ascend into upper layers; all axons of spindle cells enter white matter; axons from cells of other layers synapse here
Cerebellum I	Molecular (outer)	Few small basket, stellate, and Golgi type II cells	Their dendrites arborize in layer; extensive Purkinje cell dendritic ramifications dominate area; T-shaped axons of granule cells synapse here
II	Purkinje (middle)	Single row of very large, flask-shaped Purkinje cells associated with a few small, basket cells	Massive, treelike dendrites extend into molecular layer; Purkinje axons extend through the inner granular layer to enter white matter
III	Granular (inner)	Very numerous, closely packed dark-staining, small granule cells; some Golgi type II cells in upper part of layer	Thin, unmyelinated axons of granule cells ascend into molecular layer; their short dendrites terminate in glomeruli near cell bodies; dendrites of Golgi cells terminate in molecular layer
Spinal Cord I	White matter	Virtually none	Parallel bundles of myelinated axons fill field; essentially no dendrites or synapses present
II	Gray matter	Three types of multipolar neurons: (a) Large, stellate motor cells in ventral horn; (b) small, stellate, internuncial cells between ventral and dorsal horns; (c) medium-sized stellate sensory cells in dorsal horn	Abundance of fine unmyelinated axons; frequent axonic synaptic terminals; very extensive dendritic plexuses surround nerve cell bodies

Table 12.2 *NEUROGLIAL CELLS*

	PROTOPLASMIC ASTROCYTE (MOSSY CELL)	FIBROUS ASTROCYTE (SPIDER CELL)	OLIGO-DENDROGLIA	MICROGLIA (MESOGLIA)	EPENDYMA
Origin	Ectoderm	Ectoderm	Ectoderm	Mesoderm	Ectoderm
Distinctive LM features	Large, round, light-staining nucleus with meager heterochromatin; abundant granular cytoplasm; many freely branching, thick, rough-surfaced processes; size 8–10 μm	Same, except long, slender, nonbranching, smooth processes	Smaller, pear-shaped cell body; often eccentric, smaller, darker nucleus with abundant heterochromatin; few, slender processes relatively free of branches; less cytoplasm but more granular; size 6–8 μm	Smallest nucleus, irregular shape, deeply staining; very limited, granular cytoplasm; few (2–4) short, twisted, processes; cells probably have ameboid motion; size 5–7 μm	Simple cuboidal or columnar epithelial cells with basal extensions that project into and interweave with the underlying astrocytes; some cells have cilia, especially in lower mammals
Distinctive EM features	Relatively organelle-poor cytoplasm; most distinctive organelles are bundles of microfilaments which extend into processes; glycogen present	Same	Considerable rER and free ribosomes; active Golgi apparatus; numerous mitochondria and lysosomes; prominent microtubules; no microfilaments or glycogen	Long, narrow rER cisternae; active Golgi apparatus often next to nucleus; lipofuscin inclusions congregate in extremities of cell	Abundant small, slender mitochondria in apex of cell; bundles of microfilaments, small Golgi apparatus, limited sER and rER; few free ribosomes and lysosomes
Location	Largely in gray matter; many processes end on capillaries as expanded end plates (perivascular feet)	Chiefly in white matter; processes also end on blood vessels	Closely associated with neurons of CNS; cell bodies often rest on capillaries	Found throughout CNS	Line ventricles of brain and central canal of spinal cord; cover choroid plexuses of brain
Function(s)	Provide scaffolding or structural support for neurons; assist in regulating cellular metabolism, especially ionic flow (K^+); insulator of receptor surfaces	Same	Myelin formation in CNS	Phagocytic cells of CNS	Secretin of cerebrospinal fluid (CSF); act as selective barrier between nervous tissue and CSF; if ciliated, may aid in circulation of CSF

Chapter

13

CIRCULATORY SYSTEM

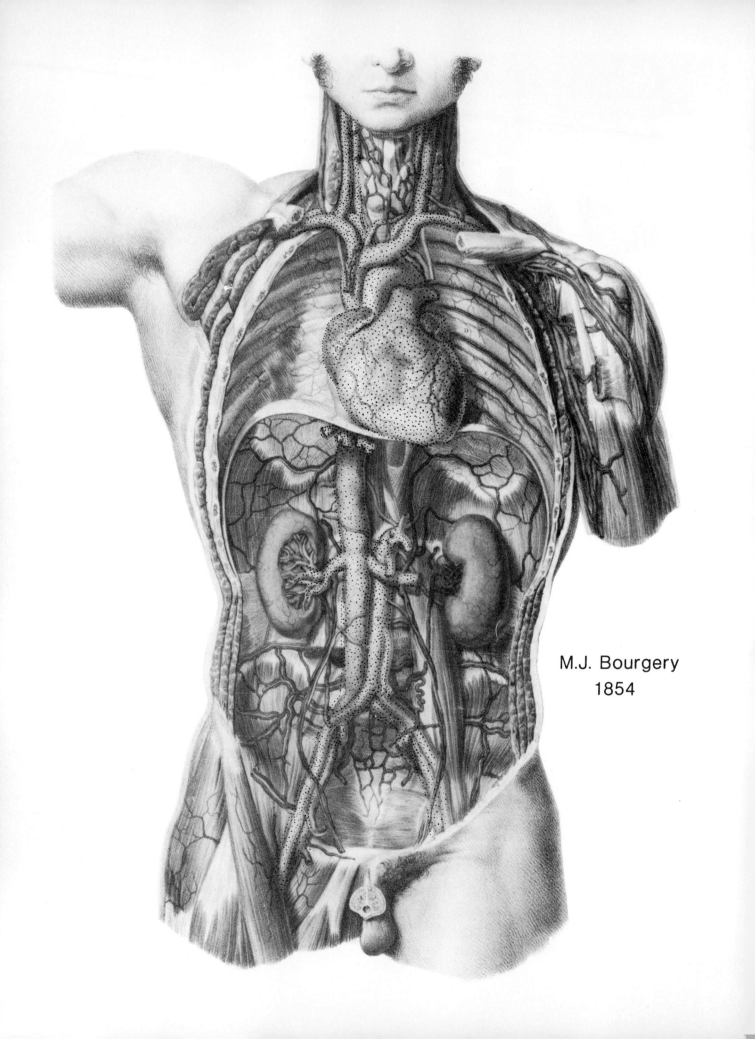

M.J. Bourgery
1854

OBJECTIVES

STUDY OF THIS CHAPTER WILL ENABLE ONE TO DIFFEREN-
TIATE THE COMPONENTS OF THE CIRCULATORY SYSTEM AT
THE LIGHT AND ELECTRON MICROSCOPIC LEVELS AND DE-
DUCE THEIR FUNCTIONS FROM THEIR MORPHOLOGY, SUCH
AS:

1. The tubular formation of the embryonic heart and its transition
   to the adult structure.

2. The tunics of the heart and why the myocardium varies in thickness in the various chambers.

3. The types of arteries, veins, and capillaries and how they differ
   with function.

4. The variations in blood vessels in certain organs to meet unusual vascular requirements.

5. The distinguishing characteristics of lymph vessels compared
   to blood vessels.

The circulatory system includes **two major subdivisions:** (1) the extensive **cardiovascular (CV) system** consists of the heart and blood vessels, and (2) the lesser subdivision is the **lymph vascular system,** composed of blind lymphatic capillaries that collect lymph from tissue spaces and drain it into lymphatic vessels. These channels anastomose with larger lymphatic vessels or trunks that empty into large veins in the neck, where the two systems merge.

CARDIOVASCULAR SYSTEM

All elements of the cardiovascular system are **tubes.** Even the heart is a tube reflected on itself, with four dilated segments, i.e., two atria and two ventricles. The walls of the system vary in thickness and composition depending on the pressure exerted on them by the circulating blood.

All components of the system, the heart, arteries, veins, and capillaries are lined with a continuous layer of **endothelial cells.** Arteries and veins have in common **three tunics** or layers: (1) the innermost **tunica intima** is composed of endothelium and a small amount of underlying connective tissue; (2) the **tunica media** is usually a circular layer of smooth muscle; and (3) the outer **tunica adventitia** consists largely of longitudinally arranged connective tissue fibers. In the heart, layers analogous to these tunics are called the endocardium, myocardium, and epicardium.

Heart

In the early embryo the heart is a **straight tube** inside the primitive pericardial cavity. During development, the tubular heart grows faster than the walls of the cavity. Such differential growth forces the tube to bend and fold on itself to form an **S- or U-shaped loop.** The ends of the loop come to lie together superiorly and become the great vessels of the heart. The rest of the tube undergoes a series of dilations and fusions that results in the formation of two small **atrial chambers** superiorly and two larger **ventricular cavities** inferiorly.

The heart, acting as a **pump,** supplies the principal **propelling force** for the circulation of the blood. The **elasticity of the large arteries** dampens the force of the heartbeat and causes the blood to flow rather evenly and continuously, instead of moving in spurts. The smaller **distributing arteries** carry the blood to all organs and tissues of the body where they terminate generally in **capillary beds.** Here the semipermeable endothelium lining the capillaries allows the exchange of O_2, CO_2, hormones, nutrients, and the disposal of metabolic wastes.

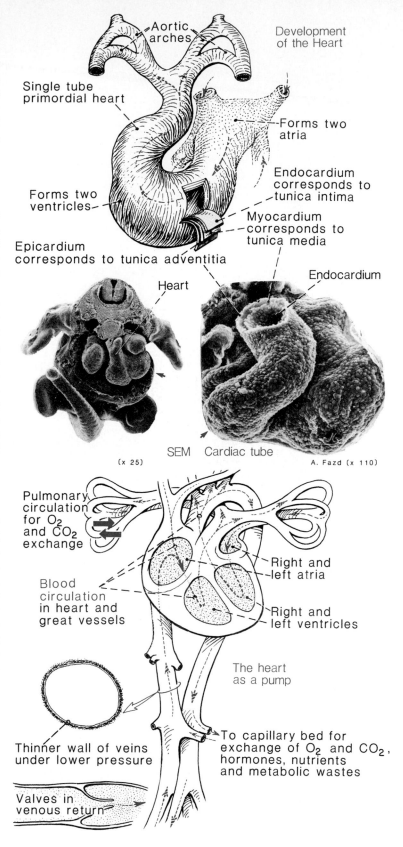

Development of the Heart

Aortic arches

Single tube primordial heart

Forms two atria

Endocardium corresponds to tunica intima

Myocardium corresponds to tunica media

Forms two ventricles

Epicardium corresponds to tunica adventitia

Heart

Endocardium

SEM Cardiac tube

(x 25)

A. Fazd (x 110)

Pulmonary circulation for O_2 and CO_2 exchange

Blood circulation in heart and great vessels

Right and left atria

Right and left ventricles

The heart as a pump

Thinner wall of veins under lower pressure

To capillary bed for exchange of O_2 and CO_2, hormones, nutrients and metabolic wastes

Valves in venous return

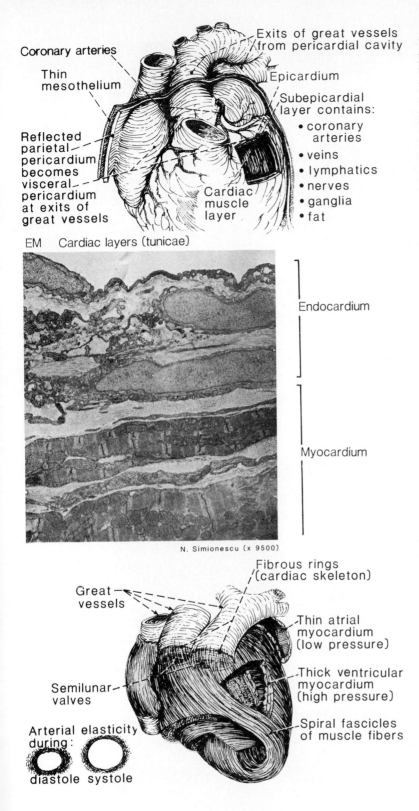

Coronary arteries

Thin mesothelium

Reflected parietal pericardium becomes visceral pericardium at exits of great vessels

Exits of great vessels from pericardial cavity

Epicardium

Subepicardial layer contains:
• coronary arteries
• veins
• lymphatics
• nerves
• ganglia
• fat

Cardiac muscle layer

EM   Cardiac layers (tunicae)

Endocardium

Myocardium

N. Simionescu (x 9500)

Fibrous rings (cardiac skeleton)

Great vessels

Thin atrial myocardium (low pressure)

Thick ventricular myocardium (high pressure)

Semilunar valves

Spiral fascicles of muscle fibers

Arterial elasticity during:

diastole   systole

The blood returns to the heart via the **thinner-walled veins,** which function under much lower pressure. They are assisted in certain areas of the body, especially the limbs, by strategically placed **valves** along their course which open to allow blood to pass toward the heart but close to prevent backflow. The force driving the venous blood towards the heart is generated largely from the contraction of the skeletal muscles, as in the extremities, which compress the thin walls of the adjacent veins, forcing the blood towards the heart.

HISTOLOGICAL FEATURES

Epicardium The three-layered heart is suspended in the **pericardial cavity** by its great vessels as they exit from the cavity. The internal lining of this fibroelastic sac is a layer of flattened, mesothelial cells (**parietal pericardium**) that reflects onto the outer surface of the heart, as the **visceral pericardium,** at the site of exit of the vessels. This serous secreting layer of cells is the outermost layer of the **epicardium.** Underlying the serous cells is a thin, supportive layer of connective tissue containing many elastic fibers. A deeper, loose connective tissue layer, sometimes called the **subepicardial layer,** is of variable thickness, depending on the amount of adipose tissue present. Embedded in this fatty layer are the coronary arteries, veins, lymphatics, nerves, and ganglia. It is within this layer that large amounts of adipose tissue accumulates in the obese individual that may compromise the action of the heart.

Myocardium The middle layer, the **myocardium,** consists of: (1) contractile fascicles of **cardiac muscle** fibers, and (2) noncontractile modified muscle fibers called **Purkinje fibers.** The cardiac muscle fibers, described in Chapter 10, are arranged in sheets in a complex, spiral manner. Many of the fibers have their origin in central, thick, fibrous rings located at the sites of origin of great vessels and valves of the heart, collectively known as the **cardiac skeleton.**

The **thickness** of the myocardium varies depending on the **pressure** within the various cavities. It is thinnest in the low-pressure atria and thickest in the high-pressure left ventricle. The thickness of the myocardium, especially in the ventricles, increases when the walls of the chambers of the heart are contracting. This phase of the cardiac cycle is called **systole.** In **diastole,** when the chambers are at rest, the myocardium is thinner.

SEM   Smooth intima of a normal coronary artery

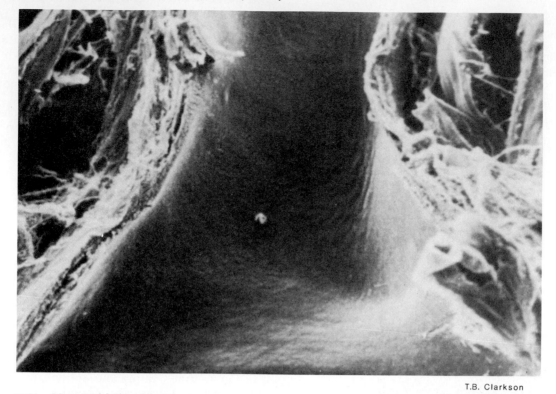

T.B. Clarkson

SEM   Disrupted intima of a coronary artery showing athrosclerotic
      plaques and early degenerative lesions

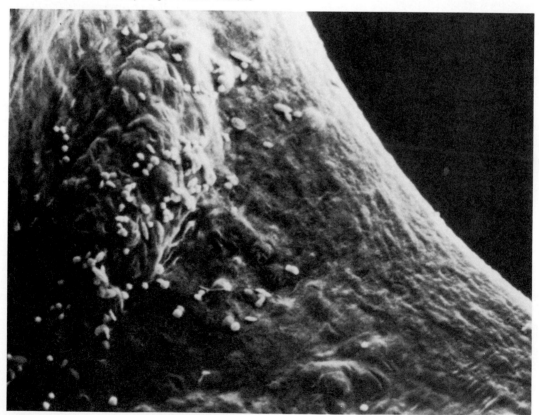

T.B. Clarkson

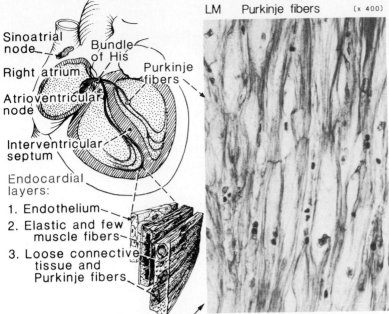

Sinoatrial node
Bundle of His
Right atrium
Purkinje fibers
Atrioventricular node
Interventricular septum

LM   Purkinje fibers   (x 400)

Endocardial layers:
1. Endothelium
2. Elastic and few muscle fibers
3. Loose connective tissue and Purkinje fibers

Faintly striated noncontractile myofibrils generate and conduct nervous impulses

Endocardium

Ventricular cavity

Endothelial cell nucleus
Basal lamina
Mitochondria
Intercalated disks

Endothelium
Connective tissue
Nucleus of fiberblast
Collagen & elastic fibers
Cardiac muscle

Atria Removed to Show Valves of Heart

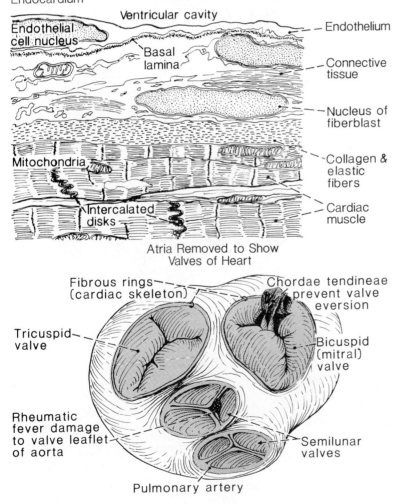

Fibrous rings (cardiac skeleton)
Chordae tendineae prevent valve eversion
Tricuspid valve
Bicuspid (mitral) valve
Rheumatic fever damage to valve leaflet of aorta
Semilunar valves
Pulmonary artery

The **Purkinje fibers** are found scattered along the innermost part of the myocardium **next to the endocardium.** These fibers are found especially along the interventricular septum and the internal surface of the ventricular walls covered by the endocardium. These modified muscle cells have the potential to **generate nervous impulses** and to conduct them throughout the myocardium. These impulses synchronize the heartbeat. Purkinje fibers are the **conduction system of the heart,** discussed in Chapter 10.

Endocardium The endocardium, the thinnest layer of the heart, has **three components:** (1) a glistening, continuous layer of **endothelium** resting on a basal lamina and a layer of loose collagenous fibers; (2) a deeper, denser layer composed mostly of **elastic fibers** and a few smooth muscle fibers; and (3) a **subendocardial zone** of loose connective tissue containing small vessels, nerves and, in the ventricles and their common septum, scattered Purkinje fibers.

The endocardium varies in thickness in reverse proportion to the thickness of the underlying myocardium. It is thickest lining the left atrium and thinnest in the left ventricle.

VALVES OF THE HEART Four fibrous **valves guard the orifices** of the heart. They are (1) the **tricuspid** located between the right atrium and right ventricle, (2) the **pulmonary semilunar,** (3) the **aortic semilunar,** and (4) the **bicuspid or mitral,** between the left atrium and left ventricle. These valves have three triangular **cusps,** except the mitral which has two. The bases of all cusps are centrally located in a dense, fibrous ring, the **annulus fibrosis,** which contributes to the heavy connective tissue core common to all valves. All cardiac valves are **folds of endocardium** enclosing a **central core** of dense collagenous and elastic fibers. A few smooth muscle fibers penetrate into the thicker valves, i.e., the tricuspid and bicuspid.

Fibrous cords, the **chordae tendineae,** extend from the inner surfaces of the ventricular wall to connect the ventricular surface of each valve leaflet. These cords serve to restrict the extent the valves can be everted towards the atria when the ventricles contract. In other words, they prevent the valves from being blown inside out during ventricular contraction.

Rheumatic fever, especially in children, often **damages the heart valves.** In their subsequent healing, the valves may become deformed or shortened due to scar formation. The result is a valve that does not open or close properly, causing the valve to leak, hence, the lay term "leakage of the heart" to describe this condition.

4636

Arteries

The layers of the heart are continuous with the **walls of the arteries.** The innermost arterial coat, the **intima,** is composed of a single layer of **endothelial cells** resting on a thin bed of connective tissue. The middle muscular layer, the **media,** consists of **circular bands of smooth muscle** with varying amounts of elastic and collagenous fibers. The external coat or **adventitia,** is a **connective tissue investment** but is not covered by mesothelium, as is the epicardium.

Arteries decrease in size and increase in number as they proceed distally from the heart. They are usually **classified** according **to size** or the **predominant tissue** component. The usual classification is (1) large or elastic, (2) medium or muscular, and (3) small or arterioles.

ELASTIC ARTERIES Large **elastic arteries** include the **aorta** and its larger branches. The wall is relatively thin as compared to the wide lumen. The **intima** is rather thick and the internal elastic lamina may not be prominent and is often replaced by the first elastic lamella of the media. The **thick media** is composed mostly of **elastic fibers** arranged in 40–60 laminae, each about 2–3 μm thick with some collagenous fibers, while the **muscle fibers** are greatly reduced. The **adventitia** is relatively thin, usually has no external elastic lamina, and contains **vasa vasorum,** a small system of vessels to nourish the heavy arterial wall, since it is too thick to be nourished by diffusion from the blood. The adventitia keeps under control the expansible media, similar to a tire casing acting on an inner tube.

MUSCULAR ARTERIES Muscular or **medium arteries** function as **distributing vessels.** They also **regulate blood flow** to various regions by either constriction or relaxation of their walls. They may be as large as the femoral or brachial arteries or as small as unnamed arteries, just visible to the unaided eye. Upon demand they have the capacity to increase greatly in size. For example, in an occlusion of the principal arteries to a region, the smaller collateral, **muscular arteries enlarge** sufficiently to effectively carry the needed blood to the ischemic area. Furthermore, when injured, these arteries contract spastically, which may prevent fatal hemorrhage.

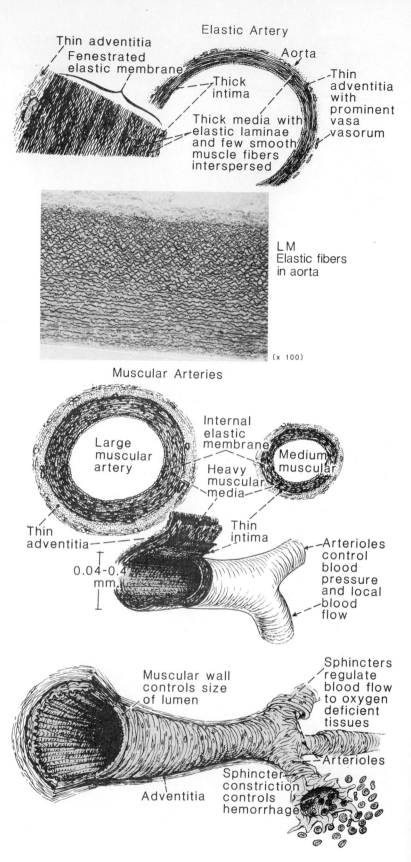

Elastic Artery

Thin adventitia
Fenestrated elastic membrane
Aorta
Thin adventitia
Thick intima
Thin adventitia with prominent vasa vasorum
Thick media with elastic laminae and few smooth muscle fibers interspersed

LM Elastic fibers in aorta

(x 100)

Muscular Arteries

Large muscular artery
Internal elastic membrane
Medium muscular
Heavy muscular media
Thin adventitia
Thin intima
0.04–0.4 mm.
Arterioles control blood pressure and local blood flow

Muscular wall controls size of lumen
Sphincters regulate blood flow to oxygen deficient tissues
Arterioles
Sphincter constriction controls hemorrhage
Adventitia

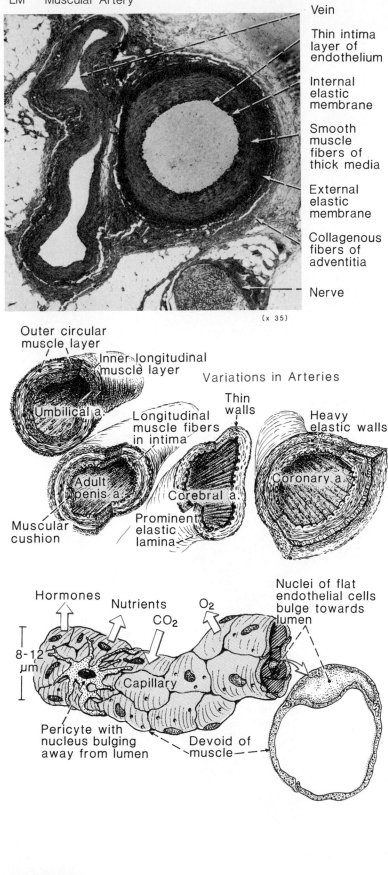

LM Muscular Artery

Vein

Thin intima layer of endothelium

Internal elastic membrane

Smooth muscle fibers of thick media

External elastic membrane

Collagenous fibers of adventitia

Nerve

(x 35)

Outer circular muscle layer

Inner longitudinal muscle layer

Variations in Arteries

Umbilical a.

Longitudinal muscle fibers in intima

Thin walls

Heavy elastic walls

Adult penis a.

Cerebral a.

Coronary a.

Muscular cushion

Prominent elastic lamina

Hormones   Nutrients   O₂

CO₂

Nuclei of flat endothelial cells bulge towards lumen

8-12 μm

Capillary

Pericyte with nucleus bulging away from lumen

Devoid of muscle

The thin **intima** consists of a layer of **endothelium** and a flattened **subendothelial layer** of collagenous and elastic fibers. An **internal elastic lamina** is a prominent feature. The thick **media** is predominantly **circular layers** (30–40) of smooth muscle fibers. In the larger arteries, elastic laminae form the external elastic lamina. The robust **adventitia** is usually thinner than the media and is composed mostly of **collagenous fibers.** Near the media its elastic fibers are numerous and some of them contribute to the external elastic lamina (L–A, plate 11).

ARTERIOLES Arterioles are the **smallest muscular arteries.** Their diameters are about 0.04–0.4 mm. The intima is thin; the **media** is relatively **thick;** and the adventitia is fairly prominent. These vessels are the prime **controllers of systemic blood pressure** and local blood flow.

Metarterioles (precapillaries) are interposed between the capillary bed and the arterioles. They are less than 40 μm in diameter and are encircled by a **few smooth muscle fibers.** They act as **sphincters** for control of blood flow into the capillary bed.

VARIATIONS IN ARTERIES Cerebral arteries resemble veins in having a thin wall but a prominent internal elastic lamina. **Coronary arteries** have thick walls with considerable elastic tissue. They are functionally equivalent to vasa vasorum of large veins and arteries and anastomose with the vasa vasorum of the great vessels of the heart. At puberty, the **arteries of the penis** develop longitudinal muscle fibers in the thickened intima called a cushion. **Umbilical arteries** have an inner longitudinal and an outer circular layer of smooth muscle in the media.

Capillaries

A **true capillary** is essentially an **endothelial lined tubule** usually about 8 μm in diameter, although some may be much larger (12 μm) or smaller (5 μm). They are devoid of muscular and connective tissue coats. The endothelial cell boundaries can be revealed by silver impregnation. Since a capillary is a very thin tube, it is often collapsed and may be unnoticed in histological sections. However, the **nuclei** of the endothelial cells bulge into the lumen, thus aiding in the identification of the capillary.

Because capillaries have no smooth muscle in their walls, they cannot actively contract. However, the basal lamina of capillaries splits to enclose **pericytes (myoepithelial cells)** that may contract and perhaps constrict the capillaries. Capillary beds are found in almost every tissue of the body. They are the **sites for exchange** of CO_2, O_2, nutrients, and hormones between the blood and the cells of the body. By diffusion through the capillary wall, oxygen is conveyed from the blood plasma into adjacent cells.

EM   Arteriole

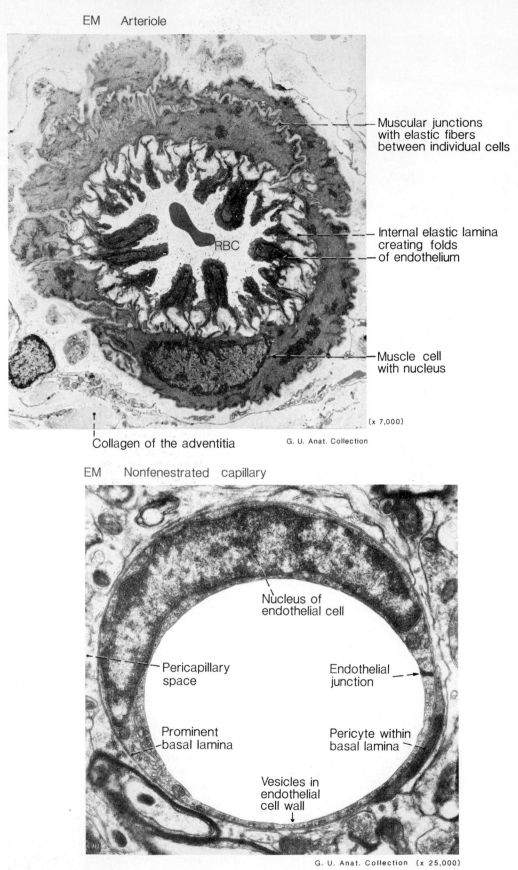

Muscular junctions
with elastic fibers
between individual cells

Internal elastic lamina
creating folds
of endothelium

RBC

Muscle cell
with nucleus

(x 7,000)

Collagen of the adventitia

G. U. Anat. Collection

EM   Nonfenestrated capillary

Nucleus of
endothelial cell

Pericapillary
space

Endothelial
junction

Prominent
basal lamina

Pericyte within
basal lamina

Vesicles in
endothelial
cell wall

G. U. Anat. Collection (x 25,000)

In this upper EM micrograph of an arteriole the luminal surface is distorted by abnormal
folds of endothelium, created by agonal contraction of the internal elastic membrane. The
media consists of two or three layers of smooth muscle.

The lower EM micrograph of a continuous capillary reveals an uninterrupted,
continuous lining that contains no pores. The endothelial lining cells are joined by tight
junctions. Observe that the basal lamina splits to enclose a pericyte, which may constrict
the capillary.

252

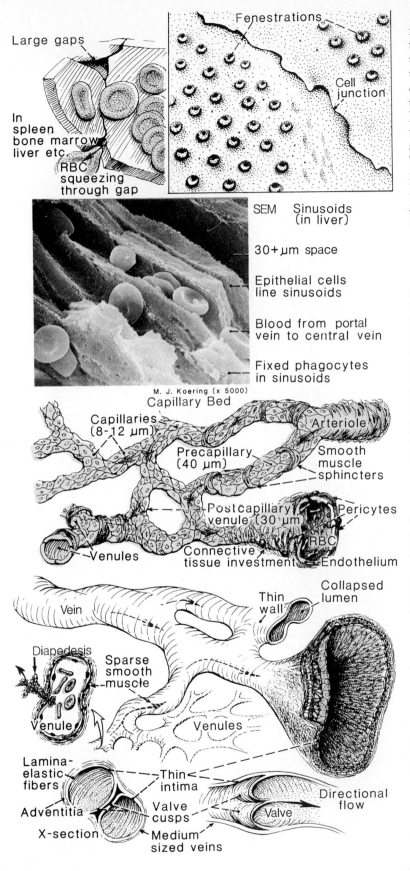

Fenestrations

Large gaps

Cell junction

In spleen bone marrow liver etc.

RBC squeezing through gap

SEM Sinusoids (in liver)

30+ μm space

Epithelial cells line sinusoids

Blood from portal vein to central vein

Fixed phagocytes in sinusoids

M. J. Koering (x 5000)

Capillary Bed

Capillaries (8-12 μm)

Arteriole

Precapillary (40 μm)

Smooth muscle sphincters

Postcapillary venule (30 μm)

Pericytes

RBC

Venules

Connective tissue investment

Endothelium

Vein

Collapsed lumen

Thin wall

Diapedesis

Sparse smooth muscle

Venule

Venules

Directional flow

Lamina-elastic fibers

Thin intima

Adventitia

Valve cusps

Valve

X-section

Medium sized veins

Most capillaries are **continuous,** that is, the flat, endothelial cells are connected by cell junctions and overlapping, serrated margins. Another type of capillary, found principally in the intestinal villi and the glomeruli of the kidney, has endothelium with minute pores, called **fenestrations,** through the cells, not between them; hence, they are called fenestrated capillaries. A third type, **discontinuous (sinusoidal)** capillaries, are found in the spleen, bone marrow, and liver. These differ from the other types by their larger, irregular lumina, and the cells are separated by large gaps through which blood cells may pass. Junctional complexes are absent, except in the spleen.

Sinusoids

Sinusoids resemble capillaries but possess certain **distinctive features.** Since the basal lamina may be deficient or absent, the endothelial cells may rest directly on connective tissue. They have relatively **wide, uneven channels** (30 μm or more), and the blood flow is sluggish. The **endothelium is incomplete,** consisting of flat endothelial cells and fixed phagocytic cells that often project into the lumen. Sinusoids may connect arterioles with venules, as in the bone marrow, spleen, or adrenal cortex; or they may link venules to venules, as in the liver and adenohypophysis (Table 13.1).

Veins

Veins are subject to more variation in structure than arteries, and therefore a rigid classification is difficult. Nevertheless, the same categories are identified as for arteries, i.e., large, medium, and small (venules). The **lumen** of a vein is always proportionally **larger,** often collapsed or **usually filled with blood,** as contrasted with the open, empty lumen of an artery.

VENULES Postcapillary **venules** may have a diameter of 30 μm or more. Their thin walls consist of **endothelium,** an incomplete layer of **pericytes,** and a thin, **connective tissue investment.** Functionally, they are similar to capillaries.

Venules are the smallest veins, about 0.2–1.0 mm in diameter. Their **intima** has continuous endothelium with a thin basal lamina. Their thin **media** has only a few smooth muscle fibers. As the vessel becomes larger, the amount of muscle increases and a rather thick adventitia develops, yet the wall continues to allow passage of blood cells through it. For example, by a process called **diapedesis,** leukocytes pass between the endothelial cells to escape into the surrounding connective tissue. Even though the space between the endothelial cells is smaller than the diameter of the leukocyte, a small portion of the cell squeezes through the opening, momentarily constricted to the size of the opening.

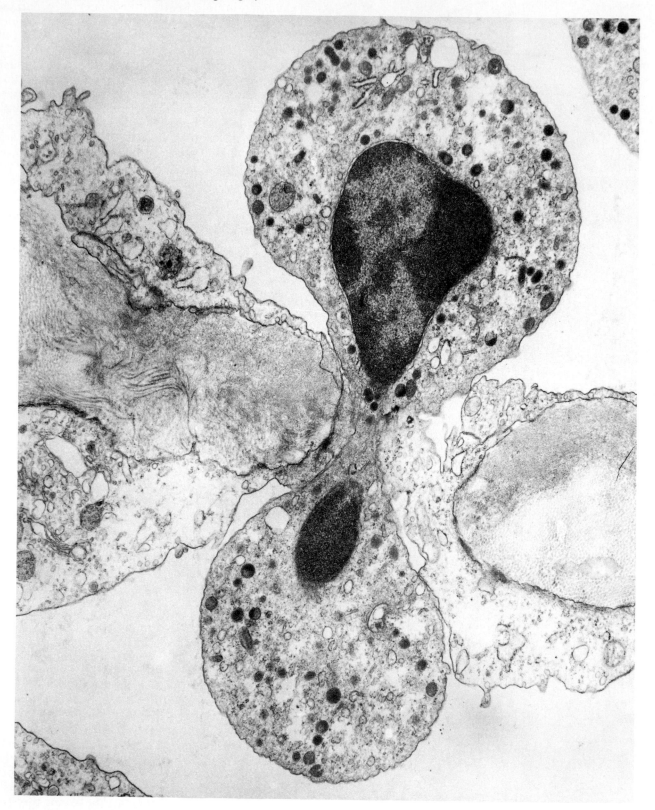

L. V. Leak (x 17,000)

In this EM micrograph of the inferior (peritoneal) surface of the diaphragm, a neutrophil is observed passing through a stoma (an opening between the mesothelial cells) to enter the lumen of a lymphatic vessel within the diaphragm. Such a view dramatically demonstrates the extreme plasticity of leukocytes which enables them to traverse openings much smaller than their normal diameter.

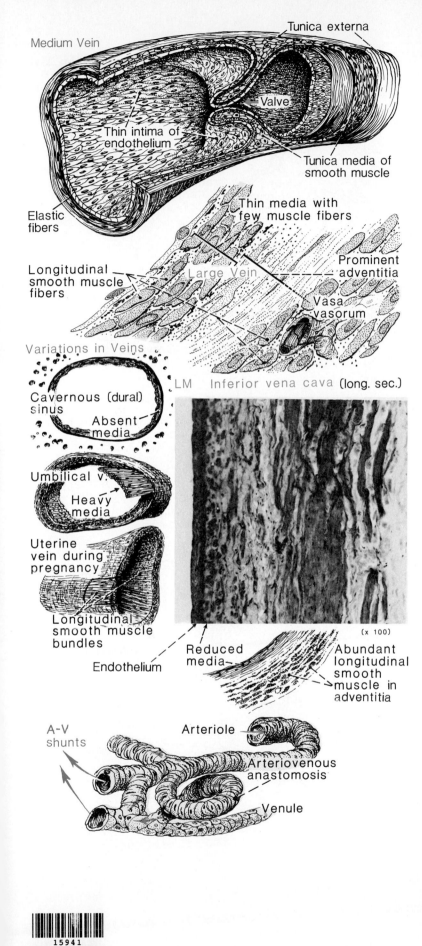

Medium Vein

Tunica externa

Valve

Thin intima of endothelium

Tunica media of smooth muscle

Elastic fibers

Thin media with few muscle fibers

Prominent adventitia

Large Vein

Longitudinal smooth muscle fibers

Vasa vasorum

Variations in Veins

Cavernous (dural) sinus

Absent media

LM   Inferior vena cava (long. sec.)

Umbilical v.

Heavy media

Uterine vein during pregnancy

Longitudinal smooth muscle bundles

Endothelium

Reduced media

(x 100)

Abundant longitudinal smooth muscle in adventitia

A-V shunts

Arteriole

Arteriovenous anastomosis

Venule

MEDIUM VEINS Medium-sized (muscular) veins include most of the **named veins** in the body, except the largest. The **tunica intima** is thin, similar to venules. **Valves** are found in the extremities as folds of the intima, with endothelium covering both sides of a core of elastic fibers. A clear boundary between intima and media is often lacking. The **media** is thin in contrast to corresponding arteries. The **adventitia** is **well-developed** and forms the bulk of the wall of the vein.

LARGE VEINS Large veins, such as the venae cavae, have a **thicker intima** but a **poorly developed media** with smooth muscle largely replaced by fibrous tissue. However, the **adventitia** is **very prominent** and makes up most of the wall. It is composed of prominent bundles of longitudinally arranged **smooth muscle fibers,** interposed with considerable amounts of collagenous fibers. A system of **vasa vasorum** is best developed in large veins.

VARIATIONS IN VEINS Veins, with special functions or with unusual surroundings, **vary greatly** in their structure. For example, veins enclosed in a hard, unyielding enclosure or tissue **lack valves** and smooth muscle, and therefore **have no media.** These include veins of the brain and its meninges and the dural sinuses. Also included are the veins of bones, retina, placenta, and trabeculae of the spleen. In contrast, a few veins have an unusually **heavy media,** e.g., veins of the **pampiniform plexus** of the spermatic cord and the **umbilical vein.**

Other variations include longitudinal smooth muscle bundles that may occur in **uterine veins** during pregnancy. Smooth muscle is also found in the intima of the **internal jugular vein** and in some veins of the limbs. As mentioned above, longitudinal smooth muscle fibers constitute most of the adventitia in large veins. In fact, the **media may be absent** in the **inferior vena cava** and replaced with an abundance of longitudinal muscle bundles in the thick adventitia (Table 13.2).

Arteriovenous Anastomoses

In certain regions of the body, there are alternate channels that permit blood to pass directly from arterioles into venules, bypassing the capillary beds. These are **arteriovenous anastomoses or A-V shunts,** which are present mostly in the skin of the finger tips, toes, nail beds, and face. A-V shunts in such areas exhibit vasomotor activity and are acutely involved in **regulation of heat loss** through the skin. Other anastomoses are found in the liver, thyroid, placenta, erectile tissue, intestinal tract, and carotid and aortic bodies. The latter two structures are specifically responsive to chemical stimuli, e.g., blood pH and CO_2 tension.

LYMPH VASCULAR SYSTEM

The lymph vascular system is a **secondary route** for intercellular fluid to return to the heart. This fluid is **lymph**, a blood ultrafiltrate derived from the blood plasma that has escaped from capillaries into the interstitial spaces. It contains many **lymphocytes and fat droplets** (chylomicrons).

The lymphatic system begins in blind-beginning **capillaries in connective tissue spaces** in nearly all organs and tissues of the body. The exceptions, which contain no lymphatics, are the brain, spinal cord, bone marrow, fetal placenta, and coats of the eyeball. Centrally, the lymph capillaries anastomose to form lymph vessels that pass through **lymph nodes** where the lymph is filtered and additional lymphocytes and antibodies are added to the lymph stream. These vessels ultimately join two large lymphatic ducts, i.e., the **large thoracic duct** and the much **smaller right lymphatic duct** that empty into large veins in the neck. Unlike the blood vascular system, the lymph system **flows only in one direction,** from the periphery to the heart. Also it has no pump and is largely dependent upon the compression of the walls of the lymph vessels by surrounding structures for the movement of the lymph centrally toward the heart.

An important **function** of the lymph is to **carry away** from the tissue spaces **particulate matter and proteins** of high molecular weight, neither of which can be absorbed into the blood capillaries.

Discussions of the lymphatic organs, i.e., lymph nodes and nodules, spleen, tonsils, and thymus are found in Chapter 14.

Lymph Capillaries

Lymph capillaries resemble blood capillaries except that they are **not as uniform in caliber** and often have dilations and constrictions. They are delicate **endothelial-lined tubes, void of muscle** fibers, and embedded in loose connective tissue. They form extensive networks by profuse branching and anastomoses, especially near their origin. They are roughly coextensive with blood capillaries.

TEM micrographs reveal that **endothelial cells** of lymph capillaries overlap each other and have only a **few junctional complexes.** The cells have no fenestrae (pores) but have **intercellular clefts** between the cells. These clefts provide ingress of large proteins and particulate matter that cannot be absorbed by the adjacent blood capillaries.

Lymph Vessels

Large lymphatic vessels (0.3 mm in diameter) resemble veins, having **three tunics.** However, these coats are not as distinctly demarcated as in veins of comparable size. The **tunica intima** consists of flat, endothelial cells resting on a delicate

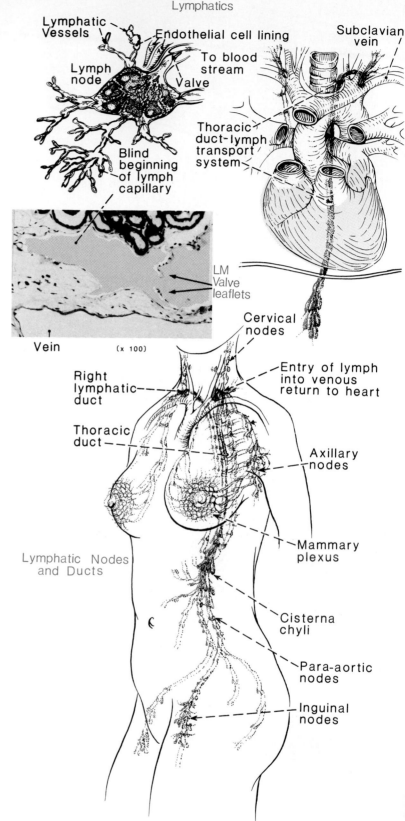

Lymphatics

Lymphatic Vessels
Endothelial cell lining
Subclavian vein
Lymph node
To blood stream
Valve
Thoracic duct-lymph transport system
Blind beginning of lymph capillary
LM Valve leaflets
Vein   (x 100)
Cervical nodes
Right lymphatic duct
Entry of lymph into venous return to heart
Thoracic duct
Axillary nodes
Mammary plexus
Lymphatic Nodes and Ducts
Cisterna chyli
Para-aortic nodes
Inguinal nodes

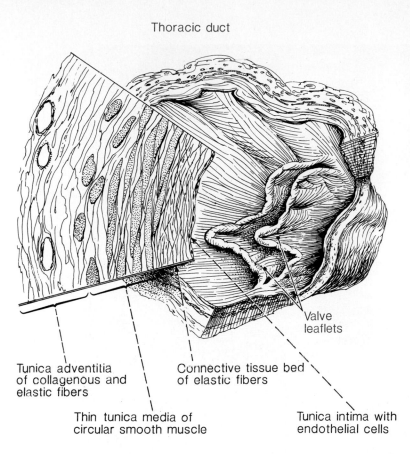

Thoracic duct

Tunica adventitia
of collagenous and
elastic fibers

Thin tunica media of
circular smooth muscle

Connective tissue bed
of elastic fibers

Valve
leaflets

Tunica intima with
endothelial cells

network of connective tissue, mostly elastic fibers. The **tunica media** is a thin layer of largely circular smooth muscle fibers with a few elastic fibers interposed between the muscle bundles. The **tunica adventitia**, the thickest coat, consists of interlacing collagenous and elastic fibers. A few longitudinally oriented smooth muscle cells are also present.

Like veins, the larger lymphatic vessels have **valves**, often more numerous than in veins.

Lymphatic Ducts

All lymphatic vessels eventually drain into two main ducts: the large and longer **thoracic duct** and the less extensive **right lymphatic duct**. The histological structure of these ducts is similar to a vein of comparable size; however, the tunics are less distinctly delineated.

The well-developed **intima** has a continuous endothelial lining, with a few muscle fibers and elastic fibers in the subendothelial layer. It is well-supplied with **valves**. The **media** is the thickest coat, with even more circular smooth muscle fibers than a vein of comparable size. The **adventitia** is poorly defined and blends with the adjacent connective tissue.

LM   Comparison of artery, lymphatic and vein

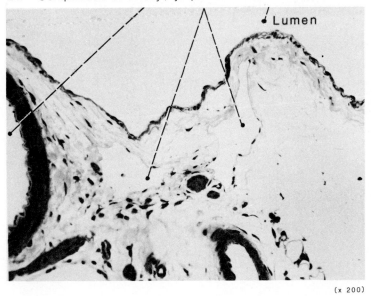

Lumen

(x 200)

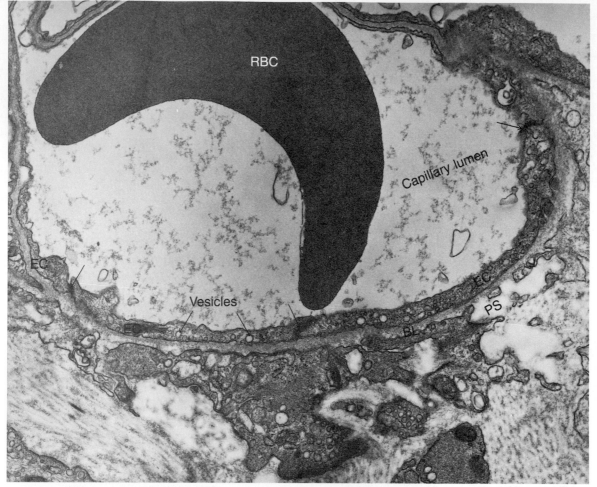

Capillary lumen

RBC

EC

EC

PS

Vesicles

EC

BL

G. U. Anat. Collection

Sinusoids

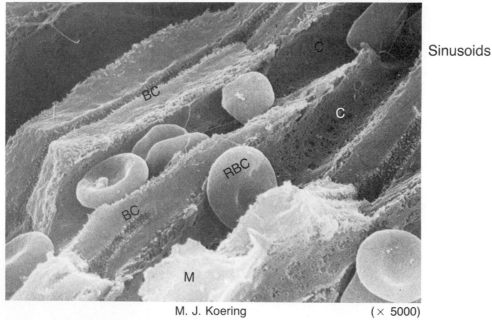

C

BC

C

RBC

BC

M

M. J. Koering   (× 5000)

Upper EM micrograph of a continuous capillary with nonfenestrated endothelium. Also indicated are endothelial junctions (at arrows), and erythrocyte (RBC), basal lamina (BL), plasmalemmal vesicles, and the pericapillary space (PS).

    The lower SEM view is a series of liver sinusoidal capillaries (C) containing erythrocytes (RBC), fenestrated endothelium (with pores), bile capillaries with microvilli (BS), and macrophages (M) that partially line a sinusoid.

Table 13.1 *COMPARISON OF CAPILLARIES, SINUSOIDS, AND SINUSES*

DIAGNOSTIC FEATURES	CONTINUOUS CAPILLARIES	FENES-TRATED CAPILLARIES	LYMPH CAPILLARIES	SINUSOIDS[a]	VENOUS SINUSES	LYMPH SINUSES
Typical location	Muscle	Most viscera	Lymph nodes	Liver, spleen, bone marrow	Spleen	Lymph nodes
Endothelium	Continuous	Continuous	Contiguous but not continuous	Discontinuous, many macrophages	Discontinuous, many macrophages	Discontinuous, with many macrophages
Fenestrations in endothelium	None	Many, small (0.07–0.1 μm)	Only in lacteals	Variable, larger (0.1–0.2 μm)	None	None
Phagocytic endothelium	None	None	None	Active	Limited activity	Very active
Diameter of lumen	Small (6–10 μm), regular	Small (6–10 μm), regular	Larger (10–50 μm), irregular	Variable (5–30 μm), irregular	Largest, irregular	Large, irregular
Basement membrane	Well developed, continuous	Well developed, continuous	Scanty or absent	Scanty or absent	Scanty, discontinuous	Absent
Intercellular spaces	None	None	None	Present 0.1–0.5 μm	Variable	Present
Junctional complexes	Present	Present	Usually absent	Absent, except in spleen	Absent	No data
Pericytes	Present	Present	Absent	Maybe present in liver	Absent	Absent

[a] Also called sinusoidal capillaries

Table 13.2 *DISTINGUISHING FEATURES OF HUMAN BLOOD VESSELS*

	ARTERIES				
	LARGE (ELASTIC)	MEDIUM (MUSCULAR)	ARTERIOLES	PRECAPIL-LARY ARTERIOLES	CAPILLARIES
Diameter of lumen Range Average	>1 cm 2.5 cm	0.5 mm − 1 cm 0.4 cm	<0.5 mm 30 μm	10–40 μm 25 μm	5–12 μm 8 μm
Wall thickness (average)	2 mm	1 mm	20 μm	No data	1 μm
Smooth muscle (relative amount)	+ +	+ + +	+ + + +	+	−
Elastic fibers	+ + + +	+ +	+	±	−
Pericytes	−	−	−	−	+
Vasa vasorum	+ + +	+	−	−	−
Nerve supply	+ + + (esp. sensory)	+ +	+ + + (esp. motor)	+ + + (esp. motor)	−
Lymphatics	+ +	+	−	−	−
Blood pressure, adult (average mm Hg)	100	95	35	No data	22
Blood flow velocity (average cm/sec)	45	12	1.0	No data	0.1
Function	Elastic recoil maintains flow in diastole	Distribution of blood	Regulate blood pressure by changes in diameter	Capillary sphincters	Exchange of O_2, CO_2, nutrients, waste products, etc.

VEINS				
POST-CAPILLARY VENULES	COLLECTING (PERICYTIC) VENULES	MUSCULAR VENULES	MEDIUM	LARGE
12–30 μm 20 μm	30–50 μm 40 μm	50 μm–3 mm 1.0 mm	3 mm–1 cm 0.5 cm	>1 cm 3 cm
2 μm	No data	0.1 mm	0.5 mm	1.5 mm
−	−	±	+	+ + (largely in adventitia)
−	±	±	+	+ +
+ + (incomplete layer)	+ + + + (complete layer)	−	−	−
−	−	−	+ +	+ + + +
−	−	+	+ +	+ + + (esp. in adventitia)
−	−	−	±	+ + +
No data	No data	12	5	3 (maybe negative near heart)
No data	No data	0.5	5	15
Similar to capillaries	Highly permeable, important in blood–tissue exchange, e.g., inflammation	Transport venous blood	Collect venuous blood	Carry venous blood to heart

LYMPHATIC SYSTEM

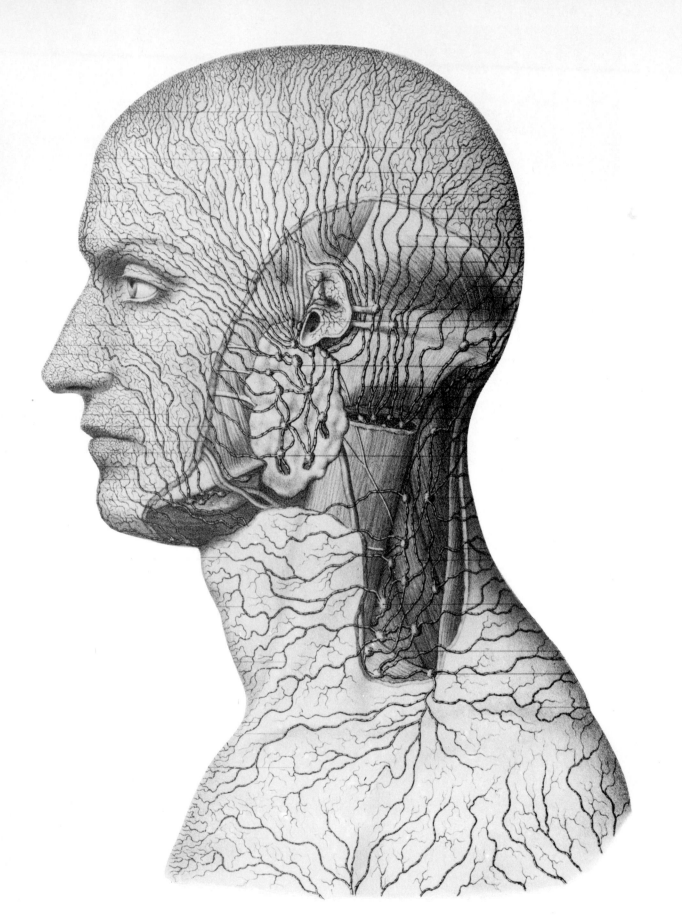

M.P.C. Sappey   1874

OBJECTIVES

TO BE ABLE TO:

1. Locate in the body the various types of lymphoid tissue.

2. Differentiate between lymphatic nodules and lymph nodes; pharyngeal and palatine tonsils; spleen and thymus.

3. Explain how the structure of the spleen is built around its blood supply.

4. Interpret the role of the thymus in the establishment of the immune system in the body.

5. Outline the functions of each type of lymphoid tissue and identify the cellular and vascular elements that make possible these varied functions.

Although lymphoid tissue is widely distributed in the body, it is not a primary tissue but rather a special type of connective tissue. As the term is generally used it connotes the **parenchyma** of lymphoid organs and the diffuse, delicate reticular connective tissue network in which the **lymphocyte,** the principal cell type, is enmeshed.

The organs and tissues of the lymphoid system are the source of **immunocompetent cells,** i.e., **lymphocytes** and **plasma cells** that function primarily to protect the body from damage from foreign substances (antigens). As discussed in Chapter 8, these immunologically competent cells have the unique capacity to recognize any substance in the body as **self or nonself** (foreign). If the material is alien, it is an **antigen** (a substance that provokes an immune response) and, whether harmful or beneficial, the cells will **destroy or neutralize** it by either of two methods: (1) by the cells, e.g., T-lymphocytes, attaching to and inactivating the antigen, called the **cell-mediated response;** or (2) by the use of **antibodies,** which are humoral products of plasma cells. Antibodies are released into the bloodstream, lymph, or tissue fluid, where they circulate until they combine with and destroy foreign antigens. This is called the **humoral response.**

The **sources of antigens** are legion, but to name a few: pathogenic bacteria; viruses; pollens; protozoa; fungi; venoms; certain foods; some drugs, e.g., penicillin; tissue and organ transplants; and certain tumor cells and their toxins.

COMPONENTS

Lymph vessels have been discussed with the circulatory system (Chapter 13). Lymphoid tissue and organs, each with distinctive morphological features and functions, will now be examined.

Lymphoid tissue is present in the body in five distinct forms: (1) as **diffuse, unencapsulated** collections of lymphocytes usually subepithelial in position; (2) as dense, discrete nonencapsulated **solitary nodules** located especially in the tunica propria, the subepithelial loose connective tissue layer of the gastrointestinal and respiratory tracts; nodules are also arranged in **aggregates,** such as Peyer's patches in the ileum, and in the tonsils; (3) as **encapsulated lymph nodes** (often incorrectly called glands) located in special sites of the body, such as axilla, groin, and neck; (4) in the **thymus as nodules** containing a cortex and medulla; and (5) in the spleen largely as the white pulp (**splenic nodules**).

Lymphocytes so dominate lymphoid tissues that they largely obscure the extensive **stroma.** All **small lymphocytes** are morphologically similar, but functionally two distinct types are recognized, i.e., the **T-lymphocyte** nurtured in the thymus, and the **B-lymphocyte** that probably has its origin in the bone marrow. These important cell types have been discussed in Chapter 8.

Other free cells in lymphoid tissues are other leukocytes, plasma cells, macrophages, and lymphoblasts. Fixed cells are mostly reticular cells which, with the reticular fibers, form the stroma where the free cells are enmeshed. Also, many fixed macrophages are attached to the stromal network.

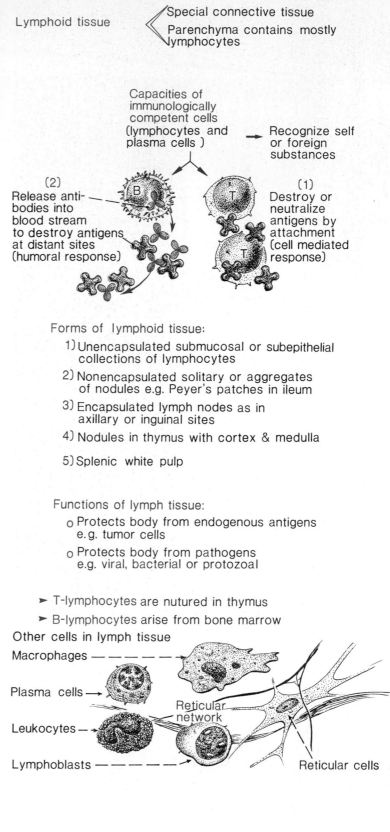

Lymphoid tissue
⟨ Special connective tissue
Parenchyma contains mostly lymphocytes

Capacities of immunologically competent cells (lymphocytes and plasma cells) → Recognize self or foreign substances

(2) Release antibodies into blood stream to destroy antigens at distant sites (humoral response)

(1) Destroy or neutralize antigens by attachment (cell mediated response)

Forms of lymphoid tissue:

1) Unencapsulated submucosal or subepithelial collections of lymphocytes
2) Nonencapsulated solitary or aggregates of nodules e.g. Peyer's patches in ileum
3) Encapsulated lymph nodes as in axillary or inguinal sites
4) Nodules in thymus with cortex & medulla
5) Splenic white pulp

Functions of lymph tissue:

o Protects body from endogenous antigens e.g. tumor cells
o Protects body from pathogens e.g. viral, bacterial or protozoal

► T-lymphocytes are nutured in thymus
► B-lymphocytes arise from bone marrow

Other cells in lymph tissue

Macrophages

Plasma cells →

Leukocytes →

Reticular network

Lymphoblasts

Reticular cells

Diffuse Lymphoid Tissue

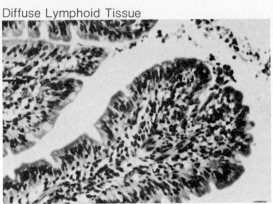

Diffuse Lymphoid Tissue

LM
Small lymphocytes caught in reticular network of tunica propria in respiratory and gastrointestinal tracts

T.G. Merrill (x 660)

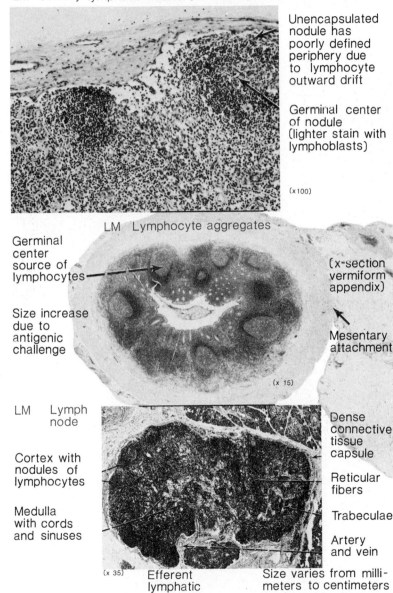

LM Solitary lymphatic nodule (0.2 -1mm)

Unencapsulated nodule has poorly defined periphery due to lymphocyte outward drift

Germinal center of nodule (lighter stain with lymphoblasts)

(x100)

LM Lymphocyte aggregates

Germinal center source of lymphocytes

Size increase due to antigenic challenge

(x-section vermiform appendix)

Mesentary attachment

(x 15)

LM Lymph node

Cortex with nodules of lymphocytes

Medulla with cords and sinuses

Dense connective tissue capsule

Reticular fibers

Trabeculae

Artery and vein

(x 35) Efferent lymphatic

Size varies from millimeters to centimeters

Diffuse lymphoid tissue is the least organized of the lymphoid structures. It is a loose concentration of **small lymphocytes** caught in a **reticular network**. Diffuse lymphoid tissue is found chiefly as an infiltration of lymphocytes into the **tunica propria** of the respiratory and gastrointestinal tracts. Except **macrophages**, other free cells are infrequently seen. With time, the lymphocyte population increases in certain areas and collects into clusters called lymphatic nodules.

Lymphatic Nodules

These nodules have several synonyms, e.g., primary nodule and lymphatic follicle. Where they occur singly, they are called **solitary nodules;** when in clusters, they are known as **aggregates** or **patches.**

They are also found as **isolated, unencapsulated bodies** in the loose connective tissue (especially in the **tunica propria**) of all organs of the digestive and respiratory systems and, to a lesser extent, in the urinary passageways. The individual nodule may be a transient structure and varies greatly in size, from 0.2 to 1.0 mm in diameter. The periphery of the roughly spherical nodule is poorly defined because the lymphocytes blend into the surrounding loose connective tissue. The center of the nodule may be quite dense and homogeneous in the primary nodule, or may show a lighter-stained central area called the **germinal center,** in which case the nodule is called a **secondary nodule.** The lighter staining of the central area results from the presence of many large, activated lymphocytes called **lymphoblasts** or immunoblasts. They have ample, light-staining cytoplasm with a large, pale, euchromatic nucleus, as contrasted to the small, heterochromatic nuclei of the small lymphocytes in the periphery of the nodule.

Aggregates of lymphoid nodules principally occur in the tunica propria of (1) the ileum opposite the mesenteric attachment, as **Peyer's patches;** (2) the vermiform appendix; and (3) the tonsils. Many of the nodules show germinal centers. They are the sites for multiplication of the **immunocompetent lymphocytes** that respond to antigenic challenges that arrive via the blood and lymph. In fact, their presence and numbers depend on the degree and frequency of these **antigenic stimulations.** For example, in localized inflammatory conditions, nodules with germinal centers greatly increase in size and number, while in the newborn infant and gnotobiotic (germ-free) animals, nodules are rare.

Lymph Nodes

Lymph nodes are oval or bean-shaped **encapsulated bodies** that are always interposed along the course of **lymphatic vessels.**

3208

The node is surrounded by a dense connective **capsule,** which sends delicate trabeculae (projections) into the node. The **trabeculae** support a **reticulum** of reticular fibers and cells which extends throughout the structure. This is the **stroma** of the node, which provides a network to hold in suspension the innumerable lymphocytes.

Each node has two distinct zones: (1) a dense, **outer cortex** just beneath the capsule composed of numerous **lymphoid nodules** usually with germinal centers, and (2) a less dense, **central medulla** with lymphocytes arranged in widely spaced strands called **medullary cords.** The cords are ropes of lymphocytes caught in a reticulum radiating from the cortex toward the **hilus,** which is an indentation of the capsule where small arteries enter, and veins and lymphatics leave the node. In addition to myriad small lymphocytes, many **macrophages and reticular cells** are also found in the cords.

Between the cortex and medulla is a poorly defined zone called the **paracortical region, or the thymic dependent zone.** It contains many densely packed lymphocytes that are primarily **T-lymphocytes,** involved in cell-mediated immune responses. The fact that these cells are migrants from the thymus or descendants of thymic cells is evident from the observation that in animals that are thymectomized at birth, this region is depleted of lymphocytes. Most of the other lymphocytes in lymph nodes are the **B-type,** concerned with the production of **specific antibodies** through **plasma cells,** to be discussed later.

LYMPH VESSELS AND SINUSES Numerous **afferent lymph vessels** with valves convey lymph from a drainage area in the body to the convex outer surface of a lymph node. Here, the vessels obliquely pierce the capsule to empty into the large marginal or **subcapsular sinus** which separates the capsule from the cortical parenchyma. Because it is a large, relatively cell-free zone, the marginal sinus is the **unique structure** that enables one to distinguish the lymph node from other "look-alike" lymphoid organs.

The subcapsular sinus drains radially into **cortical sinuses,** which lie between the lymph nodules within the lymph node. The sinuses then follow along the trabeculae to empty into the wide, expansive **medullary sinuses** that border the medullary cords. The medullary sinuses coalesce and converge towards the hilus where they pierce the capsule as the **efferent lymphatic vessels** that exit at the hilus. Efferent lymphatics are wider but less numerous than the afferent vessels. The efferent vessels are guarded by valves which direct the lymph away from the nodes. Thus the **lymph flows only in one direction** through a lymph node, the only lymphoid structure that has both afferent and efferent lymph vessels.

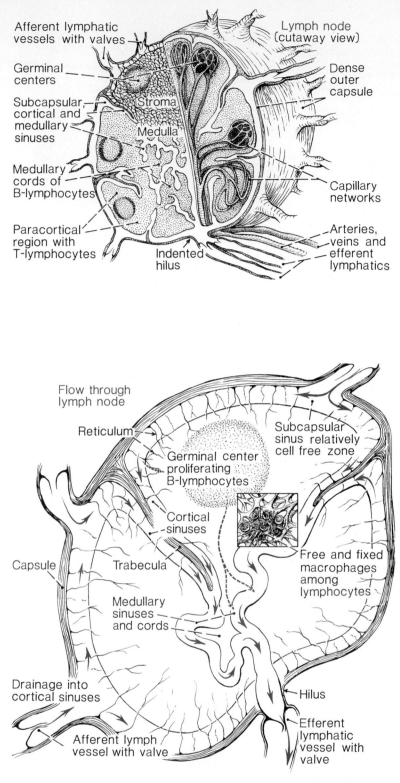

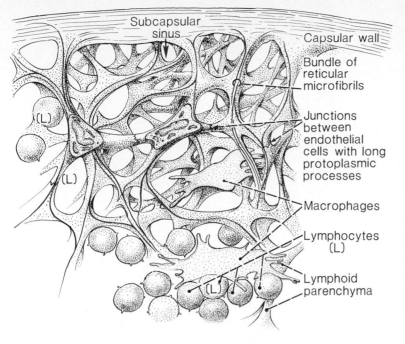

Subcapsular sinus

Capsular wall

Bundle of reticular microfibrils

Junctions between endothelial cells with long protoplasmic processes

Macrophages

Lymphocytes (L)

Lymphoid parenchyma

Function of lymph nodes in defenses against infections:

o filtration of lymph

o sites of phagocytosis (especially by macrophages)

o sites for production of antibodies (by plasma cells)

o production and recirculation of lymphocytes

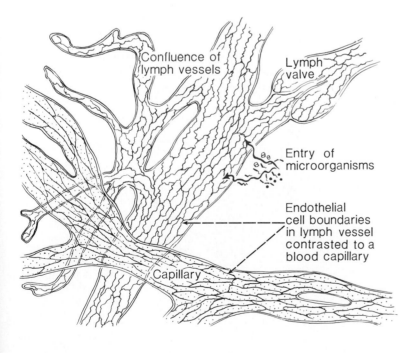

Confluence of lymph vessels

Lymph valve

Entry of microorganisms

Endothelial cell boundaries in lymph vessel contrasted to a blood capillary

Capillary

Endothelial cells, macrophages, and reticular cells line the lymphatic sinuses. The **endothelial cells** may be **discontinuous** and flat, with gaps between them, or **stellate with irregular processes** that may attach to adjacent endothelial cells by specialized junctional complexes. Also these processes may extend across the sinus for attachment. These projections function to create turbulence and a deceleration of the lymph flow, which increases the lymph node's filtration efficiency. These endothelial cells are slightly phagocytic. Fixed **macrophages** take up residence along the walls of the sinuses.

The **reticular cells**, especially in the germinal center, have long protoplasmic processes and are therefore often called **dendritic reticular cells.** The dendritic cells in the germinal centers are a cell type distinct from reticular cells. Their long dendritic processes also extend across the sinuses to impede the lymph flow. They are not phagocytic cells, as was previously believed.

FUNCTIONS OF LYMPH NODES Lymph nodes are a major component of the body's **defense mechanism** against infection. In fact, all of their various functions are involved in the control of pathogens. One of these control measures is the **filtration of lymph** as it passes through a node. The walls of the delicate lymph capillaries are easily penetrated by **pathogenic bacteria** that have breached the epidermal and mucosal barriers of the body to reach the omnipresent lymphatic system. There is no completely effective barrier to prevent the entrance of any endogenous or exogenous immunogenic substances from entering the body. However, since lymph must pass through **lymph nodes,** they act as an effective **filtration barrier** against the spread of these microorganisms and their toxins. The extensive meshwork within the lymph sinuses, composed of processes of the lining cells and reticular fibers, constitutes an effective, mechanical filter. Turbulence is set up in the lymph flow through the meshwork. This greatly decreases the flow rate, making the **filtration process more effective.** Also entrapped in the meshwork is **particulate matter,** e.g., carbon and dye particles, and cellular debris. However, the barrier is not perfect. Malignant cells, for example, may continue through the node to metastasize in an organ or tissue distal to the node.

Closely associated with filtration is the node's second action, **phagocytosis.** Fixed and free macrophages are plentiful in the lymph sinuses. The slow lymph flow favors phagocytosis of antigens, e.g., particulate matter and bacteria and their toxins.

A third function of lymph nodes is the **production of antibodies,** principally by **plasma cells** concentrated in medullary cords. These cells are descendants of large **B-lymphocytes** (lymphoblasts). Their antibodies carry a **humoral immune response** to the antigen, especially bacteria, from the regions drained by the lymph node. For example, an antigen from an infection of the hand elicits an antibody response in the axillary nodes. As the nodes react to a **tissue inflammation** in their drainage area, there is a marked increase in number of germinal centers, an enlargement (**hypertrophy**) of the lymph nodes, and proliferation (**hyperplasia**) of lymphocytes and reticular cells in the cortical lymph nodules. Thus, lymph nodes become swollen, tender, and are more easily palpable.

The **production and recirculation of lymphocytes** is a fourth function of lymph nodes. Frequent mitotic figures are seen in the large lymphocytes of the germinal centers, yet only about 5% of lymphocytes leaving the lymph nodes are newly formed cells; the remainder are **recirculating small lymphocytes.** Both T- and B-lymphocytes recirculate but usually not the large lymphocytes (lymphoblasts). As the T- and B-cells enter a node, via the afferent lymph vessels in the capsule, or by passing through the walls of blood vessels in the paracortex, they go separate ways. **B-lymphocytes** congregate in the **lymphoid nodules** in the cortex, while the **T-cells** settle out in the **paracortical region,** the thymic-dependent zone.

Regional Differences

Recall that lymph nodes are widely distributed in the body, especially in the axilla, groin, superficial neck, along the larger blood vessels, and mesenteries. There are considerable **histological variations** in these regional nodes. For example, in one region the nodes may have a **well-developed medulla** with prominent medullary cords. Nodes from another region may show an **expansive cortex,** richly populated by abundant, active germinal centers but with a very limited medulla. One should be constantly aware of these variations and seek out typical sections for study with both cortex and medulla adequately represented.

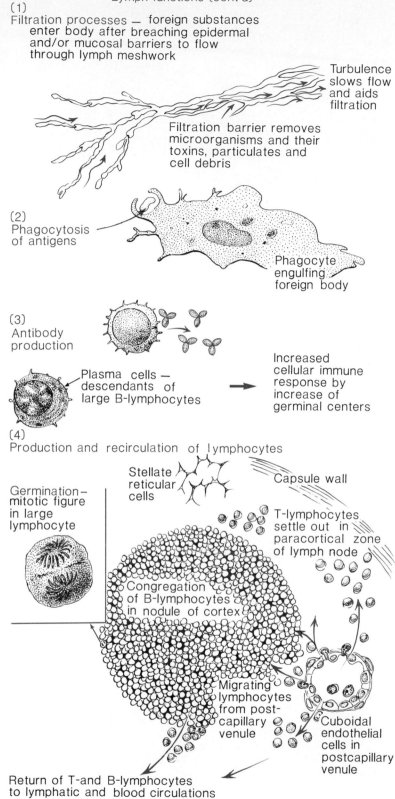

Lymph functions (cont'd)

(1) Filtration processes — foreign substances enter body after breaching epidermal and/or mucosal barriers to flow through lymph meshwork

Turbulence slows flow and aids filtration

Filtration barrier removes microorganisms and their toxins, particulates and cell debris

(2) Phagocytosis of antigens

Phagocyte engulfing foreign body

(3) Antibody production

Plasma cells — descendants of large B-lymphocytes

Increased cellular immune response by increase of germinal centers

(4) Production and recirculation of lymphocytes

Germination—mitotic figure in large lymphocyte

Stellate reticular cells

Capsule wall

T-lymphocytes settle out in paracortical zone of lymph node

Congregation of B-lymphocytes in nodule of cortex

Migrating lymphocytes from post-capillary venule

Cuboidal endothelial cells in postcapillary venule

Return of T-and B-lymphocytes to lymphatic and blood circulations

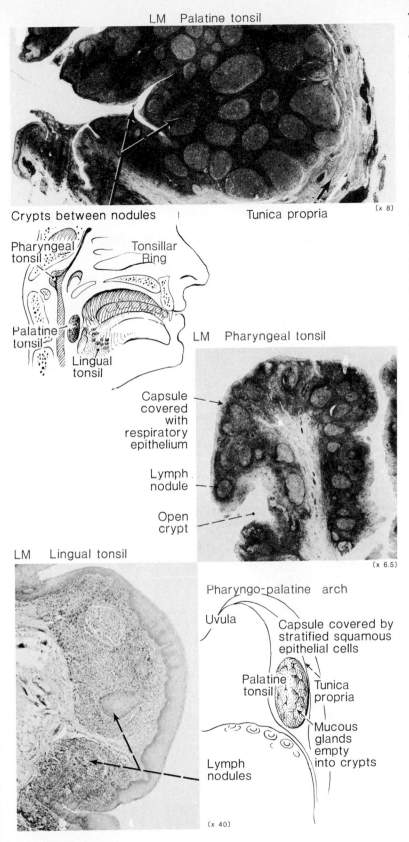

LM Palatine tonsil

Crypts between nodules   Tunica propria   (x 8)

Pharyngeal tonsil

Tonsillar Ring

Palatine tonsil

Lingual tonsil

LM Pharyngeal tonsil

Capsule covered with respiratory epithelium

Lymph nodule

Open crypt

(x 6.5)

LM Lingual tonsil

Pharyngo-palatine arch

Uvula

Capsule covered by stratified squamous epithelial cells

Palatine tonsil

Tunica propria

Mucous glands empty into crypts

Lymph nodules

(x 40)

TONSILS

The various tonsils are structures that form a ring of lymphoid tissue, called **Waldeyer's ring,** around the pharynx where the oral and nasal passageways are joined. Tonsils are named from their location, i.e., pharyngeal (in nasopharynx), palatine (in oropharynx near the palate), lingual (in root of tongue), and tubal [encircling the auditory (eustachian) tube].

Pharyngeal Tonsil

The pharyngeal tonsil is a **single mass** of lightly **encapsulated lymphoid tissue,** attached to the superoposterior wall of the nasopharynx behind the nasal cavity. It is normally covered by pseudostratified columnar ciliated eipthelium, i.e., typical **respiratory epithelium.** However, patches of stratified squamous epithelium may be found. The surface epithelium is folded into pleats, forming shallow, **open crypts** that extend into the tunica propria. The tunica propria contains many **lymph nodules.** Especially in children with frequent nasal infections, this tonsil may become inflamed causing marked **hypertrophy** with resulting obstruction of the nasal passageways, a condition clinically called **adenoids.** In chronic nasal infections, the respiratory epithelium covering the tonsil may undergo dedifferentiation into stratified squamous epithelium, commonly seen in pathological specimens.

Palatine Tonsils

The **two palatine tonsils** are ovoid structures with many lymphoid nodules. They are located at the entrance of the throat, one on each side. They have an **incomplete robust capsule** attaching them to the deeper structures of the throat. The tonsils are covered with **stratified squamous epithelium** that penetrates deeply into the parenchyma to form many invaginations or **crypts.** This gives the tonsils a wrinkled, irregular appearance. The deep crypts may contain masses of bacteria, desquamated epithelial cells, and many lymphocytes. Normally, the crypts are kept reasonably clean by the flushing action of secretions of **mucous glands** located in the submucosa. Some of their ducts empty into the crypts. However, if the crypts become clogged and infected, the tonsil becomes enlarged, inflamed, and painful, typical of an attack of **tonsillitis** (L-A, plate 12).

Lingual Tonsil

The lingual tonsil is an **aggregate of lymph nodules** buried beneath the stratified squamous epithelium at the **base of the tongue,** posterior to the prominent circumvallate papillae. It has several **wide-open crypts** with lymph nodules in the adjacent parenchyma. The crypts are seldom infected because of the excellent flushing action of underlying **mucous glands.**

Tubal Tonsils

The two small, circular **tubal tonsils** guard the pharyngeal orifice of each pharyngotympanic **(auditory) tube.** They may be considered to be lateral extensions of the pharyngeal tonsil. They are also covered by **respiratory epithelium.** Like other members of the tonsillar ring, they may enlarge during nasal and oral infections. Their enlargement can occlude the openings of the tubes, resulting in a muffled hearing sensation with some hearing loss.

VERMIFORM APPENDIX

The **vermiform appendix,** a narrow blind evagination of the cecum, is another lymphoid organ associated with the digestive tract. Because its **lamina propria** is almost entirely filled with **lymphoid nodules,** it has been called the "tonsil of the abdomen." Its functions are similar to tonsils, e.g., **production of lymphocytes** and the control of pathogenic bacteria and viruses. Its detailed histology is discussed later in Chapter 18.

PEYER'S PATCHES

Peyer's patches are **accumulations of lymphoid tissue** in the intestinal wall, mostly in the **ileum,** opposite the mesenteric attachment. Each patch may have 20–30 **lymph nodules.** Because of their functions, they are often referred to as the "tonsils of the intestine." Solitary nodules are scattered throughout the subepithelial tissues of the intestines. They **increase in number** in the more **distal gut** segments; i.e., they are sparse in the duodenum but profuse in the large intestine.

SPLEEN

The spleen is the **largest lymphoid organ** in the body. It is located beneath the left portion of the diaphragm under shelter of the lower ribs. Unlike lymph nodes, it has **no afferent lymphatic vessels.** Because it is interposed within the circulatory system, it acts as a **discriminatory filter,** screening out blood-borne foreign matter, effete blood cells, pathogenic organisms, and cellular debris. These materials are destroyed or immobilized by the myriad **macrophages** that are permanent residents of the spleen. As lymph nodes react to lymph-borne antigens by an appropriate immune response, so does the spleen **react to blood-borne antigens.** It is perhaps the most important site for **antibody production** in the body.

Structure

The capsule of the spleen consists of a dense, **robust, collagenous capsule** that has considerable **elastic fiber** and **smooth muscle** components. Many branching **trabeculae** of the capsule divide

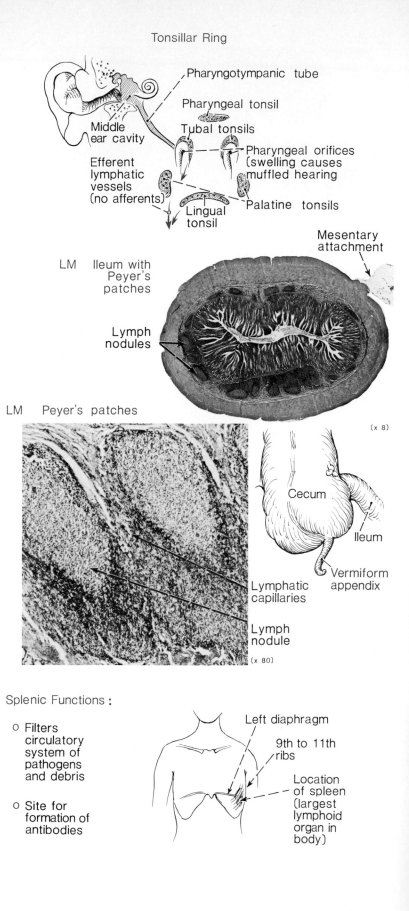

Tonsillar Ring

Pharyngotympanic tube
Pharyngeal tonsil
Tubal tonsils
Middle ear cavity
Efferent lymphatic vessels (no afferents)
Pharyngeal orifices (swelling causes muffled hearing
Palatine tonsils
Lingual tonsil

LM Ileum with Peyer's patches
Lymph nodules
Mesentary attachment
(x 8)

LM Peyer's patches
Cecum
Ileum
Vermiform appendix
Lymphatic capillaries
Lymph nodule
(x 80)

Splenic Functions :

o Filters circulatory system of pathogens and debris

o Site for formation of antibodies

Left diaphragm
9th to 11th ribs
Location of spleen (largest lymphoid organ in body)

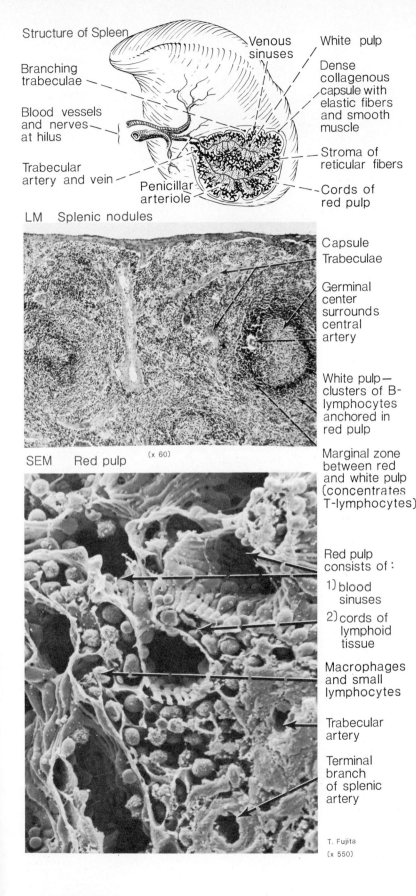

Structure of Spleen

Branching trabeculae

Blood vessels and nerves at hilus

Trabecular artery and vein

Penicillar arteriole

Venous sinuses

White pulp

Dense collagenous capsule with elastic fibers and smooth muscle

Stroma of reticular fibers

Cords of red pulp

LM Splenic nodules

Capsule

Trabeculae

Germinal center surrounds central artery

White pulp — clusters of B-lymphocytes anchored in red pulp

Marginal zone between red and white pulp (concentrates T-lymphocytes)

(x 60)

SEM Red pulp

Red pulp consists of:

1) blood sinuses

2) cords of lymphoid tissue

Macrophages and small lymphocytes

Trabecular artery

Terminal branch of splenic artery

T. Fujita

(x 550)

the spleen into incomplete compartments. Entering at the hilus, blood vessels and nerves follow along these incomplete partitions.

It is the contraction of the **smooth muscle** fibers in the capsule and trabeculae that gives the spleen its feeble, **rhythmical contractions** that result in changes in splenic volume. These variations may be considerable, especially in animals under stress, causing a **small blood transfusion** to be delivered into the bloodstream with each contraction. Such "transfusions" are probably negligible in humans.

The **stroma** is composed of a fine mesh of **reticular fibers** that attach to and blend with the walls of blood vessels, trabeculae, and the inner surface of the capsule. These fine reticular fibers hold the **cellular elements** that make up the splenic pulp in suspension, e.g., reticular and plasma cells, macrophages, RBCs and lymphocytes.

Splenic Pulp

The parenchyma is the lymphoid and erythroid tissue that comprise the **splenic pulp.** A freshly cut spleen reveals two distinct areas, i.e., small islands of greyish white, the **white pulp,** which are anchored in a blood-filled stroma, the **red pulp.**

Under the LM, the **white pulp** consists of small clusters of **lymphocytes** arranged in nodules with germinal centers called **splenic nodules** or **Malpighian corpuscles.** They contain varying numbers of large and medium lymphocytes, monocytes, plasma cells, and macrophages. These nodules are organized around a small arteriole called the **central artery,** which is usually eccentric in position, located at the edge of the germinal center. Also in the white pulp are small trabeculae arranged in a delicate reticular network.

The **red pulp** is the major component of the parenchyma. It consists of large, thin-walled **sinuses filled with blood** and thin plates or cords of lymphoid tissue, the **splenic cords** (of Billroth) wedged between the sinuses. In addition to all circulating blood cells, these cords contain many **macrophages,** which destroy senile RBCs and granulocytes, and effete plasma cells. Postnatally, the red pulp is a **storage depot** for red blood cells, while in the early fetus it is a temporary site of **hemopoiesis.**

The **marginal zone** is a poorly defined area (20–30 μm) between the red and white pulp where most of the arterioles from the white pulp terminate. It is an important area for **filtering** out antigens.

Blood Supply

The structure of the spleen is built around its blood supply. Therefore, for an understanding of this organ, one must be able to visualize its vasculature.

The terminal branch of the splenic artery divides into several branches before entering the spleen at the hilus. These **splenic branches** subdivide into muscular arteries that course along the trabeculae, as the **trabecular arteries.** As these arteries leave the trabeculae to enter the red pulp, they acquire **periarterial lymphatic sheaths,** which enclose the **central arteries** that penetrate the splenic nodules. The muscular coat of these central arteries has been replaced with a reticular sheath that is highly infiltrated with lymphocytes. Their lining **endothelial cells** are **cuboidal,** not squamous, in shape. As the central artery proceeds through the pulp, lymphatic nodules in reticular sheaths force the artery to occupy an **eccentric position** in respect to the node; yet it is still called the central artery.

Breaking out of the white pulp, the central artery enters the red pulp at the marginal zone to divide into several branches that lie close together like bristles of a brush. These are the **penicilli** (L. penicillus, brush) **arterioles** about 25 μm in outside diameter, each with three successive, distinctive regions. The longest and most proximal segment is called the **pulp arteriole.** It has a thin, smooth muscle wall with cuboidal endothelial lining cells resting on a thick basal lamina. When the pulp arteriole is thickened by a reticular, spindle-shaped sheath, it is called the **sheathed arteriole.** Its sheath is infiltrated with macrophages and lymphocytes; its endothelium is continuous, but the basal lamina is discontinuous. When the sheathed arteriole loses its sheath distally, it is called the **terminal arteriole or capillary,** which has a flat, continuous endothelium with an intact basal lamina.

The terminal capillaries may transport blood by one of two routes: (1) The blood is delivered **directly into the venous sinuses** located in the red pulp between the splenic cords, the so-called **closed circulation** concept. (2) The blood drains into the spaces **between the sinuses** to be collected later into the sinuses, the **open circulation** route. Probably both systems exist. For example, if the spleen is distended with blood (storage phase), the circulation would be open. If the organ has limited blood, the capillaries then would have direct communications with the sinuses, i.e., a closed circulation exists.

The venous return consists of **venous sinuses** that anastomose freely throughout the **red pulp** dividing it into the **pulp cords.** These are true blood sinuses. They have irregular lumina that are easily distended and have discontinuous endothelial lining. The slightly phagocytic lining cells are **atypical endothelium,** being fusiform, elongated cells, arranged parallel to each other like staves of a barrel. Incomplete strips of **basal laminae** of variable thickness encircle the sinusoids like hoops of a wooden barrel.

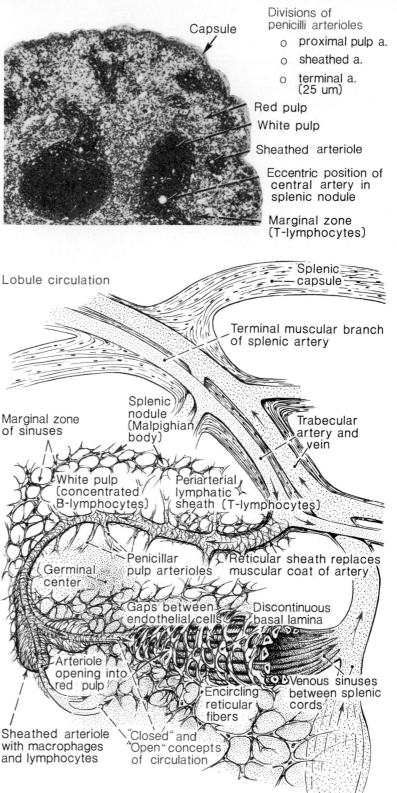

Splenic blood supply

Capsule

Divisions of penicilli arterioles
o proximal pulp a.
o sheathed a.
o terminal a. (25 um)

Red pulp

White pulp

Sheathed arteriole

Eccentric position of central artery in splenic nodule

Marginal zone (T-lymphocytes)

Lobule circulation

Splenic capsule

Terminal muscular branch of splenic artery

Trabecular artery and vein

Splenic nodule (Malpighian body)

Marginal zone of sinuses

White pulp (concentrated B-lymphocytes)

Periarterial lymphatic sheath (T-lymphocytes)

Reticular sheath replaces muscular coat of artery

Penicillar pulp arterioles

Germinal center

Gaps between endothelial cells

Discontinuous basal lamina

Arteriole opening into red pulp

Encircling reticular fibers

Venous sinuses between splenic cords

Sheathed arteriole with macrophages and lymphocytes

"Closed" and "Open" concepts of circulation

Splenic Sinuses

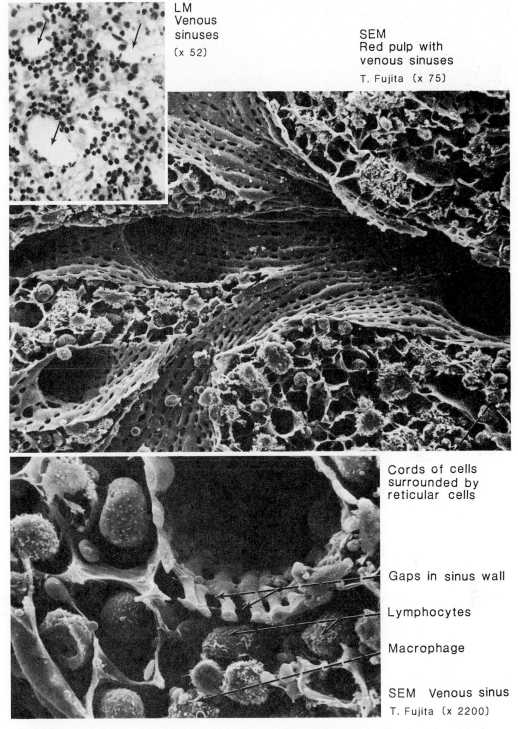

LM
Venous
sinuses
(x 52)

SEM
Red pulp with
venous sinuses

T. Fujita (x 75)

Cords of cells
surrounded by
reticular cells

Gaps in sinus wall

Lymphocytes

Macrophage

SEM   Venous sinus

T. Fujita (x 2200)

Upper view: Light microscopic view of several splenic sinuses lined with a thin layer of endothelical cells.

Middle view: This is a SEM longitudinal view of a confluence of several splenic sinuses. Junctional complexes are present where elongated lining cells are in contact. Between these contact points are many slitlike spaces that permit cells in the surrounding red pulp to squeeze through the wall to enter the lumen of the sinus.

Lower view: SEM micrograph of a transverse section of a sinus. Note that the rod-shaped endothelial cells resemble staves of a wooden barrel. These cells are partly surrounded by widely spaced, circular bands of basement membrane, which resemble hoops of a barrel. A network of reticular fibers, the extracellular reticulum, entraps free cells, e.g., lymphocytes (with microvilli), macrophages, monocytes, plasma cells, and especially erythrocytes.

Confluence of the various sinuses form the **pulp veins,** which enter the trabeculae to become the larger **trabecular veins.** At the hilus these veins unite to form the **splenic veins** that empty into the **portal vein.** All of these veins are lined with typical, simple squamous endothelium; however, only the splenic veins have a smooth muscle tunica media.

Lymphatics and Nerve Supply

In man, the lymphatic drainage of the spleen is poorly defined. **No afferent vessels** exist and the **efferent lymphatics** begin in the white pulp but are largely limited to the **capsule** and the **larger trabeculae.** However, a few lymph vessels may follow the larger arteries. The meager lymphatic vessels coalesce and exit at the hilus.

Axons of unmyelinated **sympathetic neurons,** originating from the celiac plexus, follow the branches of the splenic artery to enter the spleen at the hilus. These nerves terminate on the **smooth muscle** of the capsule and trabeculae. A few nerve fibers penetrate into the red and white pulp to supply the smooth muscle of the central and pulp arterioles. Stimulation of the sympathetic fibers causes contraction of the smooth muscle. This results in **constriction** of the spleen, which discharges stored blood into the systemic circulation. Sympathetic inhibition causes **relaxation** of the capsule, and the splenic sinuses are again filled with blood.

Functions

Most of the **functions** of the spleen deal with its relationships to the blood, e.g., it filters, stores, produces, modifies, destroys, and protects the **blood elements.** There is no component of the blood that escapes the impact of the spleen on its life-span and well-being.

The functions of the spleen include:

1. It is a **filter** strategically placed across the bloodstream. The many macrophages, housed in the spleen, protectively cleanse the blood of cellular debris, parasites, pathogenic bacteria, and senile, rigid blood cells, especially erythrocytes.

2. The **destruction of erythrocytes** that have spent about 120 days in the circulatory blood is accomplished by special macrophages principally found in the splenic cords of the red pulp. The eradication is so effective that the spleen has been called the "graveyard" of the RBC.

3. The spleen is a **hemopoietic organ,** i.e., it produces blood cells, principally lymphocytes and monocytes in the adult, and in addition, for a short duration in the fetus, granulocytes and erythrocytes. Postnatally, the germinal centers of the white pulp are sites of origin of lymphocytes. These cells migrate into the venous sinuses of the red pulp and finally into the general blood circulation.

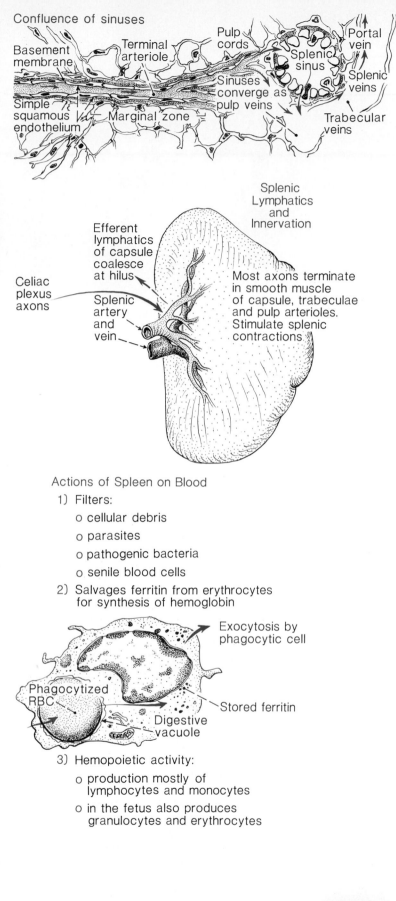

Confluence of sinuses

Basement membrane — Terminal arteriole — Pulp cords — Portal vein — Splenic sinus — Splenic veins — Simple squamous endothelium — Marginal zone — Sinuses converge as pulp veins — Trabecular veins

Splenic Lymphatics and Innervation

Efferent lymphatics of capsule coalesce at hilus — Celiac plexus axons — Splenic artery and vein — Most axons terminate in smooth muscle of capsule, trabeculae and pulp arterioles. Stimulate splenic contractions.

Actions of Spleen on Blood

1) Filters:
   o cellular debris
   o parasites
   o pathogenic bacteria
   o senile blood cells

2) Salvages ferritin from erythrocytes for synthesis of hemoglobin

Exocytosis by phagocytic cell — Phagocytized RBC — Stored ferritin — Digestive vacuole

3) Hemopoietic activity:
   o production mostly of lymphocytes and monocytes
   o in the fetus also produces granulocytes and erythrocytes

(Cont'd Actions of Spleen on Blood)

4) Blood reservoir:

   o storage of large quantities in red pulp sinuses   → expelled by contraction of capsule

   o 1/3 of platelets stored   → expelled on demand

5) Body defenses:

   o T-lymphocytes in periarterial sheaths   → enter bloodstream to invoke immune responses

   o B-lymphocytes in germinal centers   develop into)

   o antibody-producing plasma cells   → enter blood steam to combat antigens

   o macrophages ingest particulate matter

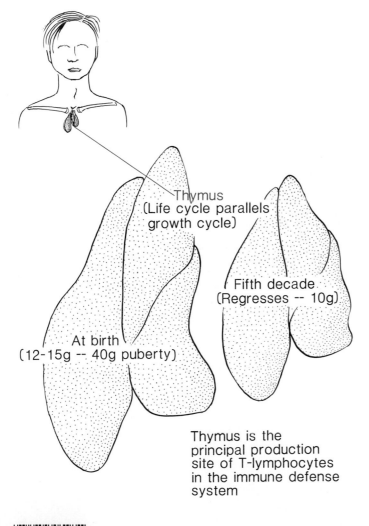

Thymus
(Life cycle parallels growth cycle)

Fifth decade
(Regresses -- 10g)

At birth
(12-15g -- 40g puberty)

Thymus is the principal production site of T-lymphocytes in the immune defense system

4. The spleen is a **reservoir for blood.** Because of the spongy character of the red pulp, it can store large quantities of blood cells to be expelled when needed into the general circulation, principally by the contraction of the heavy, fibromuscular capsule. It also stores about one third of the **platelets** of the body.

5. The spleen is very important in **body defense.** It contains large populations of B- and T-lymphocytes, antibody-producing plasma cells, and macrophages. In the spleen, the B- and T-lymphocytes leave the blood and separate. The **T-cells** enter the **periarterial sheaths** of the white pulp where they proliferate. Later they reach the bloodstream where they invoke cell-mediated immune responses. The **B-cells** are held primarily in the **germinal centers** of the splenic nodules; there they multiply and transform into plasma cells, which produce antibodies to combat foreign antigens.

Although the spleen has many important functions, none is essential to life, since splenectomy does not cause death in the normal, healthy individual. The implication is clear that other cells or tissues, e.g., lymph nodes, very rapidly take over the splenic functions.

THYMUS

The thymus is primarily a lymphoid organ of infancy and early childhood. At **birth**, it is a relatively large (**12–15 g**), well-developed, bilobed, greyish white body located in the superior part of the chest. It rests on the great vessels of the heart and extends into the root of the neck. By the second year, it has doubled in size and, by **puberty**, reaches its maximum size of about **40 g.** Then it regresses and is largely replaced by adipose tissue until, at the fifth decade of life, it probably weighs less than **10 g.** Its interesting life cycle suggests that it has some undefined role in development, since it reaches its greatest development during the body's most active growth period and then begins to atrophy about the time the growth of the body levels off.

It was assumed earlier that the thymus was not essential to life since **thymectomy,** in the adult animal, has little or no effect. However, it was discovered in the 1960s that **thymectomized newborn mice** fail to develop immunological competence, and they usually **die early** from infections. **Lymph nodules** and the lymphoid tissue in these animals also **fail to develop.** In the absence of the thymus, these structures cannot be populated with immunocompetent T-lymphocytes. A thymic implant restores this function to the thymectomized animals. Since the thymus is the principal **production site of T-lymphocytes,** it is a cardinal factor in the immune defense mechanism of the body. The thymus also produces **humoral factors** important to the establishment of the immune system in general.

Structure

A thin, connective tissue **capsule** surrounds each of the two lobes of the thymus. Thin **septa** from the capsule penetrate the gland to divide it into **incomplete lobules** uneven in size. Blood vessels, efferent lymphatic vessels, and nerves follow the septa deep into the gland. From the larger trabeculae, small extensions penetrate the parenchyma to contribute to the formation of a **stromal network.** The other components of the meshwork are long cytoplasmic processes of the large, stellate epithelial-reticular cells, to be discussed later.

The **parenchyma** of each lobule is divided into an outer, dark-staining **cortex** composed mostly of closely packed, **small lymphocytes** (thymocytes) and an **inner medulla** with a looser texture. The medulla is lighter staining because it has fewer lymphocytes, more light-staining **epithelial-reticular cells,** and contains large blood vessels. In most sections, the medulla of each lobule appears to be separate. However, the **medulla** is actually **continuous** from lobule to lobule. Some of the epithelial-reticular cells in the medulla form **Hassall's (thymic) corpuscles.** These are very large (30–150 μm), concentrically lamellar, cellular masses, with deeply eosinophilic, hyaline, central cores. They are more common in older individuals and are not present in all lobules. Their function is unknown. They are an excellent clue for distinguishing the thymus from other "look-alike" lymphoid organs.

The cellular elements of the cortex and medulla are similar; however, they vary greatly in distribution. For example, the **cortex** has large numbers of small, dark-staining T-lymphocytes with fewer epithelial-reticular cells. The opposite is true for the lighter staining **medulla,** where large lymphoblasts and epithelial-reticular cells, with large euchromatic nuclei, predominate. In addition, both regions have a scattering of macrophages, mast cells and, with aging, a great increase in adipose cells.

The **epithelial-reticular cell** warrants a brief comment. As its name suggests, this cell has features of epithelial cells as well as connective tissue (reticular) cells. Morphologically these cells closely resemble **reticular cells** of mesenchymal origin. However, they arise from endoderm, which is the origin of many types of epithelium. Furthermore, unlike reticular cells, they are not involved in reticular fiber formation. In fact, there are very few, if any, reticular fibers in the thymus. The interconnecting meshwork, or **reticulum,** is largely formed by the interlocking of long, slender cell **processes of the epithelial-reticular cells.** Like epithelial cells elsewhere, these processes are held together by **desmosomes. Tonofibrils** are found at these junctional sites, another epithelioid feature. Finally, TEM

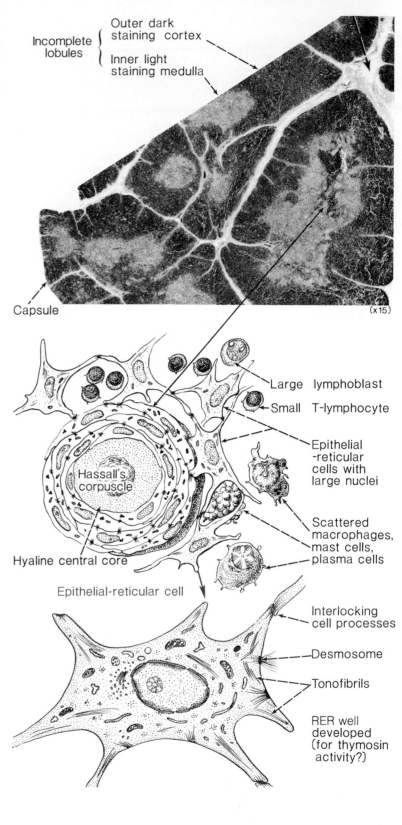

LM Thymus (x-section)

Septa containing blood vessels, nerves and efferent lymphatics

Incomplete lobules {
Outer dark staining cortex
Inner light staining medulla
}

Capsule

(x15)

Large lymphoblast

Small T-lymphocyte

Epithelial-reticular cells with large nuclei

Hassall's corpuscle

Scattered macrophages, mast cells, plasma cells

Hyaline central core

Epithelial-reticular cell

Interlocking cell processes

Desmosome

Tonofibrils

RER well developed (for thymosin activity?)

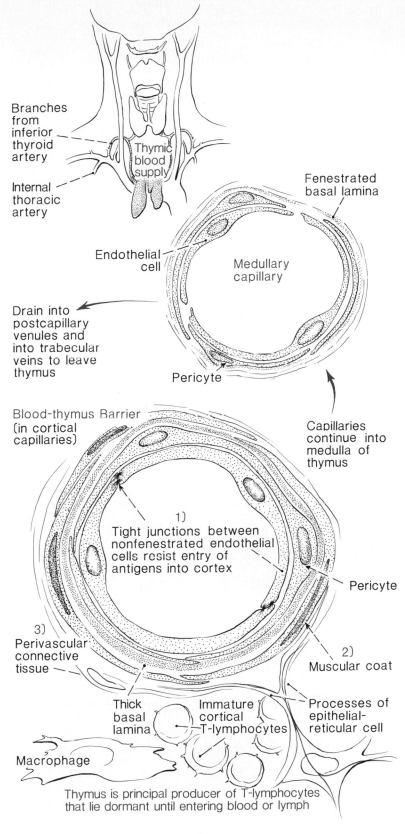

Branches from inferior thyroid artery

Internal thoracic artery

Thymic blood supply

Fenestrated basal lamina

Endothelial cell

Medullary capillary

Drain into postcapillary venules and into trabecular veins to leave thymus

Pericyte

Blood-thymus Barrier (in cortical capillaries)

Capillaries continue into medulla of thymus

1) Tight junctions between nonfenestrated endothelial cells resist entry of antigens into cortex

Pericyte

3) Perivascular connective tissue

2) Muscular coat

Thick basal lamina

Immature cortical T-lymphocytes

Processes of epithelial-reticular cell

Macrophage

Thymus is principal producer of T-lymphocytes that lie dormant until entering blood or lymph

studies of these cells reveal a well-developed **rER** with many **electron-dense granules**, suggestive of secretory activity, perhaps the site for the synthesis of **thymosin**—a postulated thymic hormone.

Blood Supply

The **branches** of the internal thoracic and inferior thyroid arteries penetrate the thymic **capsule** where they branch and follow along the **interlobular septa**. At the corticomedullary junction, only **capillaries** ensheathed by epithelial-reticular cells **pass into the cortex**. They take an arching course through the cortex to drain into **venules** that penetrate the medulla. Coalescence of these vessels forms veins that follow the trabeculae to exit as several veins which penetrate the capsule.

Both capillaries and arterioles enter the **medulla** in the junctional area. However, unlike the cortical capillaries, the medullary vessels do not have an enveloping sheath and therefore are permeable to circulating antigens and blood cells (L-A, plate 10).

Blood-Thymus Barrier

The cortical capillaries and venules are lined with **nonfenestrated, continuous endothelium** with a **thick basal lamina**. Pericytes, together with epithelial-reticular cells, form a sleeve around blood vessels of the cortex. Such a layer essentially **separates the circulating blood from the lymphocytes** housed in the thymus, creating a physical barrier. Enveloped by epithelial-reticular cells, cortical **capillaries** are impenetrable to other cells or very large molecules; thus, they do not allow antigens to enter the cortex. Those antigens that may reach the medulla are quickly engulfed by macrophages before they can diffuse into the surrounding cortex.

These investments of epithelial-reticular cells that surround the cortical blood vessels, and the endothelium lining them, constitute only a part of the **blood-thymus barrier** that separates the thymus (T) lymphocytes from blood-borne cells and molecules. The other barrier components include: (1) tight junctions of the endothelial cells, (2) the **muscular coat** of the larger vessels, and (3) the perivascular connective tissue investments. This barrier allows the immature cortical T-lymphocytes to multiply and differentiate in an enviroment **free of foreign antigens** before they migrate to the medulla and exit the thymus to enter the bloodstream. The blood-thymus barrier is important in that it **prevents the young T-lymphocytes** from being prematurely **exposed to foreign antigens** that they are being programmed to recognize. Such premature contact may destroy the T-lymphocytes.

Functions

Although the thymus has no germinal centers, **T-lymphocyte production** is its principal function, especially during late fetal life and early childhood. These **cells are seeded** by the lymph and bloodstreams into other **lymphoid organs** where they proliferate. These cells are mostly long-lived T-lymphocytes that recirculate through definite regions of lymphoid organs, e.g., the deep cortex or paracortical region of lymph nodes and the periarterial sheaths in the white pulp of the spleen.

Most T-lymphocytes are not immunocompetent in the thymus. They **become immunocompetent** only when they are **in the blood, lymph, or connective tissue,** including other lymphoid structures. In these locations they are responsible for **cell-mediated immune responses,** e.g., homograft rejection and delayed hypersensitivity.

Certain T-cells, called **helper cells,** provide a factor that stimulates B-lymphocytes to clonal division and differentiation. Thus, T-lymphocytes do not produce antibodies per se but stimulate the B-lymphocytes to differentiate into **plasma cells** that synthesize antibodies directed against specific antigens. Another possible function of the thymus is the production by the epithelial-reticular cells of a hormonal factor called **thymosin.** This hormone appears to promote maturation of the T-lymphocytes and stimulate lymphocyte production in other lymphoid organs. (Table 14.1)

Helper T-cells stimulate B-lymphocytes to divide and differentiate into plasma cells that synthesize antibodies

Epithelial-reticular cells of thymus produce thymosin?

Locations of T & B-lymphocytes (from H. N. Claman)

	B-lymphocytes	T-lymphocytes
Thymus	rare	+++
Bone marrow	++++ (as precursors)	+
Circulating blood	+	+++
Lymph nodes	++ (germinal centers)	+++ (deep thymus dependent cortex)
Spleen	++ (germinal centers)	+++ (periarterial lymphatic sheaths)
Thoracic duct	+	+++

SEM of T- and B- lymphocytes

EM of lymphocyte

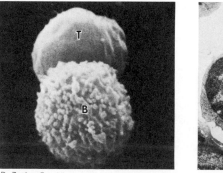

D. Zucker-Franklin

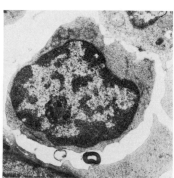

L.S. Lessin

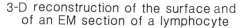

3-D reconstruction of the surface and of an EM section of a lymphocyte

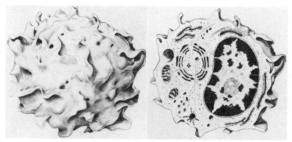

M. Bessis

Activated Lymphocyte

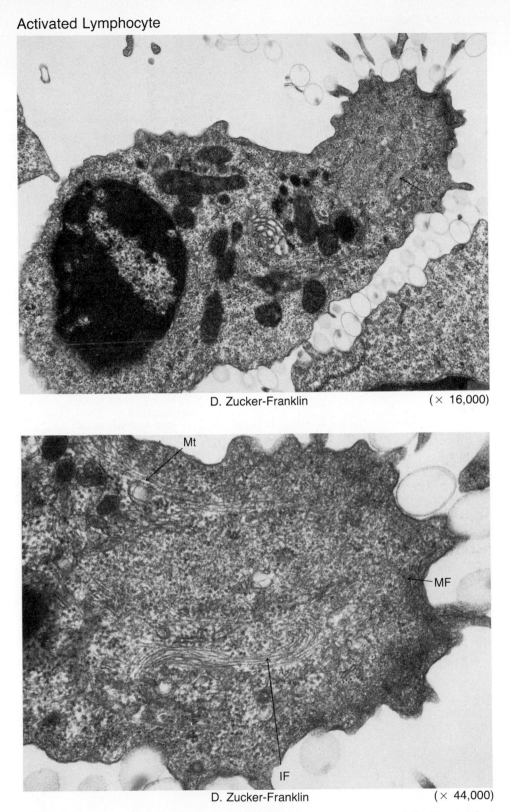

D. Zucker-Franklin   (× 16,000)

D. Zucker-Franklin   (× 44,000)

Upper EM micrograph. Activated lymphocytes show prominent modification in their normal shape. A change from a spherical to a "hand mirror" profile may occur, as seen in the upper micrograph of an activated B-lymphocyte. Also a marked increase in filaments is noted (at arrows).

Lower EM micrograph. This view is a higher magnification of the newly formed extension of the activated B-lymphocyte in the upper figure. Especially revealed are bundles of prominent 10 mm intermediate filaments (IF) running roughly parallel with clusters of microtubules (Mt). Some microfilaments (about 7 mm in diameter) intermingle with the microtubules and the intermediate filaments.

Table 14.1 *COMPARISON OF LYMPHOID ORGANS*

	LYMPH NODE	HEMAL NODE	SPLEEN	THYMUS
Lymph nodules	In cortex	In cortex	In white pulp as splenic nodules	None
Lymph vessels	Afferents enter at capsule; efferents exit at hilus	None	No afferents; efferents in capsule and trabeculae	No afferents; few efferents along septa
Blood vessels	Arteries in trabeculae; diffuse capillaries elsewhere	Sinuses	Arteries in trabeculae and splenic nodules; extensive venous sinuses elsewhere	Arteries enter medulla, spread into cortex
Capsule	Consists of thin collagenous connective tissue	Thin connective tissue	Robust—has collagenous, elastic, and smooth muscle fibers	Thin connective tissue
Cortex and medulla	Present	Present	Absent	Present
Hilus	Present	Present	Present	Absent
Epithelium	None	None	Covered with mesothelium	None
Diagnostic features	1. Subcapsular sinus 2. Medullary cords	Blood in sinuses	1. Eccentric central arteries 2. Heavy fibromuscular capsule 3. Red and white pulp 4. Abundant venous blood sinuses	1. Hassal's bodies 2. No germinal centers

TONSILS			
PALATINE	PHARYNGEAL	LINGUAL	TUBAL
Subepithelial in position			
No afferents; blind origins of efferents			
Arteries enter along attached surfaces			
Prominent connective tissue	Less definite	Thin or absent	Absent
Absent	Absent	Absent	Absent
Absent	Absent	Absent	Absent
Stratified squamous	Respiratory	Stratified squamous	Respiratory
Deep crypts lined with stratified squamous epithelium	Shallower crypts lined with respiratory epithelium	Located in root of tongue. Wide, shallow crypts	Associated with pharyngotympanic tube

Chapter

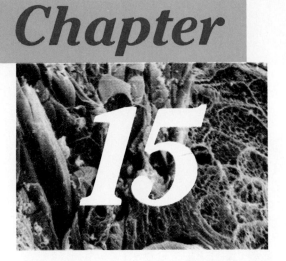

15

THE INTEGUMENTARY SYSTEM

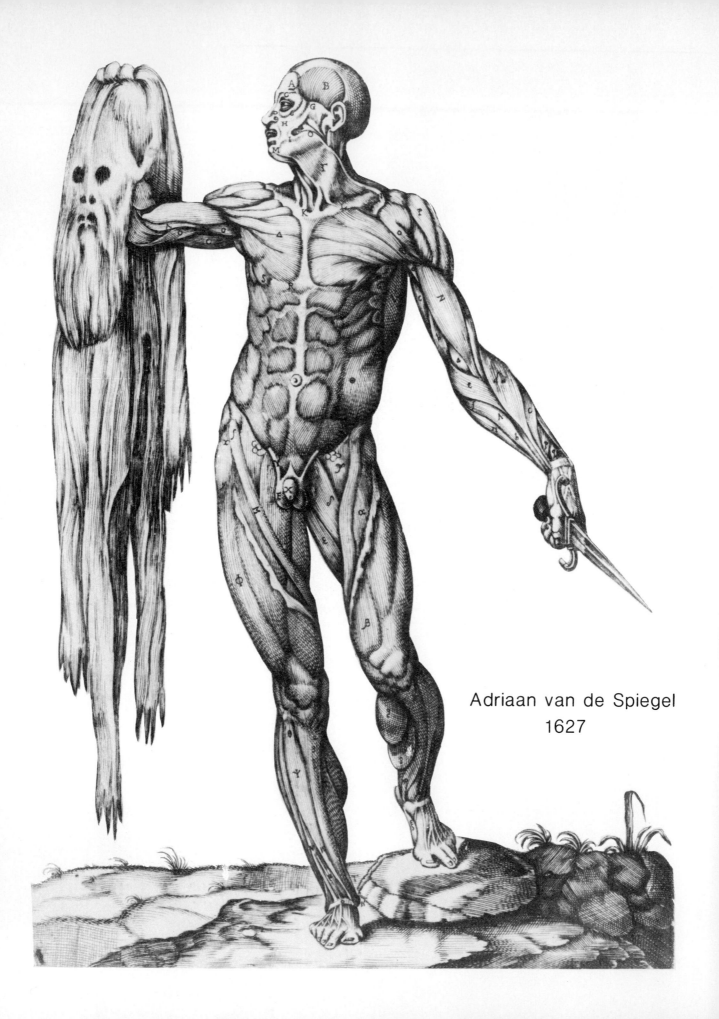

Adriaan van de Spiegel
1627

OBJECTIVES

THE READER SHOULD BE ABLE TO EVALUATE:

1. The histologic components of the various layers in thick and thin skin.

2. The varied functions of skin and how the various cells accomplish them.

3. The concept of melanogenesis and the role melanin plays in hair and skin color and protection against ultraviolet light irradiation.

4. The development, growth, and cellular morphology of hair and nails.

5. The functions of sebaceous and sweat glands in maintaining the health and comfort of the individual.

The integumentary system includes the **skin** and its **appendages** (derivatives), which consist in man of hair, nails, and several types of glands. In other animals the skin may have additional derivatives, such as feathers, beaks, spines, scales, hooves, horns, and claws.

SKIN

Professor R. D. Lockhart, an eminent Scottish anatomist, in his textbook, *Anatomy of the Human Body*, comments: "There is no magician's mantle to compare with the skin in its diverse roles of waterproof, overcoat, sunshade, suit of armor and refrigerator, sensitive to the touch of a feather, to temperature and to pain, withstanding the wear and tear of three score years and ten, and executing its own running repairs."

This remarkable structure is the **largest organ** of the body. In the adult human, the skin covers about 18 square feet of area and is responsible for about 15% of the body weight. It varies in thickness from ½ to 3 mm, depending on the body region, i.e., thinnest over the eyelids and thickest over the heels.

Functions

The skin is a true organ having all of the primary tissues organized to accomplish a wide variety of **functions**:

1. It has a **protective** function. It is a very efficient barrier against the invasion of pathogenic organisms, certain poisons, and harmful ultraviolet rays.

2. It is a **waterproof** covering of the body. All tissues of the body are in a fluid medium. The waterproof skin prevents loss of this vital fluid, a role which is grossly compromised following **severe burns**. For example, burns over one third of the body may be fatal, due to fluid loss. In the first few hours, 50–75% of the patient's plasma volume may be lost, a condition that prevents the red blood cells from functioning properly since their transport mechanism is seriously impaired. The skin is essentially **impervious to water**; therefore, we do not become waterlogged when immersed in fresh water nor shrunken when submerged in salt water.

3. The skin **regulates the temperature** of the body. A reduction in body temperature is accomplished by heat loss through the skin by radiation, convection, and evaporation. About 95% of total **body heat is dissipated** through the skin. For example, in hot, dry climates the body is cooled by the evaporation of sweat from its surface.

4. The skin is an **excretory organ**. Through its **sweat glands**, waste products, e.g. sodium and urea, are constantly being excreted. If the sweat is copious, about 1 g of nonprotein nitrogen is

Integumentary System

➤ Skin

➤ Appendages

  o hair

  o nails

  o glands

Roles served by skin

  Acts as:

    o raincoat

    o overcoat

    o sunshade

    o armor

    o refrigerator

    o general sensory organ

  Unusual features:

    o is self repairing

    o resists wear by increasing thickness

    o area is about 18 sq. ft. in adult

    o is about 15% of body weight

Functions

1) Protection from:

  o pathogens

  o poisons

  o ultraviolet rays

2) Waterproof:

  o retains tissue fluids

  o impervious to H_2O

3) Regulates temperature:

  o heat lost by radiation, convection, and evaporation

  o heat conserved by reduction in blood flow to skin

4) Excretory:

  o sweat glands for nitrogenous wastes & sodium salts

  o sebaceous glands for sebum secretion (mostly oil)

5) Selective absorption:

  o most substances do not penetrate

  o certain drugs, hormones and vitamin D are absorbed

6) Regenerative:

  o epidermis and dermis effect repairs

7) Source of sensations:

  o pain, **pressure**, touch and temperature

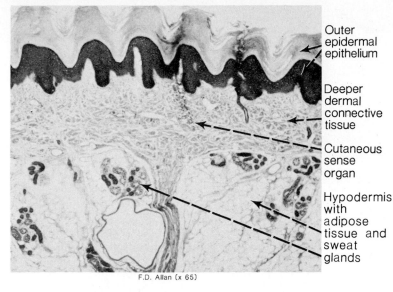

Outer epidermal epithelium

Deeper dermal connective tissue

Cutaneous sense organ

Hypodermis with adipose tissue and sweat glands

F.D. Allan (x 65)

Skin as an organ contains:

1) several varieties of epithelium

2) different types of connective tissue

3) limited muscle tissue

4) considerable nervous tissue

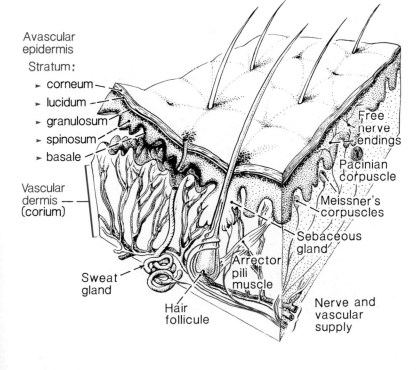

Avascular epidermis

Stratum:

▸ corneum

▸ lucidum

▸ granulosum

▸ spinosum

▸ basale

Vascular dermis (corium)

Sweat gland

Hair follicule

Arrector pili muscle

Nerve and vascular supply

Sebaceous gland

Meissner's corpuscles

Pacinian corpuscle

Free nerve endings

excreted each hour as well as relatively large amounts of sodium salts.

5. It has a selective **absorptive** function. Although most noxious gases and poisons are not absorbed through the skin, certain drugs, hormones, and vitamin D are readily absorbed.

6. The skin has tremendous **regenerative potential.** Since its outer **epidermal layer** is epithelial and its deeper **dermal layer** is connective tissue, both of these primary tissues can quickly and completely **repair** themselves.

7. The skin is an extensive **sensory organ** with many **nerve endings** mediating pain, pressure, touch, and temperature. It is the principal source of our general sensations. It keeps us constantly informed about our external environment.

The Skin As an Organ

Consider the concept of the skin as an organ:

1. Skin has varieties of epithelia. Most of the epidermis is **stratified squamous.** The blood vessels of the dermis are lined with **endothelium.** The sweat and oil glands are **glandular epithelium.**

2. There are several types of **connective tissues,** such as collagenous and elastic fibers, and fat cells in the dermis.

3. Muscle fibers are found in the dermis. For example, **smooth muscle** fibers are associated with the arrector pili muscles of oil glands and the walls of blood vessels.

4. Considerable **nervous tissue** is associated with the skin as nerve fibers and nerve endings. **Tactile sensation** through Meissner's corpuscles and **deep pressure** mediated by Pacinian corpuscles are found in the dermis, while **free nerve endings** for pain are found in the basal layer of the epidermis.

Histology of the Skin

The skin is the outermost component of the integumentary system. Histologically, it consists of two distinctively different layers: (1) a superficial, epithelial, waterproof, avascular layer, the **epidermis;** and (2) a deeper, vascular, connective tissue layer, the **dermis** or corium, which supplies support for the overlying epidermis. It contains parts of the **appendages** of the skin, i.e., hair follicles and nail beds, and vascular and nervous structures. The dermis rests on the **hypodermis,** a layer of loose connective tissue with pads of fat cells, sweat and oil glands, and blood vessels.

The histological pattern of skin is similar throughout the body. However, the thickness of its layers varies in different regions of the body, resulting in two types of skin, **thick and thin.**

Epidermis

The epidermis, derived from **ectoderm**, is a **stratified squamous epithelium** consisting of various types of cells. They vary in shape from the flat, dead, superficial cells constantly being shed on the skin surface, to a single layer of rapidly multiplying columnar cells in the deepest layer.

THICK SKIN The epidermis of **thick skin**, such as found in the palms of the hands and soles of the feet, has **several layers.** They are named from the deepest layer outward: (1) stratum basale (cylindrical), (2) stratum spinosum (prickle cell layer), (3) stratum granulosum, (4) stratum lucidum, and (5) stratum corneum (horny cell layer). Confusion exists in naming these various strata. For example, **strata basale and spinosum** are often combined into a single layer called either **stratum Malpighi or stratum germinativum** because the cells of both layers are mitotically active. Also some authorities use the terms stratum basale and stratum germinativum as synonyms, since this is the basal layer and is also the most active layer in mitosis.

Since the epidermis is essentially all epithelium, it has **no blood or lymph vessels.** Therefore, it must secure all of its nutrients and oxygen by diffusion from capillaries in the dermis. **Free nerve endings**, mediating **pain** sensations, terminate on the basal cells.

Stratum basale, the deepest layer, is a single layer of basophilic, **columnar or cuboidal cells.** It is darkly stained with H&E because of the basal row of closely packed, large, **basophilic nuclei**, surrounded by a less basophilic cytoplasm rich in ribosomes. Frequent mitotic figures are present. The cells rest on a **basal lamina,** which separates the epidermis from the deeper dermis. On the lateral and upper cell surfaces, multiple **desmosomes** bind the cells together. On their basal surfaces, **hemidesmosomes** attach the cells to the underlying basal lamina. Associated with all of these junctional complexes are prominent concentrations of **tonofilaments** (7–9 nm in diameter) which, when assembled into bundles, are the **tonofibrils** seen with the light microscope. **Ribosomes,** in the basal region, are largely responsible for the **basophilia** of the cells and suggest a metabolically active, polarized cell.

Stratum spinosum consists of several layers of polygonal, somewhat flattened, lightly basophilic cells, called **prickle cells.** As their name implies, they have **short spines** or extensions bristling from their external surfaces. These extensions terminate as **desmosomes** on spines of adjacent cells. These connections are the **intercellular bridges** of light microscopy, so called because it was formerly believed that they were passageways (bridges) for the movement of protoplasm from one cell to another, a concept no longer tenable. Desmosomes and tonofibrils increase in number in areas of abrasion and pressure, e.g., the heels and palms. **Tonofilaments,** terminating

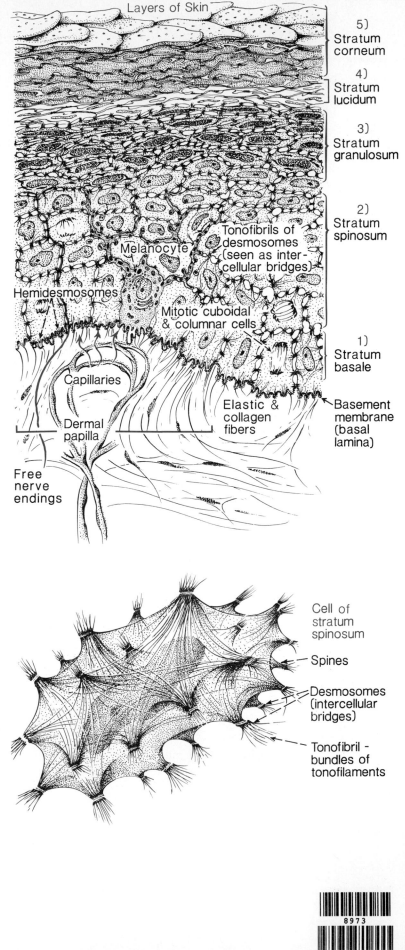

Layers of Skin

5) Stratum corneum

4) Stratum lucidum

3) Stratum granulosum

2) Stratum spinosum

Tonofibrils of desmosomes (seen as intercellular bridges)

Melanocyte

Hemidesmosomes

Mitotic cuboidal & columnar cells

1) Stratum basale

Capillaries

Basement membrane (basal lamina)

Dermal papilla

Elastic & collagen fibers

Free nerve endings

Cell of stratum spinosum

Spines

Desmosomes (intercellular bridges)

Tonofibril - bundles of tonofilaments

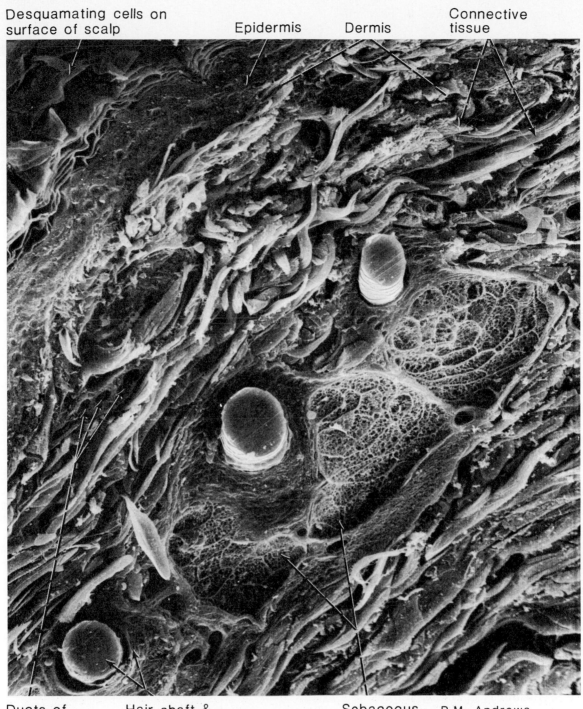

Desquamating cells on surface of scalp   Epidermis   Dermis   Connective tissue

Ducts of sweat glands   Hair shaft & root sheath   Sebaceous glands   P.M. Andrews

This SEM micrograph reveals primarily the dermis of the scalp which houses the hair follicles and their associated structures. Three hair shafts are seen cut transversely. Surrounding each shaft is a root sheath consisting mostly of epidermal, leaflike cells which, when desquamated, contribute to the formation of dandruff. Two of the hair shafts are intimately associated with spongy-appearing sebaceous glands. These are holocrine-type glands, i.e., their cells become part of the secretion. For oil to be produced, the mature cells nearest to the hair shaft undergo necrosis and become part of the secretion (sebum), which lubricates the surface of the scalp and moistens the hair shafts as they emerge from the hair follicles. Sweat glands and ducts are less closely associated with the hair shafts. Observe that the dermis is characterized by abundant, dense irregular connective tissue, consisting largely of collagen fibers, while the epidermis consists of stratified squamous epithelium whose superficial layers are desquamating.

on the desmosomes, are prominent in TEM micrographs.

The stratum granulosum consists of two to four layers of **flattened cells** containing many prominent basophilic granules called **keratohyalin granules.** Waldeyer (1882) coined the term for these granules because he believed they were hyaline in nature and possibly involved in keratinization. Little is known about their origin, chemical nature, or functions, except that they are neither hyaline-like nor keratin, yet the name persists. EM studies reveal the granules to be closely packed, **amorphous particles** not enclosed in a membrane but surrounded by **ribosomes. Microfilaments,** which extend across the granules, may attach to the surfaces of the granules.

The stratum lucidum (clear layer) is formed by two to three layers of **translucent,** poorly stained, or slightly eosinophilic **squamous cells.** No nuclei or organelles are present. Although a few desmosomes persist, it is a layer with reduced cell adhesion and a cleavage line often appears that artificially separates the outer stratum corneum from the deeper strata.

The outermost stratum corneum consists of many layers of **dead, flattened, anucleate cells** whose cytoplasm is replaced by **keratin,** a birefringent, filamentous scleroprotein. The most **superficial cells** are dehydrated, horny scales that are constantly being shed. Normally a balance is maintained between the number of cells produced in the stratum germinativum and those lost at the stratum corneum. Such a parity is essential since the young, mitotically active cells of the basal layers are gradually crowded toward the superficial layer to replace the desquamating, dead cells of the stratum corneum. (For summary of features of thick skin, see Table 15.1.)

THIN SKIN Thin skin covers the rest of the body. Its **epidermis** differs from that of thick skin in that the **stratum lucidum is absent** and the stratum granulosum is also frequently missing. Furthermore, the **stratum corneum** is greatly **reduced in thickness,** having only a few sheets of heavily keratinized, desquamating, dead cells. The **stratum spinosum** is generally limited to a few inconspicuous cell layers. However, the **stratum basale** is quite **similar to thick skin.** Thus, only the deep stratum germinativum (strata basale and spinosum) and the superficial, thin stratum corneum are constantly present in the epidermis of thin skin.

Cells of the Epidermis

There are **four cell types** in the epidermis, i.e. keratinocytes, melanocytes, Langerhans cells, and Merkel cells. Their relative proportions vary with the body regions. However 85–95% of the cells are keratinized epithelial cells called **keratinocytes,** derived from surface **ectoderm.** The next most populous cell is the **melanocyte.**

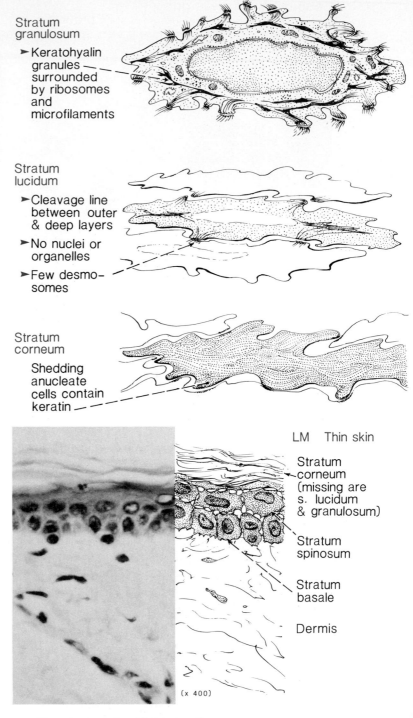

Stratum granulosum
► Keratohyalin granules surrounded by ribosomes and microfilaments

Stratum lucidum
► Cleavage line between outer & deep layers
► No nuclei or organelles
► Few desmosomes

Stratum corneum
Shedding anucleate cells contain keratin

LM   Thin skin
Stratum corneum (missing are s. lucidum & granulosum)
Stratum spinosum
Stratum basale
Dermis
(x 400)

Four types of epidermal cells

► Keratinocytes from ectoderm

► Melanocytes from neural crest (synthesize melanin)

► Langerhans cells from mesoderm

► Merkel cells from ectoderm

8889

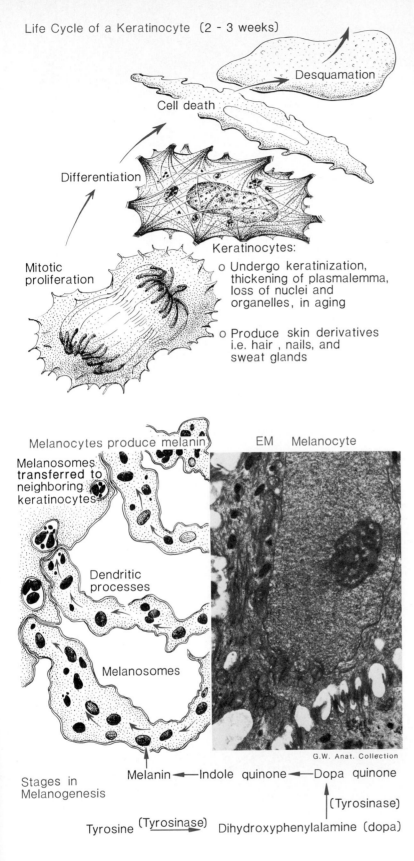

Life Cycle of a Keratinocyte (2 - 3 weeks)

Desquamation

Cell death

Differentiation

Mitotic proliferation

Keratinocytes:

o Undergo keratinization, thickening of plasmalemma, loss of nuclei and organelles, in aging

o Produce skin derivatives i.e. hair , nails, and sweat glands

Melanocytes produce melanin

EM   Melanocyte

Melanosomes transferred to neighboring keratinocytes

Dendritic processes

Melanosomes

G.W. Anat. Collection

Stages in Melanogenesis

Melanin ← Indole quinone ← Dopa quinone

(Tyrosinase)

Tyrosine (Tyrosinase) → Dihydroxyphenylalamine (dopa)

KERATINOCYTES Keratinocytes are epithelial cells that **undergo keratinization,** which results in creating a waterproof, protective armor for the body. In the production of keratin, a fibrous scleroprotein, the keratinocytes undergo a brief life cycle of about two to three weeks. The cycle includes mitotic proliferation, differentiation, and cell death, followed by desquamation.

Classification of these cells depends on their **location** and degree of **differentiation.** For example, (1) nucleated keratinocytes are found in the germinating layers (strata basale and spinosum); (2) senile, effete cells in the strata granulosum and lucidum; and (3) exfoliated cells, sheets of dead cells, in the stratum corneum. In the final stages of differentiation of these cells, **aging sets in,** as evidenced by the thickening of the plasmalemma and loss of nuclei and other organelles.

Keratinocytes function primarily as the **stem cells** for further keratinized epithelial surface cells. They may also be involved in the development of the **skin derivatives,** i.e., hair, nails, and oil and sweat glands.

MELANOCYTES Melanocytes, comprising about 7–10% of the epidermal cells, have small cell bodies with many long, thin, **dendritic processes** that terminate on **keratinocytes** in the strata basale and spinosum. They are found mainly among the cells of the stratum basale, hair follicles, and to a limited extent in the dermis.

Melanocytes are very difficult to identify with conventional stains. However, they can be easily identified if a section of epidermis is incubated with the reagent, 3,4-dihydroxyphenylalanine (**dopa**). The resulting dopa reaction selectively **blackens melanocytes.** In EM micrographs they can be identified from keratinocytes by the presence of many electron-dense bodies called **melanosomes,** a translucent cytoplasm, the absence of desmosomes, and a paucity of tonofibrils. They may represent 10–25% of the total number of cells in the basal layer.

Melanin formation occurs in the **melanocyte** within the cell organelle, the **melanosome,** which contains the amino acid **tyrosine** and the enzyme **tyrosinase.** Through a series of complex reactions, tyrosine is oxidized to **dopa** by tyrosinase. Dopa is then converted to **dopa quinone** by tyrosinase which, after several reactions, yields **indole 5,6-quinone.** The latter is **polymerized** to **yield melanin.** When the melanosome is filled with pigment, the **melanin is transferred** by the dendritic processes of the melanocyte to **adjacent keratinocytes.** Here melanin functions to screen out and scatter harmful ultraviolet radiation (L-A plate 34).

To recapitulate this concept of melanogenesis, the following simplified formula may be helpful:

8567

$$\text{Tyrosine} \xrightarrow{\text{Tyrosinase}} \text{Dihydroxyphenylalanine}$$

$$\text{(Dopa)} \xrightarrow{\text{Tyrosinase}} \text{Dopa quinone} \longrightarrow$$

$$\text{Indole quinone} \longrightarrow \text{Melanin}$$

CELLS OF LANGERHANS Langerhans cells, a small population of **stellate-shaped cells,** are found principally in the **stratum spinosum.** They resemble keratinocytes that stain poorly with H&E, but are sharply outlined when impregnated with **gold chloride.** From EM micrographs, these cells can be readily distinguished from other cells of the skin by the presence of many **rodlike or racket-shaped membrane-bound granules** scattered throughout the clear cytoplasm. Additional EM features include no desmosomes or tonofilaments, an indented nucleus, and a limited Golgi complex, mitochondria and endoplasmic reticulum. Their origin and function are obscure. The best evidence suggests that they are probably **mesodermal** in origin and are perhaps a special type of **macrophage** that entraps exogenous antigens in the skin. Thus they may be involved in the primary immune body response.

MERKEL CELL The fourth type and least numerous of all cells in the epidermis is the **clear Merkel cell.** These cells are **neural crest** migrants to the basal cells of thick skin, hair follicles, and the oral mucous membrane. They are rather large, poorly stained, oval or round cells with **short cytoplasmic processes (horns)** that interdigitate with the smaller adjacent keratinocytes. Their processes are attached to the neighboring cells by desmosomes. **Unmyelinated sensory nerve fibers** penetrate the stratum basale to terminate as expanded disks on the bases of the Merkel cells. These structures are **Merkel nerve endings,** whose functions are unclear. Probably they act as mechanoreceptors or touch receptors.

TEM studies on Merkel cells reveal many osmiophilic electron-dense, membrane-bound **granules,** 70–180 nm in diameter, concentrated in the basal regions of the cell near nerve terminals. They resemble **neurosecretory granules,** which supports the theory that Merkel cells, as APUD cells, may secrete **polypeptide hormones** similar to the catecholamines of the adrenal medulla. The cytoplasm is clear and free of tonofilaments. However, some free ribosomes, mitochondria, lysosomes, and vacuoles are present. Occasionally melanosomes are present in the cytoplasm. (See Table 15.2 for comparison of epidermal cells.)

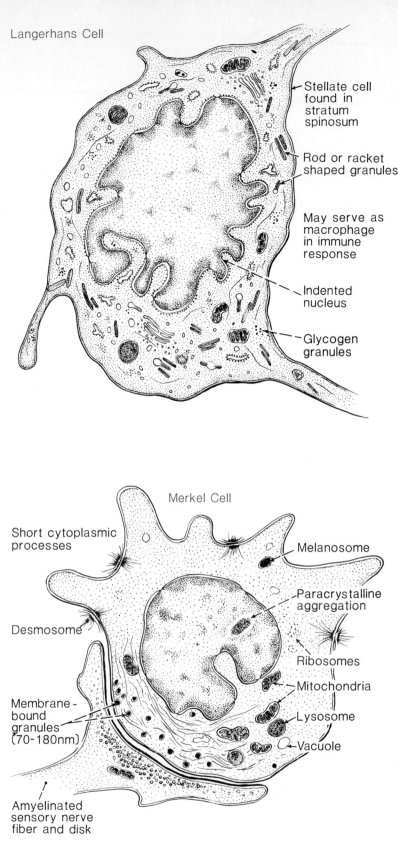

Langerhans Cell

- Stellate cell found in stratum spinosum
- Rod or racket shaped granules
- May serve as macrophage in immune response
- Indented nucleus
- Glycogen granules

Merkel Cell

- Short cytoplasmic processes
- Desmosome
- Membrane-bound granules (70-180nm)
- Amyelinated sensory nerve fiber and disk
- Melanosome
- Paracrystalline aggregation
- Ribosomes
- Mitochondria
- Lysosome
- Vacuole

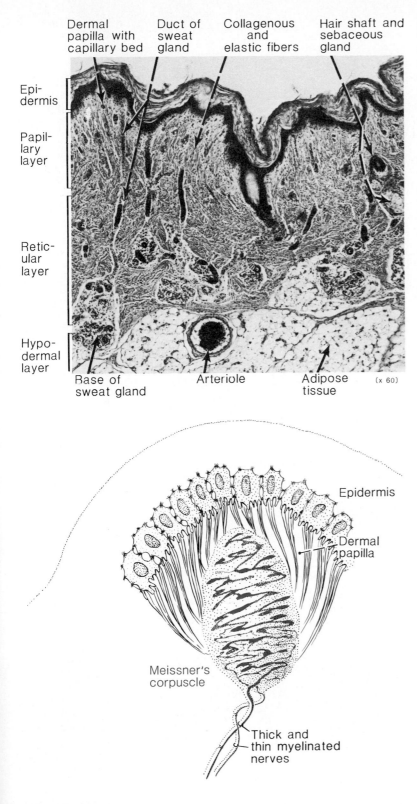

Dermal papilla with capillary bed   Duct of sweat gland   Collagenous and elastic fibers   Hair shaft and sebaceous gland

Epi-dermis

Papil-lary layer

Reti-cular layer

Hypo-dermal layer

Base of sweat gland   Arteriole   Adipose tissue   (x 60)

Epidermis

Dermal papilla

Meissner's corpuscle

Thick and thin myelinated nerves

Dermis

The vascular dermis (corium) is **mesodermal** in origin. It consists of several **irregular, feltlike layers of collagenous fibers** with a scattering of elastic fibers. It is anchored to the epidermis by numerous connective tissue conical projections, called **papillae.** Although the dermis is divided into **papillary** (subepithelial) and **reticular** (deep) layers, their fibers tend to intermingle without a clearly marked boundary between the layers.

PAPILLARY LAYER The papillary layer is characterized by the presence of **dermal papillae,** which vary in number from 50 to 250/mm^2. They are most numerous and tallest in regions where the liability of shearing stresses is greatest, i.e., soles of the feet. Most of these papillae contain a **capillary bed** which nourishes the overlying, avascular epithelium. Others are **tactile papillae,** which house encapsulated, delicate, sensory nerve endings that mediate touch sensation, called **Meissner's corpuscles.** Adjacent to the epidermis, the collagenous fibers are closely packed, giving a smooth, even texture to the outer surface of the papillary layer.

RETICULAR LAYER The thicker and deeper **reticular layer** comprises most of the dermis. Coarse, collagenous bundles and a few elastic fibers form an irregular, dense, interlacing network or **reticulum,** an excellent example of dense, irregular, connective tissue. At the deeper levels, the network becomes more open. Its spaces contain **adipose tissue, sweat and oil glands,** and **hair follicles.** Smooth muscle fibers are present in certain regions, such as hair follicles, scrotum, prepuce, and nipple. In the skin of the neck and face, **skeletal muscle fibers** insert on connective tissue bands in the dermis. These are the muscles of facial expression. The reticular layer merges with the underlying fatty, loose connective tissue, the superficial fascia or **hypodermis.**

CELL TYPES AND LEATHER Cells in the dermis are relatively scarce. They are the cells that are found in most connective tissues, e.g., mostly **fibroblasts** and **fat cells,** a few macrophages and mast cells, and, in pigmented areas, melanocytes.

In the leather tanning process, the epithelium is discarded. It is the **dermis**, when tanned, that becomes **leather**. If the hair or grain side (papillary layer) of the hide is finished, it is **grain leather**. It is the flesh or deeper side (reticular layer) that is finished as **suede leather**.

APPENDAGES OF THE SKIN

The epidermis of mammals has several **derivatives or appendages,** each with special functions. For example, hair, horn, nails, and claws function uniquely because of their gross morphology, while sebaceous and sweat glands synthesize specific secretions. All appendages of the epidermis are **epithelial derivatives,** but they develop and reside within the **dermis** and often in the **hypodermis** (the loose connective tissue layer beneath the dermis, often infiltrated with abundant adipose tissue).

Hair

One of the unique features of man is his relative hairlessness. What hair he has is largely ornamental and, except possibly for the scalp and beard, his hair offers little protection against a hostile environment. In certain regions of the body hair provides some protection, such as those that guard the external anogenital orifices, the external auditory meatuses, nostrils, and eyes (eyelashes). In addition to these minor functions, hair functions as a part of the cutaneous sensory apparatus, especially adapted for the modality of light touch.

HAIR FOLLICLES Hairs are **hard keratin** structures produced by delicate, saccular epithelial structures called **hair follicles.** They arise in the embryo as **thickenings of the epidermis** that proliferate as **cords** and penetrate the dermis. Each cord pushes ahead of it a mass of mesenchymal cells that differentiate into the vascular **dermal papilla.** The base of each cord expands and encloses a **papilla,** forming the **bulb,** which is divided into an upper region and a lower, or **matrix,** portion. The dermal papilla has a rich capillary investment that is essential to the vitality of the hair follicle.

The cells covering the papilla produce the **shaft** of the hair that erupts from the skin. The cells covering the hair bulb are continuous with the cells of the strata basale and spinosum. They are constantly undergoing mitosis and give rise to the various **cellular coverings** of the mature hair. During early development, all cells of the follicle are **mitotically active.** Later, when the follicles are fully differentiated, mitosis is re-

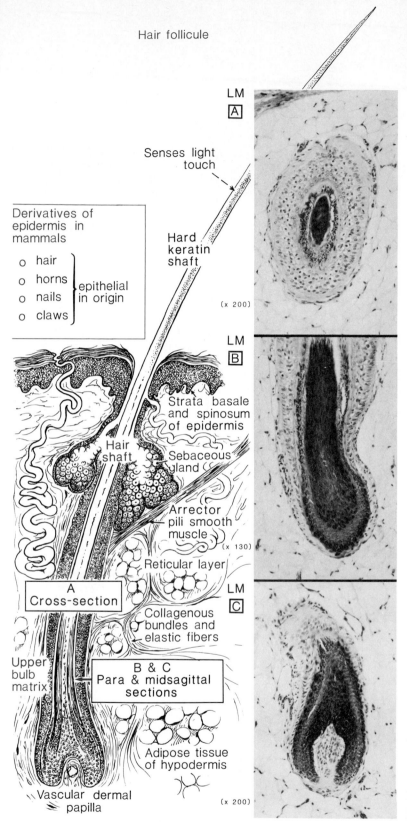

Hair follicule

LM A

Senses light touch

Hard keratin shaft

(x 200)

Derivatives of epidermis in mammals

o hair
o horns
o nails
o claws
} epithelial in origin

Hair shaft

LM B

Strata basale and spinosum of epidermis

Sebaceous gland

Arrector pili smooth muscle

Reticular layer

(x 130)

A Cross-section

Collagenous bundles and elastic fibers

LM C

Upper bulb matrix

B & C Para & midsagittal sections

Vascular dermal papilla

Adipose tissue of hypodermis

(x 200)

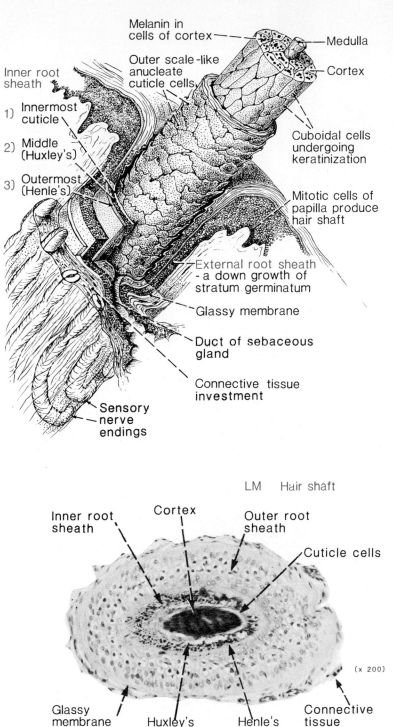

Hair follicle and shaft

Melanin in cells of cortex

Medulla

Cortex

Outer scale-like anucleate cuticle cells

Cuboidal cells undergoing keratinization

Inner root sheath

1) Innermost cuticle

2) Middle (Huxley's)

3) Outermost (Henle's)

Mitotic cells of papilla produce hair shaft

External root sheath - a down growth of stratum germinatum

Glassy membrane

Duct of sebaceous gland

Connective tissue investment

Sensory nerve endings

LM Hair shaft

Inner root sheath

Cortex

Outer root sheath

Cuticle cells

Glassy membrane

Huxley's layer

Henle's layer

Connective tissue

(x 200)

stricted to the cells of the lower bulb region, called the **matrix cells.** These cells are the progenitors of the cells that eventually populate the various regions of the hair, i.e., the medulla, cortex, and cuticle.

REGIONS The central core of the hair is the **medulla.** It is best seen near the base of a hair and does not extend to the tip of the hair shaft. It consists of **two or three layers** of large, vacuolated, **cuboidal cells** that eventually undergo keratinization. The intercellular spaces are usually filled with air.

The largest region of the hair is the **cortex,** consisting of several concentric layers of heavily keratinized, elongated cells. **Melanin** is usually sequestered between or within these cells, giving color to the hair. The cells become more flattened in the distal regions of the hair.

More peripherally are the thinnest cells of the hair root and shaft, called the **hair cuticle.** This is a single layer of very flat, scalelike, **clear anucleate cells** on the outer surface of the shaft. They are disposed in a shinglelike fashion over the surface of the cortex with their free, serrated edges projecting upward away from the base.

ROOT SHEATHS The inner (internal) root sheath is formed of the most peripheral of the matrix cells. The **sheath** is a sleeve of cells that completely surrounds the bulb and the initial part of the shaft. It consists of three layers: (1) The **cuticle** of the sheath, the **innermost zone,** is made up of simple **squamous, overlapping cells** that abuts onto the cuticle of the hair shaft. Their downward projecting edges interdigitate with the upward projecting edges of the hair cuticle cells, thus creating a firm bond between the **hair shaft** and its **inner root sheath.** Therefore, when a hair is plucked from the scalp, it carries with it some of the cells of the inner root sheath. (2) The **middle, Huxley's layer,** has several layers of elongated cells containing modified keratohyalin granules called **trichohyalin.** (3) The **outermost Henle's layer** is a single band of flat, clear cells, containing **keratin fibrils.**

The outer (external) root sheath, peripheral to Henle's layer, is the **downgrowth of the strata basale and spinosum.** The outermost cells are a single row of **columnar cells,** the continuation of the stratum basale, and several layers of **polygonal cells** with small spinous processes, the continuation of stratum spinosum. Peripheral to the outer root sheath is a loose, poorly defined **connective tissue investment,** derived from the dermis, that surrounds the hair follicle and shaft. A thin hyaline, modified basement membrane, the **glassy membrane,** separates this connective tissue sheath from the outer root sheath.

8392

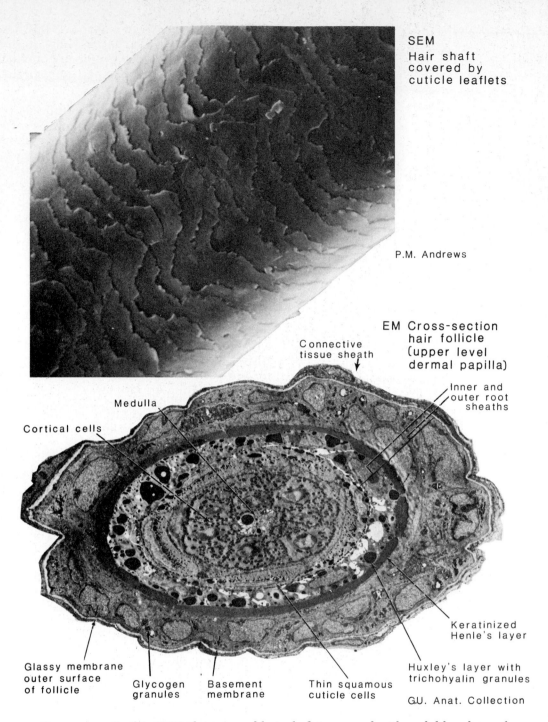

SEM
Hair shaft
covered by
cuticle leaflets

P.M. Andrews

EM Cross-section
hair follicle
(upper level
dermal papilla)

Connective
tissue sheath

Inner and
outer root
sheaths

Medulla

Cortical cells

Keratinized
Henle's layer

Glassy membrane
outer surface
of follicle

Glycogen
granules

Basement
membrane

Thin squamous
cuticle cells

Huxley's layer with
trichohyalin granules

G.U. Anat. Collection

Upper view: In this SEM, the exposed hair shaft is covered with scalelike plates, the cuticle. These are very flattened, keratinized, parallel, epithelial cells that partially overlap each other like shingles. Their wavy, scalloped edges probably result from the wear and tear of the surface of the hair. At the tip of the hair, the shaft often becomes fragmented.

Lower view: This EM micrograph shows a cross section of a hair shaft within a dermal papilla. It is enclosed in a tubular hair follicle that consists of several epidermal and dermal components. The epidermal structures include, from within outwards: (1) the central medulla containing soft keratin, (2) the extensive cortex, and (3) the very thin cuticle (both have hard keratin); (4) the inner root sheath is subdivided into Huxley's layer of several layers of columnar cells with abundant trichohyalin granules, and Henle's layer, a single layer of clear, squamous, keratinized cells, and (5) the outer root sheath which has several layers of cuboidal cells with considerable glycogen. The only dermal component is the outer connective tissue sheath, a heavy investment that surrounds the entire follicle. Separating the connective tissue sheath and the outer root sheath is a clear, hyaline, modified basement membrane, the glassy membrane.

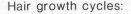

Hair growth cycles:

  o of scalp
    - active 2-3 years
    - resting 3-4 months

  o of eyebrows
    - active 1-2 months
    - resting 3-4 months

Effects of male sex hormones:

  o androgens stimulate facial hair growth

  o adrenal cortex tumors may stimulate beard growth in females

Follicular growth patterns

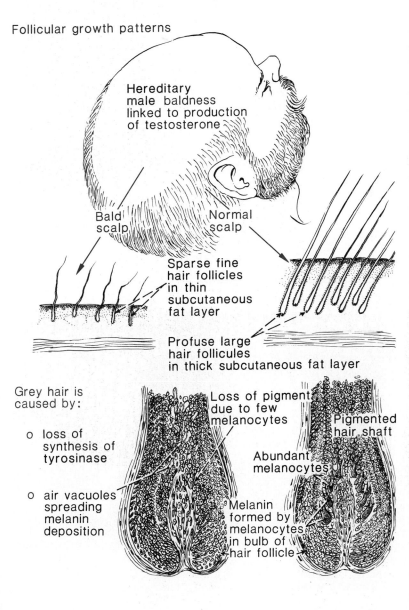

Hereditary male baldness linked to production of testosterone

Bald scalp

Normal scalp

Sparse fine hair follicles in thin subcutaneous fat layer

Profuse large hair follicules in thick subcutaneous fat layer

Grey hair is caused by:

  o loss of synthesis of tyrosinase

  o air vacuoles spreading melanin deposition

Loss of pigment due to few melanocytes

Pigmented hair shaft

Abundant melanocytes

Melanin formed by melanocytes in bulb of hair follicle

HAIR GROWTH Hair growth and replacement are **cyclical,** not constant. Also, the periods of growth and rest vary depending on the regions of the body. For example, in the scalp, the **growth cycle** may last for two to three years before entering the resting periods of three to four months. In other parts of the body, e.g., eyebrows, the growth cycle is much shorter (one to two months) and the resting period longer (three to four months).

Male sex hormones, **androgens** from the testis and the adrenal cortex, directly **affect hair growth** in certain regions of the body, such as the face, axilla, and pubis. Certain tumors of the adrenal cortex cause beard growth in females and precocious sexual development in boys because of the production of abnormally large amounts of male androgens. Boys who are castrated before puberty do not develop normal masculine hair distribution on the face or elsewhere. The frequency of shaving or cutting of hair has no observable effect on hair growth.

Upon cessation of follicular growth, the **hair ceases to grow,** becomes detached from the bulb, and eventually falls out. After a quiescent period, the **hair is replaced** by a return of mitotic activity to the remaining **matrix cells** of the new follicle, or mitotic activity is reestablished in the old, degenerating papilla. In either case, a new hair is formed in a new or regenerated follicle.

Baldness occurs when **follicles cease to be formed** and hair replacement cannot occur. Since it rarely occurs in women, it is generally assumed that **baldness** results from the presence of **testosterone,** the principal male sex hormone. However, baldness is **hereditary,** and the genetic predisposition toward baldness manifests itself only in the presence of **male sex hormones,** since eunuchs are not bald even though they may carry the genes for baldness. Nevertheless, it does not follow that bald-headed men have more testosterone and therefore are more virile than men well-endowed with scalp hair. Male sex hormones do not cause baldness unless the person carries the **baldness gene** or genes.

Like skin color, the color of the hair is due to the presence of the pigment **melanin,** formed by melanocytes in the bulb of the follicle. The cells destined to produce the cortex of the hair receive melanin from the **melanocytes,** which is tightly incorporated into the **hair cortex.** The **various shades** of natural hair results from **different amounts** of melanin and various **types of melanin,** i.e., eumelanin and pheomelanin. The **greying of the hair** is due largely to two factors: (1) the **melanosomes** in the bulb lose their capacity to synthesize tyrosinase, the enzyme essential for melanin formation; and (2) the hair shaft and bulb contain more **air vacuoles,** which spread out the melanin granules.

Nails

Nails are protective, **keratinized, hard plates of cells** that cover the dorsal surfaces of the distal ends of digits of all primates. They **resemble hair,** having a mitotically **active matrix** in the dermis that produces the nail bed, which is continuous with the stratum germinativum of the skin. The most proximal part of the nail is covered by a fold of thin skin called the **eponychium** (Gk. ep + onyx, nail) or **cuticle,** as it is commonly known. The nail plate grows out of the nail bed as a protective, keratin shield over the distal phalange. Since the **nail bed** is a continuation of the deeper layers of epidermis, it is composed of two to three layers of **prickle and basal cells** resting on a basement membrane. Projecting under the proximal part of the nail is a white, crescentic area called the **lunula** (L. luna, moon), because of its shape. It is the distal tip of the matrix projecting beyond the cuticle. The hardened stratum corneum, under shelter of the free edge of the nail, is the **hyponychium.**

Unlike hairs, **growth of nails** is not cyclic but **constant.** In addition to being aids in grasping and holding objects, nails may be subtle **indicators of the health** of an individual. For example, furrows and opacities of the nail frequently accompany infections. Thin, concave, or spoon nails are often present in chronic anemias, syphilis, and rheumatic fever. Dry and brittle nails may suggest vitamin deficiencies or a hypothyroid condition.

Glands of the Skin

SEBACEOUS GLANDS Sebaceous (oil) glands, with few exceptions, are found embedded in the **dermis** or hypodermis in association **with hair follicles.** They empty their oily secretions by a duct into the upper portion of the hair follicle next to the shaft. Morphologically, it is a simple or branched **alveolar (acinar) gland.** Each gland is ovoid in shape, resembling a cluster of grapes with a thick stem as the duct.

On the periphery of the oil gland are undifferentiated, low cuboidal cells that proliferate and differentiate into **large, spherical cells** containing many **lipid droplets** within their cytoplasm and shrunken nuclei. As these droplets continue to accumulate, the cells finally rupture, releasing the lipid secretion, **sebum,** into the large excretory duct. **Replacement of cells** lost in the secretion is accomplished by mitotic activity of the remaining **undifferentiated cells** on the periphery of the exhausted gland.

Sebaceous glands are **holocrine**-type glands **under hormonal control,** i.e., testosterone in man, and ovarian and adrenal androgens in women. These **glands enlarge during puberty,** with a substantial increase in sebum production, one explanation for the development of **acne** in many adolescents.

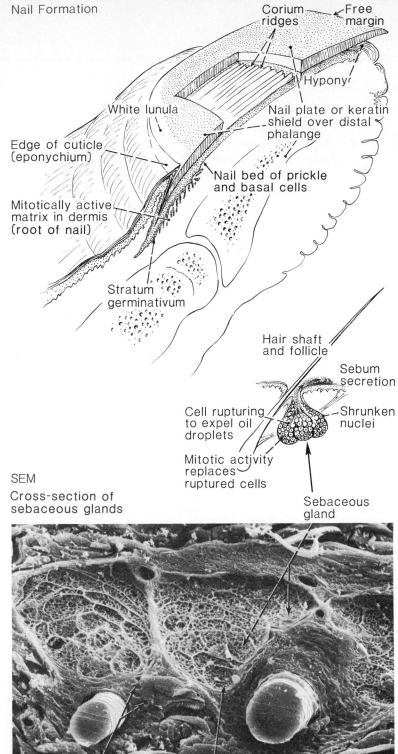

Nail Formation

Corium ridges — Free margin

White lunula

Hypony[?]

Edge of cuticle (eponychium)

Nail plate or keratin shield over distal phalange

Mitotically active matrix in dermis (root of nail)

Nail bed of prickle and basal cells

Stratum germinativum

Hair shaft and follicle

Sebum secretion

Cell rupturing to expel oil droplets

Shrunken nuclei

Mitotic activity replaces ruptured cells

Sebaceous gland

SEM
Cross-section of sebaceous glands

Hair shaft and follicle adjacent to excretory ducts

Low cuboidal cells differentiate into large lipid cells

P.M. Andrews

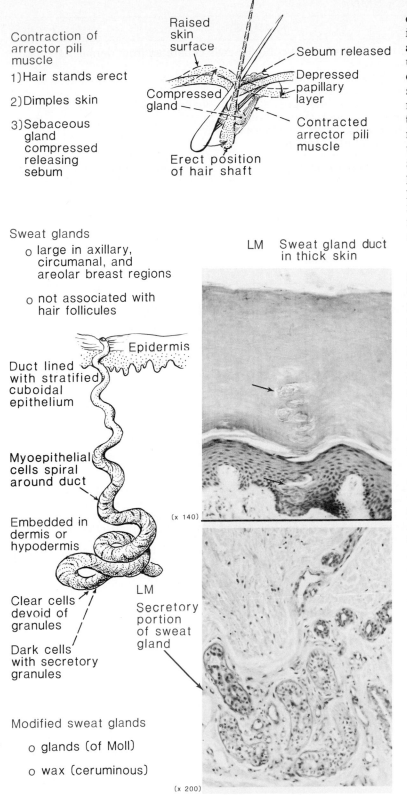

Contraction of
arrector pili
muscle

1) Hair stands erect

2) Dimples skin

3) Sebaceous
gland
compressed
releasing
sebum

Raised
skin
surface

Sebum released

Depressed
papillary
layer

Compressed
gland

Contracted
arrector pili
muscle

Erect position
of hair shaft

Sweat glands

o large in axillary,
circumanal, and
areolar breast regions

o not associated with
hair follicules

Duct lined
with stratified
cuboidal
epithelium

Epidermis

Myoepithelial
cells spiral
around duct

Embedded in
dermis or
hypodermis

Clear cells
devoid of
granules

Dark cells
with secretory
granules

(x 140)

LM   Sweat gland duct
in thick skin

LM
Secretory
portion
of sweat
gland

(x 200)

Modified sweat glands

o glands (of Moll)

o wax (ceruminous)

Attached to the connective tissue sheath of each hair, except in the face and pubic regions, is a small, oblique bundle of smooth muscle, the **arrector pili muscle.** This tiny muscle is directed upwards to attach to the papillary layer of the dermis near the emergence of the hair from the skin. Thus, the sebaceous gland lies between the muscle and the hair shaft. When the **muscle contracts,** three events occur: (1) The **hair becomes more vertical** to the skin surface, i.e., it stands up. (2) A dimple appears on the skin over the site of attachment of the muscle, i.e., "**goose pimples**" appear. (3) The **sebaceous gland is compressed** against the hair follicle, and its secretion is released onto the neck of the follicle and finally reaches the skin by following along the hair shaft.

SWEAT GLANDS With few exceptions, sweat glands are widely distributed throughout the skin. They are either merocrine or apocrine, depending on the mode of secretion. The **merocrine (eccrine)** type is found throughout most of the skin. The gland is a simple, coiled, **tubular gland** with its tightly coiled, secretory portion surrounded by myoepithelial cells. It is embedded in the dermis or hypodermis. The **secretory cells** are of two types, **clear cells** void of granules, and **dark** serouslike cells with secretory granules. The spiraling excretory duct, lined with two layers of **stratified cuboidal epithelium,** opens onto the epidermal surface.

Large **apocrine sweat glands** are limited in distribution to the axillary, circumanal, and areolar breast regions. Like sebaceous glands, they are usually **associated with hair follicles** and release a **viscous secretion,** which gives off a distinct, often offensive, odor. This odor enables animals, e.g. bloodhounds, to detect the presence of other animals, including man. Except for the increase in size, the histology of the eccrine and apocrine sweat gland is similar.

The glands of Moll, on the margins of the eyelids, and the **wax (ceruminous) glands** of the external auditory canals are also **modified sweat glands.** The **mammary glands,** highly modified **apocrine sweat glands,** are discussed with the female reproductive system in Chapter 25.

CLINICAL COMMENTS

For the physician, the skin holds a mirror to age and health. Skin is firmly elastic in youth but loosely wrinkled in the aged. It has a delicate, pink blush in health and in the young, but a greyish blue pallor in the sick and old. It heralds the onset of fever, jaundice, nutritional deficiencies, and metal poisoning. The skin, hair, and nails reveal much to the perceptive physician concerning the physical and mental health of the patient, even before the first question is asked.

8882

Table 15.1 *HISTOLOGICAL FEATURES OF THICK SKIN*

DIVISIONS	LAYERS	FEATURES
Epidermis (epithelium)	Stratum basale	1. Single layer of columnar or tall cuboidal cells separated from dermis by basement membrane 2. Marked basophilia due to row of large, deeply stained nuclei and basal cytoplasm packed with ribosomes 3. Desmosomes on lateral and upper surfaces; hemidesmosomes on basal surface, both associated with many tonofibrils 4. Active mitosis provides cells for other layers 5. Contains free (pain) nerve endings
	Stratum spinosum	1. Several layers of polyhedral, lightly basophilic cells with spines on surfaces 2. Desmosomes attach cells together at spines (formally called intercellular bridges) 3. EM reveals distinctive, small, lamellated, membrane-coated granules 4. Mitotic figures much less frequent
	Stratum granulosum	1. Fewer (2–4) layers of flattened cells with pale, indistinct nuclei 2. Cytoplasm filled with coarse, basophilic, keratohyalin granules 3. Desmosomes present
	Stratum lucidum	1. Two to three layers of flattened, anucleate cells 2. No organelles except closely packed tonofibrils in slightly eosinophilic cytoplasm 3. Few desmosomes 4. Contains eleidin, a clear, refractile substance related to keratohyalin
	Stratum corneum	1. Many layers of anucleate, dead cells 2. Keratin fills cytoplasm 3. Outer, dehydrated, horny scales are constantly shed, singly or in sheets
Dermis (connective tissue)	Papillary layer	1. Outer, thinner layer of irregular, dense connective tissue 2. Distinguished by many dermal papillae that project into epidermis, some contain Meissner's sensory nerve endings 3. Collagenous fibers closely packed next to epidermis
	Reticular layer	1. Inner, thicker layer with coarse collagenous fiber bundles forming a loose, irregular network 2. Contains oil and sweat glands, hair follicles, Pacinian sensory nerve endings, blood and lymph vessels, nerves, fine arrector pili (smooth) muscles and limited skeletal muscles in scalp and face

Table 15.2 COMPARISON OF EPIDERMAL CELLS

	KERATINOCYTES	MELANOCYTES	LANGERHANS CELLS	MERKEL CELLS
Origin	Surface ectoderm	Neural crest	Mesoderm	Neural crest
Location	All strata	Mostly in stratum basale	Scattered throughout stratum malpighii, esp. stratum spinosum	Mostly in or adjacent to stratum basale
Shape	Columnar, cuboidal, or squamous depending on stratum	Spherical or stellate with many dendritic cytoplasmic processes	Stellate with several dendritic processes; nucleus often indented	Usually spherical with short, blunt processes terminating on basal cells; nuclei clear
EM Features	St. basale—rich in ribosomes and tonofilaments; poor in rER, Golgi, and mitochondria St. spinosum—short spines of adjacent cells joined together by desmosomes St. granulosum—many large non-membrane-bound keratohyalin granules among abundant tonofilaments; small membrane granules (keratinosomes) also present	Not attached to other cells by desmosomes; melanosomes prominent; no tonofilaments	Not connected to other cells by desmosomes; Golgi well developed; rER and microtubules limited; many distinctive racket-shaped granules	Attached to other cells by desmosomes; numerous osmophilic electron-dense granules (70–180 nm); no tonofilaments
Relative number of cells	Most numerous—comprise about 90% of all cells	Next numerous—comprise about 8% of cells	Only a few cells	Only a few cells
Melanin	Limited amount, mostly in distal ends of basal cells	Large amounts distributed throughout cytoplasm and dendritic processes in melanosomes	None	An occasional melanosome
Dopa reaction	Negative	Positive	Negative	Negative
H&E staining reaction	Deeply stained; cytoplasm rather basophilic	Lightly stained	Poorly stained; specifically stained with gold chloride	Poorly stained
Keratin	Present in all cells, especially concentrated in more superficial layers	Traces	Absent	Absent
Mitotic activity	Very active in st. basale; diminishes in st. spinosum; absent in other strata	Rare	No data	No data
Neoplasia	Basal and spinous cells may become malignant	Melanocarcinoma, highly malignant	No data	No data
Functions	Produce keratin, an insoluble scleroprotein, which provides a waterproof covering	Synthesize the pigment melanin which protects the body from ultraviolet radiation	Perhaps phagocytosis since they ingest ferritin; also may be involved in body immune responses	Sensory nerve endings probably as mechanoreceptors; as potential APUD cells, may produce catecholamines
Fate	Gradually migrate to surface where they desquamate as cornified scales	Most cells endure throughout life-span of organism	Unknown	Unknown

Chapter

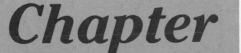

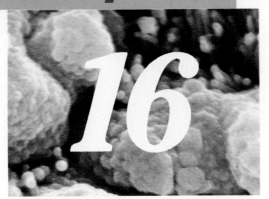

16

RESPIRATORY SYSTEM

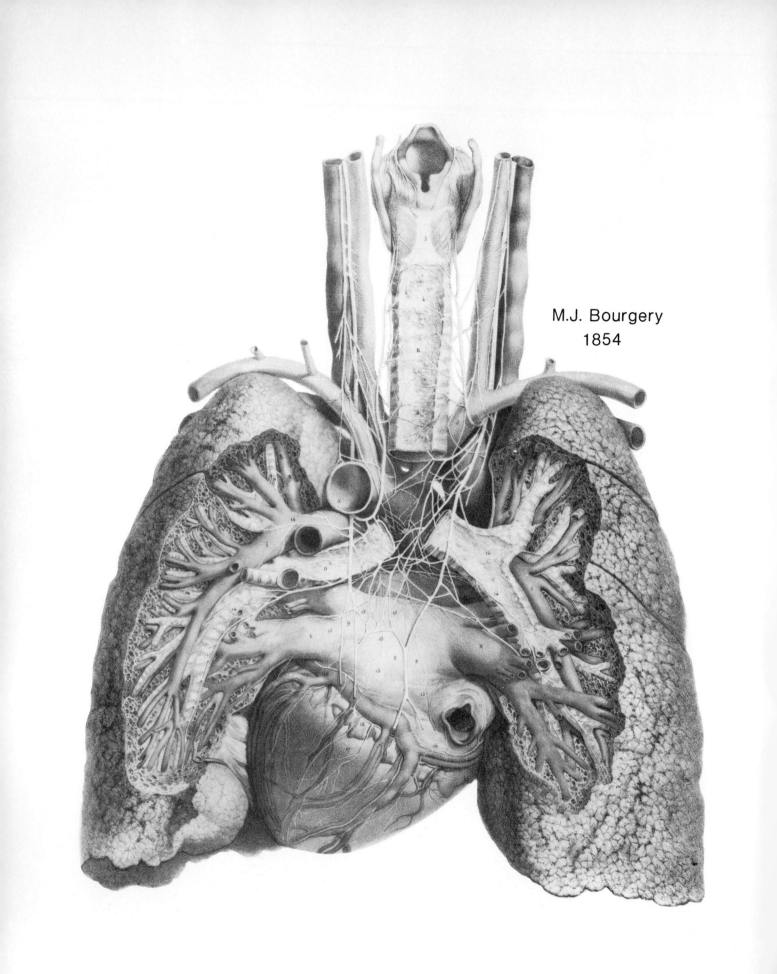

M.J. Bourgery
1854

OBJECTIVES

LEARNING OBJECTIVES OF THIS CHAPTER ARE TO ENABLE THE STUDENT TO:

1. Describe the conduction zone of the respiratory tract and analyze the function(s) of each segment.

2. Identify the transitional area separating the conduction from the respiratory zone.

3. Expound on the fine structure and functions on pulmonary alveoli and the role they play in creating a blood-air barrier.

4. Appraise the role of surfactant in preventing respiratory distress syndrome in premature infants.

5. Comment on the various units of the lung as espoused by the surgeon, the histologist, or the physiologist.

Venus, the ancient Roman goddess of love, is fabled to have had an immaculate birth, that is, without stain or blemish she arose from the foam of the sea. She is depicted by artists as being full-grown at birth. Supposedly, her respiratory system was fully mature since she rode a scallop shell over the waves to the shore where she frolicked and danced.

Mortal man is also born of an **aquatic environment**, but his lungs at birth are not fully capable of functioning. In fact, the **lungs of the newborn** are filled with **amniotic fluid** that must be forcefully expelled before the infant can draw its first breath. Furthermore, the infant's lungs must undergo considerable **growth and differentiation** before they reach full functional and histological **maturity.**

That the **fetal lung** can, at the moment the umbilical cord is severed, provide even limited **gaseous exchange** for the newborn, is a wondrous event. Other organs, such as the kidneys, heart, pancreas, and liver are operational in early fetal life and have continuously developed their functional capacities throughout fetal existence. Not so with the lungs. Since these organs have been housed in a completely aquatic milieu, they have had no opportunity to test their capacity to perform the vital task of gaseous exchange that we call respiration.

The climax of delivery is the first breath, which signals the end of fetal life and the beginning of postnatal existence. Haltingly at first, only a few, then many, tiny **air sacs** (respiratory alveoli) of the unproven lung are expanded. The **oxygen** in the inspired air passes through the very thin walls of the alveoli to enter capillaries. **Carbon dioxide** in the capillary blood reverses direction and is transported into the air sacs. On expiration, it is expelled and the first **respiratory cycle** is completed.

The primary function of the respiratory system is to **provide molecular oxygen** for cellular oxidation and to **remove excess carbon dioxide** from the blood that is generated as the principal waste product of bodily metabolism. These functions are accomplished by the bloodstream acting as the transport system for these gases to and from the lungs.

SUBDIVISIONS

The respiratory system consists of three morphologically and functionally distinct subdivisions: (1) The **air conditioning part or zone** is a series of patent tubes for the movement of air in and

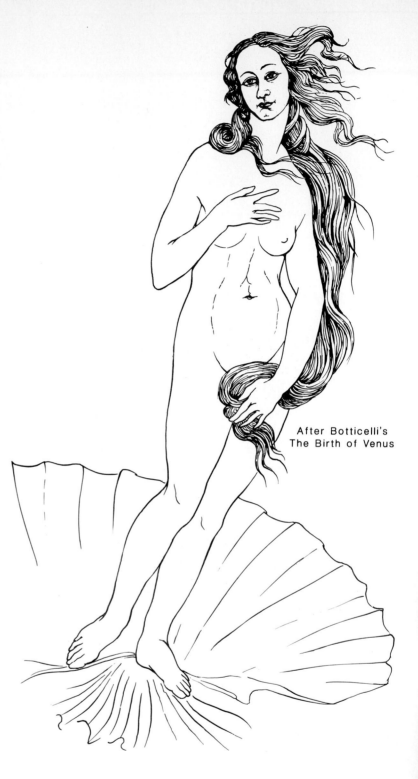

After Botticelli's
The Birth of Venus

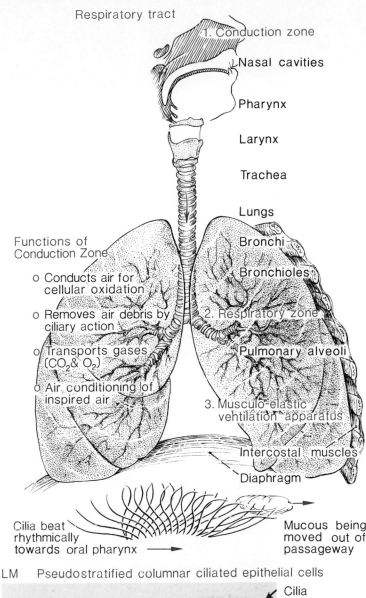

Respiratory tract

1. Conduction zone

Nasal cavities

Pharynx

Larynx

Trachea

Lungs

Bronchi

Bronchioles

2. Respiratory zone

Pulmonary alveoli

3. Musculo-elastic ventilation apparatus

Intercostal muscles

Diaphragm

Functions of Conduction Zone

o Conducts air for cellular oxidation

o Removes air debris by ciliary action

o Transports gases (CO_2 & O_2)

o Air conditioning of inspired air

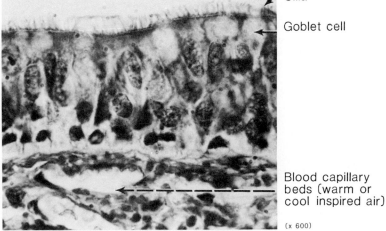

Cilia beat rhythmically towards oral pharynx →

Mucous being moved out of passageway

LM   Pseudostratified columnar ciliated epithelial cells

Cilia

Goblet cell

Blood capillary beds (warm or cool inspired air)

(x 600)

out of lungs. It includes the nasal cavities, pharynx, larynx, trachea, bronchi, and their multiple branchings deep in the lung called bronchioles, culminating in the terminal bronchioles. (2) The **respiratory portion** is where the CO_2 and O_2 exchange actually occurs across the delicate, very thin walls of the pulmonary alveoli that only appear in airways distal to the terminal bronchioles. (3) The third subdivision is largely a subject for gross anatomy and will be only superficially covered. It is a **musculoelastic ventilation apparatus** composed of the muscles of respiration, e.g., the intercostals and diaphragm, which act as bellows, and abundant elastic fibers that provide the elastic recoil of the lung in expiration.

AIR CONDUCTING ZONE

The main function of the **conduction portion** is to **conduct air** to the pulmonary alveoli for **exchange** of CO_2 dissolved in the blood with O_2 in the inspired air. **Other functions** include improving the quality of the inspired air, such as warming or cooling, moistening, cleansing by removal of particulate matter, detoxification by absorption of harmful gases, and entrapment of potentially harmful bacteria and viruses. Most of these latter functions result from the presence of **pseudostratified columnar ciliated epithelial cells** and many **goblet cells** that line nearly all of the air passageways. The **cilia** beat rhythmically in one direction only, i.e., toward the oropharynx. Thus, the cilia move the debris and pathogen-laden mucus to the oral region where it is expectorated or swallowed.

Mucus can also absorb water-soluble, **harmful gases,** such as ozone and SO_2. Concurrently, subepithelial **mucous and serous glands** pour their secretions over the mucosal surface. This greatly augments the mucous secretions of the goblet cells and aids in the **entrapment of particulate matter and bacteria,** as well as moistening the inspired air.

Another factor is **air temperature control.** This is accomplished by profuse capillary beds beneath the epithelium that warm or cool the inspired air. In the nasal cavities, capillaries are largely replaced by extensive, venous plexuses that very effectively modify the air temperature.

Nasal Cavities

The air enters the conduction portion of the respiratory system through the nostrils (anterior nares). It passes through these two hollow, irregularly shaped **nasal cavities** to exit into the nasopharynx by way of two large openings, the posterior nares. The cavities are separated by a midline septum of hyaline cartilage in its inferior extent and by the vertical plate of the ethmoid bone superiorly.

The nasal cavities are divided into several distinct regions, namely, (1) **the vestibule,** a narrow area restricted to the nostrils; (2) a **respiratory area,** occupying most of the cavity; (3) a limited **olfactory zone** in the roof of the nasal cavity; and (4) the **paranasal sinuses** in neighboring bones, which are lined by extensions of the nasal mucosa. The sinuses drain into the nasal cavity.

VESTIBULE The dilated vestibular region is lined with **stratified squamous epithelium,** a direct extension of the thin skin of the upper lip. Its opening into the respiratory cavity is guarded by short, stiff hairs, called **vibrissae,** which are associated with sebaceous glands. Sweat glands are also in the area. Embedded in the lateral exterior wall of the vestibule are one or two small plates of hyaline cartilage, the **alar cartilages,** and a few skeletal muscle fibers (**dilator nares**) that dilate the nostrils allowing more air to enter during stress.

RESPIRATORY CAVITY The respiratory cavity proper is separated from the oral cavity by the hard and soft palates. It is lined with pseudostratified columnar ciliated (**respiratory**) **epithelium,** also called the **Schneiderian membrane.** In contrast to its smooth medial (septal) surface, its lateral surface is interrupted by three overhanging, curved shelves of bone, the superior, middle, and inferior **conchae** (L., concha, a spiral mollusk shell), also called turbinate (scroll-like) bones. Beneath the respiratory epithelium, covering especially the middle and the much larger inferior turbinates, the lamina propria contains extensive, thin-walled **venous plexuses** that function for warming or, less frequently, cooling of the inspired air. When these plexuses become engorged with blood, as in certain allergies and head colds, the mucous membrane is greatly distended and swollen so as to block the nasal passageways. Because of this turgidity, this tissue is called **erectile tissue.** It is similar to the erectile tissue of the penis except that the blood is venous, while in the penis, the blood is arterial. In some individuals, this tissue reacts to erotic stimuli by engorgement that causes fits of sneezing and even nose bleeding. If a relationship exists between these two types of erectile tissue, it may be that lower animals are largely dependent on olfactory stimulation for sexual arousal.

The mucosal surface of the nasal cavity is kept moist by the secretions of abundant **goblet cells** dispersed in the lining epithelium, as well as **mucous and serous glands** embedded in the tunica propria. The beating of the cilia moves the layer of mucus posteriorly into the nasopharynx for disposal.

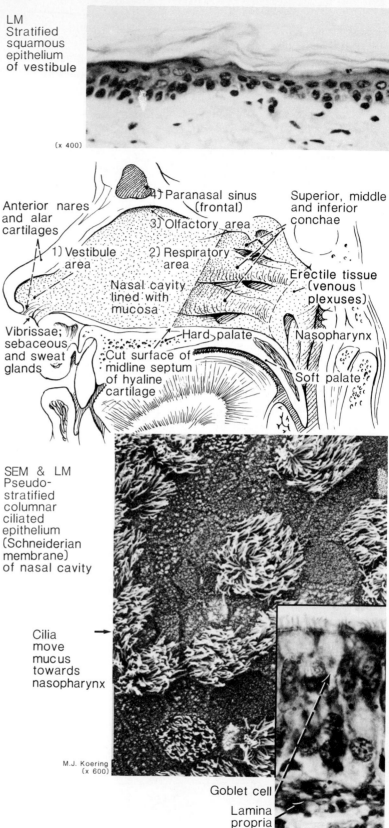

LM
Stratified
squamous
epithelium
of vestibule

(x 400)

Anterior nares and alar cartilages

4) Paranasal sinus (frontal)

3) Olfactory area

Superior, middle and inferior conchae

1) Vestibule area

2) Respiratory area

Nasal cavity lined with mucosa

Erectile tissue (venous plexuses)

Vibrissae; sebaceous and sweat glands

Hard palate

Nasopharynx

Cut surface of midline septum of hyaline cartilage

Soft palate

SEM & LM
Pseudo-stratified columnar ciliated (Schneiderian membrane) of nasal cavity

Cilia move mucus towards nasopharynx

M.J. Koering
(x 600)

Goblet cell

Lamina propria

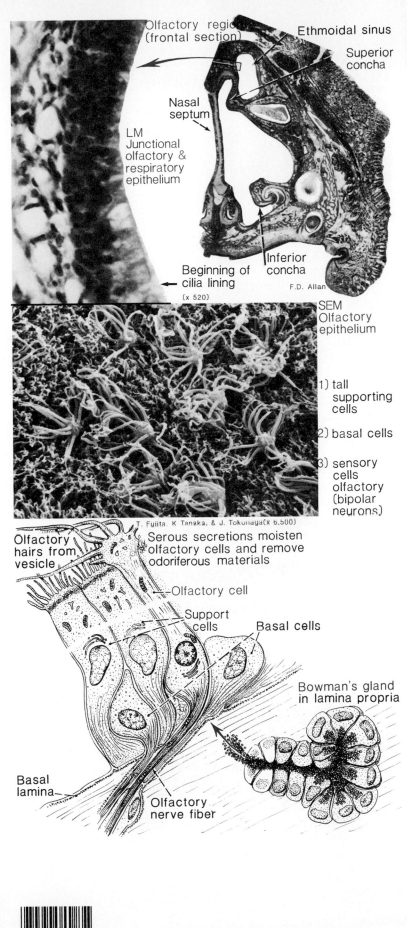

Olfactory region
(frontal section)

Ethmoidal sinus

Superior concha

Nasal septum

LM
Junctional
olfactory &
respiratory
epithelium

Inferior concha

Beginning of
cilia lining

F.D. Allan
(x 520)

SEM
Olfactory
epithelium

1) tall
supporting
cells

2) basal cells

3) sensory
cells
olfactory
(bipolar
neurons)

T. Fujita, K Tanaka, & J. Tokunaga(x 6,500)

Olfactory
hairs from
vesicle

Serous secretions moisten
olfactory cells and remove
odoriferous materials

Olfactory cell

Support
cells

Basal cells

Bowman's gland
in lamina propria

Basal
lamina

Olfactory
nerve fiber

OLFACTORY AREA The olfactory region is limited to the narrow **roof of the nasal cavities** and extends over the superior concha and onto the adjacent septum. When viewed with a naso-scope, the area appears as a yellow or reddish brown zone, in sharp contrast to the adjacent pink respiratory epithelium. The olfactory epi-thelium mimics respiratory epithelium, except that it lacks goblet cells and its pseudostratified columnar cells are taller, with cilia greatly re-duced in number.

There are three cell types in the olfactory ep-ithelium: (1) supporting or sustentacular, (2) basal, and (3) sensory or olfactory. The tall sup-porting, **sustentacular cell** has a broad apex, a narrow base, and an ovoid nucleus in its apex. On its apical free surface, the cell has long, slen-der **microvilli** embedded in the serous fluid that covers the entire olfactory area. **Lipofuscin pig-ment** in these cells is responsible for the brown-ish color of the olfactory epithelium. The **basal cells** are small, rounded, or cone-shaped cells that form a single layer resting on a basal lamina. They are undifferentiated **stem cells** capable of giving rise to support cells and also possibly to sensory cells.

The **olfactory** or sensory cells are **bipolar neu-rons** wedged between the sustentacular and basal cells. They are **spindle-shaped cells** with lightly stained, **central nuclei** usually located more basally than the darker-staining support cell nuclei. Their pointed apices are dilated to form small bulbs, the **olfactory vesicles,** which extend to the surface between the sustentacular cells. From each vesicle emerges 6–10 long, **non-motile cilia** that lie flat on the mucosal surface. They are called olfactory hairs and function as **odor receptors.** The basal segments of the cells narrow greatly to become **efferent axons** that form small bundles, the **fila olfactoria,** which pass through the cribriform plate of the ethmoid bone to synapse with neurons in the **olfactory bulb.**

Odors can only be detected if they are in so-lution. Therefore, for proper functioning, the ol-factory epithelium must be kept moist. This is largely accomplished by the serous secretion of the rather extensive **Bowman's glands** within the lamina propria. This copious, watery secretion continuously flushes over the mucous mem-brane, removing the dissolved odoriferous ma-terials, leaving the sensory cells fresh to respond to new odors.

Paranasal Sinuses

Communicating by drainage ducts into the na-sal cavity are the **paranasal (accessory) air si-nuses.** They are named from the bones they oc-cupy, i.e., frontal, maxillary, sphenoid, and ethmoid. They are lined by modified **respiratory epithelium** that is continuous with the epithe-lium lining the nasal cavity. As in the nasal cavity,

12115

the thin lamina propria is firmly attached to the underlying periosteum and contains a few seromucous glands. Secretions released by these glands and by goblet cells are swept into the nasal cavity by **ciliary action.** If the passageways are blocked, as in certain allergies and head colds, pressure builds up within the cavity that may cause severe **sinus headaches.**

The functions of the sinuses in humans are obscure. Perhaps they aid in the **humidification** of the air in the nasal cavity and as **voice resonators.** Certainly the quality of the voice deteriorates if the sinuses are filled with fluid. In certain animals, olfactory epithelium extends into the frontal and sphenoid sinuses, which may enhance the animal's keen sense of smell.

Nasopharynx

The superior part of the nasopharynx is continuous with the nasal cavity anteriorly. **Respiratory epithelium** lines most of its cavity, except in areas where epithelial surfaces are frequently in contact, such as where the uvula and soft palate contact the posterior wall of the nasopharynx during swallowing. Here the epithelium is **stratified squamous,** as it is also over the poorly defined junction with the oropharynx inferiorly.

The **fibroelastic** lamina propria is infiltrated with abundant **lymphoid tissue.** On the superioposterior wall, aggregates of lymphoid nodules coalesce to form the single **pharyngeal tonsil,** commonly called the **adenoids.** Other collections of nodules surround the openings of the auditory (eustachian) tubes, as the **tubal tonsils.** Mucous glands lie in the lamina propria in areas covered by stratified squamous epithelium, while beneath the respiratory epithelium, small serous and mucous glands are prominent. It is the thin, nonviscous, serous secretion that reduces the viscosity of the mucous coat, thus enabling the cilia to move secretions and foreign matter towards the oral cavity for disposal.

The voluntary superior constrictor muscle of the pharynx is the **muscularis externa** of the nasopharynx. It is rather deficient at its attachment to the base of the skull but is the thick, circular muscle that largely forms the nasopharyngeal wall.

Larynx

Connecting the pharynx above, with the trachea below, is the **larynx.** It is a hollow, bilaterally symmetrical chamber whose walls are made rigid by a series of irregularly shaped **cartilages.** The larynx is held together by ligaments and moved by skeletal muscles. An **extrinsic group of muscles** acts to change the position of the larynx as a whole, as in **swallowing. Smaller intrinsic muscles** act singly or in concert to alter the relative position of the **vocal cords** in the production of sound.

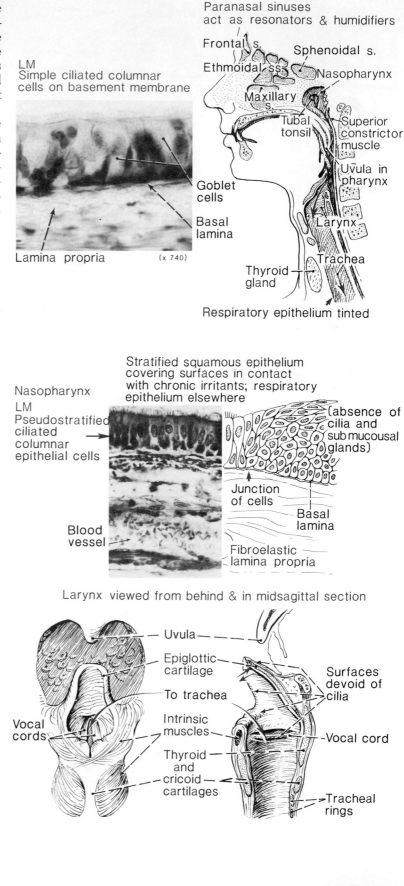

LM
Simple ciliated columnar cells on basement membrane

Goblet cells

Basal lamina

Lamina propria   (x 740)

Paranasal sinuses act as resonators & humidifiers
Frontal s.
Sphenoidal s.
Ethmoidal sss
Nasopharynx
Maxillary s.
Tubal tonsil
Superior constrictor muscle
Uvula in pharynx
Larynx
Thyroid gland
Trachea

Respiratory epithelium tinted

Stratified squamous epithelium covering surfaces in contact with chronic irritants; respiratory epithelium elsewhere

Nasopharynx LM Pseudostratified ciliated columnar epithelial cells

(absence of cilia and submucousal glands)

Junction of cells

Basal lamina

Blood vessel

Fibroelastic lamina propria

Larynx viewed from behind & in midsagittal section

Uvula
Epiglottic cartilage
To trachea
Intrinsic muscles
Vocal cords
Thyroid and cricoid cartilages
Surfaces devoid of cilia
Vocal cord
Tracheal rings

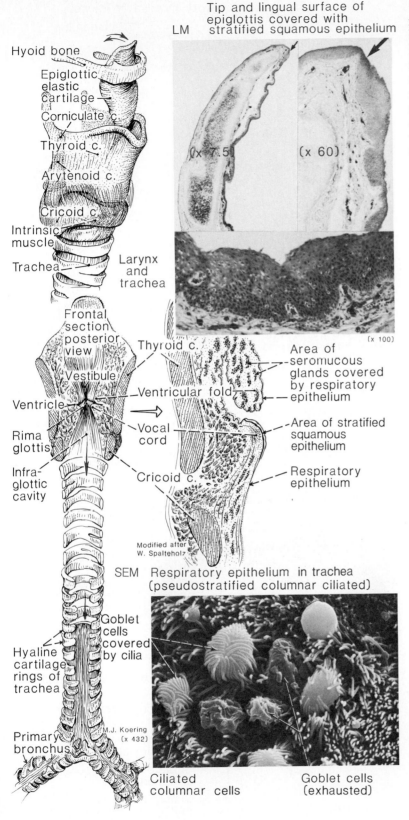

Tip and lingual surface of epiglottis covered with stratified squamous epithelium

LM

(x 7.5) (x 60)

(x 100)

Hyoid bone

Epiglottic elastic cartilage

Corniculate c.

Thyroid c.

Arytenoid c.

Cricoid c.

Intrinsic muscle

Trachea

Larynx and trachea

Frontal section posterior view

Vestibule

Ventricle

Rima glottis

Infraglottic cavity

Thyroid c.

Ventricular fold

Vocal cord

Cricoid c.

Area of seromucous glands covered by respiratory epithelium

Area of stratified squamous epithelium

Respiratory epithelium

Modified after W. Spalteholz

SEM Respiratory epithelium in trachea (pseudostratified columnar ciliated)

Goblet cells covered by cilia

Hyaline cartilage rings of trachea

Primary bronchus

M.J. Koering (x 432)

Ciliated columnar cells

Goblet cells (exhausted)

Two large, external, single cartilages, the **thyroid and cricoid, are hyaline cartilage,** as are the bodies of the largest of the paired internal cartilages, the triangular **arytenoids.** All of these cartilages tend to calcify in early life and are often ossified in later life. The much smaller, paired, internal cartilages, the corniculates (horn-shaped) and cuneiforms (wedge-shaped), the single large, spoon-shaped epiglottis, and the tips of the arytenoids are composed of **elastic cartilage.**

The large **epiglottis** guards the upper opening of the larynx. During swallowing, it is swept backward and downward to **close the larynx** like a lid, thus deflecting food or drink from entering the larynx. Since the epiglottis protrudes into the lower pharynx, it has an anterior lingual surface covered with **stratified squamous** epithelium and a posterior laryngeal surface with **respiratory epithelium.** However, the superior, free, broad tip is covered on both sides by stratified squamous epithelium.

Seen in frontal section, the cavity of the larynx **resembles a cross.** The arms of the cross are the lateral extensions of the central cavity, called the **ventricles.** The central, midline cavity above the "arms" is the **vestibule.** The long, wide cavity below is the **infraglottic cavity,** which is continuous with the trachea. At the junction of the "arms," the central cavity is called **rima glottis.** Bordering the rima inferiorly are the **true vocal cords** covered with **stratified squamous epithelium.** The cords consist of bundles of elastic fibers, the **vocal ligaments,** and the **vocalis muscle.** The latter controls phonation by varying tension and length of the cords. Above the junction are the **false vocal cords** or the protective ventricular folds which are separated from the true cords by the ventricle. The false cords are devoid of muscle but rich in mixed **seromucous glands.** They are covered by **respiratory epithelium.**

Trachea and Primary Bronchi

These extrapulmonary airways will be considered together because their histological features and functions are similar. In cross section, they present four layers, namely, a mucosa, a submucosa, an incomplete muscularis, and an adventitia.

The epithelium of the **mucosa** is typical **respiratory epithelium** (pseudostratified columnar ciliated) that rests on a **prominent basal lamina.** Four cell types are identified in the epithelial layer. **Ciliated columnar cells** are the most numerous, followed by **goblet cells.** Interspersed between these cell types are a few nonciliated columnar (**brush**) **cells** with apical microvilli. They may be immature goblet cells. The fourth cell type is the short or **basal cell** that rests on the basal lamina, and its apex does not extend to the lumen. These infrequent cells may be undifferentiated **stem cells** that give rise to the other epithelial cells and also some APUD cells.

The prominent **lamina propria** is infiltrated with lymphocytes caught in a meshwork of elastic and reticular fibers. At a deeper level a concentration of elastic fibers forms a rather distinct band, the **membrana elastica interna**, that demarcates the lamina propria from the deeper submucosa. The limited **submucosa** contains loose connective tissue and small mixed serous and mucous glands whose ducts penetrate the mucosa to reach the lumen.

The rather **dense adventitia** is the most extensive layer. In addition to thick collagenous connective tissue bands, it contains **large C-shaped hyaline cartilage rings** (16–20 in trachea; 8–10 broken rings in each bronchus). The muscularis is the involuntary **trachealis muscle** that fills the intervals between the open rings in the trachea, and the unnamed smooth muscle fibers that join the partial rings in the primary bronchi.

The presence of the rigid, horseshoe-shaped cartilage rings and the absence of complete circular smooth muscle bands almost guarantees that the trachea and primary bronchi will always be **patent,** except perhaps for crushing trauma to the neck or the inhalation of large objects.

Intrapulmonary Bronchi

As the right primary (extrapulmonary) bronchus enters the lung, it divides into three **intrapulmonary (secondary) bronchi,** one for each lobe. The left lung receives from the left bronchus two secondary bronchi, one for each of the two lobes. As these secondary bronchi plunge into the lung substance, they undergo dichotomous branching, resulting in **segmental (tertiary) bronchi** that supply each of the **bronchopulmonary segments,** i.e., the ten segments of the right lobe and eight to ten segments of the left.

The secondary and tertiary bronchi have the same general histological pattern as the primary bronchi. However, differences develop as the bronchi become smaller. These changes include: (1) The cartilage rings are reduced to irregular **plates of cartilage** that gradually diminish in size and number as the lumen of the bronchus decreases. (2) A definite circular **band of smooth muscle** develops between the cartilage plates and the mucosa. The smaller the bronchus, the relatively greater amount of muscle is present. (3) Goblet cells become less numerous. (4) The epithelium is reduced in height and becomes simple columnar with fewer cilia.

Bronchioles

Two large bronchioles arise from the final dichotomous branching of a tertiary bronchus. The distinctive histological features of bronchioles include: (1) **absence of cartilagenous plates,** (2) increase in relative size of the circular smooth muscle layers, and (3) changing of respiratory epithelium to **simple columnar ciliated epithelium** (L-A plate 11).

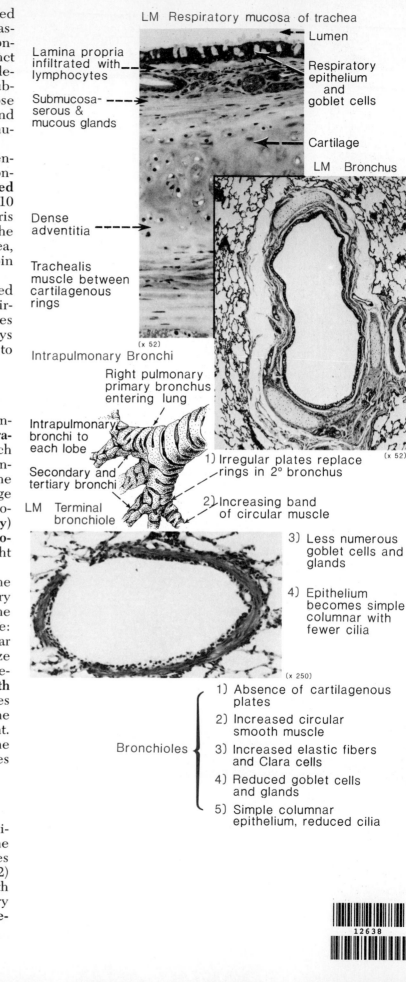

LM   Respiratory mucosa of trachea

Lamina propria infiltrated with lymphocytes

Submucosa-serous & mucous glands

Dense adventitia

Trachealis muscle between cartilagenous rings

Lumen

Respiratory epithelium and goblet cells

Cartilage

LM   Bronchus

(x 52)

Intrapulmonary Bronchi

Right pulmonary primary bronchus entering lung

Intrapulmonary bronchi to each lobe

Secondary and tertiary bronchi

LM   Terminal bronchiole

(x 52)

1) Irregular plates replace rings in 2° bronchus

2) Increasing band of circular muscle

3) Less numerous goblet cells and glands

4) Epithelium becomes simple columnar with fewer cilia

(x 250)

Bronchioles
1) Absence of cartilagenous plates
2) Increased circular smooth muscle
3) Increased elastic fibers and Clara cells
4) Reduced goblet cells and glands
5) Simple columnar epithelium, reduced cilia

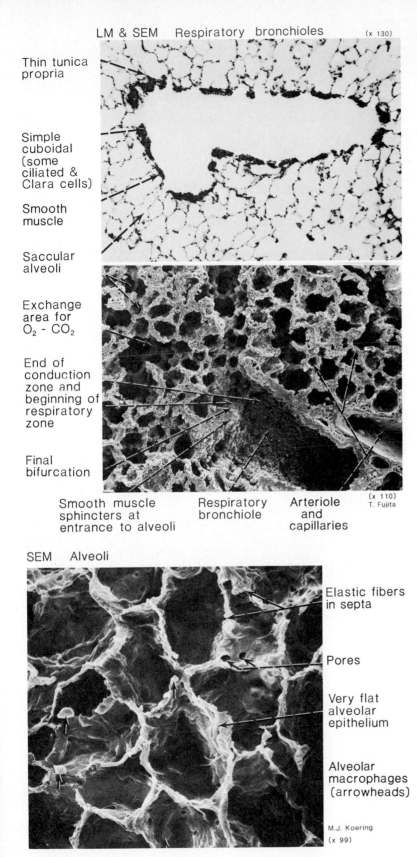

LM & SEM   Respiratory bronchioles   (x 130)

Thin tunica propria

Simple cuboidal (some ciliated & Clara cells)

Smooth muscle

Saccular alveoli

Exchange area for O_2 - CO_2

End of conduction zone and beginning of respiratory zone

Final bifurcation

Smooth muscle sphincters at entrance to alveoli

Respiratory bronchiole

Arteriole and capillaries

(x 110)
T. Fujita

SEM   Alveoli

Elastic fibers in septa

Pores

Very flat alveolar epithelium

Alveolar macrophages (arrowheads)

M.J. Koering
(x 99)

The final bifurcation of a bronchiole yields **terminal bronchioles.** They are rather distinctive air conduits showing considerable **reduction in the muscle layer** that lies directly beneath the epithelium, and the tunica propria is very thin. The epithelium is further reduced to **simple cuboidal cells;** many are ciliated, others are nonciliated **Clara cells.** Terminal bronchioles are the final air passageways of the conduction zone.

To summarize, the bronchioles of the conduction zone represent **20 or more generations** of conduits, whose diameters range from 0.5 to 1 mm. Their walls **lack cartilage** plates and respiratory alveoli but have a prominent, circular, smooth **muscle layer.** Only the larger bronchioles have mucoserous glands in the tunica propria. The **epithelium** is gradually **reduced** from ciliated columnar in the larger bronchioles to ciliated or nonciliated low cuboidal in the terminal segment. Here nonciliated **Clara cells** are plentiful but globlet cells are lacking.

RESPIRATORY ZONE

Respiratory Bronchiole

The respiratory bronchiole is the transitional structure separating the conduction zone from the respiratory part. Each terminal bronchiole divides into two or more **respiratory bronchioles.** The mucosa of the latter is very similar to the lining of the terminal bronchiole except that the wall is interrupted by **respiratory alveoli.** These small, **saccular** structures are the site for O_2 and CO_2 exchange in the lung, hence the term **respiratory bronchiole.** Other diagnostic features are the rather prominent tags of smooth muscle that persist between the alveoli, and the prominent elastic fibers in the walls of the alveoli. The bronchiolar epithelium is continuous with the attenuated, very flat, **alveolar epithelium** lining each alveolus. The **alveoli** are more numerous in the distal segments of the respiratory bronchiole, where they occupy most of the wall. Gradually, the epithelium becomes somewhat flattened, and many of the cells lose their cilia.

Alveolar Ducts and Sacs

Each respiratory bronchiole divides into several **alveolar ducts** whose walls consist entirely of alveolar openings. The very thin, attenuated alveolar epithelium that lines the alveoli also outlines the alveolar duct. Remnants of the muscle layer are seen as a thin ring of tissue surrounding the openings of the alveoli.

As an alveolar duct becomes wider in its distal segment, it terminates in a cluster of alveoli sharing a common, dilated chamber, called an **alveolar sac.** The junctional space between the alveolar duct and the alveolar sac is often called the **atrium,** a rather redundant term for the expanded terminal segment of the alveolar duct.

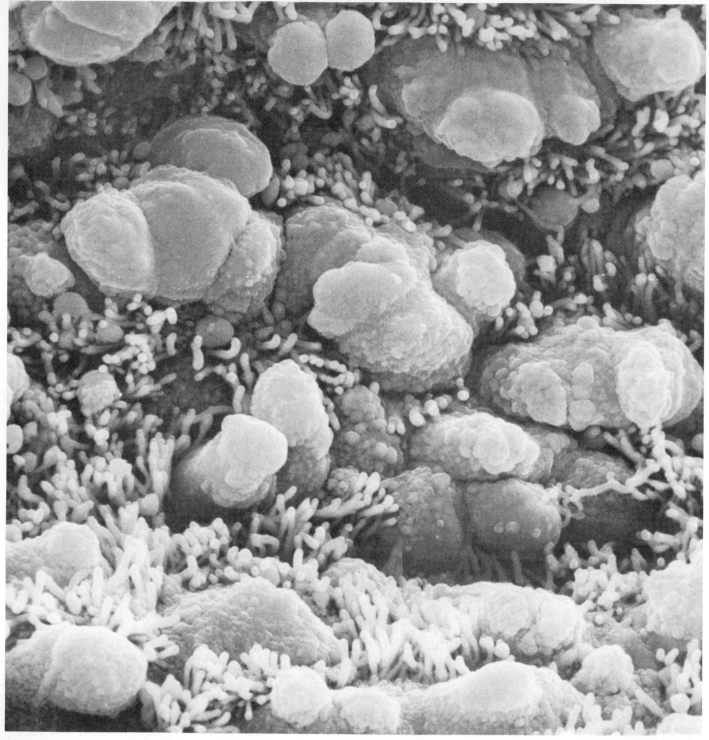

P.M. Andrews

Interspersed among the ciliated epithelial cells of the large bronchioles are the nonciliated dome-shaped Clara cells. From the abundance of rER, apical granules, and Golgi bodies, these cells appear to be secretory but their exact function is uncertain. However, they may secrete surface-active agents, e.g., aqueous, proteinaceous components of surfactant, a lung alveolar surface stabilizing agent that prevents the collapse of the alveolar walls after each expiration.

12780

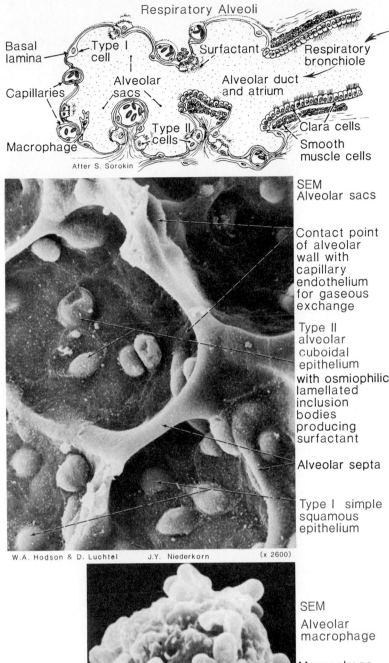

Respiratory Alveoli

Basal lamina — Type I cell — Surfactant — Respiratory bronchiole

Capillaries — Alveolar sacs — Alveolar duct and atrium

Macrophage — Type II cells — Clara cells — Smooth muscle cells

After S. Sorokin

SEM
Alveolar sacs

Contact point of alveolar wall with capillary endothelium for gaseous exchange

Type II alveolar cuboidal epithelium with osmiophilic lamellated inclusion bodies producing surfactant

Alveolar septa

Type I simple squamous epithelium

W.A. Hodson & D. Luchtel   J.Y. Niederkorn   (x 2600)

SEM
Alveolar macrophage

Macrophage (10-12 um) free in alveoli to scavenge debris esp. dust particles

Trapped spores

Microvilli and surface evaginations

(x 2600)

Respiratory Alveoli

The functional unit of the lung is the **alveolus.** Only within this tiny, polyhedral box does **gaseous exchange** occur. This respiratory chamber has the side next to the lumen missing, thus allowing easy access of inspired air. Alveoli are very thin-walled outpocketings of the respiratory bronchioles, alveolar ducts, and alveolar sacs. In the ducts and sacs, they are tightly wedged together and share very thin common walls, called **alveolar septa.** The most conspicuous feature of the alveolar wall is the presence of a tiny **capillary** lined with very flat endothelial cells with a continuous basal lamina. Unless the capillary is distended with blood, it is difficult to see with the light microscope.

Only under the EM can one clearly identify the lining cells of the alveoli. They consist of very flattened, **simple squamous epithelium** of two cell types. **Type I** are small alveolar epithelial cells (squamous pneumocytes). Although somewhat less numerous (40%), they line about 95% of the alveolar surface area. They have a **flattened, central nucleus** with many broad, thin, **winglike cytoplasmic extensions** 0.1–0.3 μm thick. In some areas, the basal lamina of the type I cells and the endothelium of the capillary are fused. These fusion sites are possible areas of gas exchange. Located near the nucleus are a few organelles. EM studies show the surfaces of type I cells are free of microvilli.

Type II, the **large alveolar cells** (granular pneumocytes), are more numerous (60%) but, because they are essentially **cuboidal cells** without wide cytoplasmic extensions, they occupy only about 5% of the alveolar surface. Under the EM, the hallmarks of these cells are the numerous osmiophilic, **lamellated inclusion bodies** and many **microvilli** on their free surface. There is good evidence connecting these lamellated bodies with the production of **surfactant,** an alveolar surface stabilizing material (to be discussed later). Other inclusions and organelles are more numerous than in type I cells. They include larger mitochondria, and more extensive Golgi bodies, rER, ribosomes, and lysosomes.

Macrophages (**dust cells**) are also associated with alveoli. These are large cells, 10–12 μm in diameter, which usually lie free in the alveoli and the air passageways. They are the principal cell type found in fluid flushed from the lungs, whose prime function is **protection**. These alveolar macrophages clean the lungs of invading **bacteria** and particularly of ingested **particulate matter,** such as carbon and other dust-borne debris. These cells are avid **scavengers.** Any deficiency or malfunction of these macrophages contributes greatly to the incidence of virulence of pulmonary infections, e.g., black lung disease, pulmonary tuberculosis, and emphysema (see Tables 16.1 and 16.2 for summary).

12745

THE UNITS OF THE LUNG

What constitutes the different units of the lung depends on one's viewpoint. To the surgeon, the **bronchopulmonary segment** is the gross anatomical **unit** of the lung. In the human, each lung is divided into eight to ten such segments, consisting of the parenchyma and airways of the lung that are supplied by a **single tertiary bronchus** and accompanying artery and nerves. Each segment is drained by veins that course along the periphery in the intersegmental plane. The bronchopulmonary segment is the **smallest topographic unit** that can be **removed surgically**, since surgery must not disturb the main blood supply or airways of the lung proper.

To the histologist, W.S. Miller's description of units of the lung has wide acceptance. This eminent lung researcher subdivided the lung into two basic lobules. His **primary lobule** arises from the branchings of a **respiratory bronchiole**, consisting of a series of alveolar ducts, atria, alveolar sacs, and alveoli, including their accompanying blood and nerve supply. His larger **secondary lobule** consists of a **large bronchiole** and all of its branches and accompanying blood vessels and nerves. This lobule is **limited by connective tissue septa** that demarcate a pyramidal-shaped lobule whose base rests on the pleura and whose apex is directed towards the center of the lung.

More recently, a third lobule has had wide currency, especially among physiologists. It is the **acinus,** so called because the **aggregates of alveoli** suggest clusters of grapes. It is defined as that part of the lung supplied by a **single terminal bronchiole** and all of its branches. [Note that the lung acinus and the primary lobule are the same except that the terminal bronchiole is not included in the primary lobule (of Miller)]. Finally, the **functional unit** of the lung is the tiny, thin-walled alveolus, the unique sac where gaseous exchange actually occurs, regardless of where it is found.

SURFACTANT

Contributing to the lining of the alveoli of the late fetus are **type II granular alveolar cells** that synthesize a special stabilizing surface-active material called **surfactant**. It contains primarily **phospholipids**, especially **lecithin**, complexed to **proteins** and **carbohydrates** in stable combinations. In TEM micrographs, surfactant is seen as osmiophilic **lamellar inclusion bodies,** a cardinal clue in the identification of type II cells. About the 24th week of human gestation, these cells appear. Shortly thereafter, the characteristic lamellar inclusions are present. By the 30th week, surfactant is detectable in the lung and amniotic fluid but not in sufficient amounts to prevent respiratory distress, if the infant is born prematurely.

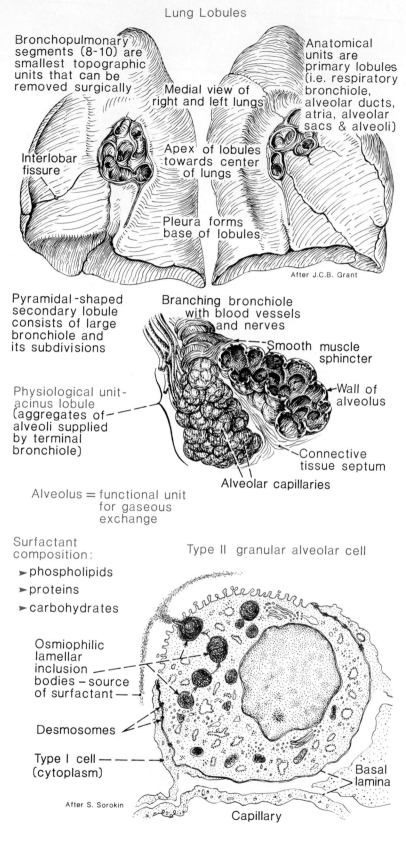

Lung Lobules

Bronchopulmonary segments (8-10) are smallest topographic units that can be removed surgically

Medial view of right and left lungs

Anatomical units are primary lobules (i.e. respiratory bronchiole, alveolar ducts, atria, alveolar sacs & alveoli)

Interlobar fissure

Apex of lobules towards center of lungs

Pleura forms base of lobules

After J.C.B. Grant

Pyramidal-shaped secondary lobule consists of large bronchiole and its subdivisions

Branching bronchiole with blood vessels and nerves

Smooth muscle sphincter

Wall of alveolus

Physiological unit-acinus lobule (aggregates of alveoli supplied by terminal bronchiole)

Connective tissue septum

Alveolar capillaries

Alveolus = functional unit for gaseous exchange

Surfactant composition:
➤ phospholipids
➤ proteins
➤ carbohydrates

Type II granular alveolar cell

Osmiophilic lamellar inclusion bodies – source of surfactant

Desmosomes

Type I cell (cytoplasm)

Basal lamina

After S. Sorokin

Capillary

12773

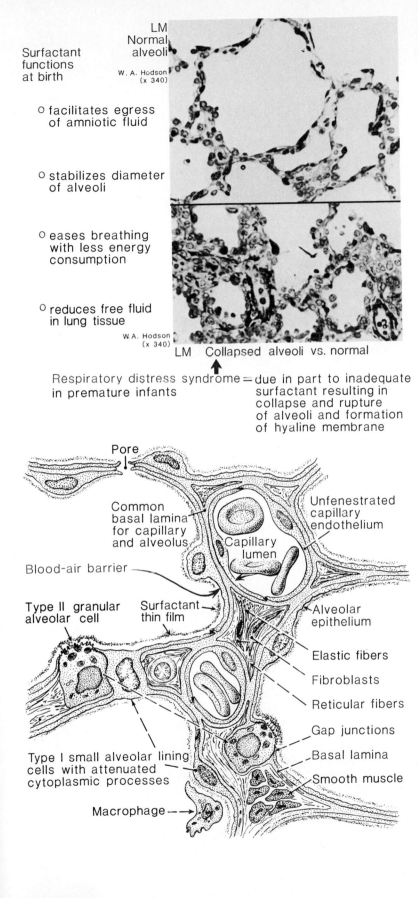

Respiratory distress syndrome = due in part to inadequate
in premature infants   surfactant resulting in
                              collapse and rupture
                              of alveoli and formation
                              of hyaline membrane

Pore

Common
basal lamina
for capillary
and alveolus

Unfenestrated
capillary
endothelium

Capillary
lumen

Blood-air barrier

Type II granular
alveolar cell

Surfactant
thin film

Alveolar
epithelium

Elastic fibers

Fibroblasts

Reticular fibers

Gap junctions

Basal lamina

Smooth muscle

Type I small alveolar lining
cells with attenuated
cytoplasmic processes

Macrophage

Surfactant is crucial to the function of the lung because:

1. It acts as a **detergent** that greatly facilitates the rapid egress of amniotic fluid from the lungs at birth, before the first breath.

2. Its high viscosity and low surface tension **stabilize the diameter of the alveoli** and prevent their collapse after each expiration, allowing some air to be retained in the alveoli after each breath. Thus, a residual air capacity is established in the lungs.

3. Because the alveoli remain partially open, they are expanded on subsequent inspirations with much less expenditure of energy, i.e., the **newborn can breathe much easier.**

4. By **lowering alveolar surface tension,** surfactant helps to keep the alveoli relatively free of fluid, thus preventing respiratory distress of the newborn.

Respiratory Distress Syndrome

Respiratory distress syndrome occurs frequently in **premature infants** and occasionally in healthy, full-term newborns. It is characterized by **cyanosis** and labored breathing, caused by failure of the alveoli to expand or to remain open after each inspiration. To counteract the collapse of the alveoli, **forced oxygen** is often administered to the cyanotic newborn. Initially the infant may improve; however, the forced ventilation tends to rupture the thin alveolar epithelial wall. Breeching of this **air-blood barrier** allows blood plasma to seep into the alveoli, causing hyaline membranes to form across the alveoli. Clinically, this is **hyaline membrane disease,** a fairly common condition in the premature infant. This disease may result from an **inadequate supply of surfactant** at birth. Unless the level of surfactant is rapidly increased to normal levels, the baby may die within 48 hours.

BLOOD-AIR BARRIER

The very thin wall between adjacent alveoli containing pulmonary capillaries represents a **blood-air barrier** that oxygen and carbon dioxide molecules must penetrate before respiration can occur. On the air surface, the barrier consists for the most part of the thin, attenuated, cytoplasmic **processes of type I** small alveolar lining cells. Surfactant covers these cells as a thin film of lipoprotein and polysaccharides that **stabilizes** the alveolar wall. The alveolar epithelium rests on a **basal lamina,** which may blend with the basal lamina of the endothelial cells lining the capillary.

12717

On the blood side, a **nonfenestrated endothelium,** held together by **gap junctions** and a prominent, **continuous basal lamina,** represents the blood portion of the barrier. If the basal laminae of the alveolar epithelium and endothelium are separated, the space is filled with many delicate **reticular and elastic fibers.** Thus, the blood-air barrier consists of these fibrous **components,** the thin cytoplasm of type I cells covered with surfactant and their basal lamina, and the basal lamina and attenuated cytoplasm of the capillary endothelium.

BLOOD VESSELS

The lung has a **dual blood supply,** i.e., functional **(pulmonary)** and nutritive **(bronchial) vessels.** Functional **pulmonary arteries** accompany bronchi and bronchioles and eventually pass through the **center of a secondary lobule.** They transport **deoxygenated** blood from the right ventricle of the heart to the lungs, where CO_2 is purged and O_2 is bound. **Pulmonary veins,** coursing in the connective tissue **septa** in the periphery of the **secondary lobules,** return **oxygenated** blood to the heart for distribution throughout the body. Since pulmonary arteries and veins resemble each other histologically, they are difficult to distinguish. However, since the **pulmonary arteries** accompany bronchi and bronchioles, they **do not occur singly** but are accompanied by some **air passageways.** In contrast, **pulmonary veins occur singly,** usually on the periphery of the secondary lung lobules, not accompanied by a segment of the air conduit system.

The nutrient bronchial arteries (branches of the aorta) also **accompany and nourish the bronchi** and the larger **bronchioles.** However, they have much smaller diameters and thinner walls than the pulmonary arteries. **Bronchial veins** also follow the larger bronchioles and bronchi to the root of the lung to empty eventually into the **azygos** system of veins or the **pulmonary** veins.

PLEURA

The pleura is a double-layer **serous, mesothelial membrane** that envelops both lungs as the **visceral pleura** and that lines the internal surface of the thoracic cavity as the **parietal pleura.** These two layers are **continuous** at the hilum of each lung and therefore form two closed sacs, the **pleural cavities.** Each sac is lined with **mesothelium** and normally contains only a **thin film** of fluid that **lubricates** the lung and pleural cavity surfaces, allowing for essentially frictionless movement of the lung over the inner chest wall during respiration.

In addition to mesothelium, the pleura consists of a layer of **fibroelastic connective tissue,** interspersed with fibroblasts, macrophages, blood capillaries, and lymphatic vessels.

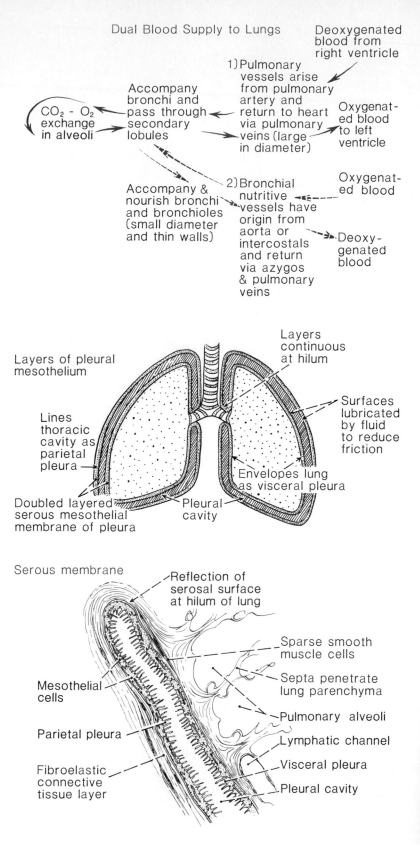

Dual Blood Supply to Lungs

$CO_2 - O_2$ exchange in alveoli

Accompany bronchi and pass through secondary lobules

1) Pulmonary vessels arise from pulmonary artery and return to heart via pulmonary veins (large in diameter)

Deoxygenated blood from right ventricle

Oxygenated blood to left ventricle

Accompany & nourish bronchi and bronchioles (small diameter and thin walls)

2) Bronchial nutritive vessels have origin from aorta or intercostals and return via azygos & pulmonary veins

Oxygenated blood

Deoxygenated blood

Layers of pleural mesothelium

Layers continuous at hilum

Lines thoracic cavity as parietal pleura

Surfaces lubricated by fluid to reduce friction

Doubled layered serous mesothelial membrane of pleura

Pleural cavity

Envelopes lung as visceral pleura

Serous membrane

Reflection of serosal surface at hilum of lung

Mesothelial cells

Parietal pleura

Fibroelastic connective tissue layer

Sparse smooth muscle cells

Septa penetrate lung parenchyma

Pulmonary alveoli

Lymphatic channel

Visceral pleura

Pleural cavity

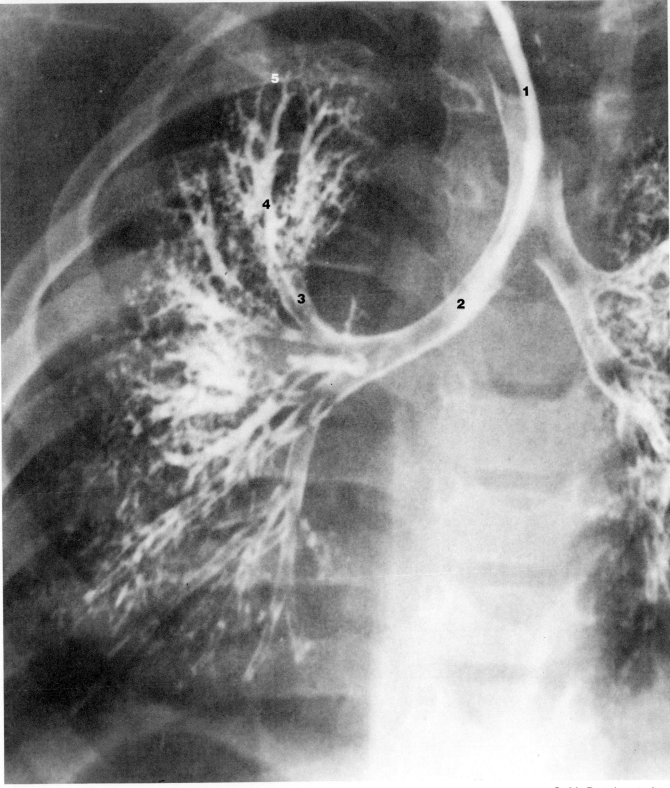

S. M. Brooks et al.

To test your mastery of the air-conduction parts of the lung, identify the numbered structures in the above X-ray. Tabulate the changes in the epithelium, cartilage, and smooth muscle that occur along the air passageways. Compare your tabulation with Table 16.2.

Table 16.1 *SUMMARY OF HISTOLOGY OF RESPIRATORY SYSTEM*

ZONE	STRUC-TURE	SUBDIVISIONS	EPITHELIUM	LAMINA PROPRIA	MUSCLE
Conduction	Nasal cavity	Vestibule	Stratified squamous (thin skin with vibrissae)	Irregular, dense connective tissue with papillae	Few skeletal muscle fibers (dilatator naris muscle)
		Respiratory	Respiratory (pseudostratified columnar ciliated)	Large venous plexuses; nerve endings	None
		Olfactory	Olfactory with neurosensory, support and basal cells	Collagenous and elastic fibers bound to periosteum; Bowman's glands	None
	Pharynx	Nasal	Respiratory	Pharyngeal and tubal tonsils; diffuse lymphoid tissue, collagenous and elastic fibers	Overlapping pharyngeal constrictor (skeletal) muscles
		Oral	Stratified squamous, nonkeratinized	Palatine tonsil; few seromucous glands	Constrictor muscles in wall
	Larynx		Respiratory, except for the superior half and anterior surface of epiglottis, and true vocal cords which have stratified squamous	Thinner layer with less collagenous and elastic fibers; few lymph nodules	Extrinsic and intrinsic muscles are all skeletal
	Trachea		Respiratory with many goblet cells	Thin, many elastic fibers, few collagenous; diffuse lymphoid tissue with occasional nodule	Smooth muscle between free ends of cartilage rings (trachealis muscle)
	Bronchi	Primary (stem or main)	Respiratory; fewer goblet cells	Same as trachea	Trachealis muscle diminished
		Secondary (lobar)	Respiratory; goblet cells diminished	Thinner layer; elastic fibers prominent	Smooth muscle forms thin complete ring internal to cartilage plates
		Tertiary (segmental)	Simple columnar, ciliated; goblet cells sparse	Reduced	Circular smooth muscle band more prominent
	Bronchioles	Large (each serve a secondary lobule)	Same as above, except cells reduced in height	Same as above	Circular smooth muscle band proportionally larger
		Terminal	Simple tall cuboidal; some cells ciliated, others (Clara cells) nonciliated	Further reduction in thickness	Layers incomplete, greatly reduced in number and lie directly beneath the epithelium
Respiratory	Bronchiole	Respiratory (serves a primary lobule)	Simple cuboidal; fewer ciliated cells; no goblet cells	Few collagenous fibers; elastic fibers dominate	Few interrupted fibers
	Alveolar duct		Low cuboidal or simple squamous	Essentially all elastic fibers	None
	Alveolar sac		Thin simple squamous	Elastic fibers with a few reticular fibers	None
	Alveolus (unit of function and structure)		Very thin, tenuous squamous cells, only recognized with EM	Occasional elastic fibers	None

GLANDS	CARTILAGE	ALVEOLI	FUNCTION
Sweat and sebaceous	Hyaline (alar cartilages)	None	Vibrissae guard nostrils
Seromucous and goblet cells	Hyaline in conchae and part of nasal septum	None	Purifies, cools, warms and moistens air
Bowman's glands (tubular alveolar serous type); no goblet cells	Superior conchae and superior part of septum (hyaline)	None	Olfaction
Few seromucous glands and scattered goblet cells	None	None	Air pasageway
Minor salivary (serous and mucous)	None	None	Air and food directed towards appropriate exit
Serous and mucous	Thyroid, cricoid, and arytenoid cartilages are hyaline; cuneiforms, corniculates, and epiglottis are elastic	None	Sound production; controls air movements in and out of lung
Tracheal (serous and mucous) in submucosa	16–20 horseshoe-shaped, hyaline cartilages with open ends directed posteriorly	None	Patent air passageway between larynx and tracheal bifurcation
Serous and mucous	Rings reduced to 8–10	None	Patent airway between trachea and lung
Reduced; serous and mucous types	Hyaline rings broken into irregular plates	None	Patent air passages into each lobe
Sparse	Small, irregular hyaline cartilage islets	None	Patent air passageways into each bronchiopulmonary segment
None except occasional goblet cells	None	None	Control diameter of airways by contraction of smooth muscle
None	None	None	Same as above
None	None	Numerous alveoli as outpocketings of walls	Exchange of O_2 and CO_2
None	None	Wall lined with alveoli	Same as above
None	None	Entire wall consists of alveoli	Same as above
None	None	Not applicable	Actual site of a gaseous exchange

Table 16.2   *CHANGES[a] IN WALL OF AIR PASSAGEWAYS*

	HYALINE CARTILAGE	SMOOTH MUSCLE	GLANDS	ELASTIC FIBERS	EPITHELIUM	GOBLET CELLS	ALVEOLI
Trachea	+ + + +	+	+ + +	+ +	Pseudostratified columnar ciliated (respiratory)	+ + +	0
Primary bronchi (to each lung)	+ + +	+	+ + +	+	Same	+ + +	0
Secondary bronchi (to each lobe)	+ +	+ +	+ +	+ +	Same	+ +	0
Tertiary bronchi (to each segment)	+	+ + +	+	+ +	Same	+	0
Large bronchioles (to each secondary lobule)	0	+ + + +	±	+ + +	Same	±	0
Terminal bronchioles	0	+ +	0	+ + +	Simple columnar ciliated	0	0
Respiratory bronchioles (to each primary lobule)	0	+	0	+ + +	Simple cuboidal, some ciliated	0	Few
Alveolar ducts	0	±	0	+ + +	Simple cuboidal	0	Many
Alveolar sacs	0	0	0	+ + +	Low cuboidal or squamous	0	Many
Alveoli	0	0	0	+ + +	Very thin simple squamous	0	300–400 million in each lung

[a] Relative amounts: + + + +, large; + + +, moderate; + +, small; +, trace.

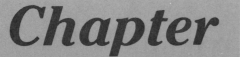

Chapter

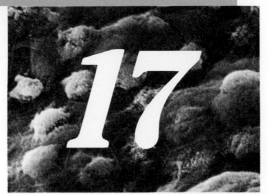

17

DIGESTIVE SYSTEM I— ORAL CAVITY AND PHARYNX

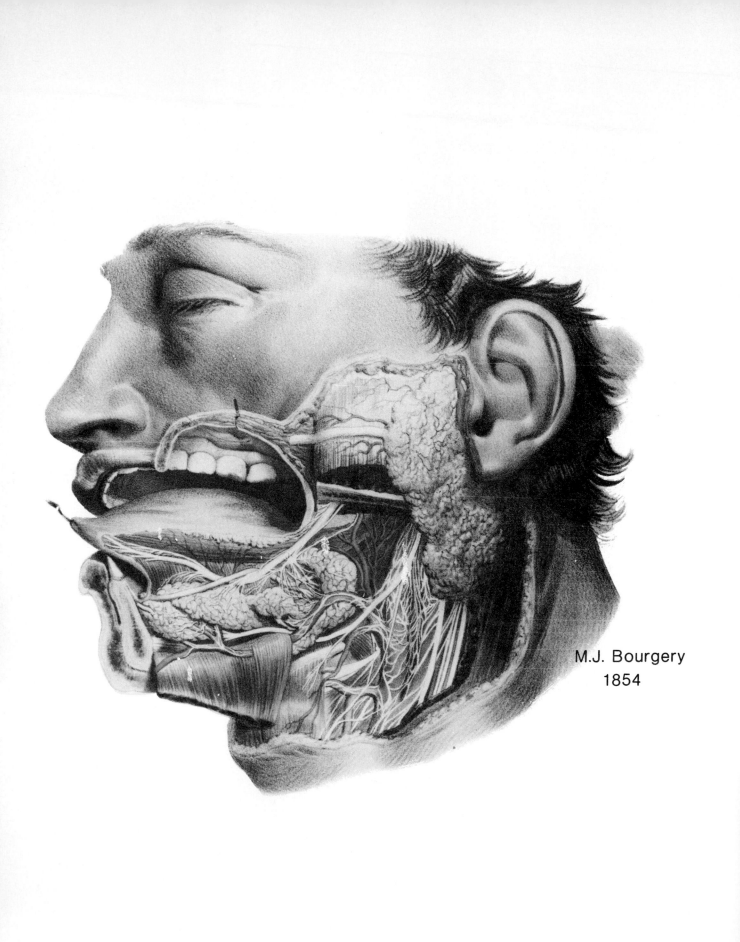

M.J. Bourgery
1854

OBJECTIVES

FROM INFORMATION IN THIS CHAPTER, ONE CAN PERCEIVE HOW THE STRUCTURES OF THE ORAL CAVITY AND PHARYNX ARE INVOLVED IN VARIOUS FUNCTIONS, SUCH AS:

1. The ingestion of food by the mouth and its related structures, e.g., lips, teeth, tongue, cheeks, and palate.

2. The mastication of food, which involves fragmenting and grinding of food, and how the teeth are adapted to perform these actions.

3. The partial digestion of food by enzymes synthesized in salivary glands that empty into the oral cavity.

4. Most pleasure of eating is derived from the sense of taste, mediated by taste buds located largely on the dorsal surface of the tongue.

5. The complex act of swallowing is partially controlled by the muscles of the pharynx.

The primitive yet self-sufficient amoeba takes care of all of its digestive, absorptive, and eliminative processes by a single food vacuole. In humans, all of these complex activities are the province of the **digestive system**. The entrance to the system is the **oral cavity** with its associated structures and glands. They are involved in the ingestion, mastication, partial digestion, and lubrication of food to form a moistened ball, called a **bolus**. In the act of swallowing, this food mass is forcefully thrust backwards by the tongue into the **pharynx**, the first segment of the long journey through 7–10 m of a hollow, muscular tube, the **alimentary** or **digestive tract.**

With the addition of **digestive enzymes** by the oral cavity, stomach, small intestine, gallbladder, liver, and pancreas, the actual digestion of the food occurs. This process converts food materials into a **soluble form** that can be readily **absorbed** largely by the **small intestine** for the eventual nutrition of every cell in the body. The elimination of the insoluble residue and other contents of the **large intestine** is controlled by **anal sphincters,** normally under voluntary control in the adult. At the anus and mouth the mucosa is continuous with the epidermis of the skin.

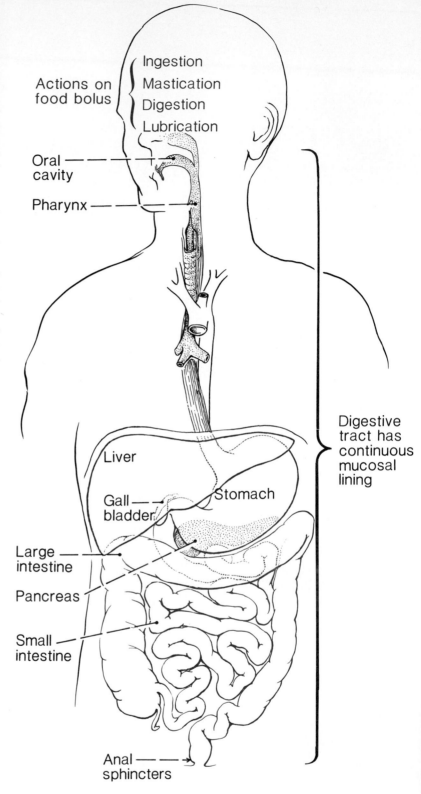

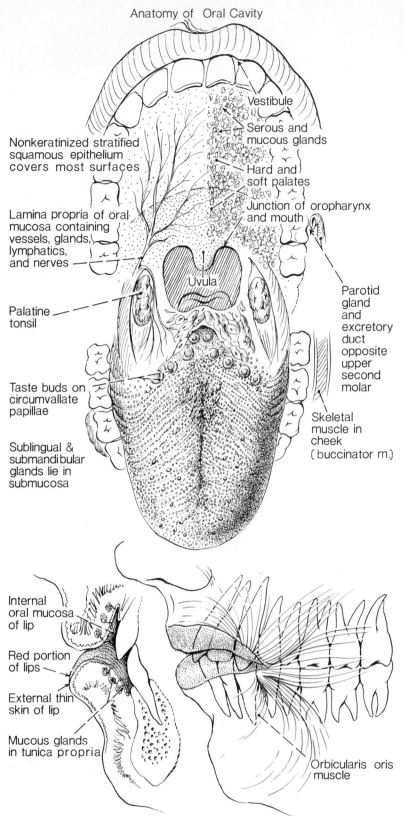

Anatomy of Oral Cavity

Nonkeratinized stratified squamous epithelium covers most surfaces

Lamina propria of oral mucosa containing vessels, glands, lymphatics, and nerves

Palatine tonsil

Taste buds on circumvallate papillae

Sublingual & submandibular glands lie in submucosa

Vestibule

Serous and mucous glands

Hard and soft palates

Junction of oropharynx and mouth

Uvula

Parotid gland and excretory duct opposite upper second molar

Skeletal muscle in cheek (buccinator m.)

Internal oral mucosa of lip

Red portion of lips

External thin skin of lip

Mucous glands in tunica propria

Orbicularis oris muscle

ORAL CAVITY

The entrance to the alimentary canal is the mouth, leading into the **oral or buccal cavity.** The cavity is divided into a **vestibule,** the space between the lips, cheeks and teeth, and the mouth cavity proper. Lying in the floor of the mouth is the large, muscular **tongue** that essentially fills the closed oral cavity. The **palatine tonsils** are located posteriorly at each side of the junction of the **oropharynx** and **mouth.** The hard and soft **palates** form the roof of the oral cavity.

Oral Mucous Membrane

The term "mucous membrane" does not necessarily presuppose that the membrane secretes mucus. In fact, the **oral mucous membrane** per se does not secrete mucus but is **kept moist** by the secretions of serous and mucous glands (**minor salivary glands**) that continuously pour their products over the oral surfaces.

Except the teeth, all structures that project into or line the oral cavity are covered by **stratified squamous epithelium,** usually nonkeratinized. The epithelium, together with the underlying **lamina propria** of loose areolar connective tissue, comprise the oral mucous membrane or **oral mucosa.** Within the lamina propria are blood vessels, small glands, lymphatics, and nerves. **Lymphocytes** also aggregate here to furnish a **line of defense** against foreign antigens that invade the body through the mouth.

The mucosa is a very sensitive membrane endowed with many **sensory endings.** That portion covering the dorsum of the tongue also contains **taste buds,** the specific end organs for the reception of taste sensations. The oral mucosa has a firm attachment to underlying structures, e.g., **skeletal muscle** as in the lips and cheek; to dense fibrous connective tissue, as in the floor of the mouth; and to bone and teeth. Large salivary glands, e.g., **sublingual and submandibular,** lying in the **submucosa,** send their excretory ducts to empty onto the oral mucosal surface. The paired **parotid glands,** the largest of the salivary glands, although located outside the oral cavity, discharge their secretions into the mouth through two large ducts that open opposite the upper second molar teeth.

Lips and Cheeks

Histologically, **lips and cheeks** are quite similar. Both are covered by thin skin externally and lined with oral mucosa internally. Between these layers, the bulk of the tissue is **skeletal muscle,** i.e., orbicularis oris muscle in the lips and buccinator muscle in the cheek. Small, predominantly **mucous glands** (labial in lips, buccal in cheeks) are embedded in the tunica propria whose secretions **keep the mucosal surface moist.** It is the attachment of the mucosa to the underlying **skeletal muscles** that provides for the wide range of movements to the lips and cheeks.

The outer margins of the lips are clearly defined by an abrupt change of the pale, rough skin, to the smooth red surface of the lips. The epithelium of the **labial surface is very translucent**, allowing the underlying profuse capillary beds to impart the red color to the lips. This transitional zone between the skin and the mucosa is called the **vermilion border.** It is present only in humans. Since this exposed area is **free of sweat and sebaceous glands** and is only lightly keratinized, it must be kept moist by the tongue to avoid drying and chapping of the lips.

Hard and Soft Palates

The roof of the mouth is a vaulted dome formed by the **hard and soft palates.** The **hard palate** is composed of horizontal bony processes covered by **oral mucosa,** which is continuous with the gingiva of the upper jaw. The mucosa is firmly attached to the adjacent periosteum and is therefore immovable. The stratified squamous epithelium is minimally keratinized. Numerous **mucous palatine glands** are situated in the tunica propria along the posterolateral areas of the palate. Irregular, transverse ridges (**rugae**) characterize its anterior region. These corrugations furnish a friction surface that aids in mastication.

The **soft palate,** the posterior fleshy extension of the hard palate, is formed by a layer of **skeletal muscle,** dense connective tissue, and **mucous glands** sandwiched between two mucous membranes. The mucous membrane on the **oral surface** has nonkeratinized, **stratified squamous** epithelium while the **nasal side** is covered by **respiratory epithelium.** In the submucosa of the oral surface are small mucous glands surrounded by many elastic fibers.

The soft palate is **highly vascular** and therefore has a reddish color in contrast to the pale pink color of the hard palate. **Skeletal muscles** occupy a large share of the tissue core between the mucous membranes. These are the small palatoglossus and palatopharyngeus muscles that extend along the lateral aspects to insert into the **uvula** (L. uva, a bunch of grapes), a small, pendulous, conical structure suspended inferiorly from the midpoint of the soft palate.

Functionally the hard and soft palates serve as a **partition between the oral and nasal cavities.** The rigid, **hard palate** provides a firm, unyielding working surface for the tongue as it mixes, crushes and **aids in swallowing** food. In contrast, the freely movable **soft palate** is drawn upward to close the nasopharynx during swallowing. This act **prevents food and drink** from entering the nasopharynx and the nasal cavities. Similarly, the nasopharynx is closed during sneezing.

In the congenital anomaly of **cleft palate,** an opening exists between the nasal and oral cavities that allows food and air to pass into the nasal cavities. If untreated, such children develop a

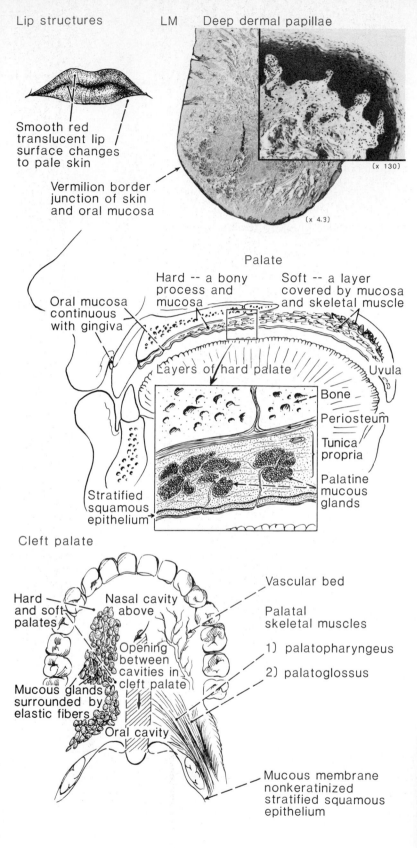

Lip structures

LM   Deep dermal papillae

Smooth red translucent lip surface changes to pale skin

Vermilion border junction of skin and oral mucosa

(x 130)

(x 4.3)

Palate

Hard -- a bony process and mucosa

Soft -- a layer covered by mucosa and skeletal muscle

Oral mucosa continuous with gingiva

Layers of hard palate

Uvula

Bone

Periosteum

Tunica propria

Palatine mucous glands

Stratified squamous epithelium

Cleft palate

Hard and soft palates

Nasal cavity above

Opening between cavities in cleft palate

Mucous glands surrounded by elastic fibers

Oral cavity

Vascular bed

Palatal skeletal muscles

1) palatopharyngeus

2) palatoglossus

Mucous membrane nonkeratinized stratified squamous epithelium

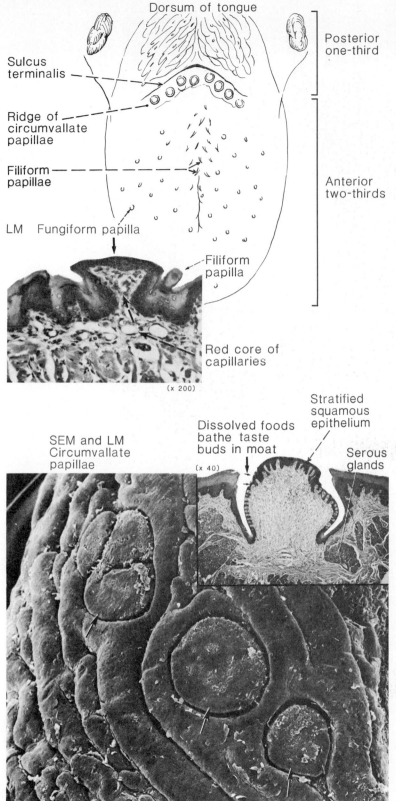

Dorsum of tongue

Sulcus
terminalis

Posterior
one-third

Ridge of
circumvallate
papillae

Filiform
papillae

Anterior
two-thirds

LM   Fungiform papilla

Filiform
papilla

Red core of
capillaries

(x 200)

SEM and LM
Circumvallate
papillae

Dissolved foods
bathe taste
buds in moat

(x 40)

Stratified
squamous
epithelium

Serous
glands

J.L. Boshell (x 72)

marked speech impediment with a pronounced nasal intonation. The condition can be corrected by early surgery before speech patterns have been established.

Tongue

The tongue is a mobile mass of muscle and mucous membrane that functions in **taste, chewing, swallowing,** and **speech.** For descriptive purposes, the tongue is divided into an anterior two thirds and a posterior one third. The demarcation between these regions is a V-shaped groove at the back of the tongue, called the **sulcus terminalis.**

PAPILLAE The anterior two thirds or **dorsum** of the tongue is covered by **stratified squamous epithelium.** Its roughened surface is caused by numerous minute projections, the **papillae,** that vary in shape and number. By far the most numerous are the small, slender, conical, pointed, **filiform** papillae (1–2 mm long). They are arranged in rows roughly parallel to the sulcus terminalis. They are the **plush** of the tongue which, under certain abnormal health conditions, becomes coated. These papillae cover the **entire dorsal surface** and are often slightly keratinized in humans but in many lower animals they are highly keratinized.

The larger but less numerous mushroom-shaped **fungiform papillae** (about 1.8 mm tall, 1 mm wide) are scattered among the filiform papillae. Because the upper, **flattened domes** are less keratinized, the **abundant capillary bed** shines through the thin epithelial surface revealing a red core. Occasionally a few taste buds may be found on fungiform papillae.

The very large (1–3 mm wide, 1–2 mm tall) circular, dome-shaped, **circumvallate** (L., to surround with a wall) papillae (9–12 in number) converge to **form a wide V** at the sulcus terminalis, with the apex of the V directed posteriorly. They resemble fungiform papillae except that they are much larger and have a deep, **circular trench** or moat surrounding their bases. It may contain dissolved food which bathes the **taste buds** that line the lateral sides of the papillae. Covering the dome of a papilla are small, **secondary papillae** formed by connective tissue cores covered by stratified squamous epithelium. Despite the large size of the vallate papillae, they do not project above the level of the epithelium of the tongue.

Leading into the trenches at the base of each papilla are ducts from **serous (von Ebner) glands** embedded in the submucosa and the underlying skeletal muscle bundles. These secretions effectively **irrigate the moats** and keep them relatively free of food and cellular debris. Just above the floor of the crypts, **ciliated cells** have been described near the bases of the circumvallate papillae.

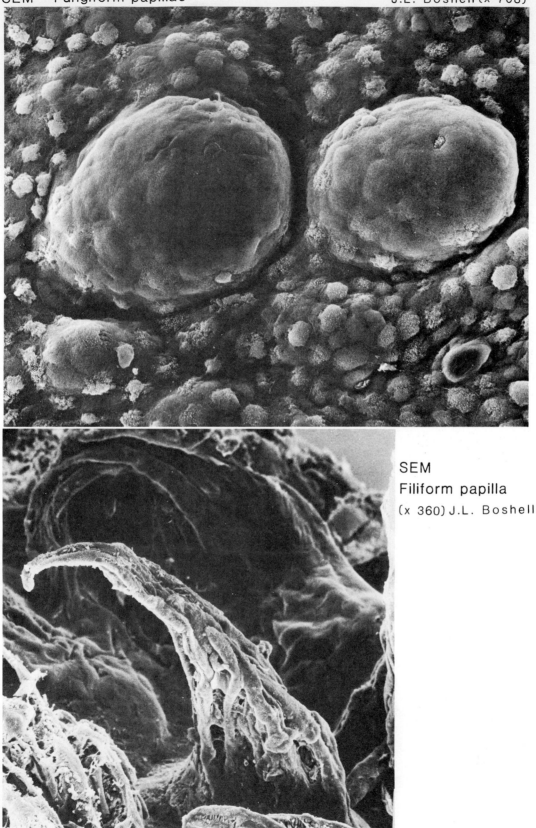

SEM
Filiform papilla
(x 360) J.L. Boshell

The very numerous, conical filiform papillae are distributed in rows across the tongue. They range from 2 to 3 mm in length. Typically in man, the tip is covered with nonkeratinized desquamating, flat cells that give the papilla its scaly appearance. The taller, but less numerous, mushroom-shaped, fungiform papillae are interspersed among the filiform papillae. They are attached to the dorsal surface of the tongue by a short stalk.

436

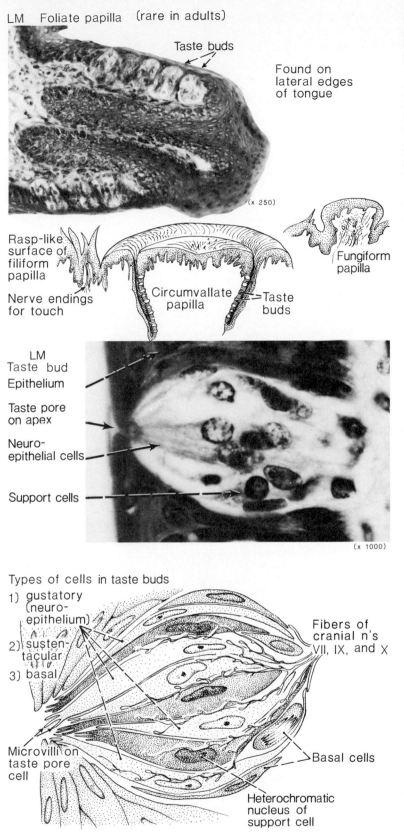

LM Foliate papilla (rare in adults)

Taste buds

Found on
lateral edges
of tongue

(x 250)

Rasp-like
surface of
filiform
papilla

Fungiform
papilla

Nerve endings
for touch

Circumvallate
papilla

Taste
buds

LM
Taste bud
Epithelium

Taste pore
on apex

Neuro-
epithelial cells

Support cells

(x 1000)

Types of cells in taste buds
1) gustatory
(neuro-
epithelium)

2) susten-
tacular

3) basal

Fibers of
cranial n's
VII, IX, and X

Microvilli on
taste pore
cell

Basal cells

Heterochromatic
nucleus of
support cell

The constant beating of the **cilia creates a microcirculation** of serous secretions and dissolved food components that wash over the taste buds in a constant renewal of various gustatory stimuli.

A fourth type, the **foliate** papillae, although present in young children, are **rudimentary** and rare in the adult human. However, they are extensive in some animals, such as the rabbit. As their name suggests, they have **leaflike, mucosal folds** or furrows. They are found on the **posterior lateral edges** of the dorsum of the tongue. Their furrows are also kept clean of debris by washings of the adjacent glands whose ducts empty into their folds. In animals, taste buds commonly line these folds.

No papillae are present on the posterior third of the tongue. However, mucosal folds and the lingual tonsil are present, discussed on page 271.

The function of the **filiform** papillae is to provide a roughened, **rasplike surface** capable of removing, by the licking action of the tongue, layers of semisolid foodstuffs. These papillae create the sandpaper-like surface of the tongue that aids in holding food on the tongue as the food is shifted from one side of the mouth to the other in the act of chewing. These papillae also contain nerve endings for **touch.** The **fungiform** papillae have a few **taste buds,** while the **circumvallate** papillae may have **200 or more taste buds** on their lateral walls.

TASTE BUDS The sensation of taste is detected by the **oval taste buds** (about 70 μm long) that resemble flower buds. At the apex of the bud is a small **taste pore** that connects the interior of the bud with the oral cavity. Through this opening, different taste modalities in solution are brought in contact with neuroepithelial cells. These cells and their supportive cells both are elongated, curved, tapering cells resembling the petals of a flower.

There are three cell types in a taste bud: (1) **taste** or gustatory cells (neuroepithelium), (2) **support** or sustenacular cells, and (3) **basal** cells (primitive stem cells). The taste and support cells resemble each other. They are long, spindle-shaped cells with their pointed distal ends covered by **long microvilli (taste hairs)** that cluster in the fluid-filled space beneath the pore. However, the **sensory cells** are **lighter staining** with oval, euchromatic nuclei, often with a dark, **distinct nucleolus.** The **support cells** are **darker staining** and have heterochromatic nuclei. Chemicals in solution diffuse through the pore to contact the plasma membranes of the microvilli. These **chemical stimuli,** received by the sensory cells, are **transduced into electrical impulses** that are transmitted to synapses formed by afferent nerve fibers at the bases of the sensory cells. (Note that these neuroepithelial cells **lack axons** and are therefore not neurons in the strictest

408

sense.) These afferent fibers of the VIIth, IXth, and Xth cranial nerves functionally replace the missing axons of the sensory cells.

The various cells of the taste bud are replaced at different rates. This renewal capacity suggests that the neuroepithelial cells are more epithelial than neural in their regenerative potential. The **life-span** of the sensory cells is short, only **about 10 days.** Therefore a continual exchange of cells is occurring, another striking deviation from typical neurons that cannot regenerate. The lost cells are replaced by new sensory cells derived from the **basal cells.** Obviously, the **synapses** between the degenerating sensory cells and the afferent nerve fibers are **disrupted** during this changeover period. Nonetheless, new **synapses are reestablished** and taste stimuli continue to flow to the brain for assessment.

There are four basic taste sensations that the taste buds respond to, i.e., **bitter, sour, sweet,** and **salty.** All taste buds do not respond the same to various taste flavors. For example, placing a drop of various flavors on different **fungiform papillae** reveals that some papillae can **detect one or two tastes** yet they are **insensitive to others.** Also, **taste buds in certain areas** of the tongue are very **responsive to a single taste** quality and unresponsive to others. Areas of the tongue have been mapped to show maximum sensitivity to various tastes. These regions of the tongue are: the **tip**— **sweet and salty;** the **sides**—**sour;** and the **base,** near the circumvallate papillae—**bitter.** Thus, functionally, taste buds differ, but morphologically they are similar.

In addition to the fungiform and vallate papillae, taste buds are also found in limited numbers on the palate, epiglottis, wall of the pharynx, posterior one third of the tongue, and the glossopalatine arches. The **regional differences** of flavor responsiveness are **clinically important.** For example, if a patient cannot taste a bitter flavor yet can taste salty, sweet, and sour, this indicates that the glossopharyngeal (**IXth cranial) nerve,** supplying the posterior back of the tongue, **is damaged.** However, the facial (VIIth cranial) nerve, supplying the anterior two thirds of the tongue, is intact and functional. Conversely, if the patient can identify **only bitter flavor,** then the **VIIth nerve is inoperative** but the IXth nerve is intact.

MUSCLES OF THE TONGUE All of the muscles of the tongue are **skeletal.** Some muscle fibers are unusual in that they **branch** as they extend forward toward the tip of the tongue. This is perhaps the only place in the body where branching of skeletal muscles occurs. There are **three intrinsic muscles** that make up the bulk of the tongue. They are named according to the direction of their fibers, i.e., **longitudinal, vertical,** and **transverse.** Histologically, these muscles are interwoven so that they reveal, in any histological section, muscle fibers in every conceivable plane of section.

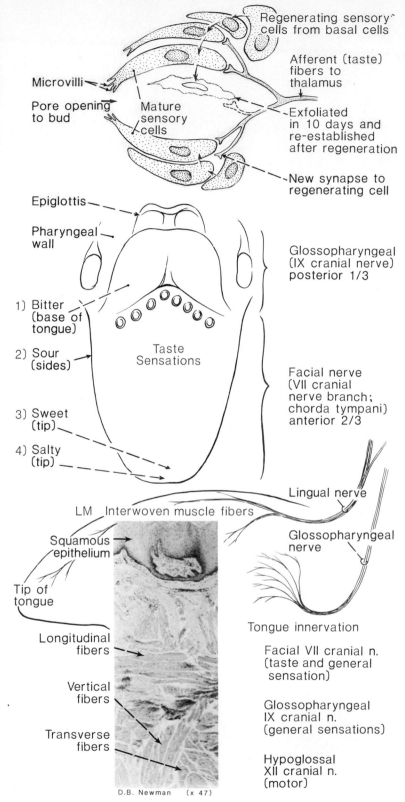

Regeneration of neuroepithelial cells of taste bud

Regenerating sensory cells from basal cells

Microvilli

Afferent (taste) fibers to thalamus

Pore opening to bud — Mature sensory cells

Exfoliated in 10 days and re-established after regeneration

New synapse to regenerating cell

Epiglottis

Pharyngeal wall

Glossopharyngeal (IX cranial nerve) posterior 1/3

1) Bitter (base of tongue)

2) Sour (sides)

Taste Sensations

Facial nerve (VII cranial nerve branch; chorda tympani) anterior 2/3

3) Sweet (tip)

4) Salty (tip)

Lingual nerve

Glossopharyngeal nerve

LM Interwoven muscle fibers

Squamous epithelium

Tip of tongue

Longitudinal fibers

Vertical fibers

Transverse fibers

Tongue innervation

Facial VII cranial n. (taste and general sensation)

Glossopharyngeal IX cranial n. (general sensations)

Hypoglossal XII cranial n. (motor)

D.B. Newman   (x 47)

OBJECTIVES

TO BE ABLE TO:

1. Conceptualize, in an illustration, the general structural plan common to all segments of the GI tract.

2. Describe the four basic layers of the alimentary canal and cite the principal functions of each layer.

3. Compare the functions and structure of: small vs. large intestine, duodenum vs. ileum, esophagus vs. stomach, and colon vs. rectum.

4. Identify the specific cells and their organelles in the mucosa of the small intestine, which enable it to digest and then absorb nutrients.

5. Rationalize in a written statement why the secretions of enteroendocrine cells, and certain other APUD cells, are essential for the normal function of the digestive tract.

GENERAL STRUCTURAL PLAN

Although each region of the digestive (alimentary) tract has specific functions, there is a general structural plan common to all segments. An understanding of the plan will greatly aid in an appreciation of the variations of this central theme that reveal the distinctive features of each organ of the digestive tract.

From the pharynx to the anus, the digestive tract consists of **four layers or tunics.** From within outwards they are the mucosa, submucosa, muscularis externa, and serosa or adventitia.

Mucosa

The tunica mucosa (**mucous membrane**) usually has three components: (1) **epithelium,** including a basal lamina; (2) **lamina propria;** and (3) **muscularis mucosae.** The **epithelium** is **stratified squamous** in the oropharynx, esophagus, and anus; and **simple columnar** throughout the remainder of the tract. All cells rest on a **basal**

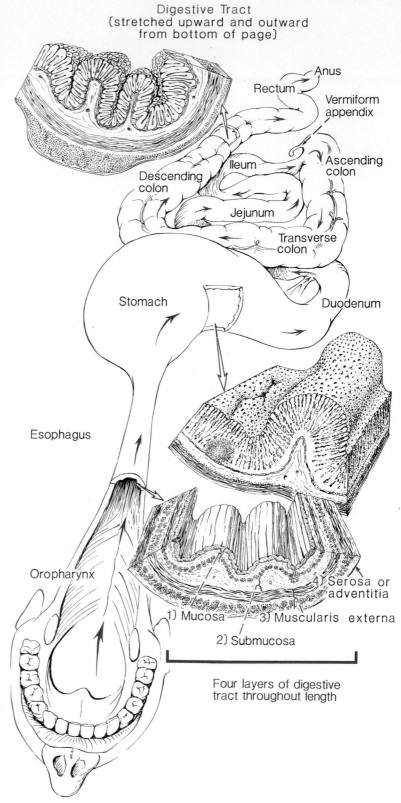

Digestive Tract
(stretched upward and outward
from bottom of page)

Anus

Rectum

Vermiform
appendix

Ileum

Ascending
colon

Descending
colon

Jejunum

Transverse
colon

Stomach

Duodenum

Esophagus

Oropharynx

4) Serosa or
adventitia

1) Mucosa   3) Muscularis externa

2) Submucosa

Four layers of digestive
tract throughout length

Digestive Tract Layers

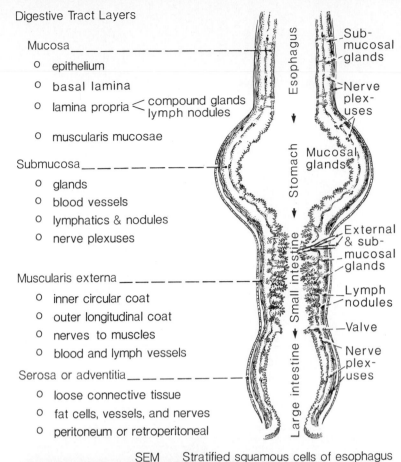

Mucosa_____

o epithelium

o basal lamina

o lamina propria < compound glands / lymph nodules

o muscularis mucosae

Submucosa_____

o glands

o blood vessels

o lymphatics & nodules

o nerve plexuses

Muscularis externa_____

o inner circular coat

o outer longitudinal coat

o nerves to muscles

o blood and lymph vessels

Serosa or adventitia_____

o loose connective tissue

o fat cells, vessels, and nerves

o peritoneum or retroperitoneal

(Diagram labels: Esophagus, Sub-mucosal glands, Nerve plexuses, Stomach, Mucosal glands, External & sub-mucosal glands, Lymph nodules, Valve, Nerve plexuses, Small intestine, Large intestine)

SEM   Stratified squamous cells of esophagus

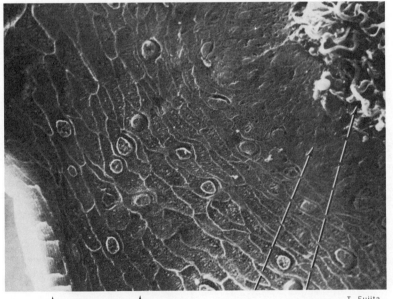

Desquamating cells | Stratified squamous epithelial cells | Basal layer | Lamina propria containing blood vessels

T. Fujita (x 1780)

723

---

lamina of variable thickness and stainability. Immediately beneath it is the **lamina propria,** an area of loose connective tissue with abundant reticular fibers and many lymphocytes. Discrete **compound glands and lymph nodules** are found in the lamina propria of certain regions of the GI tract. For example, **lymph nodules** are prominent in the **ileum** and **colon,** while **glands** are found in the **esophagus** and **stomach. The muscularis mucosae** is a thin, longitudinal or circular **sheet of smooth muscle** that separates the lamina propria from the underlying submucosa.

Submucosa

The submucosa is usually a rather **expansive,** fibroelastic, **connective tissue zone** containing glands, blood vessels, lymphatics, and nerves. Especially noteworthy is a plexus of unmyelinated, autonomic nerves, **Meissner's submucosal plexus. Compound glands (of Brunner)** are prominent in the **duodenum,** as well as deep glands in the esophagus. **Lymph nodules** are occasionally present in the upper regions, but are prominent in the lower segments.

Muscularis Externa

In most of the GI tract, the **muscularis externa** consists of two prominent layers of smooth muscle. The **inner layer is circular, the outer longitudinal.** The inner circular coat is modified in certain regions to form **sphincters and valves.** Between the layers of muscle is located a nerve plexus of autonomic nerve fibers and parasympathetic ganglion cells called **Auerbach's myenteric plexus,** which innervates the muscles.

Serosa or Adventitia

The outermost layer is the **serosa or adventitia.** It consists of **loose connective tissue,** largely of collagenous and elastic fibers, **fat cells, vessels, and nerves.** If the organ lies within the abdominal cavity, suspended by a mesentery and **covered by peritoneum (mesothelium),** the layer is called the **serosa.** If the organ is outside the abdominal cavity (retroperitoneal), it has **no mesentery or mesothelial covering** and its outer coat is termed the **adventitia.**

ESOPHAGUS

The first segment of the alimentary canal is the **esophagus.** In the human adult, it is a muscular tube about 20–25 cm long that acts solely to transport food and drink from the pharynx to the stomach by rapid peristaltic activity. Except during the passage of food, its lumen is nearly closed by **longitudinal folds** of the mucous membrane. Therefore in cross section the lumen appears collapsed or **star-shaped.** Excluding limited mucus, no secretions or enzymes are added to the food as it passes through the esophagus.

Mucosa

The mucosa has the typical structural pattern of the GI tract. The **epithelium is nonkeratinized stratified squamous** that ends abruptly at the stomach junction where it becomes simple columnar. The **lamina (tunica) propria** has a large population of **lymphocytes** and a few lymphoid nodules among the fine, interlacing connective tissue fibers. Small, branched, tubular mucous glands called **cardiac glands,** because they resemble the cardiac glands of the stomach, are found in two limited areas, i.e., the upper esophagus opposite the cricoid cartilage and near the cardiac region of the stomach. These glands are variable in size and may be absent.

The usually **well-developed muscularis mucosae** is an excellent landmark in the histological identification of the esophagus. Here it reaches its greatest development and is composed mostly of **longitudinal smooth muscle** fibers.

Submucosa

The submucosa is an extensive, rather loose collagenous and elastic **connective tissue zone.** Because of its great resiliency it **acts as a shock absorber** for the large, often rough, boluses of food that pass through the esophagus. During passage, these masses compress the mucosa causing it to bulge into the ample, pliable submucosa, thus greatly enlarging the diameter of the normally narrow lumen of the esophagus.

Compound tubuloacinar mucous glands are randomly distributed throughout the submucosa. These are the **esophageal glands** proper that empty their lubricating, mucoid secretions onto the epithelial surface and greatly facilitate the movement of food down the esophagus.

Muscularis Externa

The muscularis externa consists of prominent **inner circular** and **outer longitudinal** muscle layers. Since the **upper third** of the esophagus is involved in the voluntary act of swallowing, both muscle layers have **skeletal muscle fibers.** These fibers are progressively replaced inferiorly by smooth muscle so that, in the **lower third** of the esophagus, **only smooth muscle** is present. Both muscle types are present in the middle third.

Adventitia

The outermost tunic is the loose connective tissue **adventitia,** which attaches the esophagus to the other structures of the neck. Blood vessels and nerves course through the adventitia to supply the esophagus.

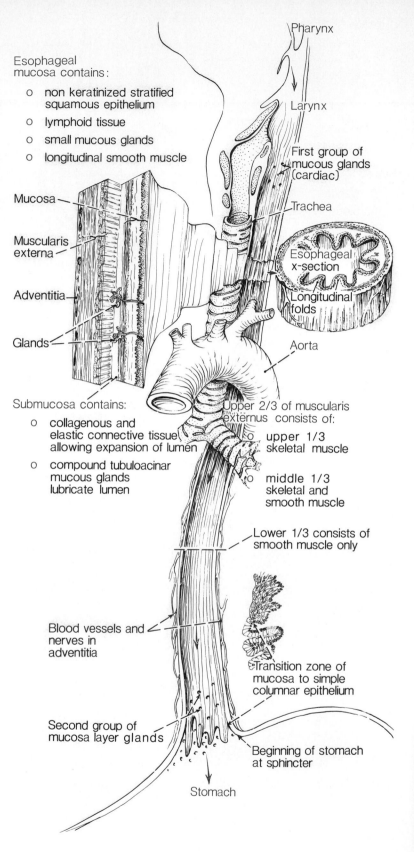

Esophageal mucosa contains:

- o non keratinized stratified squamous epithelium
- o lymphoid tissue
- o small mucous glands
- o longitudinal smooth muscle

Pharynx

Larynx

First group of mucous glands (cardiac)

Trachea

Mucosa

Muscularis externa

Adventitia

Glands

Esophageal x-section

Longitudinal folds

Aorta

Submucosa contains:

- o collagenous and elastic connective tissue allowing expansion of lumen
- o compound tubuloacinar mucous glands lubricate lumen

Upper 2/3 of muscularis externus consists of:

- o upper 1/3 skeletal muscle
- o middle 1/3 skeletal and smooth muscle

Lower 1/3 consists of smooth muscle only

Blood vessels and nerves in adventitia

Transition zone of mucosa to simple columnar epithelium

Second group of mucosa layer glands

Beginning of stomach at sphincter

Stomach

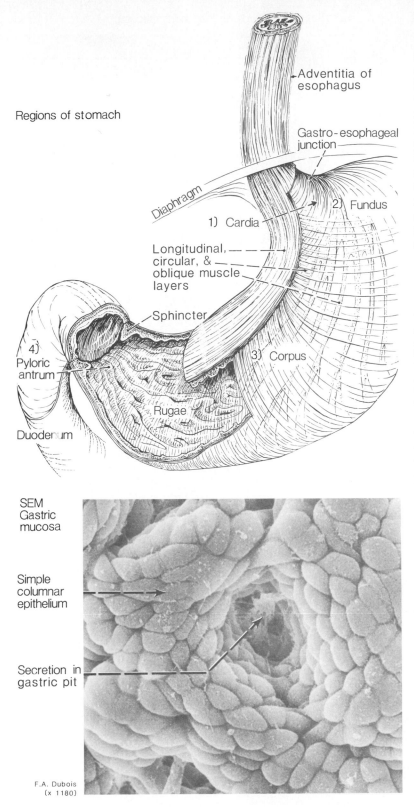

Regions of stomach

Adventitia of esophagus

Gastro-esophageal junction

Diaphragm

2) Fundus

1) Cardia

Longitudinal, circular, & oblique muscle layers

Sphincter

3) Corpus

4) Pyloric antrum

Rugae

Duodenum

SEM Gastric mucosa

Simple columnar epithelium

Secretion in gastric pit

F.A. Dubois
(x 1180)

STOMACH

The stomach is a fibromuscular bag for the mixing and partial digestion of food. Its kneading action provides that the ingested nutriments will be thoroughly mixed with the **gastric juices** which are heavily laced with digestive enzymes, mucin, hydrochloric acid, and water. While carbohydrate digestion is initiated in the oral cavity and continues in the small intestine, **protein breakdown and assimilation** begins in the **stomach** and continues in the intestine. Assimilation of **soluble nutrients** through the stomach walls into the bloodstream is limited to **simple amino acids** and **ethyl alcohol,** explaining why one feels, almost immediately, the effects of a strong alcoholic drink.

Regions

For descriptive purposes, the stomach is divided into four regions. (1) The **cardia** is a small, circumscribed zone near the gastroesophageal junction (so called because of its proximity to the heart). (2) The large, dome-shaped **fundus** projects superiorly above the level of the esophageal opening. (3) The **body or corpus** is about two thirds of the stomach, extending from the fundus inferiorly towards the pyloris. (4) The **pyloris** is the most inferior region. It is funnel shaped, with the expanded cone portion joining the body as the pyloric antrum. The stem of the funnel is the **pyloric canal,** which ends in the narrow **pyloric sphincter** at the junction with the duodenum (the first segment of the small intestine).

Histological Features

MUCOSA The mucous membrane (mucosa) of the stomach is thrown into deep, irregular, longitudinal folds called **rugae.** The **epithelium is simple columnar.** The surface cells are **mucus secreting cells** yet do not stain with some mucin dyes. The surface epithelium continues into small, deep depressions called **gastric pits or foveolae,** into which the **gastric glands** open and release their secretions. These glands comprise most of the mucous membrane. The epithelial cells differentiate into several cell types that line the gastric glands.

The **lamina propria** is largely occupied by the basal portions of gastric glands, which are surrounded by loose connective tissue and limited diffuse lymphoid tissue. The boundary between the lamina propria and the underlying submucosa is the **muscularis mucosae.** This rather delicate layer of smooth muscle is composed of longitudinally arranged fibers externally and circular fibers internally.

GASTRIC GLANDS A typical **gastric gland** is a **simple, tubular type** that may be **straight** or **coiled** depending on the region. The initial segment, **the neck**, is lined with modified surface cells called **mucous neck cells.** They are undistinguished morphologically yet functionally very important. Besides **secreting mucus,** they are the ancestral **stem cells** that give rise to probably all of the epithelial cells of the mucosa.

The intermediate gland segment is the **body,** the major **straight portion** of the gland. Here the epithelium in most of the stomach, i.e., fundus and body, is specialized into two different secretory cells: (1) the small, slightly basophilic **chief** or principal (peptic) cells that secrete **pepsinogen,** and (2) the large, eosinophilic **parietal** (oxyntic) cells that produce **hydrochloric acid.**

The rather bulbous, blind-ending terminal part of a gastric gland is the **base.** It is lined with the same cells that line the body of the gland.

SUBMUCOSA The rather extensive submucosa is composed of blood vessels and nerves (**Meissner's submucosal plexus**) freely laced with loosely arranged collagenous and elastic fibers.

MUSCULARIS EXTERNA The muscularis externa has three layers of smooth muscle: (1) an **inner oblique** layer, especially well-developed in the cardiac region; (2) a **middle circular layer;** and (3) an **outer longitudinal layer.** Auerbach's **myenteric nerve plexus** lies between the constant circular and the longitudinal muscle layers.

SEROSA The serosa, a covering of loose connective tissue surrounded by **mesothelium,** encloses the entire stomach.

Regional Differences (plate 18)

CARDIAC REGION The regions of the stomach are histologically quite different. In the small **cardiac region,** the glands are the **least numerous** since the cardia of the stomach is limited to a collar about 25 mm wide around the esophageal orifice. They have rather **wide, open, deep pits** that continue into **short,** slightly **coiled glands** lined with mucous-type cells. The glands occupy most of the lamina propria, and the bases of the glands rest on a thin muscularis mucosae.

FUNDIC AND BODY REGIONS In the body and fundus, the glands (collectively called **fundic glands**) are the **most numerous** since these regions occupy about three fourths of the stomach. Fundic glands have **narrow, shallow pits** that usually terminate by bifurcating into **two simple, straight, long tubules.** The **pits** are lined with

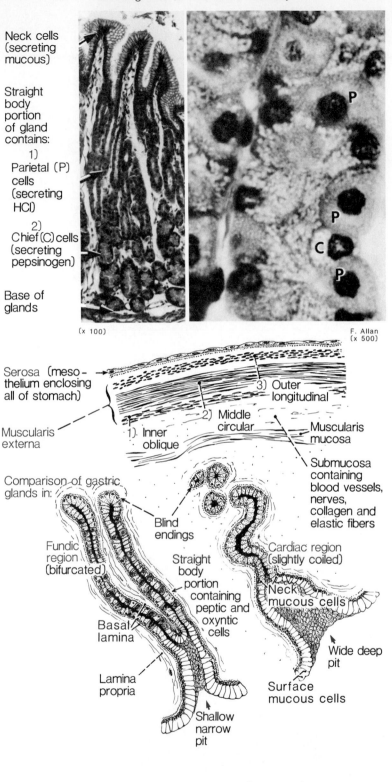

LM   Gastric glands (in the fundus mucosa)

Neck cells (secreting mucous)

Straight body portion of gland contains:
1) Parietal (P) cells (secreting HCl)
2) Chief (C) cells (secreting pepsinogen)

Base of glands

(x 100)

F. Allan (x 500)

Serosa (mesothelium enclosing all of stomach)

Muscularis externa

3) Outer longitudinal

2) Middle circular

1) Inner oblique

Middle circular

Muscularis mucosa

Submucosa containing blood vessels, nerves, collagen and elastic fibers

Comparison of gastric glands in:

Blind endings

Fundic region (bifurcated)

Basal lamina

Lamina propria

Straight body portion containing peptic and oxyntic cells

Cardiac region (slightly coiled)

Neck mucous cells

Wide deep pit

Surface mucous cells

Shallow narrow pit

Lumen of stomach

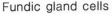

Fundic gland cells

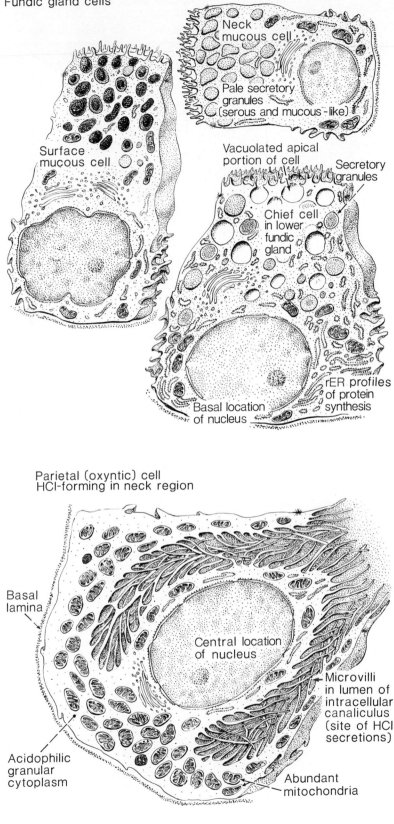

Neck mucous cell

Pale secretory granules (serous and mucous-like)

Surface mucous cell

Vacuolated apical portion of cell

Secretory granules

Chief cell in lower fundic gland

rER profiles of protein synthesis

Basal location of nucleus

Parietal (oxyntic) cell HCl-forming in neck region

Basal lamina

Central location of nucleus

Microvilli in lumen of intracellular canaliculus (site of HCl secretions)

Acidophilic granular cytoplasm

Abundant mitochondria

surface mucous-type cells. The small, irregular **neck mucous cells** have pale **secretory granules** that stain strongly with mucicarmine, distinguishing them from the stomach surface mucous cells. Mucous neck cells produce an atypical product that is somewhat intermediate between a serous and a mucous secretion, similar to the secretion of Brunner's glands of the duodenum.

The elongated **body** of a fundic gland is lined with parietal and chief cells, distinctive histological features of fundic glands. The **chief cells** are the **most numerous** hence their name, chief or principal. They are also called **zymogenic cells** because their granules contain an inactive enzyme (a zymogen) called **pepsinogen.** Chief cells are rather **cuboidal or pyramidal** in shape and are concentrated in the lower part of the fundic gland. The **apical portion** of the cell has a **vacuolated** appearance and is lightly stained because the secretory granules are poorly preserved in most common fixatives and have been largely dissolved. The **basal part** of the cell is **basophilic** due to the presence of a nucleus, abundant **ribosomes**, and extensive **rER** profiles, suggestive of active protein synthesis in the cell.

The distinctive **eosinophilic**, large, oval or polygonal **parietal cells** are most numerous in the neck region. They are intercalated between the mucous neck cells in the upper portions of the body of the gland. They are also called **oxyntic cells** because they are **acid (HCl) secreting cells.** The central nucleus is surrounded by finely granular cytoplasm that has a strong affinity for acid dyes.

Electron micrographs of parietal cells reveal a very unusual feature, i.e., unique, deep, **intracellular canaliculi.** This is a network of channels formed by the involution of the luminal surface of the cell. Such an infolding carries the **plasmalemma** of the apical surface of the cell deep into the cell proper, forming the intracellular canaliculi. Many **microvilli** project from the plasmalemma into the lumen of the canaliculus, partially occluding its lumen but greatly increasing the absorptive surface area of the cell membrane. Thus, these **invaginations** may be considered to be extensions of the lumen of the fundic gland, not a bona fide intracellular organelle.

The secretion of HCl, or its ions, probably occurs throughout these extensive intracellular **canaliculi.** Also involved in the process are the many mitochondria in the cytoplasm bordering the secretory canaliculi. There is substantial experimental evidence that the parietal cells in humans also secrete the gastric **intrinsic factor**, a glycoprotein that binds to vitamin B_{12}, facilitating the absorption of the vitamin in the small intestine. In **vitamin B_{12} deficiency**, there is a reduction in red cell production in the bone marrow, causing **pernicious anemia.**

Other cells occasionally found in the gastric glands are certain **enteroendocrine cells.** These are poorly visualized in LM studies unless they are impregnated by silver or chromate in special staining techniques. The older terms for these cells, i.e., argyrophil, argentaffin, and enterochromaffin reflect these staining reactions. When present, these cells are usually located in the bases of the fundic glands wedged between the chief cells. EM studies have identified several types of cells differing in their ultrastructure and function. One type (G) synthesizes and stores **gastrin,** a polypeptide hormone, that stimulates gastric motility, HCl production by parietal cells, and pepsinogen secretion by chief cells. Another cell type (EC) produces **serotonin,** a potent constrictor of smooth muscle. Another cell (EG) produces **enteroglucagon,** a hormone that increases blood sugar levels, the opposite action of insulin and the D cell releases the hormone **somatostatin,** which plays a local regulatory role with the EG and G cells.

PYLORIC REGION The pyloric region occupies about 20% of the stomach and is continuous with the duodenum. The **pyloric glands** resemble cardiac glands. Minor differences include deeper pits and more branching and coiling of the tubular glands. They may contain a few parietal cells and gastrin-secreting (G-cells) cells among the mucouslike cells that line the pyloric glands. (See Table 18.1 for a comparison of regions of the stomach).

SMALL INTESTINE

The small intestine extends from its junction with the stomach at the **pyloric sphincter** to its union with the large intestine at the **ileocecal valve,** a distance of about 6–8 m. Throughout the course, its typical four layers resemble the generalized pattern of the GI tract. Anatomically it is divided into **three regions.** A horseshoe-shaped **proximal loop, the duodenum,** is about 25–30 cm long. It does not have a mesentery but lies behind the peritoneum. Therefore a serosa covers only its anterior surface. An **adventitia** covers the other surfaces.

The middle segment is the **jejunum,** about 2.5–3 m long. It is surrounded by a **serosa** since it is suspended by a mesentery attached to the posterior body wall. Also suspended by mesentery and covered by **serosa** is the **distal ileum,** the longest segment, about 4–4.5 m long.

The small intestine has **two principal functions:** (1) to complete the **digestion of food** by the action of appropriate enzymes, and (2) to selectively **absorb** the finished products of digestion into the blood and lymph vessels. The small intestine also synthesizes and releases certain hormones.

EM   Enteroendocrine cells found in bases of fundic glands which synthesize:

1) gastrin   2) serotonin   3) enteroglucagon

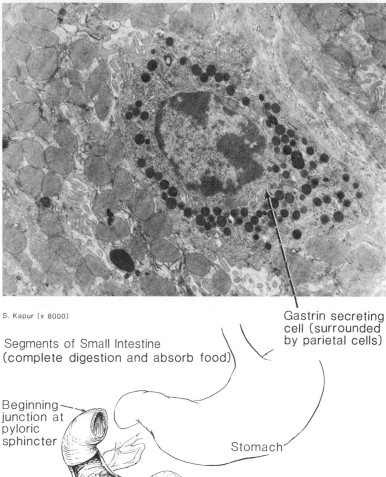

S. Kapur (x 8000)

Gastrin secreting cell (surrounded by parietal cells)

Segments of Small Intestine (complete digestion and absorb food)

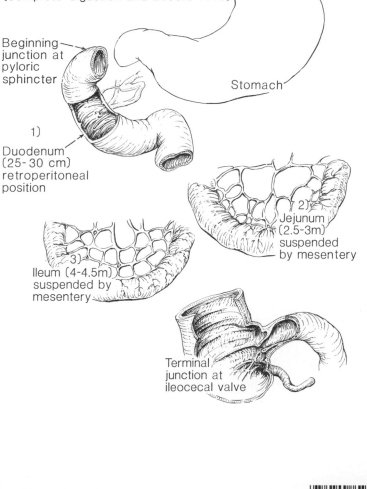

Beginning junction at pyloric sphincter

Stomach

1)
Duodenum (25-30 cm) retroperitoneal position

2) Jejunum (2.5-3m) suspended by mesentery

3) Ileum (4-4.5m) suspended by mesentery

Terminal junction at ileocecal valve

Villi of small intestine

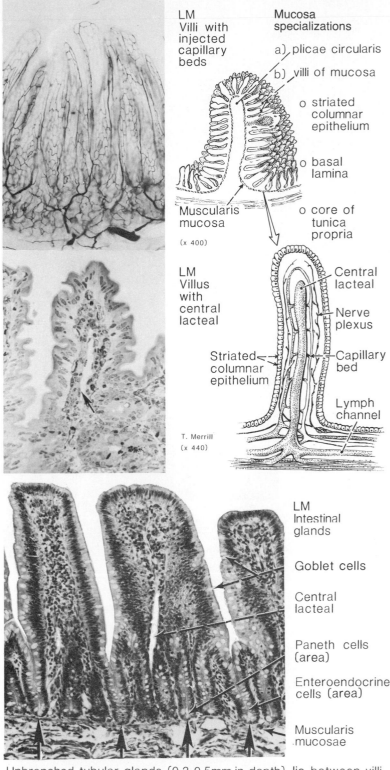

LM Villi with injected capillary beds (x 400)

Mucosa specializations

a) plicae circularis

b) villi of mucosa

o striated columnar epithelium

o basal lamina

Muscularis mucosa

o core of tunica propria

LM Villus with central lacteal

Central lacteal

Nerve plexus

Striated columnar epithelium

Capillary bed

Lymph channel

T. Merrill (x 440)

LM Intestinal glands

Goblet cells

Central lacteal

Paneth cells (area)

Enteroendocrine cells (area)

Muscularis mucosae

Unbranched tubular glands (0.3-0.5mm in depth) lie between villi

Common Histological Features

All regions of the small intestine have the typical layers of the gut, i.e., mucosa, submucosa, muscularis externa, and serosa or adventitia.

MUCOSA

Plicae Circularis The mucosal surface of the small bowel undergoes **several specializations** designed to **increase its surface area,** thereby enhancing its absorptive potential. The first of these modifications are permanent, spiral or circular mucosal folds that extend throughout most of the length of the organ, called the **plicae circularis** or the valves of Kerckring. They have a **central core of submucosa.** These structures are not true valves that effect a complete closure, as do valves of the heart or veins. These folds seldom extend completely around the gut lumen and therefore cannot occlude it. However, they greatly **increase the mucosal surface area.** They reach maximal development in the lower duodenum and upper jejunum and then gradually diminish to disappear in the lower ileum.

Villi Villi are long finger-, club-, or leaflike **projections of the mucosa** that extend into the gut lumen. They are about 0.5–1.5 mm long and are not found elsewhere in the gut. They are covered with **simple columnar epithelium** resting on a definite basement membrane (basal lamina). Interposed between the columnar absorptive epithelial cells are **goblet cells,** which become more numerous in the distal segments of the small intestine. Villi have a central core of **lamina propria,** not submucosa. The delicate reticular stroma of the lamina propria has, in addition to reticular fibers, a few fine elastic and collagenous fibers. Within it are many free cells, especially **lymphocytes,** and a scattering of neutrophils, plasma cells, and macrophages.

Immediately below the basement membrane is a **capillary network** supplied by arterioles and drained by venules. A single, large, blind-beginning lymphatic vessel, the **lacteal** (L. lacteus, milky) lies in the center of the villus. (After a fatty meal, the lymph in the lacteal has a milky appearance due to abundant fat droplets.) When dilated, its bulbous tip may occupy half the diameter of the villus. A fine nerve plexus ramifies among the blood vessels and the lacteal.

Intestinal Glands (Crypts of Lieberkuhn) Another mucosal modification that increases the surface area is the presence of myriad **intestinal glands (crypts of Lieberkuhn).** These are **straight, unbranched, tubular glands** about 0.3–0.5 mm in depth, located between the bases of the villi and extending as deep as the muscularis **mucosae.** The lamina propria of the villus extends downward to surround the glands.

The **surface epithelium** covering the villus extends into and lines the crypts. The **goblet cells** tend to be concentrated in the upper half of the gland. They may be replaced in the bases of the crypts by the large **Paneth cells** with deeply staining **eosinophilic granules**. These are zymogen granules, the precursors of the bacteriocidal enzyme, **lysozyme**, which may regulate the flora associated with the small intestinal mucosa. Also in the crypts are a few **enteroendocrine cells** that secrete intestinal hormones such as **secretin, cholecystokinin,** and others.

Microvilli The ultimate expander of the mucosal surface area is the **microvillus**. EM studies reveal that the **striated border** of the lining epithelial cells is composed of parallel rows of **microvilli** of even height. They extend from the cell border like brush bristles, hence the term **brush border** is a synonym for striated border. Each microvillus is covered by an extension of the **cell plasma membrane**. Extending beyond the microvillus is a nondescript, feltlike accumulation of fine filaments, described in Chapter 1 as the **fuzzy coat or glycocalyx**, which contains an acid mucopolysaccharide.

In the center of the microvillus are many longitudinally oriented, **fine microfilaments**, whose bases rest in the **terminal web** of the villus. Some of these microfilaments are **actin** filaments which, when contracted, may shorten and/or bend the microvilli, as discussed in Chapters 1 and 10.

Lamina Propria The loose reticular connective tissue of the **lamina propria forms the core of each villus** and fills the potential space between the intestinal glands. Collections of small lymphocytes form **solitary lymph nodules**, with or without germinal centers. Distally along the gut, the nodules increase in size and number until, in the **ileum**, they form **large aggregations** of 20 or more nodules called **Peyer's patches**.

Muscularis Mucosae The thin muscularis mucosae has two layers of smooth muscle, an **inner, circular** and an **outer, longitudinal** layer. These layers are penetrated by blood and lymph vessels, occasional ducts, and autonomic nerves from Meissner's plexus. Where lymph nodules extend between the mucosa and submucosa, the muscularis mucosae may be deficient.

SUBMUCOSA The **submucosa** is a rather large zone, composed of coarse areolar connective tissue surrounding larger blood and lymph vessels and nerve plexuses. The nerve plexuses are largely parasympathetic, i.e., **Meissner's plexus**. In addition to numerous adipose cells, the submucosa may contain lymph nodules, e.g., **Peyer's patches** in the lamina propria that are thrust, by growth pressure, through the muscularis mucosae into the submucosa. The submucosa contains no glands except **Brunner's glands** in the duodenum.

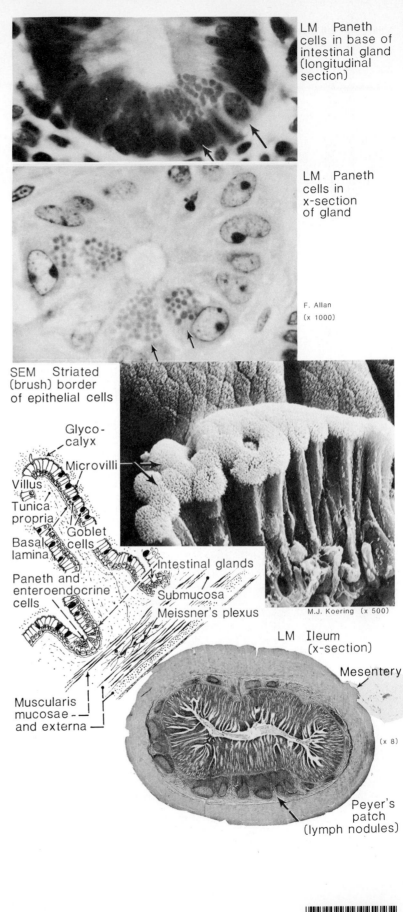

LM Paneth cells in base of intestinal gland (longitudinal section)

LM Paneth cells in x-section of gland

F. Allan (x 1000)

SEM Striated (brush) border of epithelial cells

Glycocalyx
Microvilli
Villus
Tunica propria
Basal lamina
Goblet cells
Paneth and enteroendocrine cells
Intestinal glands
Submucosa
Meissner's plexus
Muscularis mucosae and externa

M.J. Koering (x 500)

LM Ileum (x-section)

Mesentery

(x 8)

Peyer's patch (lymph nodules)

Epithelial cells in intestine

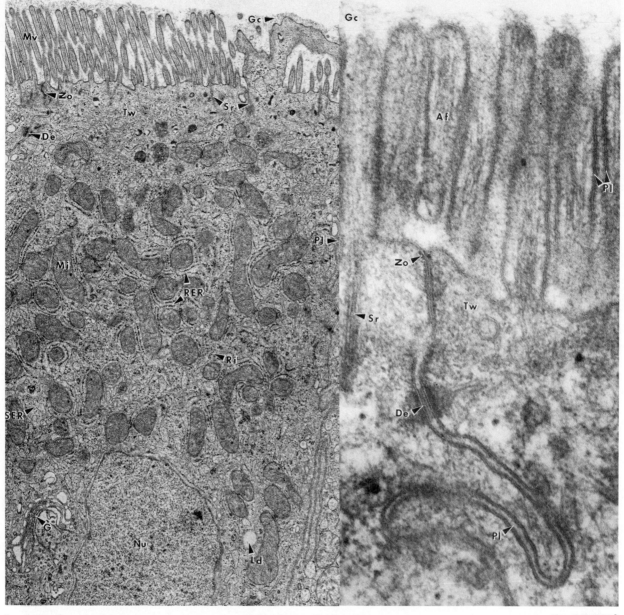

(x 5,600)

G.U. Anat. Collection

(x 97,000)

EM micrographs of a typical intestinal absorptive cell of the small intestine. Its luminal surface is composed of uniform, closely packed microvilli (Mv) embedded in the matlike surface coat, the glycocalyx (Gc). Each microvillus is anchored into the underlying terminal web (Tw) by bundles of actin filaments, called straight rootlets (Sr). Laterally the plasmalemmae of adjacent cells are united by junctional complexes, e.g., zonula occludens (Zo), zonula adherens, and desmosomes (De) (macula adherens). Clustered mostly in the supranuclear cytoplasm are cellular organelles and inclusions. They include a Golgi apparatus (G), smooth and rough endoplasmic reticulum (SER and RER), ribosomes (Ri), lipid droplet (Ld), and abundant mitochondria (Mi).

The EM micrograph on the right is a higher magnification of an absorptive intestinal cell. Shown in detail is the plasmalemma (Pl) enclosing each microvillus which is surrounded by the proteoglycan-rich glycocalyx. Actin filaments (Af) attach to the tips of the microvilli and exit the open bases of the microvilli to insert into the terminal web (Tw) as straight rootlets (Sr). Components of a junctional complex, joining contiguous cells, are seen in the center of the field.

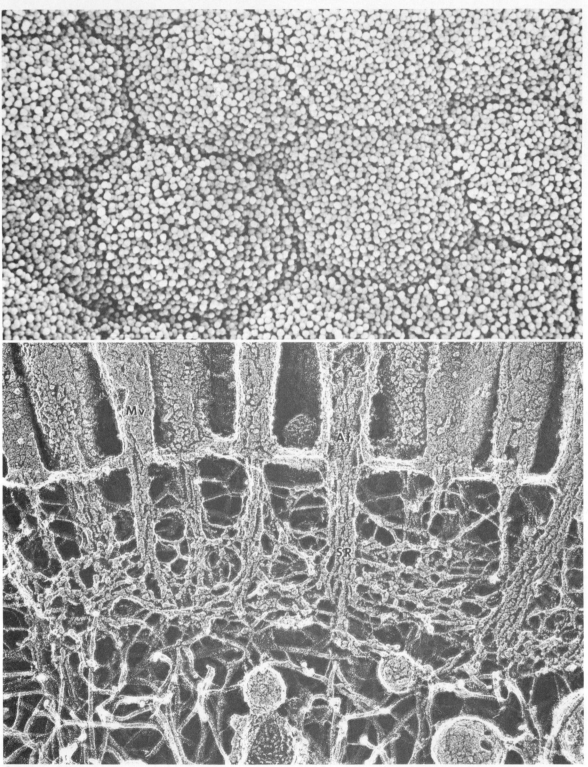

SEM   Microvilli and terminal web   N. Hirokawa (x 131,000)

The upper SEM micrograph reveals the tips of myriad closely packed microvilli that stud the luminal surface of intestinal absorptive cells. When seen in transverse TEM sections, the core of each microvillus displays 40–50 actin-containing microfilaments.

The lower SEM micrograph is a rapid-freeze, deep-etched replica of the cytoskeleton of the terminal web of the microvillus region of the mouse intestinal mucosa. Compact bundles of actin filaments (Af) project from the open bases of the microvilli (Mv) to form straight rootlets (SR) within the terminal web. The rootlets come to rest on a meshwork of thicker intermediate filaments (8 nm).

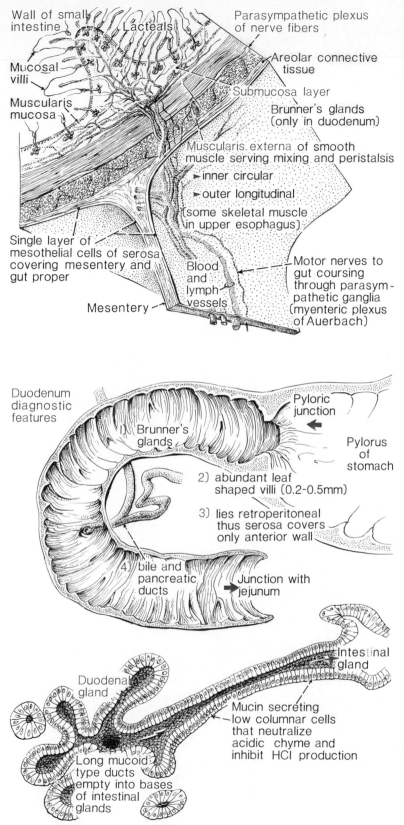

MUSCULARIS EXTERNA This large, consistent layer has an inner circular and an outer longitudinal band of smooth muscle. Nestled between the two layers are frequent parasympathetic ganglia, the **myenteric plexus (of Auerbach)**. It supplies motor innervation to the muscles of the gut that propel food along the GI tract by **peristalsis**. These muscles also provide a kneading and churning action to facilitate the mixing of food with digestive enzymes.

SEROSA Except for the retroperitoneal **duodenum**, which is covered largely by **adventitia**, all of the other regions of the small intestine are suspended by a mesentery and are therefore covered by a single layer of **mesothelial cells**, resting on a thin layer of loose connective tissue, collectively termed the **serosa**. Blood and lymph vessels and nerves traverse the serosa to serve the other layers.

Diagnostic Regional Differences

DUODENUM The name duodenum implies a structure equal in length to the breadth of 12 fingers, about 25 cm. It extends from the **pyloric end** of the stomach to its junction with the **jejunum**. It is characterized by: (1) prominent **Brunner's glands** in the submucosa, (2) abundant **leaf-shaped villi**, (3) an incomplete serosa replaced by an extensive **adventitia**, and (4) the terminations of the **bile** and **pancreatic ducts**.

The duodenal (Brunner's) glands are **mucous compound tubular**, or tubuloacinar glands restricted to the **submucosa**. Their mucin-secreting cells are low columnar type that stain weakly with H&E. The secretion is **strongly alkaline** (pH 8.8–9.3), which **neutralizes the acidic chyme** of the stomach and thus protects the duodenal mucosa from autodigestion. The epithelial cells lining the **long ducts** draining the glands are mucous secreting. The ducts penetrate the muscularis mucosae to empty into the bases of the intestinal glands. Seldom do they terminate between the villi or crypts. Recent immunofluorescence studies suggest that Brunner's glands contain **urogastrone**, a peptide hormone that **inhibits HCl production** in the stomach.

The rather short (0.2–0.5 mm) broad, leaf-shaped **villi are most numerous** (about 40/mm^2) in the duodenum. The **serosa** encloses the duodenum only for a few centimeters at its **junction with the stomach** and its **union with the jejunum**. Since the duodenum lies behind the peritoneum, the serosa covers only its **anterior wall**. Elsewhere, serosa is replaced by **adventitia**.

Goblet Cells

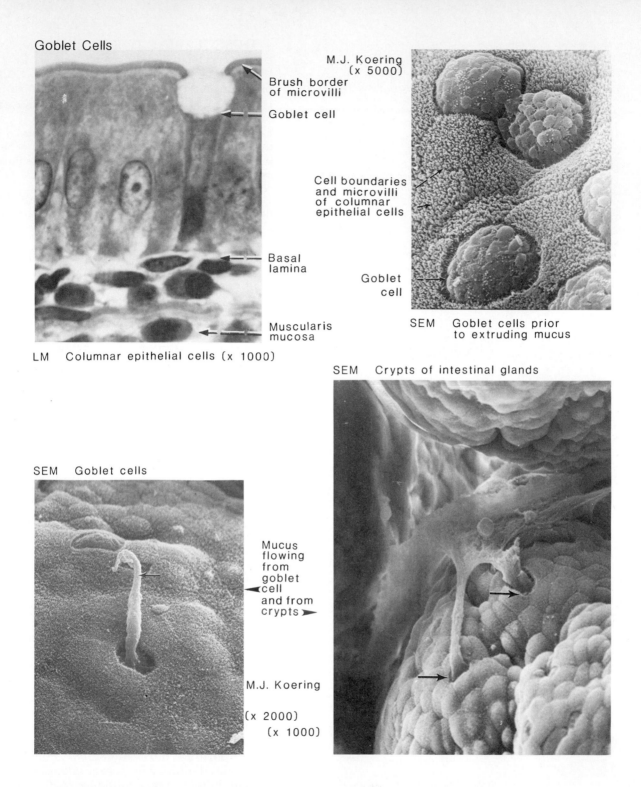

M.J. Koering
(x 5000)

Brush border
of microvilli

Goblet cell

Cell boundaries
and microvilli
of columnar
epithelial cells

Goblet
cell

Basal
lamina

Muscularis
mucosa

LM   Columnar epithelial cells (x 1000)

SEM   Goblet cells prior
to extruding mucus

SEM   Crypts of intestinal glands

SEM   Goblet cells

Mucus
flowing
from
goblet
cell
and from
crypts ➤

M.J. Koering

(x 2000)

(x 1000)

Upper left LM photomicrograph shows a typical section of the intestinal mucosa. A goblet cell is interposed between the simple columnar intestinal absorptive cells which have a distinct brush (striated) border of microvilli. The stem of the goblet cell houses an elongated, oval nucleus, while the foot of the goblet rests on the basal lamina.

The upper right SEM micrograph is a surface view of several intact goblet cells among the microvilli of the absorptive cells.

The dynamic discharge of mucus from goblet cells is seen in the lower SEM micrographs. On the left, an active goblet cell is shown at the instant a stream of mucus is projected from its ruptured apex. The slightly elevated, ovoid structures, above the mucus stream, are resting goblet cells. The micrograph to the right reveals similar events, except that the mucus secretions are flowing from intestinal crypts, generated by ruptured goblet cells located in the epithelial lining of the crypts.

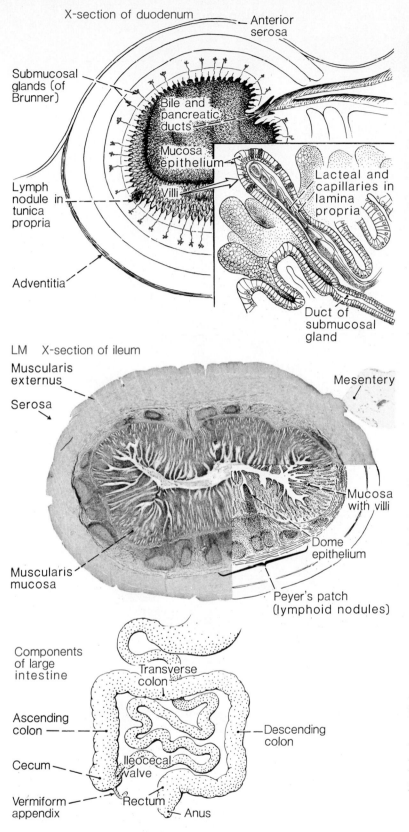

X-section of duodenum

Anterior serosa

Submucosal glands (of Brunner)

Bile and pancreatic ducts

Mucosa epithelium

Villi

Lymph nodule in tunica propria

Adventitia

Lacteal and capillaries in lamina propria

Duct of submucosal gland

LM   X-section of ileum

Muscularis externus

Serosa

Mesentery

Mucosa with villi

Dome epithelium

Muscularis mucosa

Peyer's patch (lymphoid nodules)

Components of large intestine

Transverse colon

Ascending colon

Descending colon

Cecum

Ileocecal valve

Vermiform appendix

Rectum

Anus

If present on the microscopic slide, an excellent diagnostic clue for identification of the duodenum is the presence of the **bile and pancreatic ducts** piercing the duodenal mucosa. Since this is an isolated site, only the most fortuitous sections will pass these through these structures. From a practical viewpoint, the only constant, unique histological feature of the duodenum is the presence of **Brunner's glands** in the submucosa. The other criteria are helpful if present but are not always reliable.

JEJUNUM The jejunum has no really distinctive features. While its **fingerlike villi** are the tallest and its lacteals are well-developed for maximum fat absorption, these are hardly reliable diagnostic features. Often by a process of elimination one must make a judgment. For example, if a histological section of the small intestine does not contain submucosal glands (of Brunner) or aggregates of lymph nodules in the lamina propria (Peyer's patches), then the organ is **probably jejunum.**

ILEUM The ileum has only one **unique diagnostic feature:** the presence of many aggregates of lymphoid nodules in the lamina propria. These are **Peyer's patches,** located on the side of the ileum opposite to the mesentery attachment (L-A, plate 21). The **lymph nodules, or follicles,** as they are often called, are usually pear-shaped with their rounded, dome-shaped apices directed towards the lumen. As the nodules approach the lumen, they usually are **not covered by villi** but only by a single layer of epithelium, called **dome epithelium.** There is substantial evidence that these cells are **specialized to transport antigens** from the intestinal lumen to the underlying lymphoid follicles. These cells have been designated as **follicle-associated epithelium (FAE).**

LARGE INTESTINE

Those parts of the GI tract that lie between the termination of the ileum, at the ileocecal valve, and the anus belong to the **large intestine.** In sequence they are: (1) the wide, dilated, blind pouch, the **cecum,** about 5–8 cm long; (2) the **vermiform appendix,** a blind, narrow tube about 10 cm long, an extension from the cecum; (3) the **colon** with its ascending, transverse, descending, and pelvic regions, more or less 1.3 m long; (4) the rectum, 10–12 cm long; and (5) the **anal canal,** 2.5–4.0 cm in length.

2410

SEM Intestinal villi   M.J. Koering   LM Jejunum villi T.G. Merrill
(x 200)   (x 150)

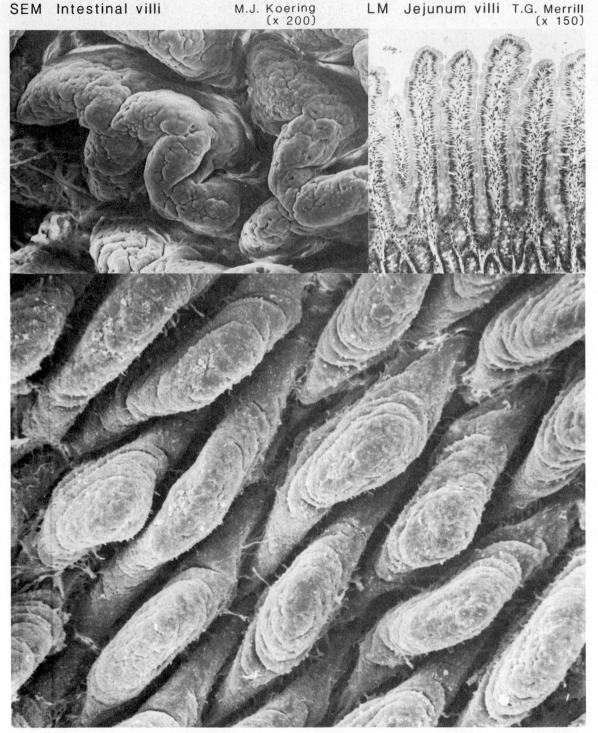

SEM Luminal surface villi of small intestine   P. Andrews (x 150)

The upper left micrograph is a SEM view of jejunal villi which are closely packed and leaf-shaped.

The upper right LM micrograph emphasizes some of the distinctive histological features of villi of the jejunum, such as their length (greatest of any intestinal region), their compactness (greatest of any region), and their leaf or tongue shape. Also present, in the cores of the villi, are plexuses of fenestrated capillaries, an arteriole, a venule, and a prominent lymph vessel (lacteal, not clearly seen at this magnification).

The lower micrograph is another SEM view of jejunal intestinal villi. Observe that the villi are tongue-shaped and closely spaced. Their surfaces are pleated from contraction of the smooth muscle fibers in the muscularis mucosae, located principally in the long axis of the villus.

2053

Wall of large Intestine

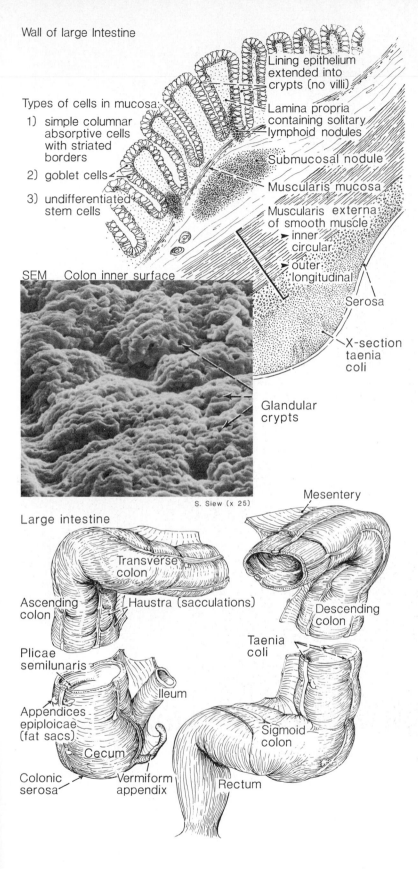

Types of cells in mucosa:
1) simple columnar absorptive cells with striated borders
2) goblet cells
3) undifferentiated stem cells

Lining epithelium extended into crypts (no villi)

Lamina propria containing solitary lymphoid nodules

Submucosal nodule

Muscularis mucosa

Muscularis externa of smooth muscle
→ inner circular
→ outer longitudinal

Serosa

X-section taenia coli

SEM   Colon inner surface

Glandular crypts

S. Siew (x 25)

Large intestine

Mesentery

Transverse colon

Ascending colon

Haustra (sacculations)

Descending colon

Plicae semilunaris

Taenia coli

Ileum

Appendices epiploicae (fat sacs)

Cecum

Colonic serosa

Vermiform appendix

Sigmoid colon

Rectum

Since the colon is the prototype for the various regions, it will be considered first; the modifications of the other regions, later.

Colon

MUCOSA The mucosa of the colon is **free of villi.** The surface epithelium consists of three types of cells. (1) **Simple columnar absorptive cells** have a thin striated border. (2) Abundant **goblet cells** intercalate between the absorptive cells. The goblet cells increase sharply in number in the more distal segments of the colon. (3) **Undifferentiated epithelial cells** in the bases of the intestinal glands are **stem cells** that give rise to the absorptive and goblet cells.

The lining epithelium is greatly increased by the myriad **crypts** that open on its surface. The epithelium extends into the openings of the crypts. These **intestinal crypts or glands** are longer than in the small intestine (0.4–0.6 mm) and are characterized by the **abundance of goblet cells** that replace most of the lining absorptive cells.

The lamina propria is similar to that in the small intestine, except that the **solitary lymph nodules** are larger and more numerous. Because of their size, they often bulge into the submucosa. The muscularis mucosae has the typical two layers of thin, smooth muscle fibers.

SUBMUCOSA Except that the submucosa contains **no glands,** it has no essential differences from the submucosa of the small intestine.

MUSCULARIS EXTERNA The **inner, circular layer** of smooth muscle is a completely encircling band, typical of the GI tract. However, the outer, **longitudinal layer** is not of uniform thickness. Most of its fibers are converted into three longitudinal, ribbonlike bands, the **teniae coli,** each about 1 cm in width. They lie at approximately equal distance from each other when viewed in cross section. Because of their tonus and also because they are shorter in length than the colon, they draw the colon into a series of puckerings or sacculations called **haustra,** an important gross anatomical diagnostic feature. Between the haustra, the gut wall is pressed into crescentic folds, the **plicae semilunaris,** that project into the lumen.

SEROSA Since the **ascending and descending colon** are pressed against the body wall by the peritoneum, the colonic **serosa** is incomplete, present **only on** their **anterior surfaces.** These regions are attached to the body wall by an **adventitia.** The other regions, i.e., the **transverse and pelvic colon,** are invested by a mesentery and therefore have a **serosa.** Scattered among the

3208

colonic serosa are rather large, pendulous sacs of fat, the **appendices epiploicae,** another unique gross feature of the colon.

Cecum

The beginning of the large intestine is the **cecum,** a **large, blind sac** that extends caudad beyond the ileocecal valve. It is similar in structure to the transverse colon, including a complete **serosa.**

Vermiform Appendix

As its name implies, the **vermiform appendix** is a small (about 10 cm long, 1 cm wide), worm-shaped tube projecting from the blind end of the cecum. It is characterized by closely spaced, multiple, large, **lymphoid nodules** in the **lamina propria.** They may also occupy the submucosa and reduce the lumen of the appendix to a narrow, stellate slit. Because many of these nodules have large germinal centers, the appendix is often referred to as the "tonsil of the abdomen."

The general structure of the appendix resembles the colon, except it has **no teniae coli** and the intestinal glands are shallower and less abundant. Because it is a blind-ending tube, the lumen may become occluded by food or cellular debris. The resulting inflammation causes the life-threatening **appendicitis.**

Rectum

The rectum is the continuation of the pelvic colon that terminates at the anal canal. Some **structural changes** gradually occur in the colon in making the transition to a rectal structure. These include: (1) the **teniae coli flatten out** to form a uniform, longitudinal, sheet of muscle; (2) the **mucosa is thicker** with prominent submucosal veins; (3) the **crypts are longer** (0.7 mm) and are lined almost entirely by goblet cells; and (4) lymphoid nodules are less abundant.

As the rectum approaches the anal canal the **crypts** become shallower, more sparse, and finally **disappear.** Its serosa is progressively replaced by an **adventitia** (L-A, plate 19).

Anal Canal

The anal canal is about 2.5–4 cm long. Its beginning is marked by the presence of 6–10 longitudinal folds, the **anal columns** (of Morgagni). These folds are formed from the mucosa, submucosa, and a few longitudinally directed smooth muscle fibers. Inferiorly the columns end abruptly by joining together into small, cup-shaped folds, the **anal valves.** At the level of the valves, the epithelium changes abruptly from the **simple columnar** to the **stratified squamous** type. Here the **muscularis mucosae** fragments and **disappears** (L-A, plate 22).

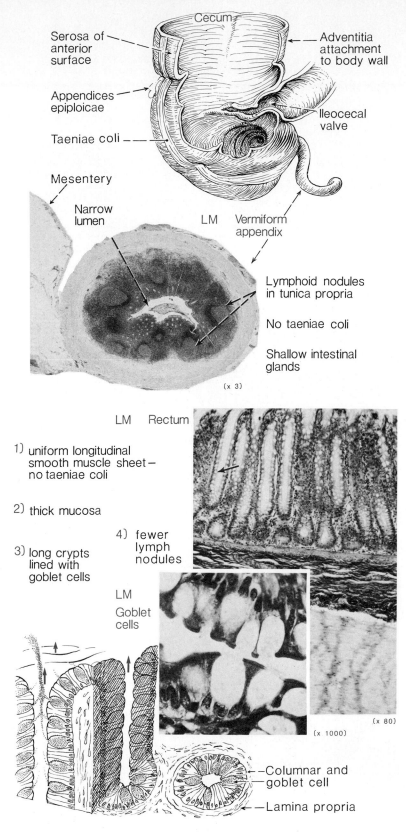

Cecum

Serosa of anterior surface

Appendices epiploicae

Taeniae coli

Mesentery

Narrow lumen

Adventitia attachment to body wall

Ileocecal valve

LM   Vermiform appendix

Lymphoid nodules in tunica propria

No taeniae coli

Shallow intestinal glands

(x 3)

LM   Rectum

1) uniform longitudinal smooth muscle sheet—no taeniae coli

2) thick mucosa

3) long crypts lined with goblet cells

4) fewer lymph nodules

LM Goblet cells

(x 80)

(x 1000)

Columnar and goblet cell

Lamina propria

Prominent Features of Anal Canal

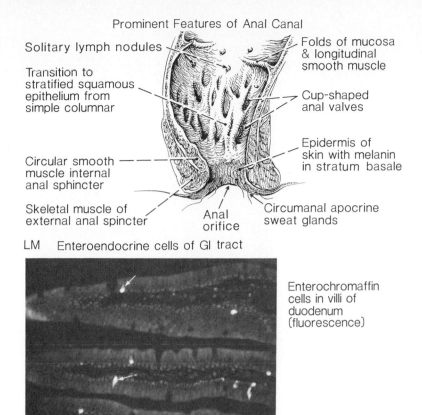

Solitary lymph nodules

Transition to stratified squamous epithelium from simple columnar

Circular smooth muscle internal anal sphincter

Skeletal muscle of external anal spincter

Folds of mucosa & longitudinal smooth muscle

Cup-shaped anal valves

Epidermis of skin with melanin in stratum basale

Anal orifice

Circumanal apocrine sweat glands

LM   Enteroendocrine cells of GI tract

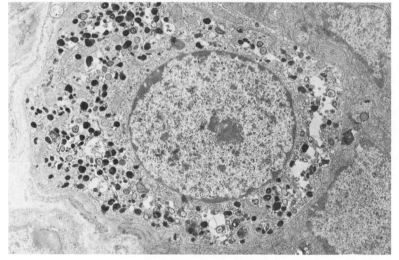

Enterochromaffin cells in villi of duodenum (fluorescence)

S. Kapur (x 125)

EM   Polypeptide synthesizing cell in pyloric antrum

S. Kapur (x 10,000)

Features in common with endocrine cells:

1) slight basophilia

2) sparse rER

3) prolific sER

4) many free ribosomes

5) sparse Golgi complex

6) small secretory granules (100-300nm)

1787

At the **anal orifice,** noncornified stratified squamous epithelium joins the epidermis of the skin of the anal region. Here the **skin** is deeply **pigmented** with many melanin granules in the stratum basale. Beneath the epithelium are enlarged, apocrine-type sweat glands, the **circumanal glands,** similar to the sweat glands of the axillae. At the anal orifice, the circular layer of smooth muscle thickens to form the **internal anal sphincter.** Somewhat more distally the superficial skeletal muscle fibers are organized into the **external anal sphincter.** (For regional differences in intestines, see Table 18.2).

ENTEROENDOCRINE CELLS

It has been noted for many years that certain cells scattered in the epithelium of the GI tract are poorly stained with H&E, yet they have granules that stain selectively with silver or chromium salts. Earlier, those cells that reacted to silver salts were called either **argentaffin** (affinity for silver) or **argyrophil** (silver loving) cells. Later it was demonstrated that both cell types stained specifically with **bichromate salts** and therefore were collectively labeled **enterochromaffin cells.**

From various histochemical and immunological techniques and EM studies, these cells can be separated into **two different groups:** those that produce a specific **polypeptide hormone,** and those synthesizing an **amine hormone.** They are collectively called the **enteroendocrine cells,** or the GI endocrine system.

This rapidly advancing area of research is producing a plethora of confusing names for these cells and their hormones. Yet reason dictates that the cell should be known by the hormone it produces, e.g., G cells are gastrin-producing cells, S cells secrete secretin, etc. However, this system of nomenclature breaks down for cells producing more than one hormone or when the same hormone is produced by several cells.

These various gastrointestinal endocrine cells have many **ultrastructural features in common.** These include: (1) slight, cytoplasmic basophilia; (2) sparse profiles of rER, (3) considerable sER; (4) many free ribosomes; (5) a poorly developed Golgi complex, and (6) small, spherical **secretory granules** (100–300 nm) in the basal region of the cell **adjacent to capillaries.** Note that these EM features are in sharp contrast to active protein-producing cells, such as the pancreatic acinar cell, which has deep cytoplasmic basophilia; an active, large Golgi apparatus; abundant rER; and large membrane-bound **granules in the apex of the cell.**

Some of these enteroendocrine cells stimulate; others inhibit certain alimentary processes. Their overlapping activities collectively **regulate and integrate** the activities of the various regions of the GI tract.

THE APUD CELLS

In the late 1960s, Pearse coined the term **APUD for enteroendocrine cells** to reflect their "<u>a</u>mine <u>p</u>recursor <u>u</u>ptake and <u>d</u>ecarboxylation" capacities. These cells are able to **take up amine precursors and decarboxylate them into amines.** They also share several common metabolic processes related to the **synthesis** of low-molecular-weight **polypeptide or protein hormones.**

However, APUD cells are also found in other sites in the body besides the GI tract. The best known include the chromaffin cells of the **adrenal medulla,** parafollicular "C" cells of the **thyroid,** the islet cells of the **pancreas,** certain cells of the **anterior pituitary,** i.e., the corticotrophs (Gk. trophe, to nourish), and melanotrophs of the pars intermedia of the pituitary. A recent spate of research reports list 30 or more cells as possible candidates for this relatively new, unique cell category. For inclusion into this special group, a cell must meet several criteria, especially (1) the capability to **synthesize** polypeptide and/or biogenic amine **hormones,** and (2) possess small, **basal, electron dense granules (100–300 nm)** for release into capillaries. A possible roster of the generally accepted members of the exclusive APUD "club" is in the adjacent column.

HISTOPHYSIOLOGY

The GI tract is a continuous muscular tube lined by a **specialized mucous membrane.** Its prime function is the preparation of food elements so they can be absorbed from the gut and utilized by the cells of the body. Regional histological variations occur along the tract that reflect its varied functions in preparing food for assimilation. These phases of food preparation include: (1) **ingestion,** in the oral cavity; (2) **fragmentation,** in the oral cavity and completed in the stomach; (3) **digestion,** initiated in the oral cavity and stomach, completed in the small intestine; (4) **absorption,** begins in the stomach, occurs mostly in the small intestine, and is finished in the large intestine; and (5) **elimination,** via the anal canal.

Generally Accepted APUD Cells

Location	Cell Types	Hormone
Anterior lobe of pituitary	Corticotrophs	ACTH
Intermediate lobe of pituitary	Melanotrophs	MSH
Pancreas - islet tissue	Alpha	Glucagon
	Beta	Insulin
	Delta	Somatostatin
Thyroid	C	Calcitonin
Stomach	G	Gastrin
	EG	Enteroglucagon
Intestines	S	Secretin
	CCK	Cholecystokinin
	EG	Enteroglucagon
	Delta-like	Somatostatin
	K	Gastric inhibitory polypeptide
	(EC) Enterochromatin	Serotonin
Adrenal medulla	Chromaffin	Epinephrine
		Norepinephrine

Histophysiology

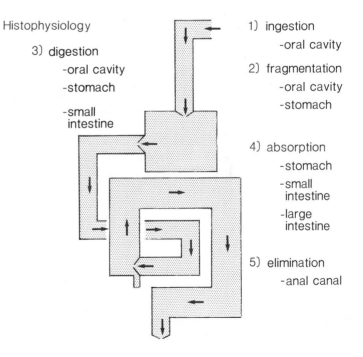

3) digestion
- oral cavity
- stomach
- small intestine

1) ingestion
- oral cavity

2) fragmentation
- oral cavity
- stomach

4) absorption
- stomach
- small intestine
- large intestine

5) elimination
- anal canal

Functions of gut layers:

1) Mucosa

    o synthesizes enzymes & hormones
    o lubricates digestive tract
    o absorbs nutrients
    o controls GI functions

2) Submucosa

    o shock absorber for mucosa

    o contains blood vessels and lymph

3) Muscularis externa

    o movement of gut contents by peristalsis

    o mixing and churning of contents

4) Serosa (or adventitia)

    o contains large vessels and nerves
      to sustain functions

Gut wall relationships

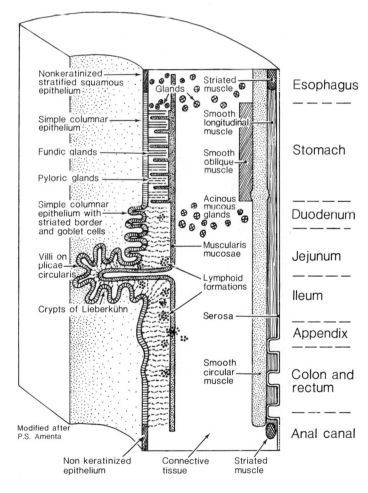

Nonkeratinized stratified squamous epithelium

Glands

Striated muscle

Esophagus

Simple columnar epithelium

Smooth longitudinal muscle

Fundic glands

Smooth oblique muscle

Stomach

Pyloric glands

Simple columnar epithelium with striated border and goblet cells

Acinous mucous glands

Duodenum

Muscularis mucosae

Jejunum

Villi on plicae circularis

Lymphoid formations

Ileum

Crypts of Lieberkühn

Serosa

Appendix

Smooth circular muscle

Colon and rectum

Modified after P.S. Amenta

Anal canal

Non keratinized epithelium

Connective tissue

Striated muscle

These varied functions are accomplished by the interplay of four constant, distinct, functional and anatomical layers or **tunics**. They are: (1) the **mucosa** whose epithelial cells may synthesize and release **enzymes and hormones** essential for digestion. Goblet cells release copious amounts of **mucus** to protect lining cells from abrasion and to lubricate the passage of material along the digestive tract. Other cells are involved in the absorption of nutrients from the gut lumen and their transportation to blood capillaries for distribution to the body tissues. And finally the gut endocrine cells, e.g., **APUD cells,** which are crucial to the control of many, if not all, GI functions. (2) The **submucosa** provides an effective shock absorber for the delicate mucosa by its abundant loose connective tissue. Also it contains blood and lymph vessels that serve the mucosa. (3) The **muscularis externa** provides peristaltic contractions for moving the contents of the gut. Also in the stomach, it produces the mixing and churning actions necessary for the fragmenting and mixing of food. (4) The **serosa, or adventitia,** contains the larger vessels and nerves that sustain the gut layers.

Table 18.1 *COMPARISON OF REGIONS OF STOMACH*

	CARDIAC	FUNDIC AND BODY	PYLORIC
Location	Area around gastro-esophageal (GE) junction (about 2.5 cm wide)	Fundus—area superior to GE junction Body—between fundus and pyloric antrum	Area extending from gas-troduodenal junction into pyloric canal and antrum
Epithelium	Simple columnar	Same	Same
Cells • Surface mucous	Cover entire luminal sur-face	Same	Same
• Neck mucous	Line neck region of mu-cosal glands	Same	Same
• Body mucous	Line body region of mu-cosal glands	Absent	Same as cardiac
• Chief (peptic)	Absent	Abundant, mostly line lu-men of lower part of body of glands	Absent
• Parietal (oxyntic)	Absent	Abundant; predominantly in upper part of body of glands and between mu-cous neck cells	Few
• Enteroendocrine	Rare	Rare	Rare
Mucosal glands	Wide, deep, gastric pits with short, slightly coiled, simple tubular glands; pits extend into less than half of mucosa	Narrow, shallow pits with straight, branched tubular glands; pits extend less than ⅕ into depth of mu-cosa	Wide, deep pits with coiled, branched, tubular glands; pits extend over half the thickness of mu-cosa
Muscularis externa	Three layers of smooth muscle; inner oblique (best developed), middle circular, and outer longitu-dinal; Auerbach's (myen-teric) nerve plexus be-tween circular and longitudinal layers	Same—except inner oblique layer inconstant	Same as fundic
Serosa	Present	Present	Present

Table 18.2 *REGIONAL DIFFERENCES OF SMALL AND LARGE INTESTINES*

	DUODENUM	JEJUNUM	ILEUM	LARGE INTESTINE
Cells • Absorptive or surface	Simple columnar with prominent striated free border (microvilli)	Same	Same	Simple columnar with reduced microvilli
• Goblet	Least numerous, interspersed among absorptive cells	Plentiful	More numerous	Most numerous, replace many columnar lining cells
• Paneth	Few cells in base of crypts	Increase in number	Most abundant	Rare
• Enteroendocrine	Scattered near or at base of crypts between absorptive cells	Same, except more numerous	Same as jejunum	Common in crypts of appendix; few in other regions
Intestinal glands (crypts of Lieberkuhn)	Very abundant; simple tubular type confined to tunica propria; populated with all cell types	Same	Same	Considerably longer and more closely packed
Submucosal glands	Brunner's (duodenal); compound tubular, mucous type with alkaline secretion	Absent	Absent	Absent
Lymphoid tissue	Diffuse; few solitary nodules	Increase in nodules	Many aggregates of lymph nodules (Peyer's patches)	Many nodules, especially abundant in appendix
Plica circularis	Absent in upper part, present in lower; medium height	Present throughout; greatest height	Lowest height; gradually disappear near ileocecal sphincter	Replaced by plicae semilunares between haustra in colon and with plicae transversales recti in rectum
Muscularis externa	Well-developed inner circular and outer longitudinal smooth muscle layers	Same	Same	Outer longitudinal layer arranged into three oval bands, the teniae coli, except in rectum and appendix, where layer is uniform in thickness
Serosa	Replaced by adventitia except at junctions with stomach and jejunum, and on anterior surface	Present	Present	Replaced by adventitia in ascending and descending colon and rectum; present in other regions
Villi	Lowest (0.2–0.5 mm) in height; abundant, leaf-shaped	Tallest (0.5–1.0 mm); less profuse, rounded, fingerlike	Medium (0.4–0.8 mm) in height; least numerous, most widely spaced, club-shaped; disappear near ileocecal valve	Absent—although appear early in development then degenerate in fetus
Functions	Maximum absorption of lipids; also assimilation of amino acids and monosaccharides	Less imbibing of lipids; absorption of amino acids and simple sugars	Maximum absorption of bile salts and vitamin B_{12}; also assimilation of amino acids and simple sugars	Absorption of water which results in formation of fecal mass; produces abundant mucus for lubrication of the mucosal surface

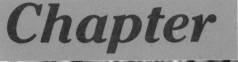

Chapter

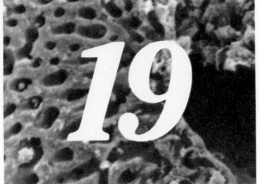

19

DIGESTIVE SYSTEM III—PANCREAS, LIVER, AND BILIARY TRACT

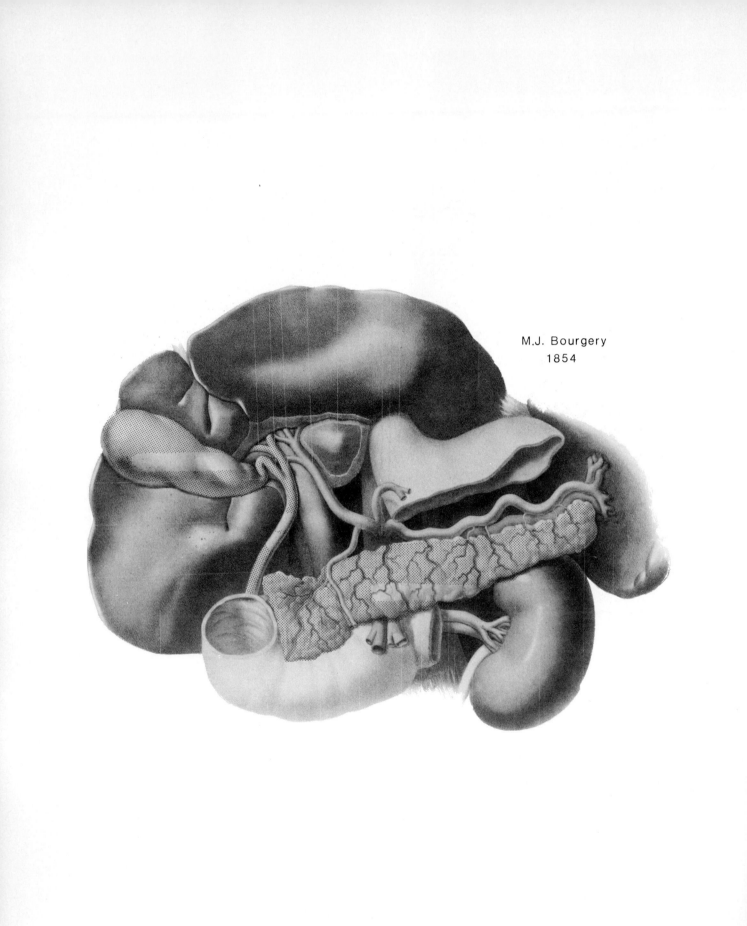

M.J. Bourgery
1854

OBJECTIVES

EXTRAPOLATE FROM THE STRUCTURE OF THESE MAJOR DIGESTIVE ORGANS THEIR VARIOUS FUNCTIONS, SUCH AS:

1. How the exocrine acinar cells of the pancreas are able to synthesize, under hormonal control, a variety of digestive enzymes.

2. How opposing roles of endocrine alpha and beta cells accomplish the control of blood sugar levels.

3. How its dual blood supply enables the liver to store and release nutrients and secrete bile.

4. How the several types of liver lobules are useful physiological concepts to explain the functions of the liver.

5. How the gallbladder can concentrate and deliver bile to the duodenum.

Major glands associated with the digestive system, discussed in this chapter, are the **pancreas, liver, and gallbladder** with its biliary system. The major salivary glands, i.e., parotid, submandibular, and sublingual, also belong in this category, but they have been described with the oral cavity in Chapter 17. Also discussed in earlier chapters are the minor glands of the digestive system, e.g., esophageal, gastric, duodenal, intestinal, and the minor salivary glands.

PANCREAS

The pancreas (Gk. pan, all; kreas, flesh) or sweetbread is a large, soft, grayish pink, lobulated, **tubuloacinar gland** that lies in the upper abdominal cavity, behind the stomach. It is shaped somewhat like a pistol with its handle (**head**) placed to the right of the abdomen, embraced by the horseshoe-shaped duodenum. The barrel (**body**) extends to the left with its extremity (**tail**) reaching the **hilus** of the spleen.

The pancreas is both an **exocrine** and an **endocrine** gland. Most of the gland consists of myriad serous, pear-shaped **acini**—the exocrine portion; small, scattered clusters of endocrine cells, the **islets of Langerhans,** comprise perhaps less than 2% of the gland.

Exocrine Pancreas

The exocrine portion of the pancreas resembles closely the parotid gland (L-A, plate 15) in that all of the glandular acini are composed of six to eight low columnar or pyramidal **serous cells** surrounding a small lumen. Delicate septa divide each gland into lobules. The exocrine pancreas **differs from the parotid** by (1) the presence of small, light-staining cells in the central area of the acinus, the unique **centroacinar cells;** (2) the **absence** of intralobular **striated ducts;** (3) the presence of a **thin,** delicate, connective tissue **capsule;** and (4) the **absence of fat cells** among the acini, except in the aged.

ACINAR CELL The pancreatic (acinar) serous cell rests on a distinct basal lamina. It has a round, dark nucleus with one or two distinct nucleoli. **Basophilic cytoplasm** fills the basal portion of the cell and surrounds the nucleus. The basophilia is due to the abundance of **rER,** which indicates extensive protein synthesis. The region often appears **striated** because of elongated **mitochondria** sandwiched between the folds of rER, richly studded with ribosomes. The cytoplasm contains many spherical acidophilic globules, the **zymogen secretory granules,** that contain inactive enzyme precursors.

TEM micrographs of the basal zone of a pancreatic cell reveal a dense accumulation of **flat cisternae of rER,** perhaps the richest such concentration of any cell in the body and an **extensive Golgi.**

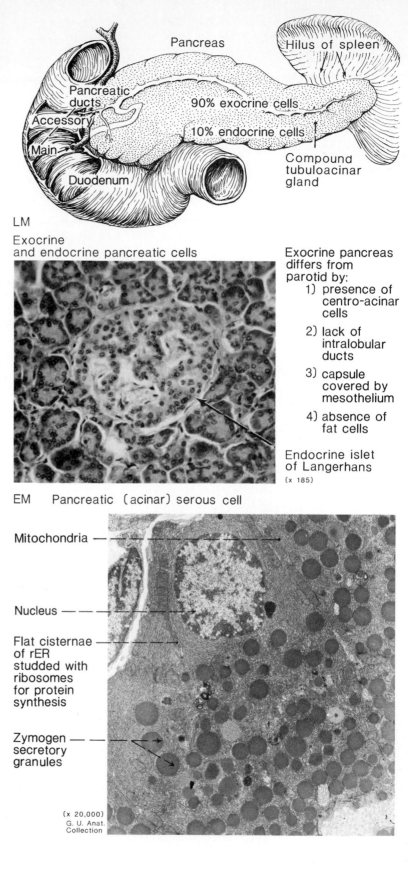

Pancreas
Hilus of spleen
Pancreatic ducts
Accessory
Main
Duodenum
90% exocrine cells
10% endocrine cells
Compound tubuloacinar gland

LM
Exocrine and endocrine pancreatic cells

Exocrine pancreas differs from parotid by:
1) presence of centro-acinar cells
2) lack of intralobular ducts
3) capsule covered by mesothelium
4) absence of fat cells

Endocrine islet of Langerhans
(x 185)

EM   Pancreatic (acinar) serous cell

Mitochondria

Nucleus

Flat cisternae of rER studded with ribosomes for protein synthesis

Zymogen secretory granules

(x 20,000)
G. U. Anat. Collection

4580

Functions of Acinar Cells

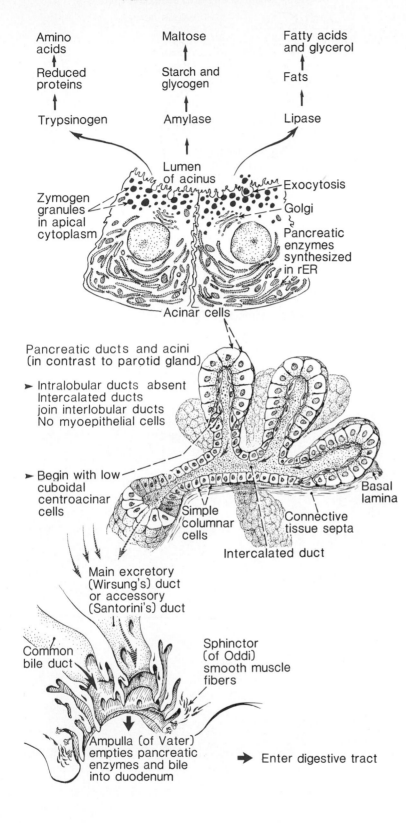

Amino acids ← Reduced proteins ← Trypsinogen

Maltose ← Starch and glycogen ← Amylase

Fatty acids and glycerol ← Fats ← Lipase

Lumen of acinus

Exocytosis

Golgi

Zymogen granules in apical cytoplasm

Pancreatic enzymes synthesized in rER

Acinar cells

Pancreatic ducts and acini (in contrast to parotid gland)

► Intralobular ducts absent
Intercalated ducts join interlobular ducts
No myoepithelial cells

► Begin with low cuboidal centroacinar cells

Simple columnar cells

Basal lamina

Connective tissue septa

Intercalated duct

Main excretory (Wirsung's) duct or accessory (Santorini's) duct

Common bile duct

Sphinctor (of Oddi) smooth muscle fibers

Ampulla (of Vater) empties pancreatic enzymes and bile into duodenum

→ Enter digestive tract

Although all **acinar cells** are morphologically similar, they secrete a variety of **enzymes** that are chemically quite dissimilar. These include proteolytic enzymes or their precursors, especially **trypsinogen**, which reduces proteins to amino acids; **amylase**, which converts starch and glycogen into maltose, which is converted to glucose by the enzyme maltase; and fat-splitting enzymes, e.g., **lipase**, which break down fats into fatty acids and glycerol. These functions may be summarized as follows: Pancreatic **enzymes** are synthesized by the abundant **rER** mostly in the basal cytoplasm of the acinar cells, where they accumulate in the cisternae of the rER. They then pass into the vesicles of the **Golgi apparatus** where they are "packaged" into membrane-bound globules, the typical **zymogen granules**. These granules then move to the apical region of the cell where they fuse with the luminal cell surface membrane and are **extruded** into the lumen of the **acinus**. This latter process is called **exocytosis**, the opposite of endocytosis (phagocytosis and pinocytosis).

DUCT SYSTEM Although the duct system of the pancreas resembles that of the parotid, it has several important differences. (1) The ducts begin with the telescoping of the flat or low cuboidal **centroacinar cells** that become the initial segment of the **intercalated ducts**. (2) Striated ducts are absent. (3) The intercalated ducts make direct connections with the larger **interlobular ducts** that are lined with low columnar cells and located in the connective tissue septa. (4) **No myoepithelial cells** are present.

The interlobular ducts coalesce to form either the **main excretory (Wirsung's)** duct, or the **accessory (Santorini's)** excretory duct, both lined with simple columnar cells and a few goblet cells. Smooth muscle cells form a thin layer beneath the epithelium. These excretory ducts join the **common bile duct** to enter the lumen of the duodenum at the dilated **ampulla (of Vater)**. This structure is nearly filled with valvular folds of mucosa that extend distally into the cone-shaped duodenal papilla. Smooth muscle fibers provide the **sphincter (of Oddi)** at the termination of the common duct. The sphincter permits intermittent flow of bile and pancreatic secretions into the lumen of the duodenum.

HORMONAL CONTROL Normally the alkaline pancreatic enzymes are released into the duodenum when the acidic gastric contents (**chyme**) enter the lumen of the gut. In fact, activation of the enzymes can occur only in a neutral solution. However, the control of these secretions is maintained by two **intestinal hormones** secreted by the duodenal mucosal cells. They are **secretin** and **cholecystokinin** (pancreozymin), which are released in response to the acid chyme in the duodenum.

Secretin stimulates the pancreas to abundant **water production** with low protein and enzyme content but **high in bicarbonate ions** which neutralize the chyme so that the enzymes can be activated. Also **secretin** is believed to stimulate selectively the **ductile tissue** to secrete these substances, not the acinar cells. In contrast, **cholecystokinin** acts on the **acinar cells** to release the enzymes, i.e., the zymogen granules from the acinar cells.

CLINICAL COMMENT In a severe **protein deficiency** of small children, called **kwashiorkor,** the pancreatic acinar cells are severely affected. Initially, they are reduced in size with marked **loss of zymogen granules.** With the concomitant disappearance of rER in the cells, **cessation of enzyme production** occurs and the breakdown of any protein in the diet to usable amino acids is arrested. The **clinical picture** of such a starving child includes massive edema, diarrhea, generalized wasting, and extensive **pancreas and liver damage.** The condition is uniformly fatal unless treated with amino acids, milk supplements, and an adequate diet.

BLOOD SUPPLY Principally from the celiac branch of the aorta, **small arteries** arise that enter the interlobular connective tissue of the pancreas. Here they give off fine branches that enter the lobules and anastomose freely to form a **vascular network** around the lobules. Veins usually parallel the arteries. The **venous blood** eventually drains into either the **portal or splenic vein** before reaching the inferior vena cava, en route to the heart.

Endocrine Pancreas

The most distinctive histological feature of the pancreas is the scattered, spherical clusters of light-staining cells called the **islets of Langerhans or islet tissue.** They account for about 1–2% of the pancreas volume. These cells are the **endocrine portion** of the pancreas and secrete two principal hormones, **insulin** and **glucagon.** Both exert a powerful influence on carbohydrate metabolism by regulating blood sugar levels. The actions of these two hormones are antagonistic, i.e., **insulin lowers the blood sugar** level, while **glucagon increases** it.

ISLET TISSUE A typical islet is spherical or ovoid in shape, containing a few to hundreds of cells. The islets are arranged in anastomosing, **irregular cords** that are penetrated by a rich network of **fenestrated capillaries,** typical of all endocrine tissue. The islet cells are **polarized** toward capillaries since their secretions will enter the bloodstream.

With H&E stain, the islets are much lighter stained than the surrounding pancreatic acinar tissue. The various cell types cannot be clearly differentiated. However, with appropriate fixation and special stains, **four cell types** are identified, i.e., alpha, beta, delta, and C cells.

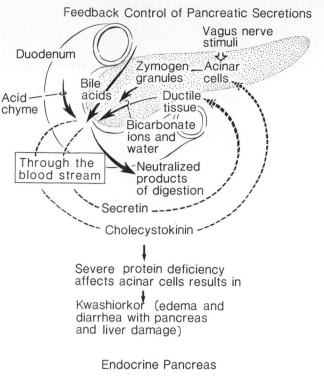

Feedback Control of Pancreatic Secretions

Duodenum — Vagus nerve stimuli — Zymogen granules — Acinar cells — Bile acids — Ductile tissue — Acid chyme — Bicarbonate ions and water — Through the blood stream — Neutralized products of digestion — Secretin — Cholecystokinin

Severe protein deficiency affects acinar cells results in

Kwashiorkor (edema and diarrhea with pancreas and liver damage)

Endocrine Pancreas
Islets of Langerhans = 1–2% of pancreas volume

LM   Islet cells of pancreas

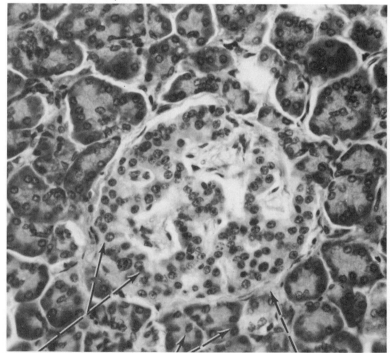

Islet cells polarized towards fenestrated capillaries

Acinar cells

Thin layer of reticular connective tissue around spherical islet (×245)

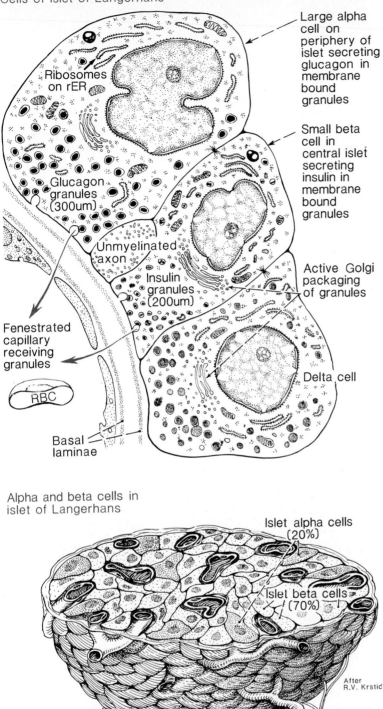

Cells of islet of Langerhans

Large alpha cell on periphery of islet secreting glucagon in membrane bound granules

Ribosomes on rER

Small beta cell in central islet secreting insulin in membrane bound granules

Glucagon granules (300um)

Unmyelinated axon

Active Golgi packaging of granules

Insulin granules (200um)

Fenestrated capillary receiving granules

Delta cell

RBC

Basal laminae

Alpha and beta cells in islet of Langerhans

Islet alpha cells (20%)

Islet beta cells (70%)

After R.V. Krstić

Nerve fibers

Blood capillaries

ISLET CELLS

ISLET CELLS The **alpha cells** are large and prominent. They are located mostly on the periphery of the islet and comprise about 20% of the cell population. They have numerous, electron-opaque, membrane-bound **secretory granules of uniform size** (about 300 nm). These granules are **not soluble in alcohol** but dissolve in water. They contain the hormone **glucagon**.

The smallest, yet the most numerous (70%), are the **beta cells**. They usually occupy the central area of the islet and secrete **insulin**. They contain **smaller** (200 nm), less electron-opaque, membrane-bound **granules** that are **alcohol soluble** but resistant to water.

Since both insulin and glucagon are polypeptides, EM studies of the two cell types show organelles typical of **protein-producing cells.** For example, they both contain a moderate amount of **rER** (much less than acinar cells), many free **ribosomes**, an **active Golgi** apparatus, and many **secretory granules** much smaller than the zymogen granules in the pancreatic acinar cell. Electron microscopic studies reveal that the sequence of events for the synthesis of these two hormones is essentially the same. **Synthesis** of their products occurs in the **rER.** The peptides are then transported to the **Golgi complex for packaging** into granules. The granules fuse with the cell membrane that lies adjacent to a **fenestrated capillary.** The granule contents eventually enter the bloodstream.

Delta cells are the **largest** and make up about 5% of the islet tissue. They contain granules similar to the alpha cells but less dense. Their function is uncertain; however, immunological studies suggest that delta cells probably secrete the hormone **somatostatin,** which inhibits the release of growth hormone.

C cells, found only in certain species, such as the guinea pig, are limited in number, are about the size of the beta cells, and contain few or no granules. They have no known function.

Historical Background

The role of the pancreas in the control of blood sugar levels was discovered rather fortuitously in 1889 by two German physiologists, von Mering and Minkosky. They were studying the effect of pancreatectomy on dogs when their animal caretaker noticed that flies were attracted to the urine of the experimental dogs but not to the unoperated control animals. Analysis of the urine revealed **high levels of glucose,** suggesting that the pancreas somehow controls blood sugar levels in the body. However, it was not until the early 1920s that two Canadians, Banting, a recent medical graduate, and Best, a third-year medical student, discovered that dogs whose pancreatic ducts had been ligated several weeks earlier suffered from total atrophy of the pancreatic acinar tissue but no damage or depletion of the islet

4685

tissue. Furthermore, **blood sugar levels were normal,** and no sugar appeared in the urine of the operated dogs. Banting and Best prepared an alcohol-soluble extract from these pancreata containing essentially only islet tissue. Injection of this preparation into pancreatectomized dogs **alleviated the diabetes.** This antidiabetic substance (hormone) was named **insulin** (L. insula, island).

Functional Considerations

Insulin reduces blood sugar by stimulating the **movement of glucose molecules** out of the blood stream and into certain cells, especially liver, muscle, and fat cells. The dynamics of this transport mechanism are: (1) an acceleration of the **conversion of glucose to glycogen** in the liver and muscle; (2) an increase in the **conversion of glucose to fat** in the liver; (3) a more **rapid utilization of glucose** by various tissues; and (4) an **inhibition** of the production of carbohydrates from fats and proteins.

An excess of insulin in the bloodstream will rapidly lower blood sugar far below normal, a condition called **hypoglycemia.** Clinically this condition is usually characterized first by the blurring of vision because of the inability to focus, then nervousness, muscular weakness, faintness, and tremors followed by **convulsions** (insulin shock) that may be fatal.

The effect of glucagon is opposite to that of insulin. A **low blood sugar level,** usually caused by fasting or an excess of insulin, **increases glucagon synthesis.** The resulting rise in blood sugar level results from (1) the acceleration of conversion of liver glycogen to glucose (**glycogenolysis**) and (2) the synthesis of new glycogen (**glyconeogenesis**) by the liver from sources other than carbohydrates. The presence of glycogen also inhibits protein production.

LIVER

Like the pancreas, **the liver** develops as an **outpocketing of the primitive gut.** Its connection to the gut is retained throughout life via the **common bile duct** that empties into the duodenum. The liver is essential for life. It is the **largest internal organ** of the body, weighing about 1200–1500 g or about 2% of the total body weight.

The liver is interposed between two important vessels: (1) the large hepatic **portal vein** carrying nutrients from the stomach and intestines, and (2) the smaller **hepatic artery** which provides the oxygen for the metabolically active liver cells (**hepatocytes**). These polygonal cells are extremely versatile, capable of **many varied functions** including synthesis and secretion of bile; storage of glucose, glycogen, fats, proteins, and vitamins; detoxification of metabolic wastes; and synthesis of blood-clotting and blood-thinning factors.

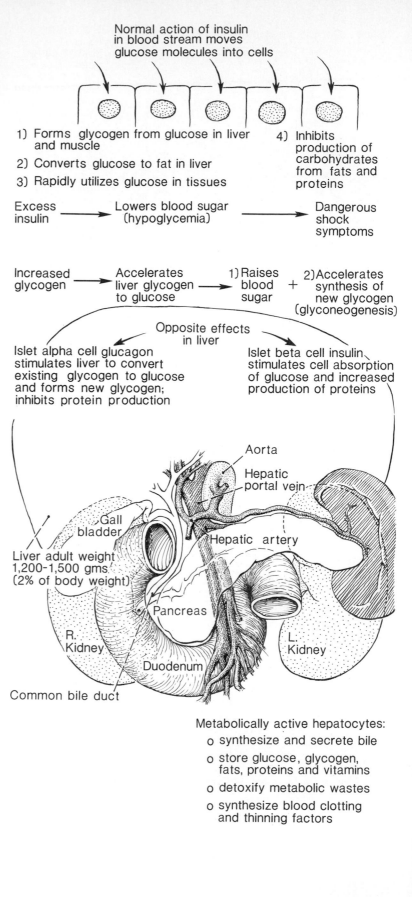

Normal action of insulin in blood stream moves glucose molecules into cells

1) Forms glycogen from glucose in liver and muscle

2) Converts glucose to fat in liver

3) Rapidly utilizes glucose in tissues

4) Inhibits production of carbohydrates from fats and proteins

Excess insulin → Lowers blood sugar (hypoglycemia) → Dangerous shock symptoms

Increased glycogen → Accelerates liver glycogen to glucose → 1) Raises blood sugar + 2) Accelerates synthesis of new glycogen (glyconeogenesis)

Opposite effects in liver

Islet alpha cell glucagon stimulates liver to convert existing glycogen to glucose and forms new glycogen; inhibits protein production

Islet beta cell insulin stimulates cell absorption of glucose and increased production of proteins

Aorta

Hepatic portal vein

Gall bladder

Hepatic artery

Liver adult weight 1,200-1,500 gms (2% of body weight)

Pancreas

R. Kidney

L. Kidney

Duodenum

Common bile duct

Metabolically active hepatocytes:
o synthesize and secrete bile
o store glucose, glycogen, fats, proteins and vitamins
o detoxify metabolic wastes
o synthesize blood clotting and thinning factors

3978

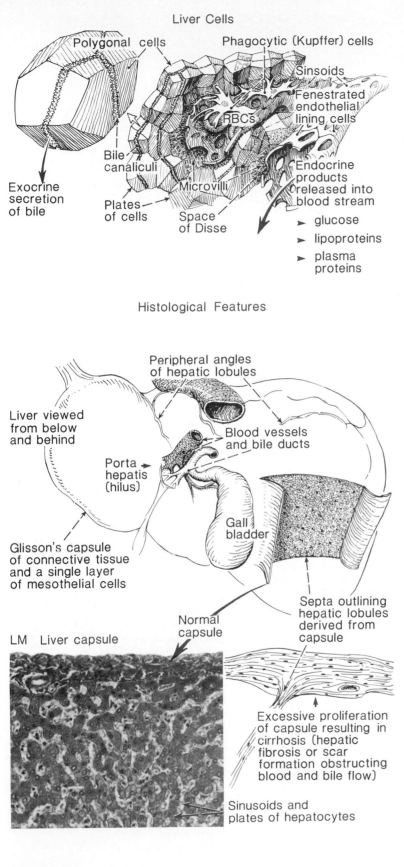

Liver Cells

Polygonal cells

Phagocytic (Kupffer) cells

Sinsoids

Fenestrated endothelial lining cells

RBCs

Bile canaliculi

Microvilli

Plates of cells

Space of Disse

Exocrine secretion of bile

Endocrine products released into blood stream

► glucose

► lipoproteins

► plasma proteins

Histological Features

Peripheral angles of hepatic lobules

Liver viewed from below and behind

Blood vessels and bile ducts

Porta hepatis (hilus)

Gall bladder

Glisson's capsule of connective tissue and a single layer of mesothelial cells

Normal capsule

Septa outlining hepatic lobules derived from capsule

LM Liver capsule

Excessive proliferation of capsule resulting in cirrhosis (hepatic fibrosis or scar formation obstructing blood and bile flow)

Sinusoids and plates of hepatocytes

Partially lining the irregular **hepatic sinusoids** that separate the plates of liver cells are the **phagocytic (Kupffer) cells.** They recognize and engulf whole and fragmented senile red blood cells. They recycle some of the red blood cell constituents, e.g., iron and copper, to be reused in blood formation.

The liver is both an exocrine and an endocrine gland. Its **exocrine secretion is bile.** Its **endocrine products** released into the bloodstream include glucose (largely derived from glycogen), lipoproteins, and plasma proteins.

That the **liver is essential to life** is mirrored by the wide range of vital biochemical processes it performs. Its complete removal is invariably fatal in experimental animals. Yet, if only one third of the liver remains in situ, no clinical signs of hepatic insufficiency appear. In a few days, the liver cells have **regenerated** and the liver has returned to its normal size.

Histological Features

CAPSULE Except where the liver is attached to the diaphragm, it is completely surrounded by **Glisson's capsule,** a thin connective tissue investment covered by a single layer of **mesothelial cells.** At the **porta hepatis,** or hilus, where blood vessels and bile ducts enter and leave the liver, the **capsule thickens** and is carried into the liver to blend with the connective tissue that surrounds blood vessels and bile ducts, especially in the **portal areas or canals.** These areas are connective tissue spaces where the **peripheral angles** or corners of the hepatic lobules come together. Also, the connective tissue **septa** outlining the hepatic lobules are derived from the capsule. The **stroma** surrounding each liver cell is a network of **reticular fibers,** only clearly demonstrable with special stains, e.g., silver impregnation.

Although the capsule is thin and inconspicuous, it functions as a tough, outer "stocking" to give **support and shape to the liver.** Its covering of mesothelial cells serves as a protective bactericidal shield against the invasion of pathogenic bacteria and other harmful organisms.

Cirrhosis When the capsule or its derivatives undergo excessive proliferation, the resulting fibrosis (scar formation) is called **cirrhosis,** a life-threatening condition. Cirrhosis of the liver (hepatic fibrosis) is a common cause of death, especially in men. It is manifested by **excessive amounts of connective tissue** forming principally around the central veins, in the portal canals, and surrounding the hepatocytes. As a result of this extensive scarring, **blood and bile flow** is **obstructed** or curtailed, and the supply of oxygen and nutrients to the liver cells is impaired. The hepatocytes, denied these nutrients, die and are replaced by scar tissue.

4055

Lobulation

HEPATIC LOBULE The classic hepatic lobule is the **anatomical unit of the liver.** It is a prismatic, polyhedral or cylindrical structure about 0.7–2 mm in diameter and surrounded by a connective tissue barrier of variable thickness derived from Glisson's capsule. **Sheets or plates of cells,** one to two cells thick, radiate outward from the **central vein** that serves as the central axis of the lobule. Because the sheets in histological sections are usually seen in profile, they appear as cords of cells. Earlier they were so described until three-dimensional reconstructions clearly revealed the cells to be arranged in **irregular, interconnecting plates.** Lying between the plates are the **blood sinusoids** fed by branches of the **hepatic artery** and the **hepatic portal vein,** both residents of the portal canals located at the corners of the lobule. The **mixed arterial and venous blood** percolates through the sinusoids to empty into the central vein. Thus the lobule is designed to maximize the exchange of nutrients between the hepatocytes and the blood flowing through the sinusoids.

Another important concept associated with the hepatic lobule is **bile production** and its direction of flow. After synthesis in the hepatocyte, the bile moves toward the lateral cell surface that abuts onto an adjacent hepatocyte. Here it enters a tiny, tubular, unlined space between the cells called a **bile canaliculus,** limited only by the plasmalemmae of the two adjacent liver cells. The canaliculi form a complex, intercommunicating network that conveys the bile toward the outer perimeter of the lobules to join the **bile ductules** (Hering's canals) at the periphery. These ductules coalesce to form the **interlobular bile ducts** in the portal canals. Thus the bile flow is opposite to the blood circulation.

Clinical Comment The arrangement of cells surrounding the central vein provides an explanation why these cells are the most severely damaged from ingested poisons, such as carbon tetrachloride and other hydrocarbons. The **cells nearest the central vein** receive the poorest oxygen supply. They are therefore always **hypoxic** since they are the farthest away from the source of oxygenated blood which is depleted by the rapid uptake of the other cells bordering the sinusoids. The central cells are therefore the most vulnerable to death, a condition called **centrilobular necrosis.**

PORTAL LOBULE Dissatisfaction with the concept that the hepatic lobule is also a unit of function has resulted in the identification of the **portal lobule** as a **physiological unit** of the liver.

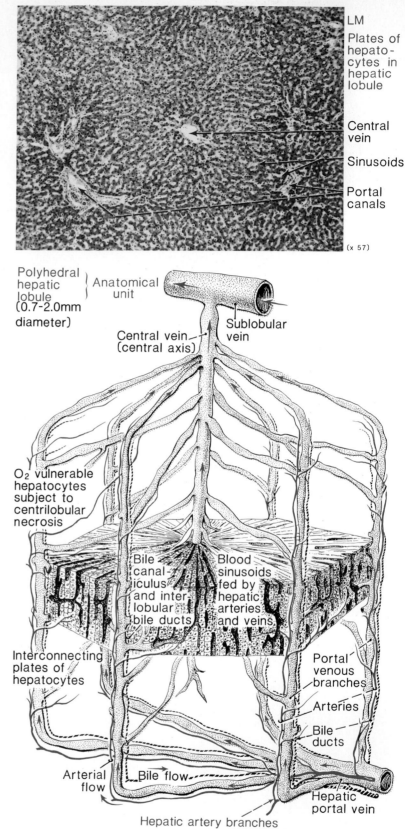

LM
Plates of hepatocytes in hepatic lobule

Central vein

Sinusoids

Portal canals

(x 57)

Polyhedral hepatic lobule (0.7-2.0mm diameter)

Anatomical unit

Central vein (central axis)

Sublobular vein

O₂ vulnerable hepatocytes subject to centrilobular necrosis

Bile canaliculus and interlobular bile ducts

Blood sinusoids fed by hepatic arteries and veins

Interconnecting plates of hepatocytes

Portal venous branches

Arteries

Bile ducts

Arterial flow

Bile flow

Hepatic portal vein

Hepatic artery branches

LM   Central vein of hepatic lobule

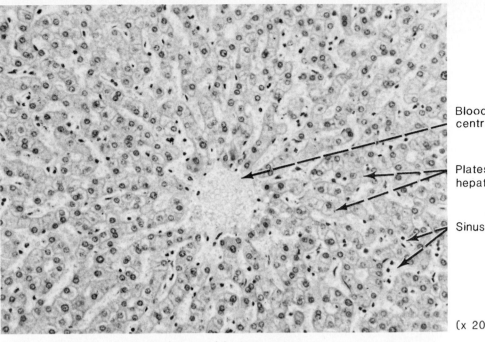

Blood cells ir
central vein

Plates of
hepatocytes

Sinusoids

(x 200)

SEM   Central vein and plates of hepatocytes

Fenestrated
wall of
central vein

Sinusoids
between
plates of
hepatocytes

M.J. Koering
(x 200)

Upper LM view: The central vein is the morphological axis of the classic polyhedral liver lobule, towards which interconnecting plates of hepatocytes radiate. The irregular, dilated hepatic sinusoids separating the plates, contain mixed blood, i.e., portal venous and hepatic arterial, which empties into the central vein. From the central vein, the blood flows into a sublobular vein, a tributary of the hepatic veins which join the inferior vena cava.

Lower SEM view: The fenestrated central vein has a very thin wall that is largely replaced by dilated, sinusoidal openings (fenestrations) which allow blood to pass into the lumen. As the vein progresses through the lobule, it acquires more fenestrations. Between each of these openings are a few endothelial cells and macrophages supported by sparse collagenous fibers, which form the thin wall of the vein.

The large portal lobule emphasizes the exocrine functional aspect of the liver, i.e., bile production and flow. Unlike the hepatic lobule, it has **the portal canal (tract)** as its morphological **axis.** From this area, all of the functional modalities of the liver radiate, e.g., branches of the hepatic artery and portal vein, lymphatics, nerves, and bile ducts.

The portal lobule is **triangular** in shape, formed by joining imaginary lines between three central veins of adjacent hepatic lobules. The triangle so enclosed contains contiguous parts of three hepatic lobules that are drained by a **common interlobular bile duct** located in the centrally placed **portal canal.** Since the bile flows from the periphery of the three portal lobules towards the center of the portal lobule (the portal canal), and the blood in the opposite direction, the flow pattern is similar to other exocrine glands.

HEPATIC ACINUS The other physiological unit is the **hepatic acinus.** It is the smallest functional unit of the liver. The acinar concept is based on the observation that the **blood supply** to cells surrounding a central vein comes from **several sources,** namely, from the branches of the hepatic artery and portal vein located in the portal canals at the corners of each hepatic lobule. Therefore, these hepatic cells, with their own blood supply, dangle from the central vein like grapes on a stem, hence the term, **liver acinus.**

By definition, a liver acinus is an irregular, **diamond-shaped,** unencapsulated mass of liver cells lying **between two central veins.** Its longitudinal **axis** (backbone) is a small radicle of the portal canal extending along the periphery of the hepatic lobule. It contains **terminal branches** of the portal vein and hepatic artery, an interlobular bile duct, lymphatics, and nerves. These structures service the cells on each side of the axis, i.e., the portions of two adjacent hepatic lobules that form a hepatic acinus.

Cells within each acinus are **segregated into concentric zones** relative to their proximity to the vascular backbone of the acinus. Those cells closest to the nutrient vessels (**zone 1**) **receive the most oxygen and nutrients.** Therefore they will survive better life-threatening episodes, e.g., poisoning and anoxia, and will regenerate faster. Cells in the intermediate area (zone 2) will receive blood of **poorer quality** and will be less able to survive damage. In zone 3, the area furthest from the oxygen and food supply, the cells will have the **poorest blood supply,** will be the first to die, and regeneration will be poor. To some extent, it is this zonation that explains the selective damage of certain liver cells to various poisons and diseases.

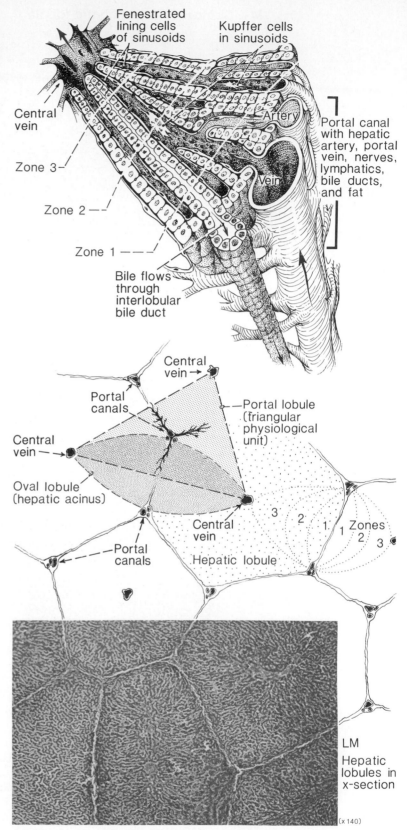

LM
Hepatic lobules in x-section

(x 140)

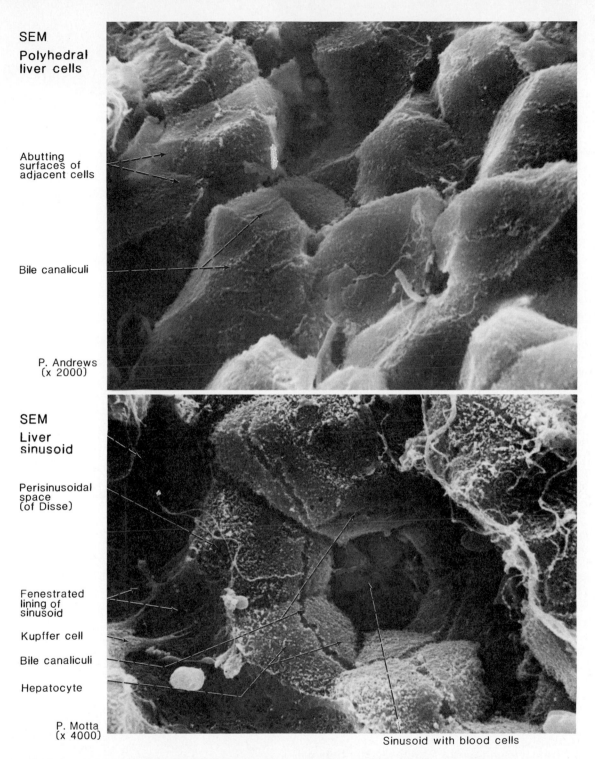

SEM
Polyhedral
liver cells

Abutting
surfaces of
adjacent cells

Bile canaliculi

P. Andrews
(x 2000)

SEM
Liver
sinusoid

Perisinusoidal
space
(of Disse)

Fenestrated
lining of
sinusoid

Kupffer cell

Bile canaliculi

Hepatocyte

P. Motta
(x 4000)

Sinusoid with blood cells

Upper micrograph. Scanning electron micrograph of mammalian liver, sectioned to demonstrate its internal structure. Plates of polyhedral hepatocytes line the alternating sinusoids. When liver cells are sectioned or fractured, numerous bile canaliculi on the opposing surfaces of the liver cells expose their irregular lumina lined with microvilli.

Lower micrograph. Scanning electron micrograph of liver sinusoids. The central, transversely sectioned sinusoid reveals a circular lumen completely lined by plates of hepatocytes and partially filled with blood cells. Branching bile canaliculi are uncovered to display irregular lining surfaces with projecting microvilli. The sinusoid on the left, sectioned longitudinally, exposes the lining cells, i.e., endothelial cells and phagocytic (Kupffer) cells. The endothelial lining cells contain fenestrations (pores) that provide a filtration barrier shielding the space of Disse from large particles in the circulating blood but permits smaller particles, such as lipoproteins, to be exchanged between the space and the sinusoidal lumen. A stellate Kupffer cell is stretched part way across the lumen.

Hepatocytes

Hepatocytes, the parenchymal cells of the liver, occupy about 60% of the organ. The other cells are the lining cells of sinusoids, cells of arteries, veins, lymphatics and bile ducts, and connective tissue cells. The **hepatocyte** is perhaps the most versatile cell in the body. Each cell **performs** practically all of the **many and varied functions** of the liver without any apparent division of labor or cell specialization. Morphologically all hepatocytes are essentially identical, except for slight variations in size and staining intensity, the latter depending largely on the relative amounts of glycogen and fats stored in the cell.

The typical liver cell is a polyhedron about 30 μm in diameter, with **six or more sides.** Each cell has **three types of surfaces.** (1) Externally, one or more surfaces **contact the wall of the sinusoid** at the perisinusoidal spaces (of Disse). (2) Internally, other surfaces **abut on adjacent liver cells.** (3) Some surface areas **face the bile canaliculi** that are located between adjacent liver cells. Opposing surfaces of two hepatic cells contribute to the formation of the canaliculus. The cells have no basement membrane.

The **cytoplasm** of hepatocytes is **granular and eosinophilic** due to the many large, round or elongated **mitochondria** and the abundance of **sER.** Within the sER occurs the detoxification of drugs, synthesis of cholesterol, and conversion of glycogen into glucose. The **rER** forms clusters of flattened cisternae dispersed throughout the cytoplasm. These structures were recognized by early light microscopists as the basophilic bodies or **ergastoplasm.** Here, blood fibrinogen (a blood-clotting protein), prothrombin (a blood anticoagulant), and blood albumin are synthesized.

Golgi complexes are numerous, perhaps 50 in a single cell. Each aggregate has three to five closely packed cisternae with bulbous vesicles, some filled with electron-dense particles. The Golgi complexes tend to cluster around the bile canaliculi and the hepatic cell nucleus.

Another prominent cytoplasmic component is **glycogen,** which is stored in large amounts in the liver. Glycogen appears in electron micrographs as dense, coarse clusters of fine granules that congregate around the sER profiles. Glycogen may appear as single tiny granules, the **beta particles,** about 30 nm in diameter, or as a berry or **rosette,** the **alpha particles,** a cluster of granules about 90–100 nm in diameter. The amount of glycogen stored at any given time in the liver depends on the nutritional state of the animal. Following a meal, deposition and removal of glycogen occurs in a few hours in a precise sequence. It is **initially deposited in the outermost cells** of the hepatic lobule. The cells surrounding the central vein are the **last to receive glycogen.**

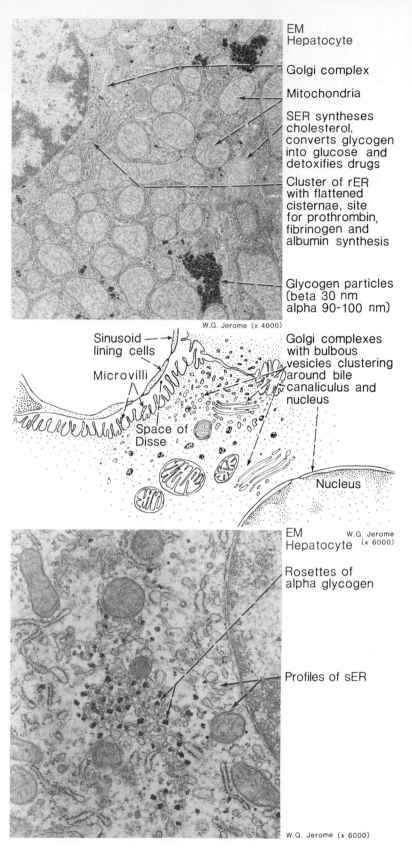

EM Hepatocyte

Golgi complex

Mitochondria

SER syntheses cholesterol, converts glycogen into glucose and detoxifies drugs

Cluster of rER with flattened cisternae, site for prothrombin, fibrinogen and albumin synthesis

Glycogen particles (beta 30 nm alpha 90-100 nm)

W.G. Jerome (x 4000)

Sinusoid lining cells

Microvilli

Space of Disse

Golgi complexes with bulbous vesicles clustering around bile canaliculus and nucleus

Nucleus

W.G. Jerome (x 6000)

EM Hepatocyte

Rosettes of alpha glycogen

Profiles of sER

W.G. Jerome (x 6000)

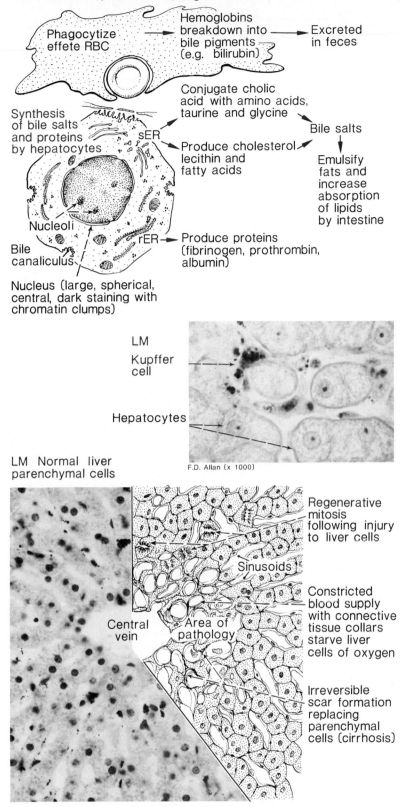

Functions of hepatic macrophages (Kupffer cells)

Phagocytize effete RBC

Hemoglobins breakdown into bile pigments (e.g. bilirubin) → Excreted in feces

Synthesis of bile salts and proteins by hepatocytes

sER

Conjugate cholic acid with amino acids, taurine and glycine

Produce cholesterol lecithin and fatty acids

Bile salts

Emulsify fats and increase absorption of lipids by intestine

Nucleoli

Bile canaliculus

rER → Produce proteins (fibrinogen, prothrombin, albumin)

Nucleus (large, spherical, central, dark staining with chromatin clumps)

LM Kupffer cell

Hepatocytes

F.D. Allan (x 1000)

LM Normal liver parenchymal cells

Regenerative mitosis following injury to liver cells

Sinusoids

Central vein

Area of pathology

Constricted blood supply with connective tissue collars starve liver cells of oxygen

Irreversible scar formation replacing parenchymal cells (cirrhosis)

Also stored in the liver are **numerous lipids,** e.g., cholesterol, fatty acids, triglycerides, and neutral fats. Neither fats nor glycogen are retained in the cell after most histological procedures since glycogen is soluble in water, and fats in alcohol. Therefore, the cytoplasm of liver cells, as seen in paraffin sections, has an empty, **spongy, flocculent appearance,** because the sites of fat and glycogen deposition are now empty.

EXOCRINE FUNCTIONS The principal exocrine function of the liver cells is the **secretion of bile** that is synthesized in the hepatocyte. The main **bile components** are bile pigments (mostly bilirubin), bile salts, cholesterol, phospholipids largely as lecithin, fatty acids, water, and electrolytes. The only components not produced in the hepatocytes are the bile pigments, especially **bilirubin.** These pigments are derived as **breakdown products of hemoglobin.** The degradation is accomplished by phagocytosis of effete RBCs, mostly in the spleen; however, the hepatic macrophages (Kupffer cells) undoubtedly play a role. The bile pigments are largely inert and are excreted with the feces.

The **bile salts** are synthesized in the sER of hepatocytes by conjugation of cholic acid with amino acids, taurine, and glycine. Also produced by sER are cholesterol, lecithin, and certain fatty acids. The bile salts are responsible for the detergent and **emulsifying actions** of bile on fats. They also increase the absorption of lipids by the intestine.

ENDOCRINE FUNCTIONS The endocrine functions of the liver are largely **related to protein synthesis.** Several proteins are produced by the hepatocytes for export into the bloodstream. These substances are produced in the **rER** but are not stored in the cell as secretory granules, as in other glands; rather, they are **released continuously** into the bloodstream. These proteins include fibrinogen, prothrombin, and albumin, the most abundant plasma protein. (Table 19.1 is a comparison of the pancreas and liver.)

LIVER REGENERATION Mitosis is rare in the normal adult liver. However, the damaged liver is **repaired very rapidly** by the mitotic activity of hepatocytes. For example, if a portion of the liver is excised in an animal, the tissue deficit is completely restored in a few days by **mitosis of hepatocytes** adjacent to the incision. Usually the regenerated tissue is identical to the excised tissue. However, repeated episodes of liver damage, e.g., certain nutritional deficiencies, alcohol abuse, and repeated liver infections may upset the ordered pattern of cellular repair. Such a derangement causes an exaggerated production of connective tissue resulting in **scar formation** that replaces the parenchymal cells. This condition is called cirrhosis, discussed on page 379.

Blood Supply

The blood that bathes the hepatocytes comes from two different sources, i.e., about two thirds of the blood is derived from the **portal vein** that drains the digestive tract rich in nutrients and from the spleen. The remaining blood, rich in oxygen, comes by way of the **hepatic artery.** Both vessels enter the liver at the porta hepatis. They divide into **interlobar** branches to serve the various lobes of the liver. Further subdivisions yield **interlobular vessels** that enter the portal areas (canals) at the periphery of the hepatic lobules, accompanied by interlobular bile ducts. These three structures, an artery, vein, and bile duct, comprise the **portal triad** of the portal canal.

Branches of the interlobular arteries do not follow the venous distribution. For example, **terminal arterioles** of the interlobular hepatic artery have **several courses.** Some supply blood to **capillaries** for the connective tissue in the **portal tract** and for the interlobular bile ducts. Others may **empty directly** into the interlobular veins, the terminal distributing veins, or directly into the hepatic vein. Some terminal arterioles **flow into the hepatic sinusoids.** About 25% of all arterial blood flows in the latter course. In contrast, the terminal branches of the interlobular portal veins, called distributing veins, divide into small, short branches, the inlet venules, that lead directly into the sinusoids.

Mixing of venous and arterial blood occurs only in the **hepatic sinusoids,** as it flows centrally into the central vein, the central axis of the hepatic lobule. The central vein has several unusual features. It has **no smooth muscle** in its walls, which contain only endothelial cells supported by a thin layer of collagen fibers. Also, its **walls** are extensively **perforated** by the sinusoids that empty into the vein.

At the base of each lobule, the central vein connects at right angles with a large **sublobular vein,** which has a distinct outer longitudinal and inner circular muscle layer, and a complete endothelial lining. Unaccompanied by other structures, such as vessels or ducts, the sublobular veins course through the parenchyma of the liver and **enter the connective tissue trabeculae.** Several sublobular veins join to form the **larger collecting veins,** which merge to form two or more **hepatic veins** that drain into the **inferior vena cava.**

Blood Supply to Hepatocytes

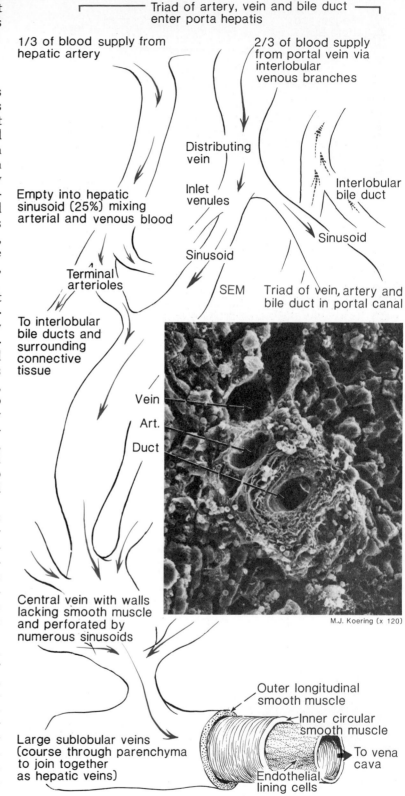

M.J. Koering (x 120)

4104

SEM   Hepatic Sinusoid

Bile canaliculi

Surfaces of hepatocytes

Microvilli from hepatocytes projecting into space of Disse

Entrapped RBCs

Phagocytic Kupffer cell

Non-phagocytic squamous endothelial cells lining sinusoid

Fenestrated wall

P. Motta (x 4000)

Hepatic lobules

Network of small lymphatic vessels

Glisson's capsule and septa

Lymphatics

Central vein of lobule

Hepatic vein

Lymph vessels

Main branches of portal vein, bile duct & hepatic artery

Connective tissue investments containing lymphatics

Lymph passes to hilus

SINUSOIDS Hepatic sinusoids meet all of the criteria for a conventional sinusoid, as discussed in Chapter 13. However, they differ from the typical sinusoids by their **larger diameter** (9–12 μm), their **lack of a continuous basal lamina,** and their sinusoidal **lining cells** consisting of two and possibly **three types of cells.** (1) The large, **stellate Kupffer cells** are avidly phagocytic, and usually have phagocytized particulate matter and fragments of red blood cells within their cytoplasm. They have protoplasmic processes that extend across the lumen of the sinusoids that slow down the movement of the blood. Kupffer cells are actually a part of the sinusoidal lining, interposed between the other lining cells. (2) Squamous, nonphagocytic **endothelial (littoral) cells** have an oval nucleus bulging into the lumen. They are **discontinuous,** that is, they are not attached to one another, as typical endothelium, but loosely overlap. Therefore gaps or **fenestrations** exist between the cells that allow passage of blood protein molecules (150–400 nm) but not blood cells or platelets. (3) Some **typical endothelial cells** may also contribute to the lining of sinusoids. (For a summary of circulation, see page 389.)

PERISINUSOIDAL SPACE OF DISSE Before leaving the discussion of the hepatic sinusoids, a brief comment about the **space of Disse** is needed. The lining cells of the sinusoids do not fit snugly over the internal surface of the liver cell that borders on the sinusoid. Between the lining cells and the hepatocytes is an unlined space of variable size, the **perisinusoidal space (of Disse)** that contains **blood plasma** but normally no blood cells. Projecting into the space are large numbers of short microvilli from the surfaces of hepatocytes bordering the space. The **microvilli,** constantly bathed in blood plasma, greatly **accelerate the exchange of metabolites** between the liver cells and the bloodstream. Within the space can be seen a few fibroblastic-like cells containing lipid granules. Their function is uncertain.

Lymphatics

The liver produces more lymph than any other organ of the body. Estimates range from 500 to 700 ml/day or from one third to one half of the body's total daily production. Yet no **lymphatics** have been demonstrated in the **lobule,** supposedly the site of synthesis for most of the lymph. However, **lymph vessels** have been described, but only among the **connective tissue elements** of the liver, e.g., the capsule and its septa that penetrate the gland, the connective tissue investments of the blood vessels and ducts that enter and leave at the **hilus,** and in the portal canals that border the lobule and supply a network of small lymphatic vessels and capillaries. Because of the high permeability of the cells lining the liver sinusoids, it has been postulated

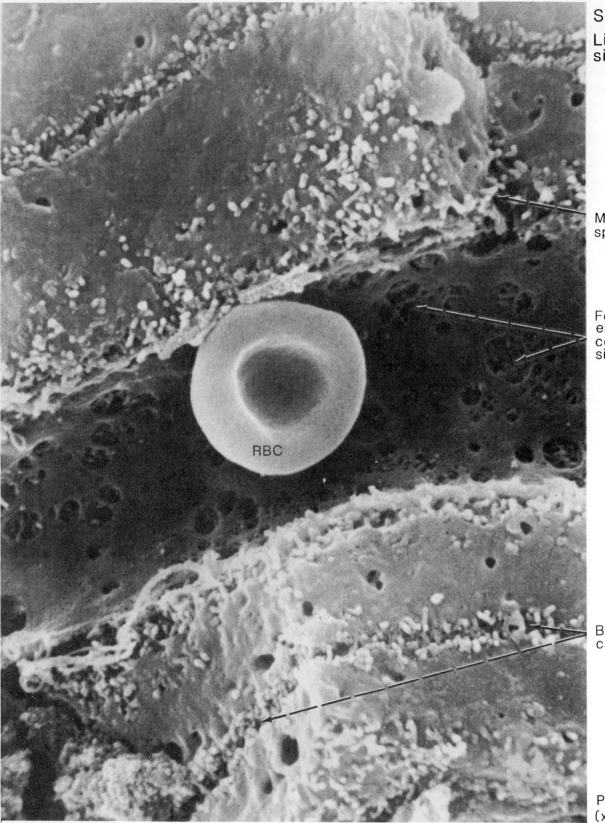

SEM
Liver
sinusoid

Microvilli in
space of Disse

Fenestrated
endothelial
cells lining
sinusoid

Bile
canaliculus

RBC

P. Motta
(x 13,000)

Scanning electron micrograph of a hepatic sinusoid. The hepatic cells have been sectioned to expose longitudinal views of bile canaliculi with many microvilli. Within the sinusoidal lumen, a single red blood cell dominates the center of the field, furnishing the clue that the lumen is about 10 μm in diameter. Fenestrated endothelial cells line the sinusoid. The fenestrations (pores) are connections between the sinusoid and the space of Disse.

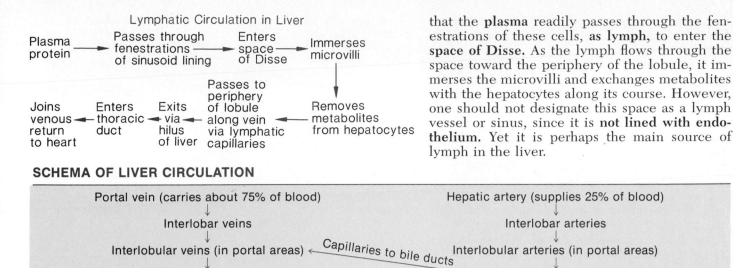

Lymphatic Circulation in Liver

Plasma protein → Passes through fenestrations of sinusoid lining → Enters space of Disse → Immerses microvilli

Joins venous return to heart ← Enters thoracic duct ← Exits via hilus of liver ← Passes to periphery of lobule along vein via lymphatic capillaries ← Removes metabolites from hepatocytes

that the **plasma** readily passes through the fenestrations of these cells, **as lymph,** to enter the **space of Disse.** As the lymph flows through the space toward the periphery of the lobule, it immerses the microvilli and exchanges metabolites with the hepatocytes along its course. However, one should not designate this space as a lymph vessel or sinus, since it is **not lined with endothelium.** Yet it is perhaps the main source of lymph in the liver.

SCHEMA OF LIVER CIRCULATION

Portal vein (carries about 75% of blood)　　Hepatic artery (supplies 25% of blood)

Interlobar veins　　Interlobar arteries

Interlobular veins (in portal areas) ← Capillaries to bile ducts → Interlobular arteries (in portal areas)

Distributing veins (in periphery of lobule) ← Terminal arterioles

Inlet venules (penetrate periphery of lobule)

Hepatic sinusoids (common terminus for venous and arterial blood)

Central (centrolobular) veins

Sublobular veins

Collecting veins

Hepatic veins (two or more)

Inferior vena cava

Bile Synthesis by Hepatocytes

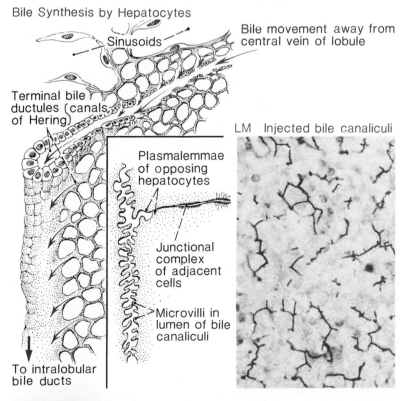

Sinusoids

Bile movement away from central vein of lobule

Terminal bile ductules (canals of Hering)

Plasmalemmae of opposing hepatocytes

Junctional complex of adjacent cells

Microvilli in lumen of bile canaliculi

To intralobular bile ducts

LM　Injected bile canaliculi

THE BILIARY TRACT

Depending on location, the passageways of the biliary tract are divided into an intrahepatic and an extrahepatic portion.

Intrahepatic Division

The components of the intrahepatic division are: (1) bile canaliculi, (2) terminal bile ductules (canals of Hering or cholangioles), and (3) interlobular bile ducts.

The **bile canaliculi,** about 0.5–1.0 μm wide, have no distinct walls of their own but are formed by the grooving of the **plasmalemmae of apposing hepatocytes.** The canaliculi form a regular, fine network that connects adjacent hepatic cells. The plasma membranes of the abutting hepatocytes are tightly bound at the canaliculus by extensive **junctional complexes,** especially occluding and gap junctions. Short microvilli from the hepatocytes project into the lumen of the canaliculus. **Bile is synthesized by the liver cells. It** is secreted into these minute passageways, which drain the bile centrifugally, from the central vein area to the periphery of the hepatic lobule where they empty into the **terminal bile ductules.**

The terminal ductules or **canals of Hering** are short, narrow connecting channels that transport the bile from the peripheral canaliculi to the **interlobular bile ducts** in the portal areas. The ductules are about 10–20 μm in diameter and are lined with simple, **low cuboidal** epithelial cells that undergo frequent mitoses. These small, clear, lining cells have many junctional complexes, a thin basal lamina, and a few cytoplasmic organelles.

In the portal areas, the conspicuous **interlobular bile duct** is a component of the **portal triad.** These bile ducts are lined with simple, **tall cuboidal** epithelium with striated apical borders and have a distinct connective tissue investment. Some of the cells may contain lipid droplets. These ducts increase in diameter by fusing together, as they proceed, with the other components of the triad (branches of the hepatic artery and portal vein) to join other interlobular ducts to eventually form the **right and left hepatic ducts** that exit the liver at the porta.

Extrahepatic Division

The extrahepatic biliary passageways are: (1) the right and left hepatic ducts, (2) common hepatic duct, (3) cystic duct, (4) gallbladder, (5) common bile duct, and (6) ampulla. These structures, especially the larger ducts, have walls consisting of three layers: (1) a **mucosa** with a prominent lamina propria, (2) a **muscularis,** and (3) an **adventitia or serosa.**

BILIARY DUCTS The right and left **hepatic ducts** join to form the **common hepatic duct** which, with the **cystic duct** (draining the gallbladder), forms the **common bile duct.** All of the various ducts have similar histological features. They are all lined with **simple columnar epithelium** with a prominent striated apical border, a few goblet cells in certain regions, and a well-developed **basal lamina. Elastic fibers** are prominent in the lamina propria as well as mucous and occasionally serous **glands.** Also, many **lymphocytes** and a few granulocytes are present in the lamina propria before they migrate through the epithelium into the lumen of the duct.

Smooth muscle fibers form a definite **muscularis,** but its layers are usually **indistinct** and freely interlace. Only in the common bile duct and gallbladder are the different layers discernible. Here most fibers are arranged longitudinally with a few directed obliquely. As the duct system nears the duodenum, the muscle **layers become more distinct** and with more circular fibers. At the junction with the **ampulla,** these muscle fibers form a **sphincter** to regulate the flow of bile into the duodenum. The adventitia of these larger ducts is largely composed of collagenous fibers.

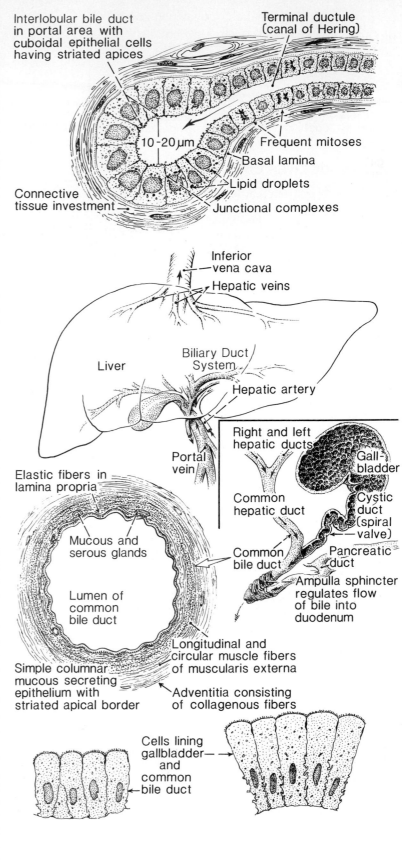

Interlobular bile duct in portal area with cuboidal epithelial cells having striated apices

Terminal ductule (canal of Hering)

10-20 μm

Frequent mitoses

Basal lamina

Lipid droplets

Junctional complexes

Connective tissue investment

Inferior vena cava

Hepatic veins

Liver

Biliary Duct System

Hepatic artery

Portal vein

Right and left hepatic ducts

Gallbladder

Common hepatic duct

Cystic duct (spiral valve)

Common bile duct

Pancreatic duct

Ampulla sphincter regulates flow of bile into duodenum

Elastic fibers in lamina propria

Mucous and serous glands

Lumen of common bile duct

Longitudinal and circular muscle fibers of muscularis externa

Adventitia consisting of collagenous fibers

Simple columnar mucous secreting epithelium with striated apical border

Cells lining gallbladder— and common bile duct

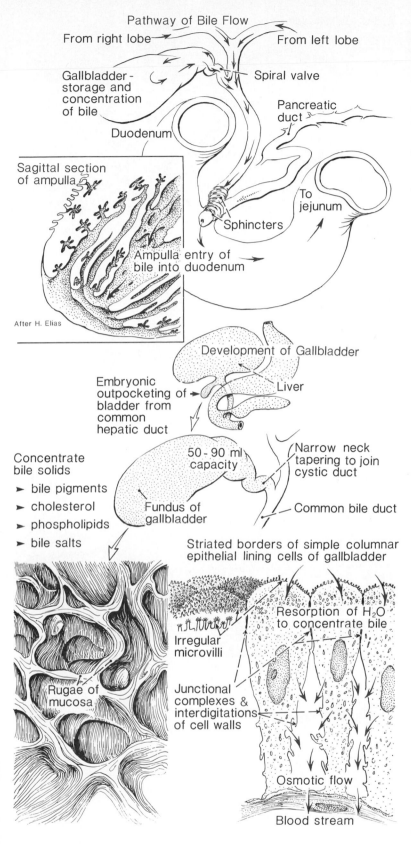

Pathway of Bile Flow

From right lobe → ← From left lobe

Gallbladder - storage and concentration of bile

Spiral valve

Duodenum

Pancreatic duct

Sagittal section of ampulla

To jejunum

Sphincters

Ampulla entry of bile into duodenum

After H. Elias

Development of Gallbladder

Embryonic outpocketing of bladder from common hepatic duct

Liver

50 - 90 ml capacity

Narrow neck tapering to join cystic duct

Concentrate bile solids

► bile pigments
► cholesterol
► phospholipids
► bile salts

Fundus of gallbladder

Common bile duct

Striated borders of simple columnar epithelial lining cells of gallbladder

Resorption of H₂O to concentrate bile

Irregular microvilli

Junctional complexes & interdigitations of cell walls

Rugae of mucosa

Osmotic flow

Blood stream

Bile flow from the common hepatic duct has **two possible pathways.** It may bypass the cystic duct and the gallbladder to empty directly into the **common bile duct.** However, the bile usually traverses the **cystic duct** to enter the gallbladder for storage and concentration. The stimulus of food in the gut causes the bile to be released from the gallbladder via the cystic duct into the common bile duct to enter the duodenum at the ampulla.

GALLBLADDER Some mammals, such as the horse and rat, do not have a gallbladder. However, they do possess the other components of the biliary system. In humans, **removal of the gallbladder** usually has little effect on the normal functioning of the digestive system, although the bile is now constantly excreted into the small intestine rather than intermittently. The gallbladder's only service is to temporarily **store and concentrate the bile,** apparently a nonessential function for the well-being of the individual.

The normal gallbladder in humans is a pear-shaped, hollow, muscular organ **arising embryonically** as an outpocketing **of the common hepatic duct.** It is divided into a large, blind-ending, rounded **fundus;** a cylindrical main portion, the **body,** which tapers into the narrow **neck** region. It is attached to the liver by the **cystic duct,** which is the continuation of the narrow neck of the gallbladder. The gallbladder has a normal capacity of about 50–90 ml, is 7–10 cm in length, and about 2–3 cm wide.

The mucosa shows many **rugae** that are subdivided into **minute folds.** As seen in histological sections, these tiny folds **resemble villi** and their bases suggest glands (L-A, plate 20). However, **neither glands or villi are present** in the fundic and body regions. However, the neck region has numerous mucous glands in the lamina propria, and many goblet cells are interspersed between the lining epithelial cells. When the bladder is distended with bile, the wall becomes thinner and all folds, except the largest, disappear. The **simple columnar** epithelial cells have a thin striated border that is poorly demonstrated with the light microscope. Yet it is very effective in the **resorption of water,** resulting in the concentration of the solids in bile, e.g., bile pigments, cholesterol, phospholipids, and bile salts, by three- to ten-fold.

Electron micrographs reveal an abundance of short, irregular **microvilli** covering the apical surface of each epithelial cell. The cell margins are bound together by junctional complexes and, laterally, the adjacent cell walls interdigitate. Therefore, the water in the bile must pass through the apices of the cells since the **zonulae occludentes** severely limit intercellular passage.

The muscularis consists of thin layers of **irregularly arranged smooth muscle** fibers richly laced with **elastic fibers** and some collagenous fibers. The innermost fibers are arranged longitudinally. The remaining larger muscle groups are circularly disposed.

The outermost layer, the serosa, consists of a rather dense connective tissue layer covered by **mesothelium** (the peritoneum). This layer is continuous with the capsule of the liver. Many blood and lymph vessels are present within the layer.

CLINICAL COMMENT Dysfunction of the biliary system, such as the insufficient synthesis of bile, failure of the release of bile from the gallbladder, or blockage of any of the bile passageways (causing jaundice), may result in **poor absorption** from the gut of fats and the fat-soluble vitamins A, D, E, and K. These individual vitamin deficiencies may precipitate a variety of **clinical disorders,** such as, respectively, night blindness, rickets, and sterility and hemophilia in animals. (See Table 19.2 for a summary of the histology of the biliary passageways.)

Wall of Gallbladder

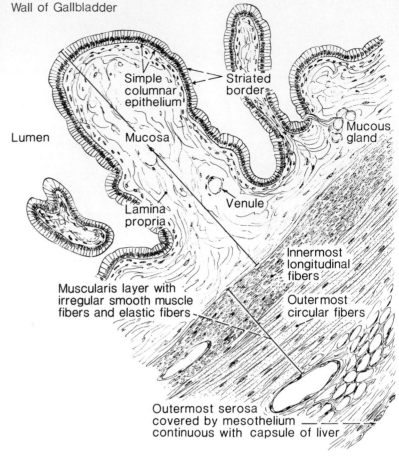

LM   Wall of gall bladder   LM

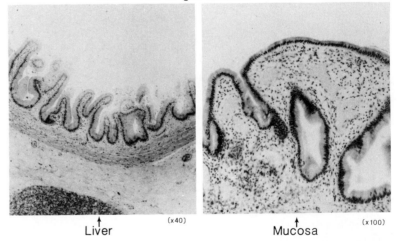

Table 19.1 *COMPARISON OF LIVER AND PANCREAS*

	LIVER	PANCREAS
Classification	Compound tubular gland	Compound tubuloacinar gland
Parenchyma • Exocrine components	Serous cuboidal cells in irregular plates, organized in radial fashion around central vein of hepatic lobule; basophilic granular cytoplasm	Serous pyramidal cells arranged in acini, resemble parotid; basal cytoplasm, basophilic; apical cytoplasm, slightly acidophilic with zymogen granules
• Endocrine components	No specific cells for synthesis of various protein endocrine secretions, e.g., albumin, prothrombin, and fibrinogen, all produced by hepatocytes	Islet tissue contains: alpha cells, produce glucagon; beta cells, insulin; delta cells, may produce somatostatin; C cells may be reserve or degenerating cells of any of the above
Stroma	Dense connective tissue capsule mostly covered by mesothelium; septa from capsule enter parenchyma to outline hepatic lobules; reticular fibers separate liver cells	Thin connective tissue capsule with septa which subdivide organ into poorly defined lobules; wisps of reticular tissue separate acini
Duct system	Intrahepatic: bile canaliculi → terminal bile ductules (cholangioles) → interlobular bile ducts; extrahepatic: right and left hepatic ducts → common hepatic duct → cystic duct → gallbladder → common bile duct empties into duodenum	Begins with centroacinar cells as origin of intercalated ducts → interlobular ducts which coalesce to form either the main excretory duct or the accessory excretory duct, both join the common bile duct to enter the duodenum
Blood supply	Afferent vessels: branches of portal vein and hepatic artery drain into hepatic sinusoids; efferent vessels (veins) begin as central veins → sublobular veins → collecting veins → two or more hepatic veins → inferior vena cava	Arterioles from branches of the aorta provide capillary network around lobules; veins accompany arteries
Secretions	Exocrine: bile; endocrine: glucose, lipoproteins, plasma proteins, fibrinogen and prothrombin	Exocrine: pancreatic juice contains enzymes trypsinogen, amylase, maltase, and lipase; endocrine: cells of islet tissue synthesize glucagon (alpha cells), insulin (beta cells), and somatostatin (delta cells)
Control of secretions	Bile secreted continuously by hepatocytes; released from gallbladder only when food entering the gut stimulates production of pancreozymin which causes gallbladder to contract	Enzymes released from acinar cells in response to intestinal hormones secretin and pancreozymin; insulin and glucagon released from islet tissue upon marked increase or decrease of blood sugar levels, respectively

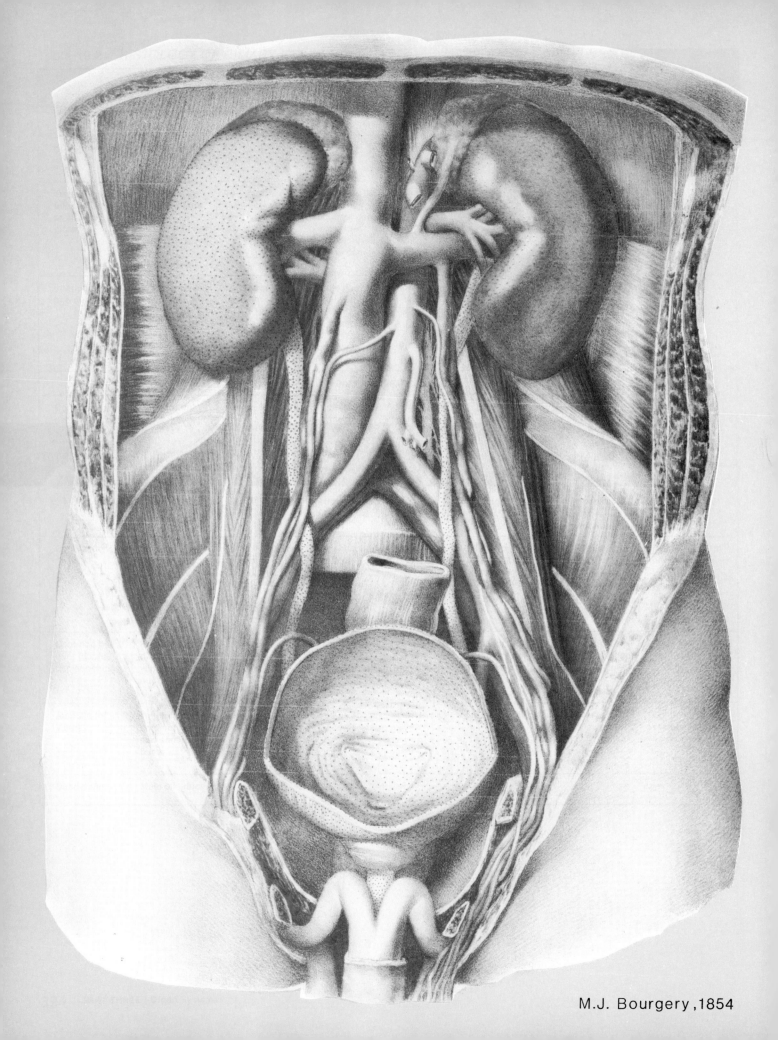

M.J. Bourgery, 1854

OBJECTIVES

FROM THIS CHAPTER THE PERCEPTIVE STUDENT WILL BE ABLE TO:

1. Appraise the kidneys as exquisite filters, designed to eliminate from the blood largely nitrogenous wastes, excess electrolytes, and water.

2. Document the role of the kidneys in the preservation of homeostasis in the body.

3. Extrapolate from its unique vasculature, how the kidney is able to concentrate the urine 100-fold.

4. Conceptualize in a sketch the nephron as the functional and anatomical unit of the kidney.

5. Contrast the function and structure of: ureter vs. urinary bladder, and male vs. female urethra.

6. Assess the kidneys as endocrine organs and how they are affected by certain hormones produced elsewhere in the body.

The urinary system is often incorrectly equated with the excretory system. They are not synonymous. In addition to the urinary system, the diffuse **excretory system** includes such diverse organs as the **skin,** which excretes sweat and oil; the **lungs,** which excrete carbon dioxide and water; and the **large intestine,** whose excrement rivals in quantity the production of urine by the **kidneys.**

The urinary system comprises two bilateral, bean-shaped **kidneys;** two muscular urine conduction tubes, the **ureters;** the **bladder,** a fibromuscular bag for temporary storage and limited concentration of urine; and the **urethra,** the passageway for urine to outside of the body.

Urinary Structures

Cortex

Medulla

Lymph vessels and nerves

Kidney

Major and minor calyces

Capsule

Renal artery and vein

Pyramids in medulla

Medullary rays

Renal pelvis

Arcuate arteries

Interlober artery

Papilla

Ureter

Ureter

Ureter-bladder junction

Bladder

Urethra

Functions of kidneys:

o Excretory
o Homeostatic
o Endocrine

Served by 1,000,000 nephrons

Eliminate nitrogenous blood impurities, electrolytes and water

Secretion of renin (increases blood pressure)

Preserves homeostasis through:

1) ultrafiltration of plasma

2) selective resorption of filtrate

Essential to life

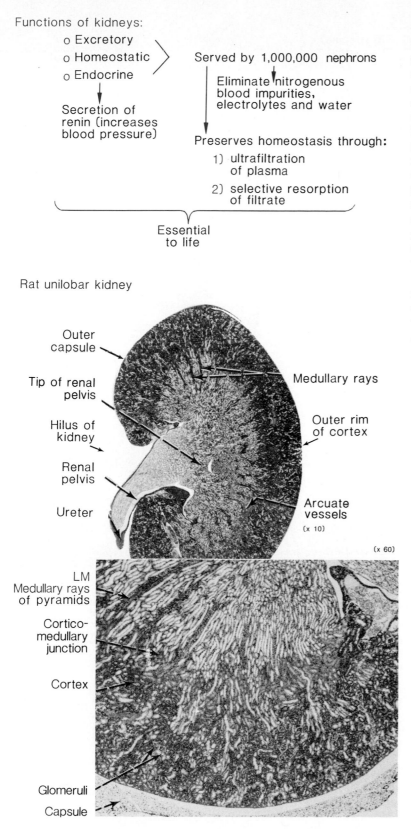

Rat unilobar kidney

Outer capsule

Tip of renal pelvis

Hilus of kidney

Renal pelvis

Ureter

Medullary rays

Outer rim of cortex

Arcuate vessels

(x 10)

(x 60)

LM Medullary rays of pyramids

Cortico-medullary junction

Cortex

Glomeruli

Capsule

KIDNEYS

The kidneys perform vital excretory, homeostatic, and endocrine functions. The first two processes are accomplished by the approximately one million functional units, called **nephrons,** in each kidney. The kidneys are exquisitely sensitive **filters.** They have an extensive array of tubules and blood vessels designed for the **elimination of impurities** from the blood, mostly nitrogenous, and certain excesses, such as electrolytes and water. Equally important, however, is the kidney's role in the preservation of a constant internal environment (homeostasis). A state of **homeostasis** is accomplished by (1) the **ultrafiltration** of the blood plasma and (2) the **resorption** of most of the ultrafiltrate which is qualitatively selective and quantitatively adjustable.

The **endocrine functions** of the kidneys are the release into the bloodstream of the proteolytic enzyme, **renin,** which indirectly increases systemic blood pressure, and **erythropoietin,** which accelerates erythropoiesis. All processes are essential to the health and life of the individual.

General Features

A longitudinal section of a fresh human kidney reveals to the unaided eye several distinctive features. (1) A thin, tough, tightly fitting **capsule** encloses the entire kidney. (2) The **cortex,** a dark brownish, granular, continuous wide outer rim of tissue, lies beneath the capsule. (3) Internal to the cortex is the extensive **medulla** with a radially striated appearance. It is composed of an interrupted series of pale, longitudinally streaked structures, the 10–15 **pyramids or lobes.** (The rat kidney [see opposite view] has only one lobe, i.e., it is unilobar.) (4) At the junction of these two zones is a number of large arched vessels, the **arcuate vessels.** (5) The tips (papillae) of the pyramids project into small epithelium-lined cups or sleeves, the **minor calyces,** that join together to form **major calyces.** (6) The **renal pelvis** is the expanded upper extremity of the ureter that receives the major calyces. (7) A marked, lateral indentation of the concave surface of the kidney is the **hilus,** which marks the site of exit of the ureter, renal vein, lymph vessels and nerves, and the entrance of the renal artery.

A low-power LM view of a hemisection of the kidney reveals additional details. The **corticomedullary junction,** marked by the arcuate vessels, is disrupted by fine streaks of tissue or extensions that issue from the bases of the medullary pyramids. These are the **medullary rays.** They are most prominent in the junctional area where they extend peripherally, fanning out into the cortex, thinning out as they go to finally disappear near the outer edge of the cortex. Their striated appearance is due to the straight tubular and vascular structures within them. These include the straight portions of the **renal tubules** that pass down into the medulla and then loop back to return to the cortex. Also the urinary **collecting tubules** and ducts pass directly from the cortex into the papilla of the pyramid.

Also seen in this section are **cortical labyrinths.** These are areas of cortex wedged between the medullary rays. These regions have a tortuous appearance because of the presence of the many convoluted tubules that are twisted among the profusion of glomeruli. Therefore, these areas are called **pars convoluta** or cortical labyrinths. A matching term, **pars radiata,** is given to the medullary rays.

Another interesting feature is the **cortical columns.** At regular intervals, plugs of cortical tissue penetrate deep into medulla, separating the individual pyramids. These displacements of cortical tissue are the cortical columns (of Bertin).

The granular appearance of the cortex in a slice of fresh kidney is determined, under the LM, to be due to the myriad **glomeruli** that populate the cortex. They function as very effective, tiny ultrafilters that separate water, ions, and nitrogenous wastes from the blood plasma, to be disposed of in the urine.

While the lobes (pyramids) of the kidney are easily seen grossly, **renal lobules** are often difficult to delineate even under the microscope. A **medullary ray** is the central core of a lobule. A ray, together with the immediate adjacent halves of **two cortical labyrinths,** constitute a renal lobule. Since these lobules are not separated from each other by connective tissue septa, as in most other glands, it may be difficult to identify their outer limits, which are the **interlobular arteries.** To locate an interlobular artery within the maze of convoluted tubules of a pars convoluta may be difficult. Nonetheless this artery is the common boundary of two adjacent lobules. In other words, a **lobule** is the tissue between two interlobular arteries, hence its name.

Blood Supply

The histology and physiology of the kidney is centered around its blood supply. The physiological processes involved in **urine production,** i.e., filtration, secretion, and reabsorption, are accomplished by very intricate and often **unique vascular structures.** Since these structures are encountered early in the study of the kidney, recognizing their position in the vascular tree is essential to an understanding of how the kidney functions.

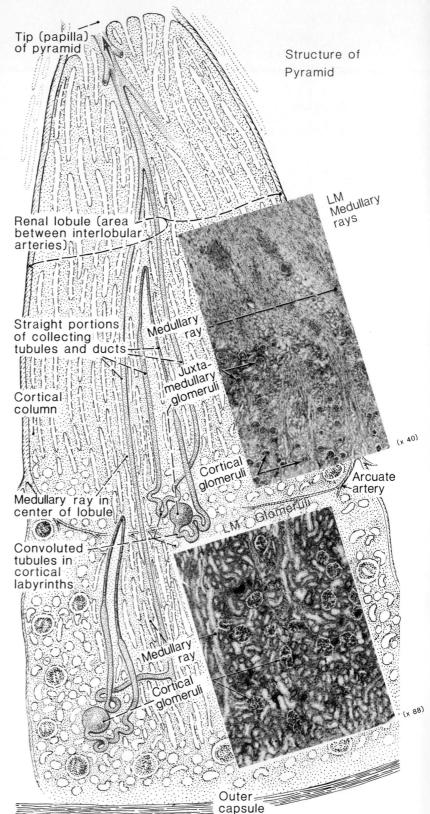

Structure of Pyramid

Tip (papilla) of pyramid

LM Medullary rays

Renal lobule (area between interlobular arteries)

Straight portions of collecting tubules and ducts

Medullary ray

Juxta-medullary glomeruli

Cortical column

Cortical glomeruli

LM Glomeruli

Arcuate artery

Medullary ray in center of lobule

Convoluted tubules in cortical labyrinths

Medullary ray

Cortical glomeruli

Outer capsule

(x 40)

(x 88)

SEM   Renal cortex and medulla

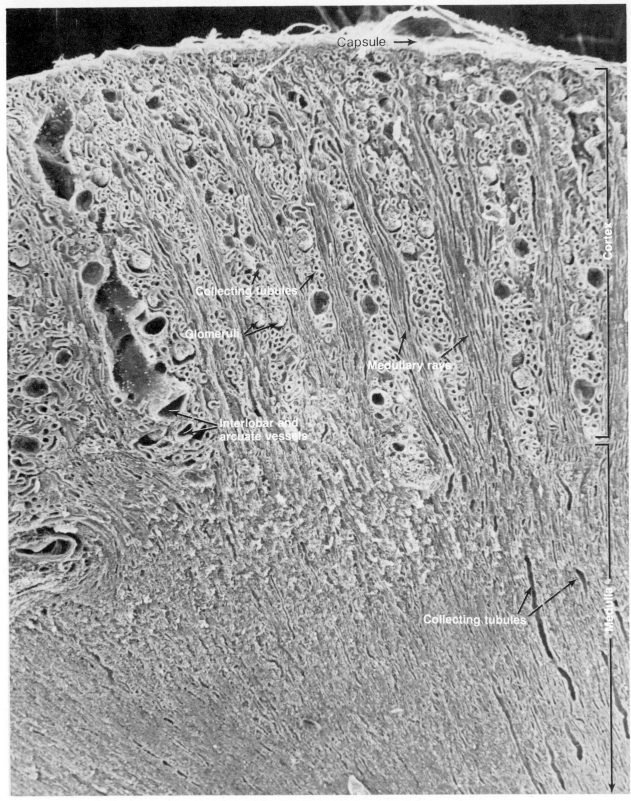

Capsule →

Cortex

Collecting tubules

Glomeruli

Medullary rays

Interlobar and arcuate vessels

Collecting tubules

Medulla

P.M. Andrews   (x 65)

A low power SEM view of the cortex and medulla of the kidney. The cortex has two distinctive features: (1) glomeruli associated with highly coiled convoluted tubules, and (2) medullary rays as parallel bundles of collecting ducts and straight portions of nephric tubules. They extend through the cortex into the medulla. A series of arcuate arteries and veins demarcate the boundary between the cortex and the medulla.

14495

Each kidney receives from the aorta a single renal artery. Near the hilus, it divides into three to five branches. As these arteries enter the adipose tissue in the hilus, they divide into several **interlobar branches,** which enter the kidney substance and ascend toward the cortex between the pyramids (lobes). Each supplies its own pyramid as it reaches the base of the pyramid at the junction of the cortex and medulla. Here the interlobular arteries end abruptly by dividing into wide branches that arch at right angles to run parallel to the cortex. These are the **arcuate arteries,** the distinctive landmark of the corticomedullary junction. There are essentially **no anastomoses** between the individual interlobar and arcuate vessels.

From the arcuate arteries arise **straight arteries** directed toward the cortex. Since they course between kidney lobules, they are called **interlobular arteries.** Each supplies adjacent lobules with a series of fine intralobular arterioles, the **afferent arterioles.** These small arteries run a short course before dividing into three or more primary branches. They further subdivide before each branch breaks up into a tuft of capillaries, the **glomerulus.** Each glomerulus has about 20–50 loops. Although numerous anastomoses occur within each loop, only a few points of anastomosis exist between the individual loops.

The afferent arteriole is a typical arteriole except in the portion next to the renal glomerulus (corpuscle). Here the prominent internal elastic layer is lost and the adventitia becomes indistinct. The typical circularly arranged smooth muscle cells of the tunica media become enlarged, glandular, **myoepithelioid cells,** which are polyhedral in shape and larger in diameter than smooth muscle cells. These are the **juxtaglomerular (JG) cells** (discussed on page 412). They are very likely the endocrine cells that produce the hormone **renin,** a powerful vasoconstrictor.

The single **efferent** arteriole draining the glomerulus has no distinctive features, except a smaller diameter than the afferent arteriole, and it has **no JG cells.** As it leaves the glomerulus, it immediately branches into a **capillary network** that nourishes the convoluted tubules clustered in the region of the glomerulus. Since the efferent arterioles **connect two capillary beds,** i.e., the glomerular capillary tufts and the peritubular capillaries, they qualify as a portal system and are therefore called the **renal portal system.** Also, the efferent arterioles give off recurrent capillary loops, the **vasa recta,** which extend, in parallel fashion, into the medulla along the medullary rays.

Venous return from both cortex and medulla empties into the **interlobular veins.** The venous blood retraces the course of the arteries to the hilus where it empties into the **renal vein.**

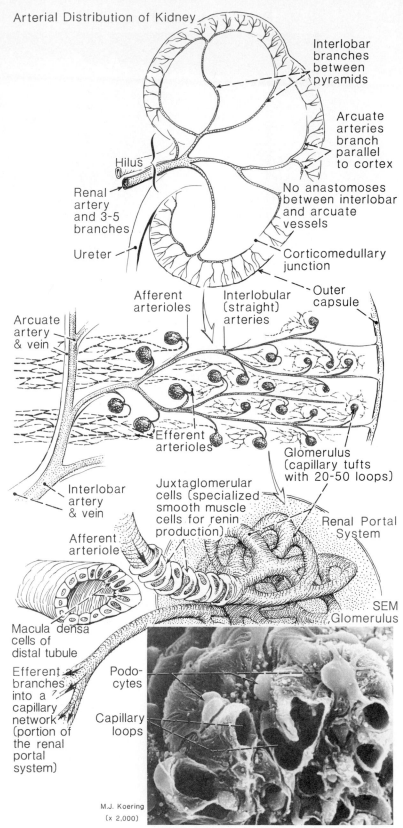

Arterial Distribution of Kidney

Interlobar branches between pyramids

Arcuate arteries branch parallel to cortex

No anastomoses between interlobar and arcuate vessels

Corticomedullary junction

Hilus

Renal artery and 3-5 branches

Ureter

Outer capsule

Afferent arterioles

Interlobular (straight) arteries

Arcuate artery & vein

Efferent arterioles

Glomerulus (capillary tufts with 20-50 loops)

Interlobar artery & vein

Juxtaglomerular cells (specialized smooth muscle cells for renin production)

Renal Portal System

Afferent arteriole

SEM Glomerulus

Macula densa cells of distal tubule

Efferent arteriole branches into a capillary network (portion of the renal portal system)

Podocytes

Capillary loops

M.J. Koering (x 2,000)

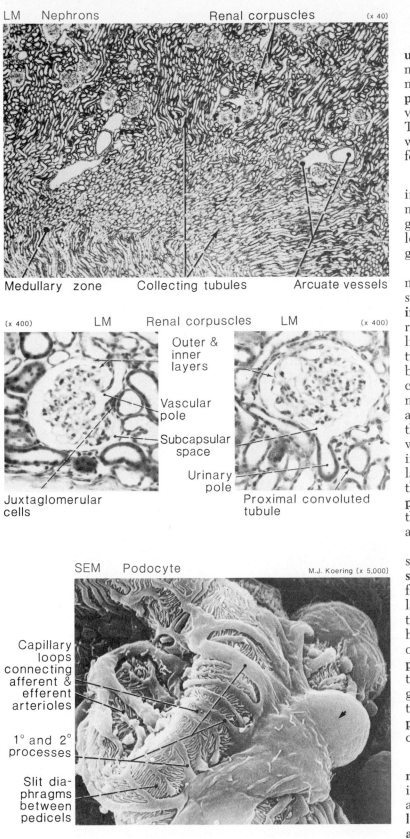

Medullary zone   Collecting tubules   Arcuate vessels

(x 400)   LM   Renal corpuscles   LM   (x 400)

Outer &
inner
layers

Vascular
pole

Subcapsular
space

Urinary
pole

Juxtaglomerular
cells

Proximal convoluted
tubule

SEM   Podocyte   M.J. Koering (x 5,000)

Capillary
loops
connecting
afferent &
efferent
arterioles

1° and 2°
processes

Slit dia-
phragms
between
pedicels

The Nephron

The nephron is a functional and anatomical **unit of the kidney.** There are approximately one million of these units in each human kidney. The nephron consists of two parts: (1) the **renal corpuscle** (glomerular or Bowman's capsule and a vascular glomerulus) and (2) the **renal tubule.** These two structures are interdependent, for with the loss of glomerulus, tubular degeneration follows.

RENAL CORPUSCLE The renal corpuscle includes: (1) the glomerular capsule (of Bowman); (2) the afferent arteriole feeding into the glomerulus; (3) the glomerulus, a tuft of capillary loops; and (4) the efferent arteriole draining the glomerular capillaries.

The **glomerular capsule** is a double-layered membrane composed of two layers of simple squamous epithelium, an **outer parietal** and an **inner visceral** layer. The latter epithelium surrounds and closely invests the capillary loops like a glove, leaving only a narrow space between the glomerular capillaries and the highly branched **podocytes** (Gk. podos + cyte, footlike cell), the cells comprising the visceral layer. The many **cytoplasmic extensions** of the podocytes are of various sizes and shapes. The smallest of the processes, called **pedicles** (L., little feet), wrap around the capillary loops by interdigitating with each other as they attach to the basal lamina of the capillary. The narrow slit between the closely packed pedicles is called the **slit diaphragm,** a barrier with pores. It is about 5 nm thick, and the pores are regularly arranged and are about 80 nm in diameter.

The outer parietal layer lines the capsule. The space between the two layers is the **subcapsular space,** where the provisional urine collects before it drains into the renal tubule. The parietal layer is continuous with the visceral layer where the capillary tuft enters the capsule. The capsule has two poles. The afferent and efferent arterioles enter and leave the capsule at the **vascular pole.** The first segment of the renal tubule leaves the capsule at the **urinary pole.** In the latter region, the squamous parietal cells abruptly thicken and become the cuboidal cells of the **proximal convoluted tubule** that drains the subcapsular space.

GLOMERULUS The glomerulus is a true **rete mirabile** (L., marvelous net) which, by definition, is a capillary network that interrupts the path of an artery. It consists of a tuft of tortuous **capillary loops** that connect the afferent and efferent **arterioles.**

As the larger **afferent arteriole** enters the glomerulus, it gives rise to several **wide capillaries,** each supplying a leaflet or lobule of the glomerulus. Between the lobules are occasional anastomoses. However, within each lobule there are

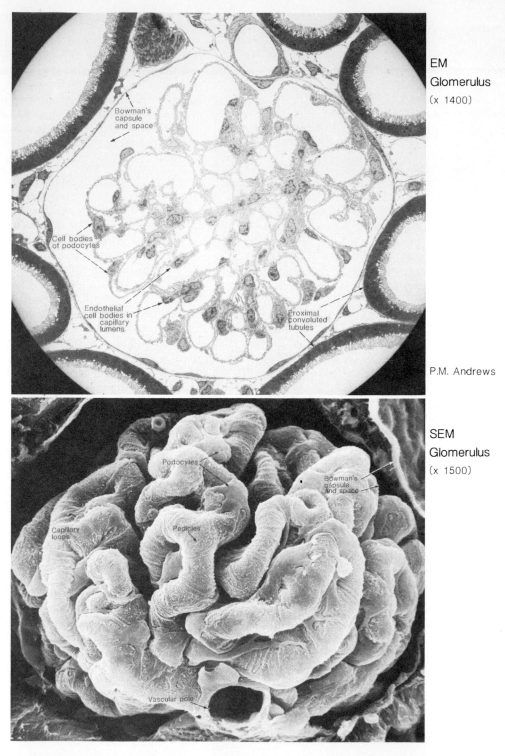

EM
Glomerulus
(x 1400)

Bowman's
capsule
and space

Cell bodies
of podocytes

Endothelial
cell bodies in
capillary
lumens

Proximal
convoluted
tubules

P.M. Andrews

SEM
Glomerulus
(x 1500)

Podocytes

Bowman's
capsule
and space

Capillary
loops

Pedicles

Vascular pole

The upper EM micrograph presents a section through a renal glomerulus, its surrounding Bowman's capsule, and adjacent proximal convoluted tubules. Note the very thin, flattened parietal epithelial cells of the capsule and the visceral epithelial cells (podocytes) closely associated with the helicoidal glomerular capillaries.

The lower SEM micrograph is of an intact renal glomerulus with portions of Bowman's capsule. The stellate cell bodies of podocytes possess cytoplasmic extensions which surround the coiled glomerular capillaries. The vascular pole of the glomerulus is seen at the base of the micrograph.

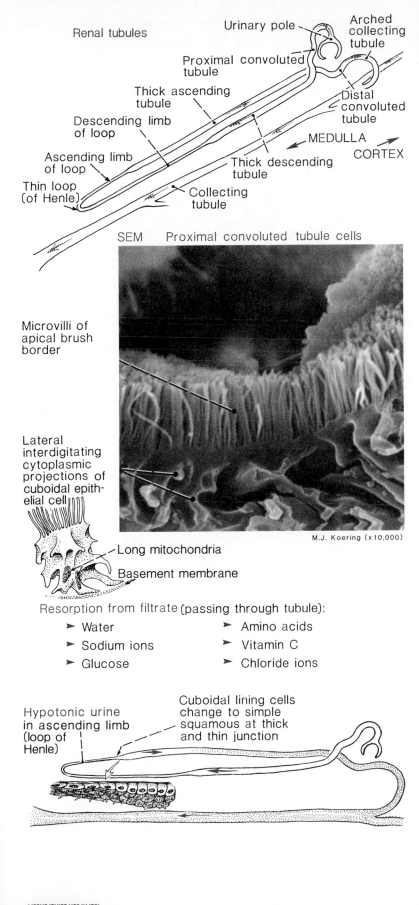

Renal tubules

Urinary pole

Arched collecting tubule

Proximal convoluted tubule

Thick ascending tubule

Descending limb of loop

Distal convoluted tubule

MEDULLA

CORTEX

Ascending limb of loop

Thick descending tubule

Thin loop (of Henle)

Collecting tubule

SEM Proximal convoluted tubule cells

Microvilli of apical brush border

Lateral interdigitating cytoplasmic projections of cuboidal epithelial cell

Long mitochondria

Basement membrane

M.J. Koering (x10,000)

Resorption from filtrate (passing through tubule):

➤ Water
➤ Sodium ions
➤ Glucose
➤ Amino acids
➤ Vitamin C
➤ Chloride ions

Hypotonic urine in ascending limb (loop of Henle)

Cuboidal lining cells change to simple squamous at thick and thin junction

many, short capillaries that join the ascending and descending segments of each wide capillary loop. All of these loops eventually unite to form the smaller **efferent arteriole.**

RENAL TUBULE The part of the nephron involved in **resorption and secretory** processes is the **renal tubule.** It is a continuous tube with varied histological features that are characteristic of its various regions. In the cortex, the tubule begins at the **urinary pole** of each glomerulus. Initially it runs a twisted, convoluted course, as **the proximal convoluted tubule.** Then, in a straight path, it passes through the cortex into the medulla as the **descending straight tubule** before it makes a hairpin loop as the **thin loop of Henle,** to return to the cortex as the ascending loop. Its wall thickens as it becomes the **thick ascending** limb of Henle's loop, which becomes tortuous again near the glomerulus of its origin, as the **distal convoluted tubule.**

Proximal Convoluted Tubule Arising at the urinary pole of a glomerulus as a direct extension of the parietal epithelium lining Bowman's capsule, the **proximal convoluted tubule (PCT)** is the longest (about 15–20 mm), the most convoluted, and hence the tubule most commonly seen in cortical sections. These tubules make up most of the cortex. The epithelium lining the lumen is **simple cuboidal** with a very distinctive, prominent, apical **brush border of microvilli** about 1 μm long. The abundant cytoplasm is acidophilic, largely because of the many, long mitochondria. The cell **boundaries are indistinct** because of the extensive interdigitations of the lateral processes. These overlapping ridges may extend the entire length of the cell. An elaborate system of **interdigitations** is also prominent in the basal part of the cell where these overlapping processes entrap a layer of longitudinally oriented, large, elongated mitochondria. Their palisade arrangement creates a pattern of **basal striations.** Only two or three round, dark nuclei are seen in the cross section of a PCT.

The main function of a PCT is the **resorption** of about 75–80% of the **water and sodium ions** from the glomerular filtrate. In addition, resorption of glucose, amino acids, vitamin C, and chloride ions also occurs. Its prominent striated border functions similarly to the brush border of the intestine in that it also **absorbs certain sugars and amino acids.** Also, by endocytosis, the brush border **removes most protein** from the urine.

The histology and functions of the **straight part of the proximal tubule** are similar to the convoluted portion. It begins in a medullary ray of the cortex and terminates in the upper part of the medulla where it ends abruptly when its lining cells change into **simple squamous epithelium** of the thin limb of Henle's loop.

14075

Loop of Henle The thin loops of Henle are the continuation of the **straight portions** of the proximal tubules. They arise at various depths in the medulla before returning to the cortex as the **ascending limbs** where they become continuous with the **thick segments** of the distal convoluted tubules. They vary in length depending on the position of the glomerulus of their origin.

Arising from **cortical glomeruli** near the capsule, the proximal convoluted tubules terminate as **thick descending** loops of Henle. These thick segments end on short, thin segments that are confined largely to the cortex and extend only a short distance into the medulla. In contrast, the **juxtamedullary glomeruli** (near the medulla) usually have **long, thick, descending** loops as well as **long, ascending,** thin loop segments. The former extend deep into the medulla before returning to the cortex as the thick ascending loop. In either case, the **thin limbs** are lined with **simple squamous epithelium,** whose oval nuclei usually bulge the lumen. Except for somewhat thicker walls and the absence of blood cells, these thin segments resemble capillaries.

The function of the thin loop is to further **concentrate the glomerular filtrate** by osmosis. In the process, the isotonic filtrate entering the loop in the cortex becomes **hypertonic** as it passes through the descending loop. About 20% of the original glomerular filtrate enters the descending loops. It is reduced to 15% by the time it enters the distal convoluted tubules. As the urine leaves the ascending segment of the loop, it is again **hypotonic** since the ascending limb is quite **impermeable to water** yet moves large amounts of sodium and chloride ions out of the lumen into the interstitial spaces. Since nearly all of the loops are in the medulla, these ions are sequestered here, producing a **hypertonic** environment surrounding the collecting ducts in the medulla. However, in the presence of the antidiuretic hormone of the pituitary, the **collecting ducts are permeable** to water, while the high osmolality of the tissue spaces surrounding the collecting ducts supplies the osmotic force to **remove water** from the lumen to dilute the hypertonic interstitial environment. The end result is **hypertonic urine** in the collecting tubules.

It is interesting that birds and mammals are the only species capable of producing hypertonic urine. They are also the only species with thin loops of Henle.

Distal Convoluted Tubules Second only in number to the PCT in the cortex are the **distal convoluted tubules (DCT).** They are shorter and less convoluted than the PCT and consist of three parts: (1) the straight, thick ascending portion, (2) the macula densa, and (3) the convoluted segment.

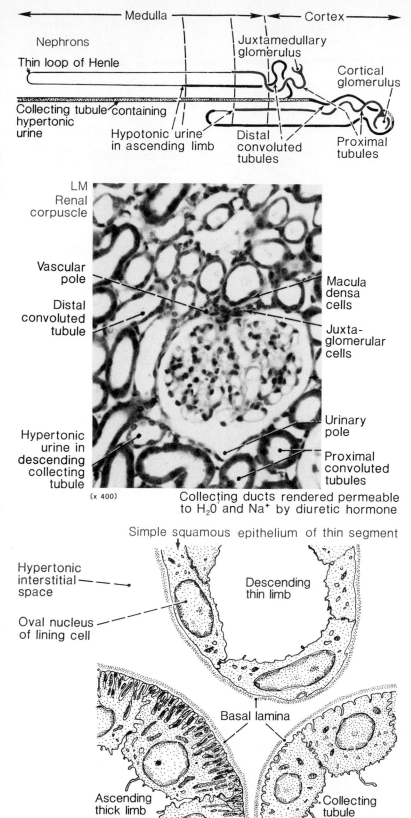

(x 400)

Collecting ducts rendered permeable to H_2O and Na^+ by diuretic hormone

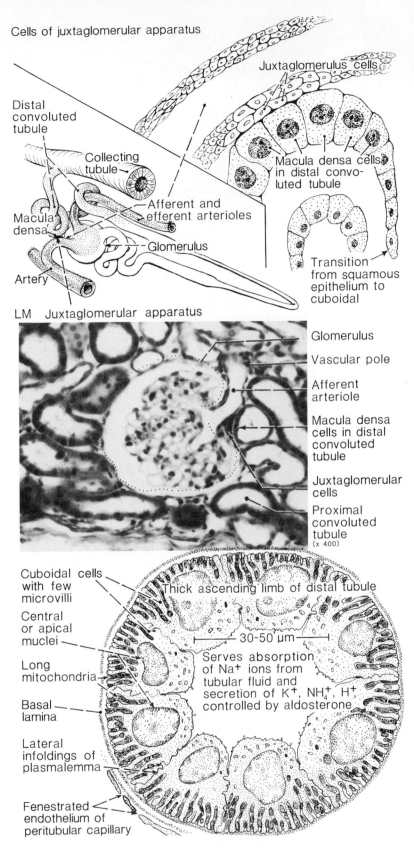

Cells of juxtaglomerular apparatus

Juxtaglomerulus cells

Distal convoluted tubule

Collecting tubule

Macula densa cells in distal convoluted tubule

Afferent and efferent arterioles

Macula densa

Glomerulus

Artery

Transition from squamous epithelium to cuboidal

LM   Juxtaglomerular apparatus

Glomerulus

Vascular pole

Afferent arteriole

Macula densa cells in distal convoluted tubule

Juxtaglomerular cells

Proximal convoluted tubule

(x 400)

Cuboidal cells with few microvilli

Thick ascending limb of distal tubule

Central or apical muclei

30–50 µm

Serves absorption of Na+ ions from tubular fluid and secretion of K+, NH4+, H+ controlled by aldosterone

Long mitochondria

Basal lamina

Lateral infoldings of plasmalemma

Fenestrated endothelium of peritubular capillary

The straight portion of the DCT is the **thick ascending segment** of the loop of Henle. It usually begins in the medulla where the squamous epithelium of the thin loop abruptly changes to cuboidal. Also its outer diameter increases to 30–50 µm with a corresponding increase in the luminal diameter. It ascends into the cortex to reach the **vascular pole** of the parent glomerulus. This limited region is specialized as the **macula densa.**

The macula densa is composed of closely packed, **modified, narrow cells** arranged in a palisade configuration that line the distal convoluted tubules. Their **dark-staining nuclei** are close together like a string of black beads. These cells have only a few mitochondria with less basal infoldings and lateral interdigitations than the other parts of the distal tubule. Its close proximity to the juxtaglomerular (JG) cells allows for the **exchange of materials** and information between them, such as the concentration of sodium ions within the DCT. When the glomerular filtrate decreases in volume, a **drop in sodium ions** follows, which probably stimulates the **release of renin** into the bloodstream from the JG cells.

The most extensive segment of the distal tubule is the **convoluted portion** that is entangled with the proximal convoluted tubules about the parent glomerulus. The **thick ascending limb** and the convoluted portion of the distal tubule **resemble** the corresponding structures of the **PCT** with the following **exceptions:** (1) The cells are shorter, more cuboidal with **no brush borders.** However, a few microvilli are noted in EM micrographs. More nuclei are seen in profile in the DCT and are usually in a central or apical position in the cell. (2) The less acidophilic cytoplasm has fewer mitochondria, lysosomes, and vacuoles. However, in the basal region, extensive lateral infoldings of the plasmalemma envelope large, long mitochondria, producing **prominent basal striations.** (3) The lumen is much **wider** (30–50 µm) and is **smooth surfaced** due to the absence of brush borders on the apices of the epithelial cells. Lumens are seen in section much less frequently because the DCT is much shorter than the PCT.

In general, all parts of the distal convoluted tubule are involved in the **resorption of sodium** ions and about 9% of the water from the tubular fluid, and especially in the secretion of potassium and hydrogen ions into the lumen. In other words, the DCT is one site for the control of **electrolyte (acid-base) balance** of the body; another is the collecting tubule. This process is controlled by **aldosterone,** a hormone of the adrenal cortex.

14376

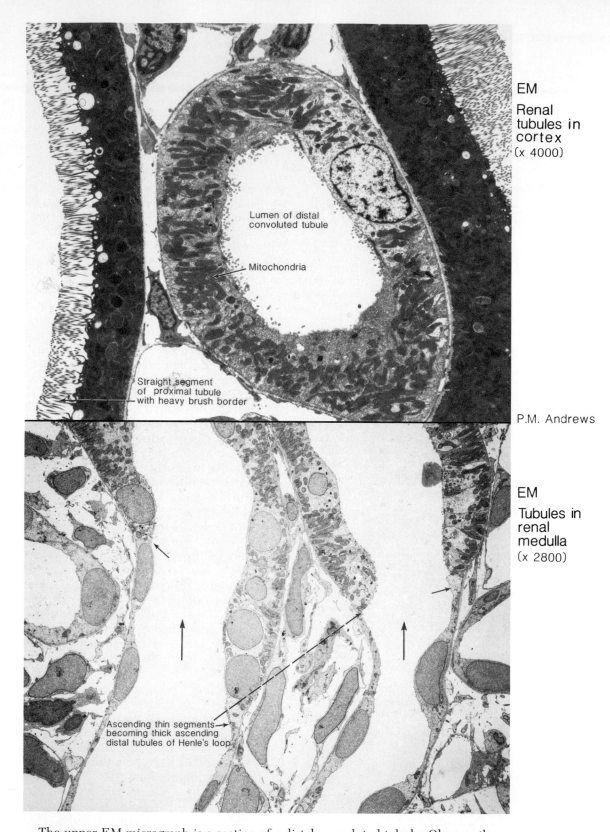

P.M. Andrews

EM
Renal
tubules in
cortex
(x 4000)

Lumen of distal
convoluted tubule

Mitochondria

Straight segment
of proximal tubule
with heavy brush border

EM
Tubules in
renal
medulla
(x 2800)

Ascending thin segments
becoming thick ascending
distal tubules of Henle's loop

The upper EM micrograph is a section of a distal convoluted tubule. Observe the abundance of elongated mitochondria, many enclosed by infoldings of the basal plasmalemma. The free apical surface has some microvilli but not sufficient to form a brush border, as seen in the adjacent descending straight segment of a proximal convoluted tubule.

The lower electron micrograph shows two thin ascending loops of Henle undergoing rather abrupt transformation into thick segments with many mitochondria and limited microvilli, both characteristics of distal tubules.

14334

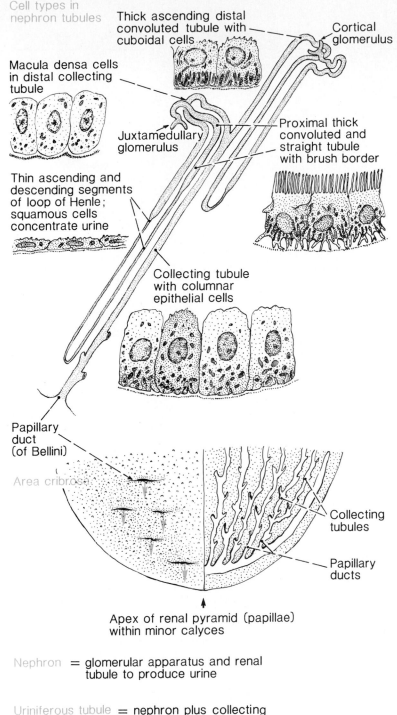

Cell types in nephron tubules

Thick ascending distal convoluted tubule with cuboidal cells

Cortical glomerulus

Macula densa cells in distal collecting tubule

Juxtamedullary glomerulus

Proximal thick convoluted and straight tubule with brush border

Thin ascending and descending segments of loop of Henle; squamous cells concentrate urine

Collecting tubule with columnar epithelial cells

Papillary duct (of Bellini)

Area cribrosa

Collecting tubules

Papillary ducts

Apex of renal pyramid (papillae) within minor calyces

Nephron = glomerular apparatus and renal tubule to produce urine

Uriniferous tubule = nephron plus collecting tubules and ducts

Kidney produces 170-180 liters/day of dilute urine by glomeruli

Urine is concentrated to 1.5-2.0 liters/day by uriniferous tubules

Collecting Tubules

The collecting tubules are the continuations of the DCT in the cortex. They begin as short, **arched tubules** that converge to form bundles of **straight tubules.** Each straight tubule is about 40 μm in diameter and is directed towards the medulla, as the principal component of the medullary rays. Here two types of lining cells exist, mostly light cells, with dark cells interspersed. The latter have abundant mitochondria and microvilli.

As the tubules approach and penetrate the medulla, their cuboidal lining cells become progressively more columnar and their lumina increase in diameter. As they traverse the medulla, these tubules join with other straight tubules to form large ducts that open onto the apex of the renal papillae as the **papillary ducts** (of Bellini) with a diameter of 200–300 μm. They empty into the **minor calyses.** The surface of renal papillae has the appearance of a sieve because of the many large, closely packed duct openings; hence it is called the **area cribrosa.**

The cells lining the collecting tubules and the collecting ducts are a **continuum,** i.e., they gradually change their shape. In the initial segment they are low cuboidal, then cuboidal to low columnar, until in the papillae they are tall columnar. In the medulla, the cells are clear, lightly staining with few organelles. The **cell borders are distinct** with few interdigitations. No basal striations are present. The nuclei are round, dark staining, and basal in position.

Uriniferous Tubule

As conduits for the urine, the collecting tubules and ducts are not parts of the nephron even though they absorb large amounts of water, while the nephron is concerned essentially with the production of urine. Together they constitute the **uriniferous tubule** of the kidney. Each has separate embryonic anlagen that unite to form a continuous uriniferous tubule, a **functional unit** of the kidney. Often the terms nephron and uriniferous tubule are incorrectly used as synonyms. In this text the nephron is presented as a part of the larger unit, the uriniferous tubule.

Concentration of Urine

The concentration of urine by the kidney is not just an interesting biological phenomenon; it is vital to our ability to survive, especially in hot, hostile environments. The kidney produces tremendous amounts of very dilute urine, the provisional urine or **glomerular filtrate,** which amounts to about **170–180 l/day,** that must be concentrated to about 1.5–2.0 l. It is the uriniferous tubule that accomplishes this task.

14327

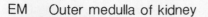

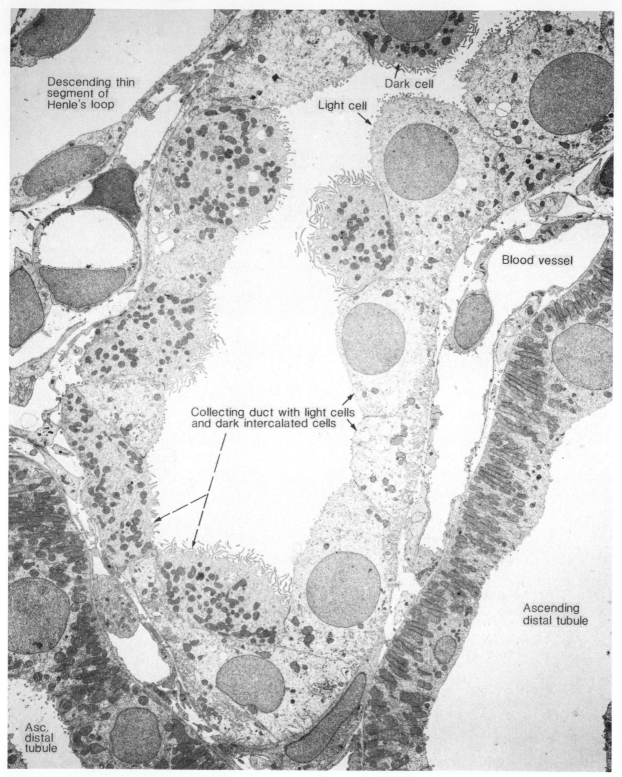

Descending thin
segment of
Henle's loop

Dark cell

Light cell

Blood vessel

Collecting duct with light cells
and dark intercalated cells

Ascending
distal tubule

Asc.
distal
tubule

P.M. Andrews   (x 12,800)

Electron micrograph of a collecting duct showing light and dark lining cells. The dark cells are electron-dense primarily because of the abundance of mitochondria. Their apical cell membranes form extensive folds and many microvilli. The light cells have only a few mitochondria and, on the apical surface, a few, short microvilli. Distinct cell boundaries are present. The lower right tubule is a segment of a thick ascending distal tubule. Note that the deep interdigitating processes of the basal plasmalemma enclose abundant, long mitochondria. The nuclei are apical in position.

14391

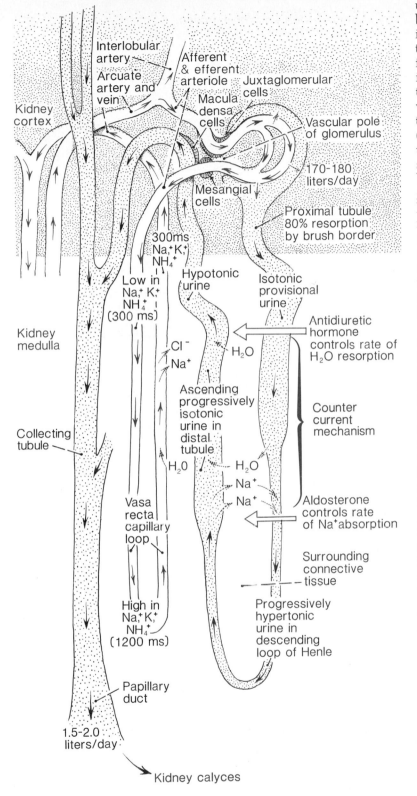

In the **proximal convoluted tubules** the volume of glomerular filtrate is **reduced about 80%** by resorption of water, the sodium and chloride ions, largely by the highly absorptive action of the microvilli in the **brush border**. As the isotonic filtrate passes into the **descending loop of Henle**, it **loses water** to the surrounding medullary interstitium and **gains sodium ions**. Thus the provisional urine becomes concentrated and **hypertonic**. When the urine reaches the **ascending (thick) limb**, sodium is actively **pumped out** of the tubule into the surrounding connective tissue. Water permeability in this region of the tubule is very low, so that the filtrate becomes progressively isotonic and finally **hypotonic, without loss of water**, as it ascends to the DCT. This repetitive process of sodium entering the descending tubule, circulating through the loop, and then being pumped out again without loss of water in the ascending limb is called the **countercurrent mechanism** because the current in the descending loop segment is moving counter to the adjacent parallel ascending segment.

The other part of the countercurrent mechanism involves loops of capillaries called the **vasa recta**. They parallel the loops of Henle as they pass down from the cortex deep into the medulla and then return to the cortex. At the beginning of their journey, the **solute concentration**, especially sodium ions and chloride ions with small amounts of potassium and ammonium ions, is quite low (**300 milliosmols**). However, as the very permeable vasa recta penetrate deeper into the medulla, their **osmolar concentration** rapidly approaches the high level found in the medullary interstitium, that is, a fourfold increase to about **1200 mOsm**. As the blood returns to the cortex, it is closely associated with the ascending limb and a rapid diffusion of solutes out of the vasa recta, especially sodium and chloride ions, with a concomitant rapid flow of water into the blood vessels, resulting in a sharp fall in the solute concentration to about **300 mOsm**. It is this rapid back-and-forth diffusion of solutes between the medullary interstitium and the capillaries that makes it virtually impossible for the blood to remove any sizable amount of solutes from the medulla. This countercurrent mechanism within the vasa recta **stabilizes** the constantly high concentration of **sodium and chloride ions** in the medullary region.

As the hypotonic provisional urine traverses the **distal convoluted tubule, water is reabsorbed** under control of aldosterone, the antidiuretic hormone (**ADH**). Sodium ions, under the influence of aldosterone, are largely replaced by hydrogen, ammonium and potassium ions, and acidification of the urine follows. Only about **15%** of the filtrate volume now remains.

Under the influence of ADH the final concentration of the urine occurs in the **collecting tu-**

bules and ducts. The capacity of these structures to concentrate the urine depends solely on the osmolality of their surroundings, i.e., the **hypertonicity** of the medullary interstitium in which they lie. The diffusion of sodium and urea from the loops of Henle into the interstitium is the cause of this hypertonicity. When urine finally reaches the calyces, it is only about **1% of the original volume** of the glomerular filtrate. (See Table 20.1 for summary of kidney tubules.)

Filtration Membrane of the Glomerulus

The exquisite filter in the kidney is the **glomerular filtration membrane,** also called the filtration barrier of the glomerulus. It has three components: (1) the **fenestrated endothelial cells** of the glomerular capillaries, (2) the glomerular **basement membrane,** and (3) the **podocytes** (visceral epithelium overlying the capillaries).

As the plasma leaves the glomerular capillaries, it passes through attenuated, **fenestrated endothelial cells.** The diameter of these fenestrations (pores) varies from 60 to 100 nm, which is only large enough to **allow passage** of noncellular elements of the blood, including **plasma proteins,** such as albumin whose molecular weight **(MW) is 65,000–70,000.** These pores greatly increase the permeability of the glomerular capillaries.

The glomerular **basement membrane,** upon which the endothelium rests, is a continuous, nonfenestrated membrane about **three times as thick (330 nm)** as basement membranes (basal laminae) elsewhere in the body. It is the only continuous layer of the three components of the filtration barrier and acts as the **principal glomerular filter.** It allows only small proteins with less than 10 nm particle size, that is, **40,000 MW or less,** to pass through but **retains** larger protein molecules, such as **serum albumin,** with a molecular weight of 68,000–70,000.

The **slits** between the podocyte pedicels average 25 nm in diameter, and each slit is bridged by a **diaphragm about 5–10 nm** in diameter. Therefore, only relatively sparse, smaller protein molecules with a molecular weight **below 50,000** pass readily through the slits but abundant larger proteins are barred.

The Juxtaglomerular Apparatus

The juxtaglomerular apparatus has three components: (1) juxtaglomerular **(JG) cells, modified smooth muscle cells** in the wall of the afferent arteriole just before it enters Bowman's capsule; (2) **modified epithelial lining cells** of the distal convoluted tubule (macula densa) where it lies adjacent to the afferent arteriole containing JG cells; and (3) **polkissen cells,** a group of small, clear cells lying between the afferent and efferent arterioles and the macula densa.

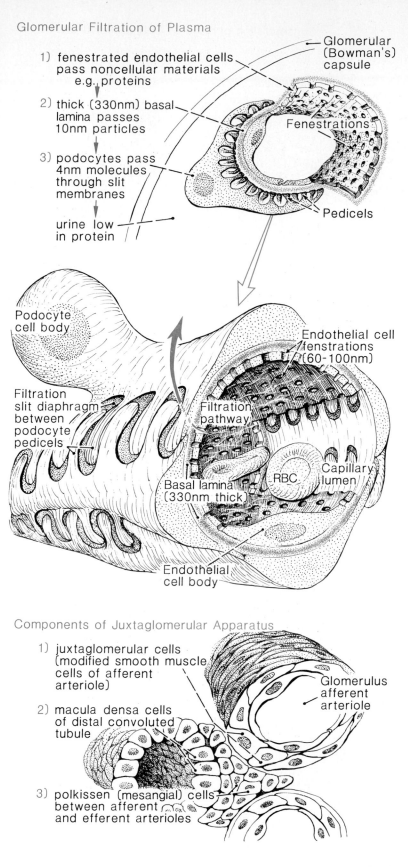

Glomerular Filtration of Plasma

1) fenestrated endothelial cells pass noncellular materials e.g. proteins

2) thick (330nm) basal lamina passes 10nm particles

3) podocytes pass 4nm molecules through slit membranes

urine low in protein

Glomerular (Bowman's) capsule

Fenestrations

Pedicels

Podocyte cell body

Filtration slit diaphragm between podocyte pedicels

Endothelial cell fenstrations (60-100nm)

Filtration pathway

Basal lamina (330nm thick)

RBC

Capillary lumen

Endothelial cell body

Components of Juxtaglomerular Apparatus

1) juxtaglomerular cells (modified smooth muscle cells of afferent arteriole)

2) macula densa cells of distal convoluted tubule

3) polkissen (mesangial) cells between afferent and efferent arterioles

Glomerulus afferent arteriole

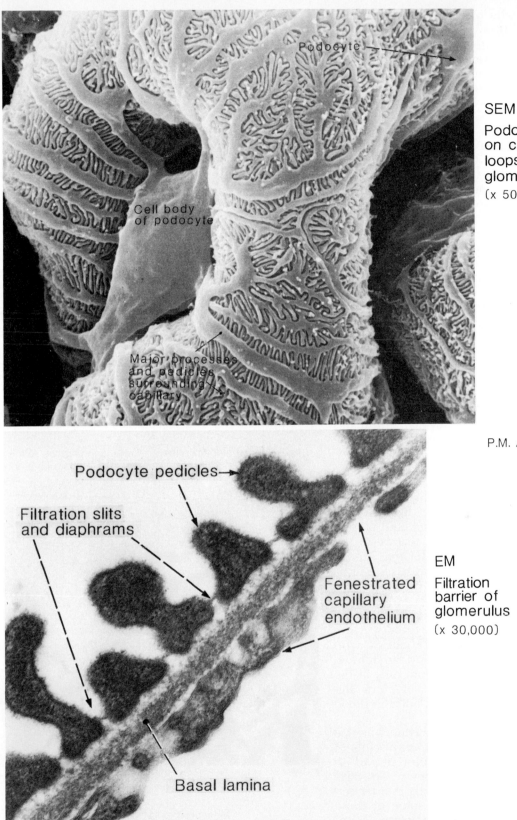

SEM
Podocytes
on capillary
loops in
glomerulus
(x 5000)

Podocyte

Cell body
of podocyte

Major processes
and pedicles
surrounding
capillary

P.M. Andrews

Podocyte pedicles

Filtration slits
and diaphrams

Fenestrated
capillary
endothelium

EM
Filtration
barrier of
glomerulus
(x 30,000)

Basal lamina

The upper SEM micrograph displays a glomerular capillary loop surrounded by interdigitating processes of podocytes, i.e., large primary, secondary, and smaller fingerlike pedicels. The small spaces between the pedicels are the filtration slits.

The filtration barrier is seen in the lower EM micrograph. Collectively, the fenestrated capillary endothelium, the fused basal lamina of the capillary and the podocyte, and the slit diaphragms form the filtration barrier. It allows the passage of some substances (MW 40,000 or less) into the tubule.

Lying in the media of the afferent arteriole, the JG cells differ from typical smooth muscle cells by a spherical, instead of an elongated, nucleus, and the cytoplasm contains PAS-positive granules instead of filaments. EM studies reveal that the JG cells have **secretory characteristics,** e.g., abundant rER, an active Golgi complex, and many secretory granules. The cytoplasmic granules contain the enzyme **renin** or its precursors.

JG cells are responsive to **changes in blood pressure** in the afferent arteriole. A decrease in pressure causes a release of **renin granules** into the bloodstream that react with a plasma globulin, **angiotensinogen,** to produce the inactive polypeptide **angiotensin I.** The latter, when subjected to a converting enzyme principally in the lung, is changed into **angiotensin II,** a powerful vasoconstrictor that initially causes arteriolar constriction and thus **increases systemic blood pressure.** However, the prime action of angiotensin II is to cause the release of the hormone **aldosterone** from the adrenal cortex. This hormone acts on the **kidney tubules** to cause them to retain more water and sodium. The retention of large amounts of fluid and sodium in the circulatory system causes an increase in systemic blood pressure. This sequence of events is called the **renin-angiotensin-aldosterone mechanism.** **Erythropoietin,** a glycoprotein that stimulates **RBC production** in the bone marrow, is probably also synthesized by the JG cells.

The **macula densa** is a group of **modified epithelial lining cells** of the distal convoluted tubule where it comes in contact with the JG cells. As compared to other regions of the distal tubule, these cells are usually taller, larger, and closely packed as flat stacks. A striking feature is the small, darkly stained, **round nuclei** that are arranged like a string of beads. The basal lamina separating the macula densa and the JG cells is very thin and inconspicuous.

The macula densa probably **monitors the sodium concentration** in the distal tubule. A decrease in systemic blood pressure causes a reduction in the output of glomerular filtrate, which precipitates a drop in sodium ions in the distal tubule. The macula densa somehow **signals the JG cells to release renin,** and the blood pressure rises to normal levels.

Polkissen cells (Ger., pole cushions), also called **mesangial cells,** are a cushion of cells in the triangular area between the afferent and efferent arterioles and the macula densa. They are lightly stained, stellate-shaped cells that resemble **pericytes.** The cytoplasm of some of these cells has fine granules. Their function is unknown; however, they may act as pericytes to support and contract the walls of the adjacent arterioles. Another interesting theory is that these cells may be **macrophages** that cleanse the basal lamina of foreign material that accumulates on the membrane during the filtration process.

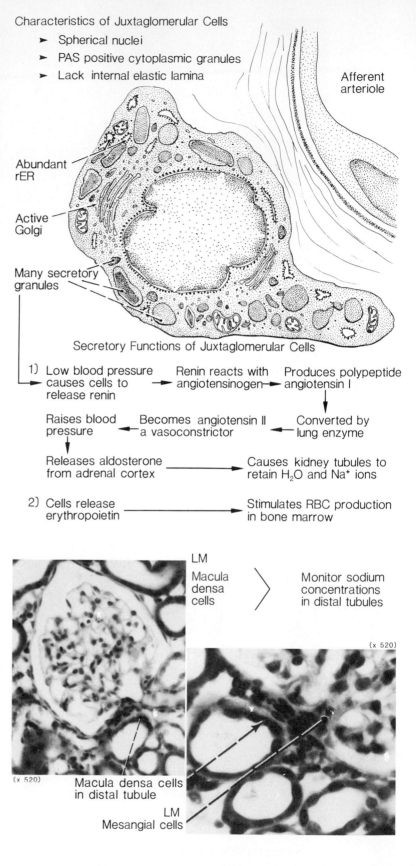

Characteristics of Juxtaglomerular Cells
- ► Spherical nuclei
- ► PAS positive cytoplasmic granules
- ► Lack internal elastic lamina

Afferent arteriole

Abundant rER

Active Golgi

Many secretory granules

Secretory Functions of Juxtaglomerular Cells

1) Low blood pressure causes cells to release renin → Renin reacts with angiotensinogen → Produces polypeptide angiotensin I

Raises blood pressure ← Becomes angiotensin II a vasoconstrictor ← Converted by lung enzyme

Releases aldosterone from adrenal cortex → Causes kidney tubules to retain H_2O and Na^+ ions

2) Cells release erythropoietin → Stimulates RBC production in bone marrow

LM Macula densa cells > Monitor sodium concentrations in distal tubules

(x 520)

(x 520)

Macula densa cells in distal tubule

LM Mesangial cells

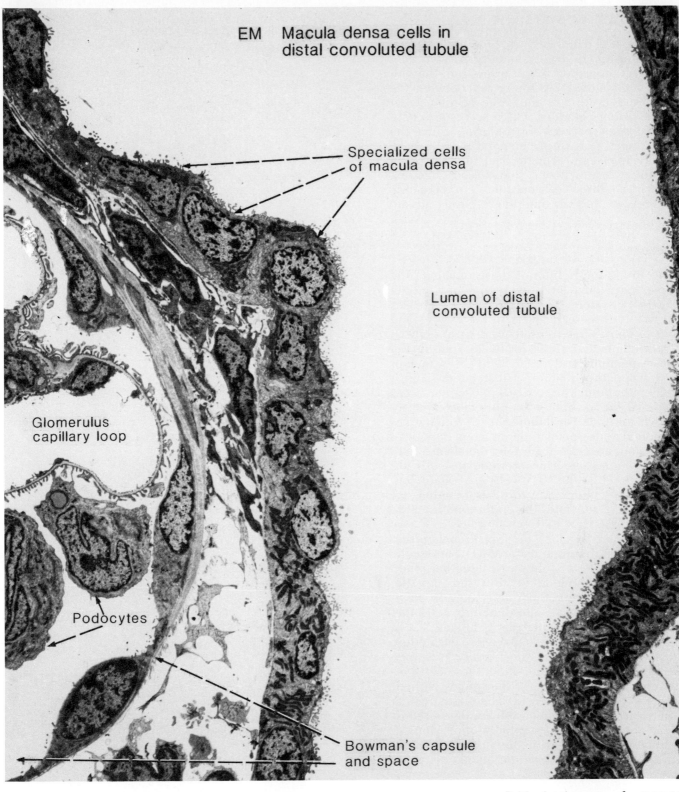

EM Macula densa cells in
distal convoluted tubule

Specialized cells
of macula densa

Lumen of distal
convoluted tubule

Glomerulus
capillary loop

Podocytes

Bowman's capsule
and space

P.M. Andrews (x 2800)

Electron micrograph of a distal convoluted tubule with macula densa cells. Note that these epithelial cells are taller than the other lining cells, have an ovoid, central nucleus, and the apical surface has numerous microvilli and a single cilium (not shown here). The basal plasmalemma has frequent interdigitations enclosing long mitochondria.

14369

URINARY PASSAGEWAYS AND BLADDER

The minor and major calyces, renal pelves, ureters, and urethrae are essentially **passive conduits** for the transport of the urine from the kidneys to outside the body. Interposed between the ureters and urethra is the large fibromuscular bag, the **urinary bladder,** which serves as a temporary **storage reservoir** for the urine. Since the calyces, renal pelves, ureters, and bladder have basically the same conventional, hollow organ structures, they will be considered together. They all have **three coats or tunics,** i.e., a mucosa, a muscularis, and an outermost fibrous adventitia.

Mucosa

The lining epithelium of these organs is the unique, **transitional stratified** type, found only in the urinary system. The stratification increases from two to three cell layers in the calyces and pelvis to four to five in ureter and six to eight in the relaxed bladder. However, the epithelium becomes **squamous** and reduced to three to four layers when the **bladder is distended.** Transitional epithelium, as described in Chapter 4, has superficial, large, lightly staining cells that are somewhat **rounded or dome-shaped,** which gives a scalloped appearance to the mucosal surface of the organ. The cells are often binucleate, with prominent nucleoli. The intermediate cells are polyhedral, while the basal cells are roughly cuboidal or low columnar. A **thin basal lamina,** not seen with LM, separates the epithelium from the lamina propria.

In the urinary bladder, the **transitional epithelium** has several unique features. (1) These cells appear to be able to **slide past each other** when the bladder is being filled, thus reducing the number of cell layers. Such movement is possible because of unusual interdigitating cell junctions, called **plaques, which act as hinges.** These attachments allow the cells to overlap each other, like an accordion, when the bladder is empty. When the bladder is being filled, these cells are extended by the opening of the hinges without damage to the cell surface. (2) The **plasmalemma** of the surface cells is much **thicker** than in most cells of the body. It is essentially **impervious** to the hypertonic, toxic urine, thus preventing any further exchanges between the blood and urine.

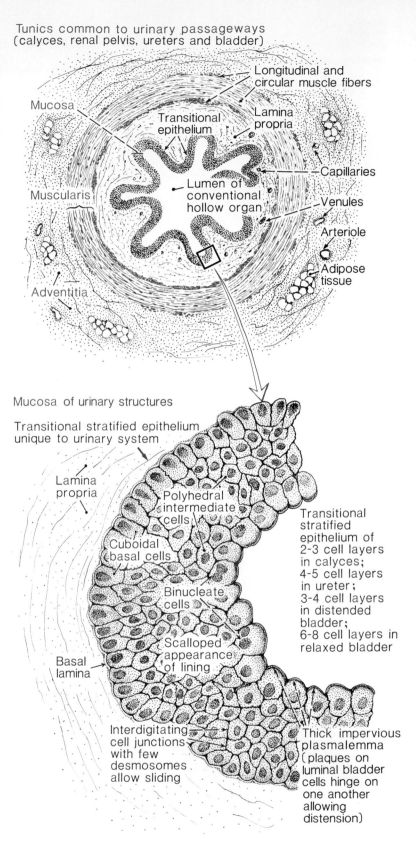

Tunics common to urinary passageways
(calyces, renal pelvis, ureters and bladder)

Mucosa
Transitional epithelium
Longitudinal and circular muscle fibers
Lamina propria
Capillaries
Lumen of conventional hollow organ
Venules
Muscularis
Arteriole
Adipose tissue
Adventitia

Mucosa of urinary structures

Transitional stratified epithelium unique to urinary system

Lamina propria
Polyhedral intermediate cells
Cuboidal basal cells
Binucleate cells
Basal lamina
Scalloped appearance of lining
Interdigitating cell junctions with few desmosomes allow sliding

Transitional stratified epithelium of 2-3 cell layers in calyces; 4-5 cell layers in ureter; 3-4 cell layers in distended bladder; 6-8 cell layers in relaxed bladder

Thick impervious plasmalemma (plaques on luminal bladder cells hinge on one another allowing distension)

Kidney

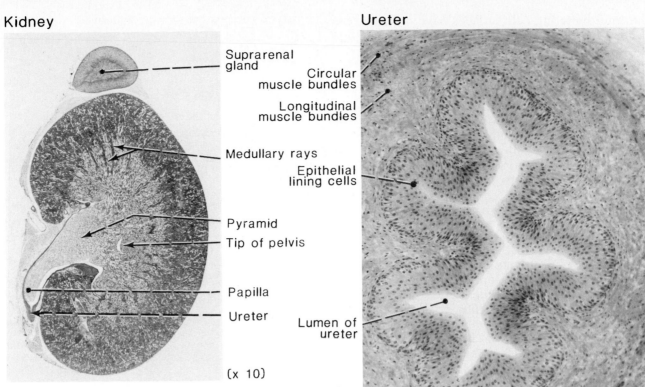

Suprarenal gland

Medullary rays

Pyramid

Tip of pelvis

Papilla

Ureter

(x 10)

Ureter

Circular muscle bundles

Longitudinal muscle bundles

Epithelial lining cells

Lumen of ureter

(x 100)

Bladder wall

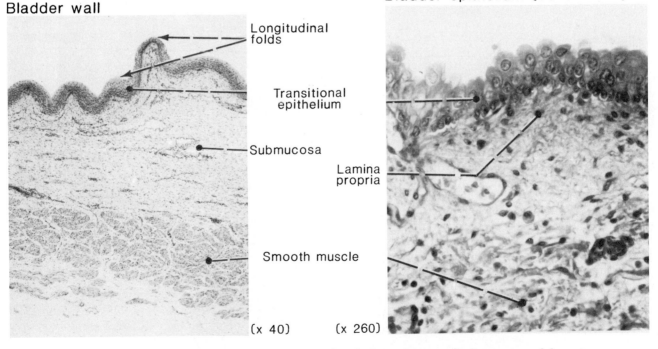

Longitudinal folds

Transitional epithelium

Submucosa

Smooth muscle

(x 40)

Bladder epithelium (contracted)

Lamina propria

(x 260)

Upper left: An LM view of a unilobar rat kidney showing the beginning of the urinary passageways, i.e., the renal pelvis which terminates as the ureter.

Upper right: A cross section of a typical ureter lined with transitional epithelium.

Lower left: A photomicrograph of the wall of a relaxed urinary bladder revealing longitudinal foldings of the mucosa and interlacing of the smooth muscle layers of the muscularis externa.

Lower right: Typical dome-shaped transitional epithelium lining the lumen of the urinary bladder.

14691

(3) The interdigitating cell surfaces have only a few desmosomes holding the cells together. However, **tight junctions** are common, which prevent passage of water across the bladder wall in spite of osmotic and hydrostatic pressure differences between the exterior and the interior of the bladder. (4) The basal layer of cells is uneven and deeply folded by strands of connective tissue that carry capillaries. Such an arrangement gives the erroneous impression that the transitional epithelium is a vascular structure, a concept held by some earlier histologists.

Tunica Propria

The tunica propria of the **calyces** and **renal pelvis** consists largely of limited **elastic and reticular fibers** and a few lymphocytes. No glands or papillae are present to indent the epithelium. Thus the junction between the tunica propria and epithelium is smooth. In contrast, the tunica propria of the **ureters and bladder** has considerable **collagenous and elastic fibers** scattered among diffuse lymphoid tissue. Many capillaries are present. Also present in the **bladder** are a few **lymph nodules and mucous glands** near the internal sphincter. In the **ureter**, the mucosa is thrown into longitudinal folds creating a **star-shaped lumen**, while in the relaxed bladder, the longitudinal mucosal folds are thick and irregular.

Muscularis

In the calyces and renal pelvis, the **muscularis** consists of a **few circularly** arranged outer smooth muscle fibers and a delicate inner **longitudinal band of muscle.** These two bands become the relatively heavy, **discrete layers** of the ureter. In the lower third of the ureter, a third layer of muscle appears that envelops the circular muscle band to become the **outermost longitudinal layer.** The ureters enter the bladder at an oblique angle, which causes their walls to collapse as the bladder is filled, thus, preventing the refluxing of urine into the ureters.

The three muscle layers of the ureter increase greatly in size as they continue onto the **urinary bladder** as the thick, robust muscularis. The middle circular layer is the largest. Its fibers thicken at the urethral orifice as the **internal sphincter** of the bladder. The muscle bundles of these three layers interlace so that the layers become quite indistinct.

Adventitia

The adventitia of these extrarenal passageways is a **fibroelastic outer covering** that blends with the surrounding connective tissue. In the renal pelvis it is continuous with the capsule of the kidney. The ureters and bladder are retro-

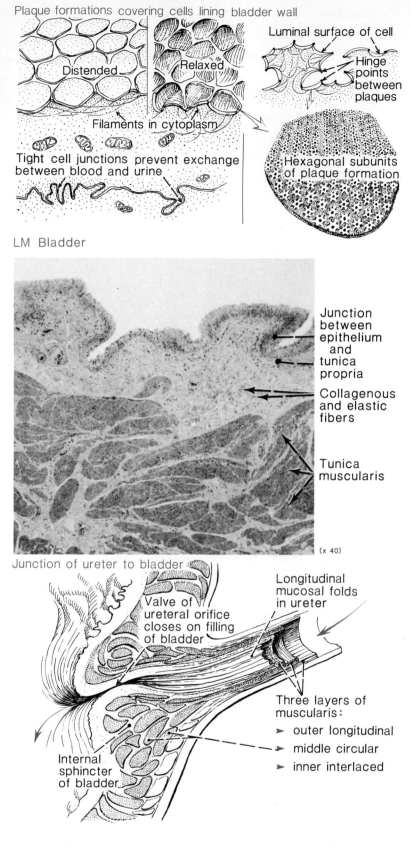

Plaque formations covering cells lining bladder wall

Distended   Relaxed

Luminal surface of cell

Hinge points between plaques

Filaments in cytoplasm

Tight cell junctions prevent exchange between blood and urine

Hexagonal subunits of plaque formation

LM Bladder

Junction between epithelium and tunica propria

Collagenous and elastic fibers

Tunica muscularis

(x 40)

Junction of ureter to bladder

Valve of ureteral orifice closes on filling of bladder

Longitudinal mucosal folds in ureter

Internal sphincter of bladder

Three layers of muscularis:
▸ outer longitudinal
▸ middle circular
▸ inner interlaced

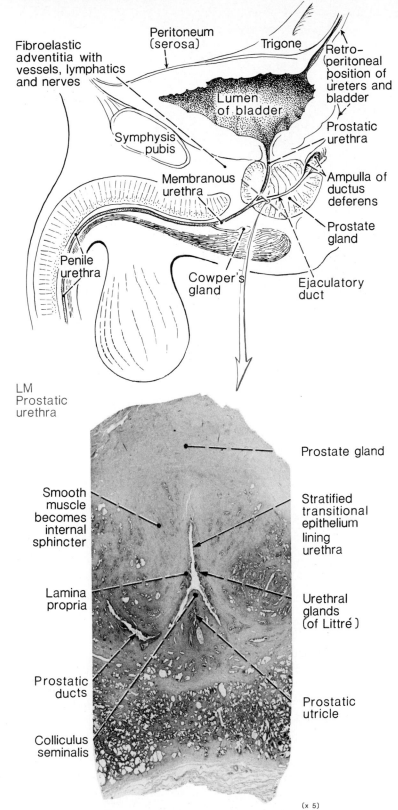

LM
Prostatic
urethra

Fibroelastic adventitia with vessels, lymphatics and nerves

Peritoneum (serosa)

Trigone

Retro-peritoneal position of ureters and bladder

Lumen of bladder

Symphysis pubis

Prostatic urethra

Membranous urethra

Ampulla of ductus deferens

Penile urethra

Cowper's gland

Prostate gland

Ejaculatory duct

Prostate gland

Smooth muscle becomes internal sphincter

Stratified transitional epithelium lining urethra

Lamina propria

Urethral glands (of Littré)

Prostatic ducts

Prostatic utricle

Colliculus seminalis

(× 5)

peritoneal, except the superior surface of the bladder which is covered with **peritoneum.** Thus the outer coat in this region is a **serosa** and not an adventitia. Blood vessels, lymphatics, and nerves course through the adventitia to serve the muscularis and mucosa.

URETHRA

The urethra, the final conducting part of the urinary tract, differs significantly from the rest of the extrarenal collecting system and therefore will be described separately.

Male Urethra

The **male urethra** is a mucous membrane tube about 20 cm long that serves a dual purpose, namely, to **transport both urine and sperm** to the outside. It is divided into three parts, a prostatic portion (3–4 cm), a membranous segment (1–2 cm), and a cavernous, spongy, or penile region (about 15 cm).

Located next to the bladder, embedded in the prostate gland, is the **prostatic urethra.** It is lined with **transitional epithelium** that becomes pseudostratified or stratified columnar distally. In its distal dorsal wall is a longitudinal swelling, the **colliculus seminalis,** with a blind dimple at its tip, the **prostatic utricle** (the vestigial homolog of the uterus). On either side are slitlike terminations of the ductus deferentes, called the **ejaculatory ducts.** The prostate gland empties its secretions into this segment.

The indistinct **lamina propria** has considerable elastic fibers that intertwine among the many small thin-walled venules. Also, a few **urethral glands (of Littré)** empty into the lumen. Wisps of smooth muscle, mostly circular, lie outside the loose lamina propria where they are reinforced to form the **internal sphincter** of the bladder.

As the urethra penetrates the urogenital diaphragm, a fibromuscular layer between the pelvic bones, it acquires an investment of skeletal muscle and becomes the **membranous urethra.** The circular muscular fibers form the **external (voluntary) sphincter.** Pseudostratified or stratified columnar epithelium lines this, the shortest part of the urethra. **Urethral glands are increased in size and number.**

18083

The cavernous or **penile urethra** is also lined with stratified or pseudostratified columnar epithelium, except near the dilated opening (**meatus**) where it becomes **stratified squamous**. **Urethral glands** are conspicuous as they empty into prominent lateral pockets in the mucosa, called the **lacunae of Morgagni**. In these deep, irregular recesses, the epithelium proliferates to form small clusters of clear, stratified columnar cells. They are **intraepithelial glands**, discussed in Chapter 5.

Female Urethra

The shorter (3–5 cm) **female urethra** is lined with **transitional epithelium** only near the bladder. The distal portion of the urethra has **stratified squamous epithelium** that is continuous with the epidermis of the skin. Patches of stratified or pseudostratified columnar epithelium may be found inserted between these areas. A few glands open onto the mucosal surface, which shows longitudinal folds.

The thin **lamina propria** has an abundance of **elastic fibers** that interlace among the prominent thin-walled, **venous plexuses**. An outer circular and an inner longitudinal layer of smooth muscle surround the urethra. The layers are irregularly arranged with some intermingling of the venous plexuses of the tunica propria. Some circular fibers condense as the **internal sphincter**. Distally, at the lower end of the urethra, other smooth muscle fibers are reinforced by **skeletal muscle** bundles to form the voluntary **external sphincter urethrae**. (See Table 20.2 and LA-, plate 28).

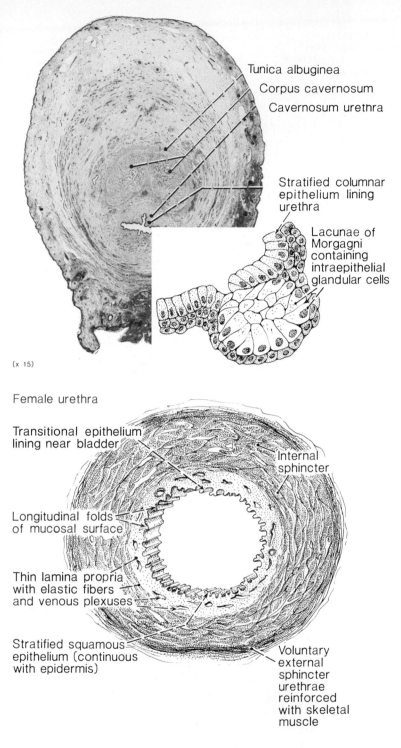

Penile urethra

Tunica albuginea
Corpus cavernosum
Cavernosum urethra

Stratified columnar epithelium lining urethra

Lacunae of Morgagni containing intraepithelial glandular cells

(x 15)

Female urethra

Transitional epithelium lining near bladder

Internal sphincter

Longitudinal folds of mucosal surface

Thin lamina propria with elastic fibers and venous plexuses

Stratified squamous epithelium (continuous with epidermis)

Voluntary external sphincter urethrae reinforced with skeletal muscle

A Retrospective View of the Malpighian Corpuscle

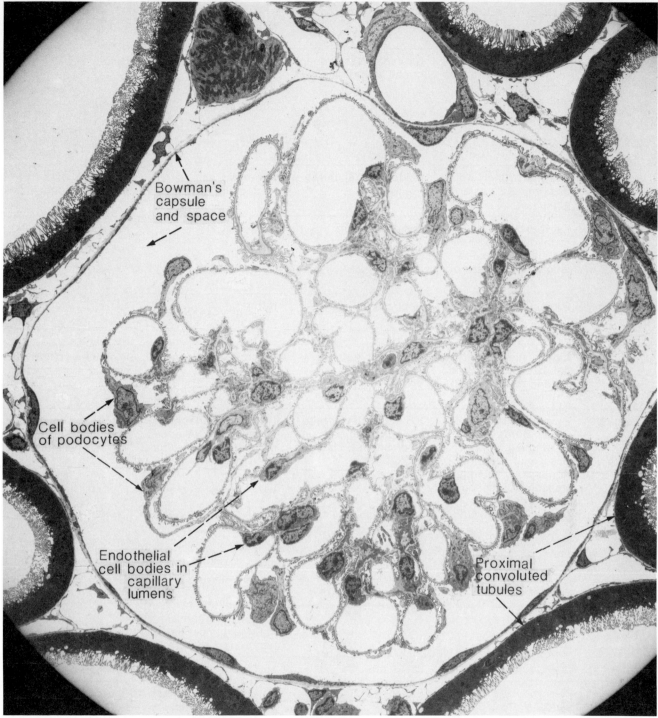

EM Glomerulus (×1400)

P. M. Andrews

In 1666 the Italian anatomist M. Malpighi was the first to describe the renal glomeruli, as seen through the microscope. He portrayed them as "very small, round bodies, like a coil of small worms, attached like apples to the blood vessels and stretched out into the form of a beautiful tree." Later these glomeruli were appropriately called *Malpighian corpuscles.*

Now, over three centuries later, let us examine the components of the renal glomerulus, as revealed by the transmission electron microscope. For example, what are Malpighi's "coils of worms"? What are the "very small, round bodies" actually attached to the vascular tree? What are the present concepts of the structure and function of Bowman's capsule? Of the glomerular filtration barrier? Identify the differences, if any, between glomerulus, Malpighian corpuscles, renal corpuscle, nephron, uriniferous tubule, rete mirabile, and tuft of capillaries.

Table 20.1 *COMPARISON OF KIDNEY TUBULES*

	PROXIMAL CONVOLUTED (PCT)	THICK DESCENDING	THIN LOOP (OF HENLE)	THICK ASCENDING
Epithelium	Tall cuboidal or pyramidal; cell borders indistinct due to lateral wall interdigitations	Cuboidal; less overlap of cell boundaries	Squamous	Cuboidal
Cytoplasm	Abundant, finely granular, markedly acidophilic	Acidophilic, slightly granular	Agranular, pale, faintly acidophilic	Some fine granules more acidophilia
Basal striations	Fairly prominent; formed from long mitochondria oriented lengthwise in base of cell	Less prominent	None	Poorly developed
Brush border	Prominent diagnostic feature (very long microvilli)	Reduced in height	None	None
Nuclei	Lightly stained, spherical; usually only 3–4 seen in cross section	Oval, light staining; 3–4 in most cross sections	Ovoid; 5–6 seen in cross section	Prominent, ovoid; 5–8 seen in cross section
EM features	Prominent microvilli (brush border) and pleated lateral and basal wall interdigitations; many vacuoles, ribosomes, lysosomes, and peroxisomes; Golgi complex with many vesicles and cisternae; many mitochondria, esp. in basal zone	Except for fewer mitochondria and basal interdigitations, similar to PCT	Reduced overlapping of cell walls; fewer cell organelles; occasional microvilli	Mitochondria conspicuous; few short microvilli and wall interdigitations
Length	14–20 mm	4–6 mm	Variable; cortical nephrons have short segments (less than 2 mm); juxtamedullary nephrons 2–10 mm	About 9 mm
Diameter	30–60 μm	25–35 μm	15–20 μm	30–35 μm
Functions	Resorbs from filtrate glucose, small proteins, amino acids, 80–85% of H_2O, and electrolytes; acts as an ion pump; excretes certain dyes and drugs, e.g., penicillin, and some metabolites	Same as PCT	Resorbs about 6% of filtrate H_2O; pumps Na^+ and Cl^- ions out of lumen into extracellular space	Acts as ion pump esp. Na^+ and Cl^-; resorbs no H_2O

DISTAL CONVOLUTED (DCT)	ARCHED COLLECTING	STRAIGHT COLLECTING	PAPILLARY DUCTS
Cuboidal often binucleate and irregular in shape; upper region, columnar cells with closely packed, dark nuclei, i.e., the macula densa	Cuboidal to columnar; mostly light-staining cells with dark cells interposed	Columnar; light cells with few dark cells	Tall columnar; only light cells
Granular considerable acidophilia	Agranular, slightly acidophilic	Agranular, slightly acidophilic	Agranular, slightly acidophilic
Prominent	None	None	None
None	None	None	None
Prominent, round, darkly stained; 5–8 seen in cross section	Round, darkly stained; 8–10 seen in cross section	Round, darkly stained; 8–10 seen in cross section	Round, darkly stained; 8–10 seen in cross section
Very extensive basal interdigitations, with long, densely packed mitochondria produce basal striations; lysosomes less numerous; short microvilli more numerous	Limited pleating of cell walls; many mitochondria in dark cells; glycogen plentiful in light cells; organelles reduced in number and size; few irregular, short microvilli	Fewer interdigitations and mitochondria; dark cells less numerous	Little or no cell overlapping; few dispersed mitochondria; some lipid and lipofuscin granules; only light cells observed
About 5 mm	Since the collecting tubule has no clear segmental boundaries, the length of various segments cannot be determined accurately; however, the entire length of a collecting tubule is about 20–22 mm		
30–50 μm	Range for all segments 40–300 μm		
Under influence of antidiuretic hormone (ADH) resorbs about 9% of filtrate H_2O; sodium pumped out; produces ammonia	Under influence of ADH they resorb about 4% of filtrate H_2O; they act as conduits for urine; only about 1% of filtrate H_2O retained in urine		

Table 20.2 *COMPARISON OF URINARY PASSAGEWAYS*

	EPITHELIUM	LAMINA PROPRIA	MUSCULARIS	ADVENTITIA	FUNCTION
INTRARENAL COLLECTING DUCTS					
Collecting tubules	Upper region—clear, simple cuboidal; lower region—clear, simple columnar	Absent	Absent	Absent	Concentration of urine by resorption of water
Papillary ducts	Clear, simple columnar	Absent	Absent	Absent	Limited concentration of urine by water resorption
Calyces	Transitional (2–3 layers of cells)	Limited elastic and reticular fibers; few lymphocytes; no glands	Few inner longitudinal and outer circular smooth muscle fibers	Delicate connective tissue	Reception of urine from papillary ducts
Renal pelvis	Transitional (2–3 layers)	Elastic and reticular fibers; more lymphocytes; no glands	Rather distinct inner longitudinal and outer circular muscle layers	Limited fibroelastic covering continuous with the renal capsule	Funnel for reception of urine from major calyces
EXTRARENAL COLLECTING SYSTEM					
Ureters	Transitional (4–5 layers)	Collagenous and elastic fibers; many lymphocytes; no glands	Two prominent layers; inner longitudinal, outer circular; in lower third another layer present, an outer longitudinal	Loose fibroelastic with adipose tissue	Conduit for urine emptying into bladder
Bladder	Transitional 6–8 layers when bladder empty; 2–3 layers when distended	Occasional lymph node and diffuse lymphoid tissue in vascular connective tissue; mucosa thrown into folds in relaxed state; few mucous glands near internal sphincter	Three layers: inner longitudinal or oblique, middle circular, and outer longitudinal; layers indistinct due to interlacing of fibers	Peritoneal serosa over superior surface; remainder covered by loose connective tissue	Temporary storage and limited concentration of urine
Male urethra ● Prostatic	Near bladder, transitional; distally, pseudostratified columnar	Replaced by prostate; very vascular, fibromuscular tissue; no distinct papillae; few glands of Littré	Delicate inner longitudinal and outer circular layers; circular fibers thickened as internal sphincter	Replaced by prostate	Conduit for urine and semen
● Membranous	Pseudostratified or stratified columnar	Limited fibroelastic tissue; no papillae; few glands of Littré	Striated muscle fibers of urogenital diaphragm form external sphincter	Replaced by external sphincter	Conduit for urine and semen
● Cavernous	Pseudostratified or stratified columnar; at meatus, stratified squamous	Replaced by corpus cavernosum urethrae (spongiosum); many glands of Littré; some papillae	Replaced by smooth muscle in septa of erectile tissue	Replaced by erectile tissue	Conduit for urine and semen

Table 20.2   *(continued)*

	EPITHELIUM	LAMINA PROPRIA	MUSCULARIS	ADVENTITIA	FUNCTION
EXTRARENAL COLLECTING DUCTS					
Female urethra	Upper part, transitional; lower part, stratified squamous	Mucosa folded longitudinally; abundant elastic fibers and venous plexuses; no papillae; few glands of Littré	Inner longitudinal; outer circular layers; circular fibers condense as internal sphincter; distally these fibers replaced by skeletal muscle fibers to form external sphincter	Poorly defined or absent	Conduit for urine

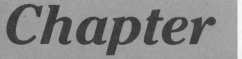

Chapter

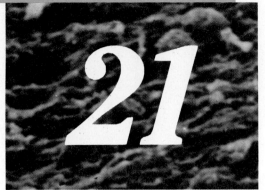

21

ENDOCRINE SYSTEM I— PITUITARY AND HYPOTHALAMUS

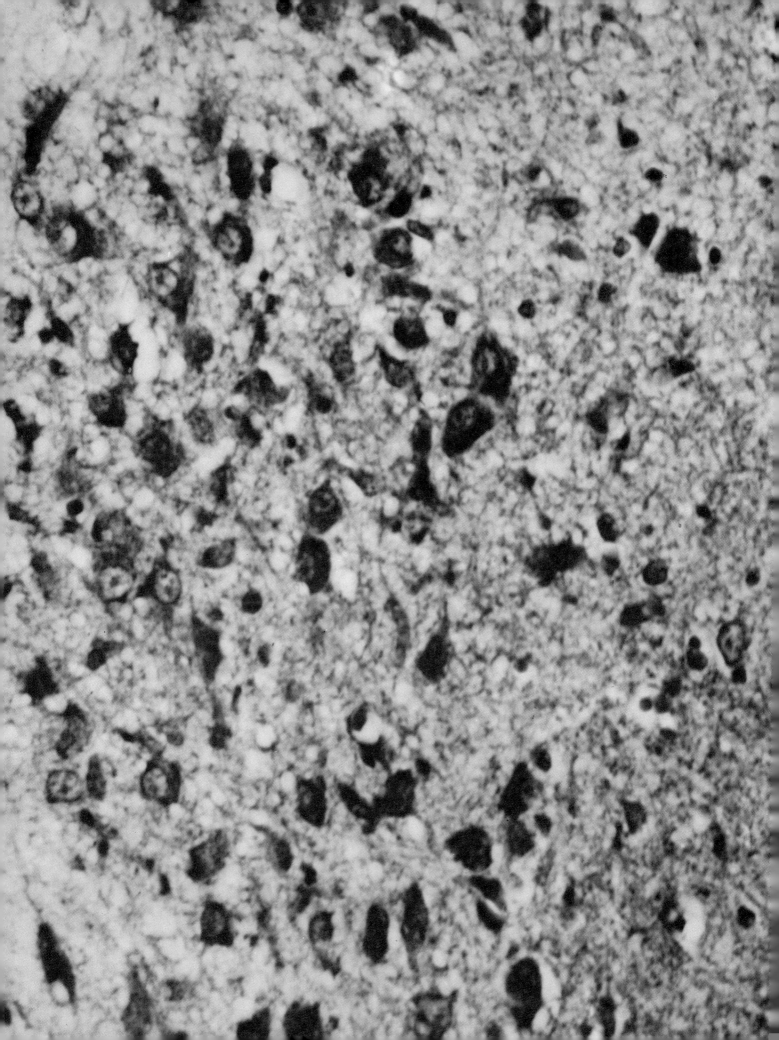

TO ENABLE THE STUDENT TO:

1. Recognize hormones as chemical messengers which may influence every cell in the body.

2. Contrast the regions of the pituitary as to origin, histology, secretions, and functions.

3. Differentiate the various cell types in the pituitary and explain their endocrine functions.

4. Accept the concept that the pituitary is largely under the control of the hypothalamus.

5. Explain the interplay that the releasing and inhibiting factors (hormones) of the hypothalamus have on the synthesis and release of the pituitary hormones.

The two great integrating forces of the body are the **nervous and endocrine systems.** Both systems respond to variations in the external and internal environments of the body. They react by sending messages to various parts of the body that cause the organism to adjust to the environmental changes. Thus, both of these systems are **homeostatic mechanisms** since they help maintain a constant, steady state in the various physiologic systems of the body.

While the nervous system can send signals at great speed, e.g., 130 m/sec, the endocrine system responds much more slowly because its messengers, the hormones, must travel via the bloodstream, usually to some distant organ or tissue. While some hormonal effects occur in seconds, others may take days before they begin and then they may continue for days, months, or even a lifetime.

Although these two systems usually act independently, there are many instances of **interdependence.** For example, certain hormones of the adrenal medulla and the pituitary gland are only released into the bloodstream in response to nervous stimuli arising in the hypothalamus.

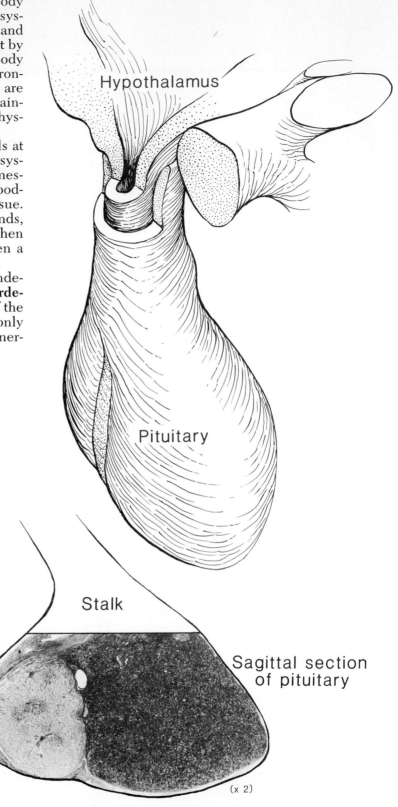

Hypothalamus

Pituitary

Stalk

Sagittal section
of pituitary

(x 2)

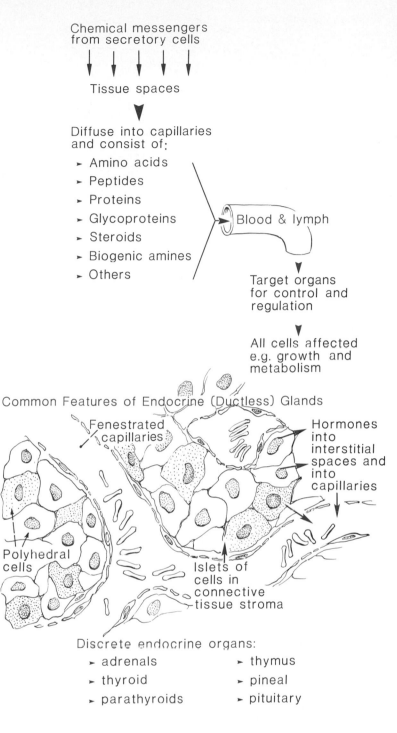

Chemical messengers
from secretory cells

↓ ↓ ↓ ↓ ↓

Tissue spaces

▼

Diffuse into capillaries
and consist of:

► Amino acids
► Peptides
► Proteins
► Glycoproteins
► Steroids
► Biogenic amines
► Others

Blood & lymph

Target organs
for control and
regulation

▼

All cells affected
e.g. growth and
metabolism

Common Features of Endocrine (Ductless) Glands

Fenestrated
capillaries

Hormones
into
interstitial
spaces and
into
capillaries

Polyhedral
cells

Islets of
cells in
connective
tissue stroma

Discrete endocrine organs:

► adrenals   ► thymus
► thyroid   ► pineal
► parathyroids   ► pituitary

Consolidated endocrine cells with other structures:

► hypothalamus   ► testes
► pancreas   ► ovaries
► GI tract   ► others

HORMONES AS CHEMICAL MESSENGERS

The secretory cells of the endocrine system synthesize organic compounds, the hormones (Gk. homaein, to set in motion, to excite), which are secreted into the tissue spaces surrounding capillaries before the hormones **enter the capillaries by diffusion.** The chemical nature of hormones may be amino acids, peptides, proteins, glycoproteins, steroids, biogenic amines, and possibly others (see Table 21.1).

Since these chemical messengers are carried throughout the body by the blood and lymph, they are accessible to all cells of the body. Yet in most instances, they influence primarily some distant organ or tissue, called the **target organ.** In other words, hormones usually do not affect all cells indiscriminately but direct their action toward the control and regulation of the functions of a specific organ. However, a few hormones influence essentially every cell in the body, such as the growth hormone of the pituitary and thyroxin of the thyroid gland. **Activities controlled** wholly or in part by hormones include smooth muscle contraction, sexual maturation, development and growth of the body, and many metabolic functions, to name only a few.

SIMILARITIES OF ENDOCRINE GLANDS

The parenchymal cells of endocrine glands have the following **features in common:** (1) They have a **rich blood supply.** At least one surface of each endocrine cell abuts onto a fenestrated capillary. Such a relationship facilitates the entry of the hormones into the bloodstream after it is discharged into the surrounding interstitial spaces. (2) They have **no functional duct system.** Therefore, endocrine glands are also called **ductless glands.** (3) Cells usually are arranged in blocks, islets, plates, or cords. (4) Except the neurosecretory cells of the hypothalamus, all endocrine cells are **epithelial in origin,** supported by delicate connective tissue stroma. (5) Cells are usually **polyhedral** in shape with a prominent spherical nucleus. (6) **Organelles are very numerous,** especially the mitochondria, Golgi complexes, secretory vesicles, and endoplasmic reticulum.

Being a diffuse system, the endocrine glands may be separate, discrete organs or they may be incorporated into other organs scattered throughout the body. Those **separate endocrine glands** include the adrenals, thyroid, parathyroids, thymus, pineal, and pituitary. These glands will be discussed in this chapter and in Chapter 22, except the thymus, which was described with the lymphoid tissues in Chapter 14. The other endocrine glands or cells are **consolidated with other structures.** These cell groups are the neurosecretory cells of the hypothalamus, islet cells of the pancreas, enteroendocrine cells of the GI tract, interstitial cells of the testes, and others.

HYPOPHYSIS OR PITUITARY GLAND

The famous Renaissance anatomist, Vesalius, named this gland the **pituitary** (L. pituita, phlegm), because he incorrectly assumed that it secreted phlegm or mucus associated with the nose and throat. Nearly two centuries later when the true function of the gland was discovered, the term **hypophysis** was coined; it means "to grow under." This is a much more appropriate term since the hypophysis is an appendage of the brain, suspended by a stalk from its inferior surface (the hypothalamus). It fits snugly into a bony fossa, the sella turcica ("Turkish saddle"), in the base of the skull.

The hypophysis is often called the "**master or chief gland**" of the endocrine system. Such a designation is no longer entirely appropriate. The pituitary is actually a servant of the brain, since nearly all of its hormonal secretions are controlled by signals emanating from the hypothalamus, i.e., the **hypothalamic releasing and inhibiting factors** or hormones. The hypophysis plays a major role in **integrating the endocrine and nervous systems** in the control of many of our physiological processes.

Types of Hormones

The pituitary hormones are divided into two general categories:

1. Some hormones **act directly** upon and modulate the function of other **endocrine glands.** These are the so-called **trophic** (Gk. trophikos, nursing) hormones that influence the growth, development, and nutrition of specific target glands. These pituitary-dependent endocrine glands include the **thyroid,** which responds to the thyroid-stimulating hormone (**TSH**); the **gonads,** which react to the follicle-stimulating hormone (**FSH**) and to the luteinizing hormone (**LH**) [identical to the interstitial cell stimulating hormone (**ICSH**) of the testis], and the **adrenal cortex,** which is stimulated by the adrenocorticotrophic hormone (**ACTH**).

2. The other classification contains those hormones that **act directly on nonendocrine tissues** or organs. They are somatotropin (**STH**) **or growth hormone (GH)**, which acts mostly on skeletal structures, e.g., bones and muscles; **prolactin** or lactogenic hormone, which triggers milk production; antidiuretic hormone (**ADH**) or **vasopressin,** which concentrates the urine in the kidney, allowing resorption of water; **oxytocin,** which aids contraction of the uterine muscles during parturition; and the melanocyte-stimulating hormone (**MSH**), which controls melanin dispersal in the skin of certain lower animals, e.g. amphibians.

Pituitary relationships:

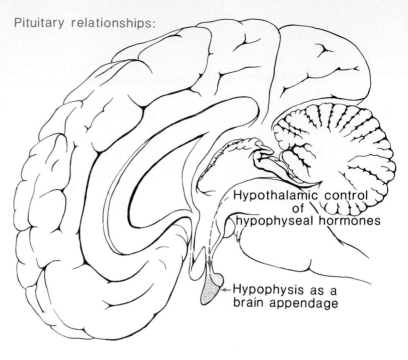

Hypothalamic control of hypophyseal hormones

←Hypophysis as a brain appendage

Hypophyseal (pituitary) hormones:

1) modulate other endocrine glands (trophic for growth, develpment and nutrition)

➤ thyroid stimulating (TSH)

➤ follicle stimulating (FSH)

➤ luteinizing (LH) equivalent to interstitial cell stimulating (ICSH)

➤ adrenocorticotrophic (ACTH)

2) Act on nonendocrine tissue and organs

➤ somatotropin (STH) or growth (GH) on skeletal structures

prolactin (milk production)

➤ antidiuretic (ADH) or vasopressin on kidneys

➤ oxytocin (uterine contraction at parturition)

➤ melanocyte stimulating (MSH) dispersal of melanin e.g. in amphibians

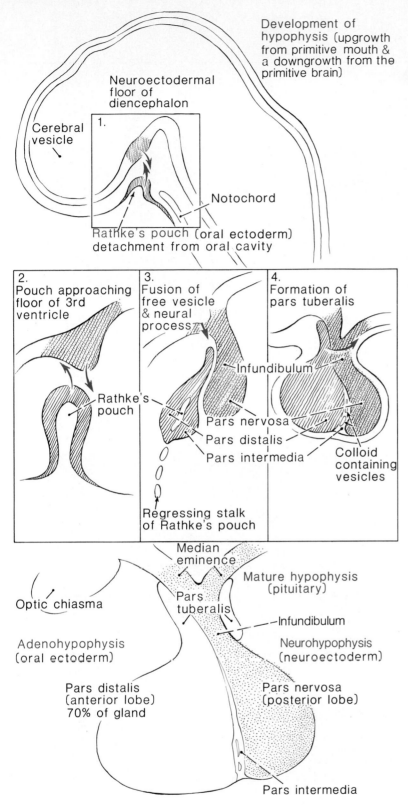

Development of hypophysis (upgrowth from primitive mouth & a downgrowth from the primitive brain)

Neuroectodermal floor of diencephalon

Cerebral vesicle

1.

Notochord

Rathke's pouch (oral ectoderm) detachment from oral cavity

2. Pouch approaching floor of 3rd ventricle

Rathke's pouch

3. Fusion of free vesicle & neural process

Infundibulum

Pars nervosa
Pars distalis
Pars intermedia

Regressing stalk of Rathke's pouch

4. Formation of pars tuberalis

Colloid containing vesicles

Median eminence

Optic chiasma

Pars tuberalis

Adenohypophysis (oral ectoderm)

Mature hypophysis (pituitary)

Infundibulum

Neurohypophysis (neuroectoderm)

Pars distalis (anterior lobe) 70% of gland

Pars nervosa (posterior lobe)

Pars intermedia

Origin

The hypophysis has a **dual origin.** The glandular part, **adenohypophysis,** is derived from **oral ectoderm** as an upward outpocketing of the roof of the oral cavity, called **Rathke's pouch.** Simultaneously, the nervous part, the **neurohypophysis,** arises from **neural ectoderm** as a tubular downgrowth (the **infundibulum**) of the floor of the third ventricle of the primitive brain.

During development, Rathke's pouch loses its connection with the oral cavity and, as a free epithelial sac, migrates towards the neural process which is still attached to the brain. These two anlagen eventually fuse.

The components of the **adenohypophysis** develop from **Rathke's pouch.** The greatly thickened anterior wall of the pouch becomes the **pars distalis** (anterior lobe). The narrow fusion region between the two anlagen develops into the **pars intermedia** (intermediate lobe), while the superior lateral extensions of the pouch wrap around the upper stalk of the infundibulum like a collar. These extensions become the **pars tuberalis,** which is actually an extension of the pars distalis.

The **neurohypophysis** develops from the **neural anlage.** The **pars nervosa** arises from the large, bulbous distal end, the **infundibulum** (pituitary stalk) from the medial portion, and the **median eminence** from the expanded proximal portion. The latter structure is a part of the **hypothalamus,** located in the floor of the third ventricle of the brain. The **posterior lobe** is formed by the fusion of pars nervosa with pars intermedia.

Between the pars distalis and the pars intermedia, the original lumen of Rathke's pouch remains as a **permanent cleft.** Anterior to the cleft is the large, glandular **anterior lobe,** and posteriorly is the smaller neural **posterior lobe.**

Components of the Hypophysis (Pituitary)

ORIGIN	PRIMARY DIVISIONS	SECONDARY DIVISIONS
Oral ectoderm	Adenohypophysis	Pars distalis Pars tuberalis Pars intermedia
Neuroectoderm	Neurohypophysis	Pars nervosa Infundibulum Median eminence

ADENOHYPOPHYSIS The prefix adeno- (Gk. adenos, glandular) indicates that the **adenohypophysis** comprises the **glandular elements** of the pituitary. They include, (1) the large **pars distalis** (anterior lobe), (2) the smaller **pars tuberalis** that is wrapped around the infundibular stalk, and (3) the rudimentary **pars intermedia,** a narrow cleft situated between the pars distalis and the nervosa.

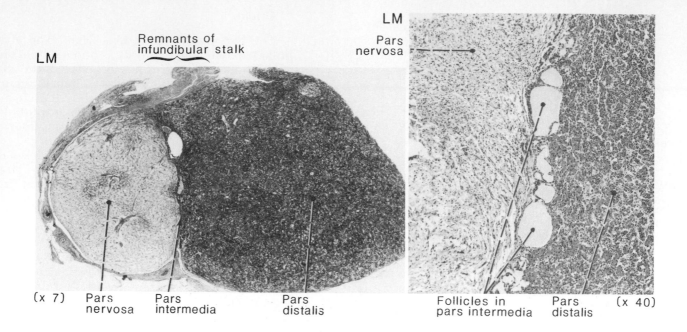

LM

Remnants of infundibular stalk

LM
Pars nervosa

(x 7) Pars nervosa Pars intermedia Pars distalis

Follicles in pars intermedia Pars distalis (x 40)

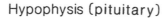

Hypophysis (pituitary)

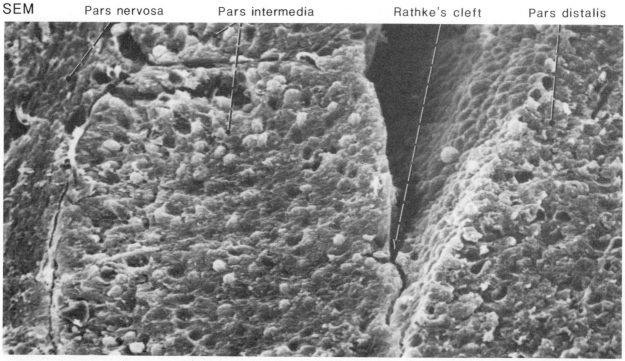

SEM Pars nervosa Pars intermedia Rathke's cleft Pars distalis

S. Correr & P.M. Motta (x 1200)

The upper photomicrographs reveal the spatial relationships of the principal divisions of the pituitary.

On the lower SEM micrograph of an adult rat hypophysis, Rathke's cleft (pouch) persists as a distinct fissure separating the pars distalis from the pars intermedia. The pouch is lined with a continuous layer of cells possessing microvillous and ciliated apical surfaces. In some specimens the cleft may be filled with colloid.

7293

Pars distalis (anterior lobe) of hypophysis synthesizes:

➤ somatotropin (STH) or growth (GH) hormone

➤ luteinizing (LH)

➤ follicle stimulating (FSH)

➤ thyrotropin (TSH)

➤ adrenocorticotropin (ACTH)

➤ prolactin

LM   Cells of pars distalis

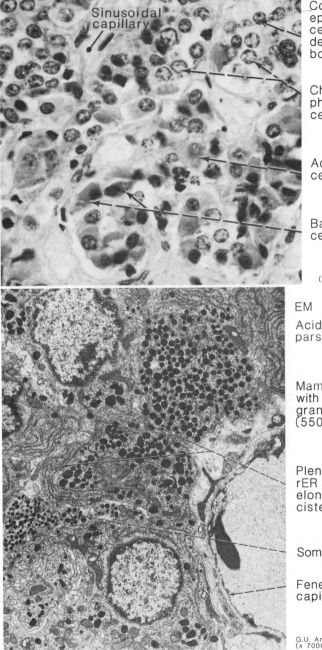

Sinusoidal capillary

Cords of epithelial cells with defined bouhdaries

Chromo-phobic cells (50%)

Acidophilic cells (40%)

Basophilic cells (10%)

(x 420)

EM

Acidophils in pars distalis

Mammotroph with secretory granules (550-700nm)

Plentiful rER with elongated cisternae

Somatotroph

Fenestrated capillary wall

G.U. Anat. Collection
(x 7000)

Pars Distalis (Anterior Lobe) The largest subdivision of the pituitary is the **pars distalis**. It occupies about 70% of the entire gland and is the site of **synthesis of six well-established hormones**, i.e., growth hormone (GH) or somatotropin (STH), luteinizing (LH), follicle-stimulating hormone (FSH), thyrotropin (TSH), adrenocorticotropin (ACTH), and prolactin.

The parenchyma of the pars distalis consists of solid, irregular **cords or blocks of epithelial cells** that abut onto the walls of fenestrated, sinusoidal capillaries. Most of the epithelial cells are polyhedral in shape, with well-defined cell boundaries. Histologically they are divided into two classes: (1) **chromophilic,** meaning color-loving; and (2) **chromophobic,** color-fearing. Those chromophilic cells, whose cytoplasm stains deeply with acidophilic dyes, are called **acidophils,** while those staining with basic dyes are **basophils.** The **chromophobes** have no special affinity for either acid or basic dyes and are therefore essentially unstained by conventional methods. However, electron microscopic and histochemical procedures reveal that there is a **specific cell type for each hormone** secreted by the pars distalis.

In the normal human adult, about 40% of the cells are acidophils, 10% basophils, and the remainder chromophobes. However, these **percentages vary** considerably depending on (1) the **region** of the gland—acidophils favor the periphery, (2) **age**—cells atrophy with age and the percentage of basophils increases with age, (3) **gonadectomy**—basophils become vacuolated and assume a signet ring appearance of the nuclei, (4) **pregnancy**—all cells undergo hypertrophy, and perhaps other conditions.

ACIDOPHILS There are two populations of **acidophils,** namely, **somatotrophs** that synthesize growth hormone (somatotropin) and **mammotrophs** that produce the lactogenic hormone, prolactin. These types cannot be distinguished with any degree of certainty with the LM using H&E stain. Granules in the cytoplasm of both types of cells stain reddish yellow (**eosinophilic**). However, under the EM the two cell types can be readily identified. For example, the most abundant ovoid or polyhedral **somatotrophs** have many homogeneous spherical or ovoid electron-dense secretory **granules about 300–400 nm** in diameter. Prominent profiles of **rER** with stacks of elongated cisternae lie parallel to the cell surface. A well-developed **Golgi apparatus** is usually present as well as a few lysosomes.

The less plentiful **mammotrophs** are characterized by the **large secretory granules.** These homogeneous, dense granules are the largest of any cell in the pituitary, ranging from **550–700 nm.** The cells are also of **various shapes,** e.g., ovoid, ellipsoidal, or spherical.

BASOPHILS The less abundant **basophils** are divided into three functional and morphological types, **gonadotrophs** (FSH and LH), **thyrotrophs** (TSH), and **corticotrophs** (ACTH). Although the granules of all basophils stain selectively with basic dyes, they often react poorly with H&E. However, they give a strong positive reaction to periodic acid-Schiff reagent (**PAS**) since these cells synthesize and release peptide hormones that contain bound carbohydrates (**glycoproteins**). Therefore, the PAS reaction is more indicative of the presence of hormones than a nonspecific basic dye, such as hematoxylin.

Functionally the gonadotrophs are divided into **two groups:** (1) those cells that synthesize and release follicle-stimulating hormone (**FSH**), and (2) those cells that secrete luteinizing hormone (**LH**). In the male, the luteinizing hormone stimulates the interstitial cells of the testis and is therefore called interstitial cell stimulating hormone (**ICSH**). It activates the interstitial cells to secrete **testosterone.** These cells are scattered singly throughout the anterior lobe and cannot be clearly distinguished under LM with conventional stains.

However, in EM studies these two cell types of gonadotrophs can be identified by differences in their cell organelles. For example, **gonadotrophs** that secrete **FSH** are **large, spherical cells** with uniform, dense, rounded **secretory granules about 200 nm** in diameter. They have an **extensive Golgi** apparatus and considerable rER characterized by distended and dilated sacs. In contrast, the **LH-** and **ICSH-**producing **cells are smaller** with **larger (250 nm) dense granules.** The Golgi body is less extensive, and the vesicular elements of the rER are flattened rather than dilated.

The thyrotrophs are basophils that are usually **smaller cells** and tend to be angular in shape rather than spherical. They frequently cluster in groups. Their **granules**, less dense and irregular, are the **smallest** of all cells of the pars distalis, averaging about **120–150 nm** in diameter. They tend to collect in the periphery of the cell. The rER consists of a few flattened cisternae of irregular distribution and limited ribosomes. They release the hormone **thyrotropin.**

Corticotrophs synthesize the hormone **ACTH** that stimulates the middle and inner zones of the adrenal cortex to secrete **glucocorticoids.** Corticotrophs are spherical cells larger than most other cells in the gland, and their **granules** are relatively **large (350–400 nm)**. There are abundant **ribosomes** in the cytoplasm and usually a small Golgi apparatus. Unusual cytoplasmic features are the presence of numerous **lipid droplets, lysosomes, and microfilaments** (6–8 nm in diameter). (L-A, plate 40)

LM   Basophils in pars distalis

(x 740)

PAS reactive indicating synthesis of glycoproteins

Groups of gonado-trophs

1) FSH

2) LH/ICSH

Gonadotrophic cell granules

FSH

LH/ICSH

200nm rounded granules   250 nm dense granules

EM   Thyrotrophic and gonadotrophic cells

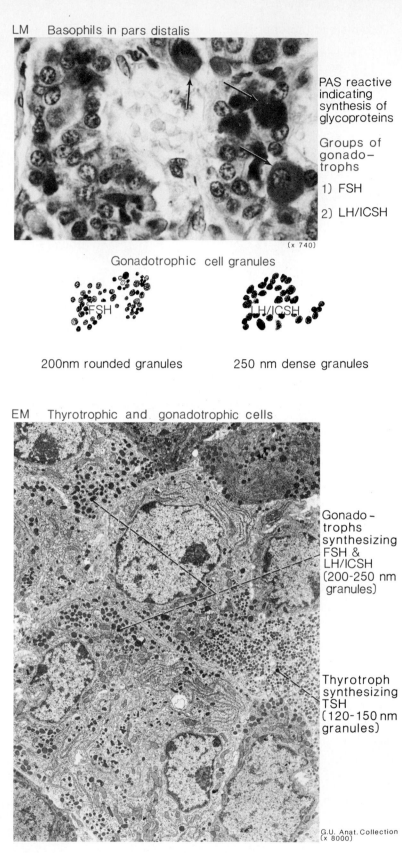

Gonado-trophs synthesizing FSH & LH/ICSH (200-250 nm granules)

Thyrotroph synthesizing TSH (120-150 nm granules)

G.U. Anat. Collection
(x 8000)

Theory:

Chromophobic cells → differentiate into chromophils
serving as a reserve population
for glandular cells

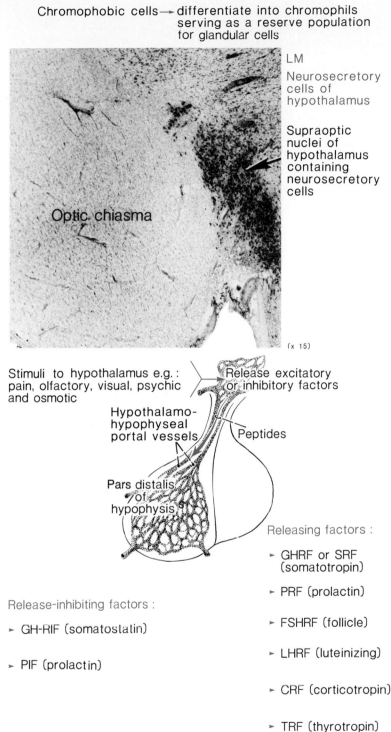

LM
Neurosecretory
cells of
hypothalamus

Supraoptic
nuclei of
hypothalamus
containing
neurosecretory
cells

Optic chiasma

(x 15)

Stimuli to hypothalamus e.g.:
pain, olfactory, visual, psychic
and osmotic

Release excitatory
or inhibitory factors

Hypothalamo-
hypophyseal
portal vessels

Peptides

Pars distalis
of
hypophysis

Releasing factors :

➤ GHRF or SRF
(somatotropin)

➤ PRF (prolactin)

➤ FSHRF (follicle)

➤ LHRF (luteinizing)

➤ CRF (corticotropin)

➤ TRF (thyrotropin)

Release-inhibiting factors :

➤ GH-RIF (somatostatin)

➤ PIF (prolactin)

CHROMOPHOBES True chromophobes, if they exist at all, are present in much smaller numbers than usually stated. The fact that these cells appear to be **agranular under the LM** is the principal reason given why they have no affinity for either basic or acidic dyes. However, when the pituitary is examined with the **EM**, it is apparent that the **chromophobes have granules**, albeit small in size (**150 nm**) and number. Thus they are too small and too few to be recognizable with the LM. Evidence supports the present theories that chromophobes are either cells that can **differentiate into any of the chromophils** or that they are really **exhausted chromophils** which are partially degranulated. If either or both of these hypotheses are accepted, it follows then that chromophobes are actually a **reserve population of cells** from which any of the various fully granulated cells can originate.

In the course of these EM studies of the unstained chromophobes, a new line of chromophobes was discovered called **follicular cells.** These are large **supportive cells** that enclose the cords of glandular cells with an extensive network. These are **nonsecretory cells,** possessing microvilli and occasional cilia. They may be phagocytic in function as well as supportive.

CONTROL OF HORMONE SECRETION
Although production of a hormone occurs within a specific cell, its **synthesis and release** are **controlled by signals** that emanate from the neurosecretory cells in the hypothalamus, especially in the **median eminence.** The hypothalamus is constantly receiving information from various parts of the nervous system, e.g., pain, olfactory, visual, psychic, and osmotic stimuli. These messengers, either singly or collectively, signal the release of **excitatory or inhibitory factors** (hormones) that are relayed to the pars distalis via the **hypothalamohypophyseal portal vessels** for the regulation of its hormonal secretions. These factors (hormones) are small peptides that are synthesized in the hypothalamus for transport to the pars distalis.

Presently there are six known **releasing factors** or hormones in mammals, i.e., growth hormone or somatotropin-releasing factor (GHRF or SRF), prolactin-releasing factor (PRF), follicle-stimulating hormone-releasing factor (FSHRF), luteinizing hormone-releasing factor (LHRF), corticotropin-releasing factor (CRF), and thyrotropin-releasing factor (TRF).

The hypothalamus also elaborates **inhibitory factors** to counterbalance the releasing factors. However, only two factors have been identified. These are the growth hormone release-inhibiting factor (**GHRIF**), also known as **somatostatin,** which is a peptide with 14 amino acids.

The **delta cells of the islet tissue** of the pancreas are perhaps a major source of this hormone, giving credence to the observation that it may control the output of the adjacent alpha and beta cells which secrete glucagon and insulin, respectively. Therefore, somatostatin may exert a multitude of physiologic effects on the body.

The other **inhibitory hormone** acts to control the secretion of prolactin, as the prolactin-inhibiting factor (**PIF**).

Pars Intermedia In most mammals, the **pars intermedia,** or intermediate lobe, is a rudimentary, diffuse, cellular zone lying between the pars distalis and the pars nervosa. It is composed mostly of slightly **basophilic cells** with **small secretory granules (200–300 nm)** that cannot be seen with the LM. These cells often surround small, **colloid-filled cysts** or follicles called Rathke's cysts. These lining cells may be ciliated and often invade the pars nervosa. **In the fetus, a distinct cleft** (of Rathke) is present between the two lobes, lined with **ciliated epithelium.** Some cells are light staining, others are basophilic. The cleft may persist in children but rarely in adults.

The basophils synthesize β-endorphin, which binds opiate receptors in the CNS. Basophils also secrete the melanocyte-stimulating hormone (**MSH**), a polypeptide especially active in amphibians where it **causes dispersion of melanin granules** causing darkening of the animal's skin. It has limited or no action in man. However, there is some evidence that **ACTH** is produced in the intermediate lobe, perhaps by these same basophils that synthesize MSH, since ACTH and MSH molecules have some identical amino acid sequences. Perhaps in man these basophils may migrate from the pars intermedia into the pars distalis where they may also manufacture ACTH and β-endorphin.

Pars Tuberalis As noted earlier, the funnel-shaped **pars tuberalis** forms a collar or tube of cells around the infundibular stalk about 25–60 μm thick. The cellular collar flares out proximally to join the floor of the **hypothalamus.**

The **parenchyma** is continuous with the **pars distalis** and includes the **three cell types** characteristic of this lobe, i.e., acidophils, basophils, and chromophobes. The cells are arranged either in cords, clusters or, at times, in follicles. All cells are separated by sinusoids.

The pars tuberalis is the **most vascular** region of the pituitary. Recall that it is traversed by the **arteries** supplying the anterior and posterior lobes, as well as the hypothalamohypophyseal **venous portal system.** Although the pars tuberalis is present in all vertebrates studied, it has **no known function.**

SEM   Pars intermedia

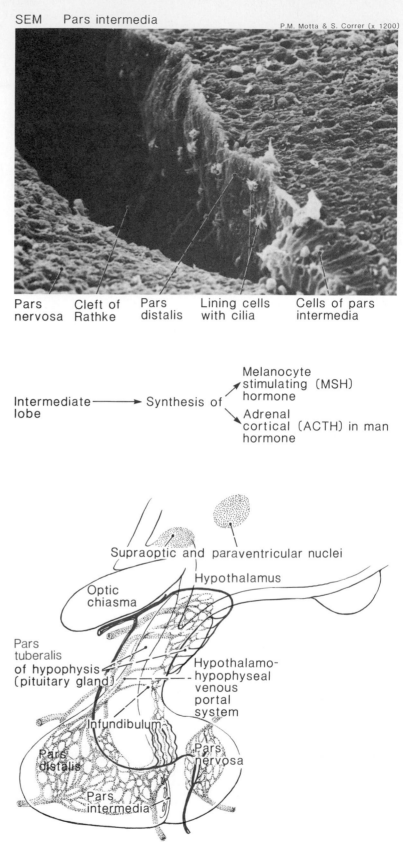

P.M. Motta & S. Correr (x 1200)

Pars nervosa | Cleft of Rathke | Pars distalis | Lining cells with cilia | Cells of pars intermedia

Intermediate lobe → Synthesis of → Melanocyte stimulating (MSH) hormone / Adrenal cortical (ACTH) in man hormone

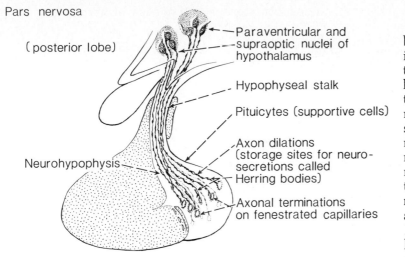

Pars nervosa

(posterior lobe)

→ Paraventricular and supraoptic nuclei of hypothalamus

Hypophyseal stalk

Pituicytes (supportive cells)

Axon dilations (storage sites for neuro-secretions called Herring bodies)

Neurohypophysis

Axonal terminations on fenestrated capillaries

LM   Neurosecretory cells in hypothalamus

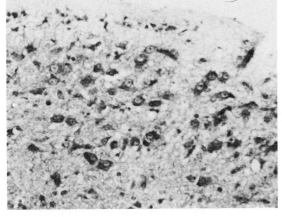

(x 200)

LM   Pituicytes (nonsecretory support cells) and Herring bodies

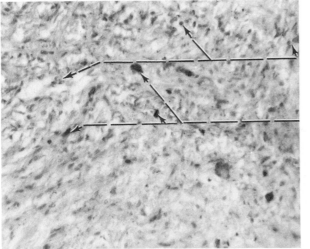

Pituicytes

Herring bodies

(x 200)

NEUROHYPOPHYSIS OR PARS NERVOSA (POSTERIOR LOBE)

The posterior lobe bears little or no resemblance to a gland. In fact, it is a mass of **neuroglial cells, called pituicytes,** that are invaded by **nerve fibers** arising from the **hypothalamus.** These pituicytes **do not secrete** the hormones oxytocin or vasopressin of the pars nervosa. They are simply a strong, **supporting structure** to accommodate the vast number of terminal nerve fibers and their endings arising mostly from the supraoptic and paraventricular nuclei in the hypothalamus. These nerve tracts traverse the **hypophyseal stalk** to enter the **neurohypophysis.** The hormones are transmitted **along the axons** in membrane-limited granules, 100–300 nm in diameter. Intermittent, axonal dilations act as temporary storage sites for the neurosecretions. These irregular, basophilic masses are called **Herring bodies.**

Upon an appropriate signal from the hypothalamus, the granules are released through the **terminal endings of the axons,** by exocytosis, to enter the fenestrated capillaries that abut on the axonal terminations. Thus the function of the neurohypophysis is not for the production of hormones, but only for their **storage and eventual release** into the bloodstream.

Neurosecretory Cells A neurosecretory cell can be defined as a neuron that also possesses **glandular activity.** This was a highly controversial concept when it was first advanced in the mid-1950s since the only function of nerve cells accepted previously was the propagation and transmission of electrical impulses. By neurosecretion is meant the **synthesis and release of hormones by specialized nerve cells** that have cytological characteristics of secretory cells. Furthermore, the **axons** of these unmyelinated nerves **transport the secretory material** to the basal lamina of capillaries or to the plasmalemma of epithelial cells. From the bulblike terminations, the secretory granules (hormones) are released by exocytosis into the extracellular space. The material then passes through thin fenestrated endothelium into blood capillaries.

Pituicytes Protoplasmic processes of the **gliallike pituicytes** invest the unmyelinated nerves and their terminations that traverse the neurohypophysis. These processes usually terminate on the walls of the fenestrated capillaries. These cells have a role equivalent to astrocytic glial cells in the central nervous system.

Pituicytes are irregular in shape and size with **many filamentous processes.** Unlike true glial cells, the limited cytoplasm of pituicytes may contain variable amounts of **lipid droplets,** golden brown pigment (probably **lipofuscin**), and particulate **glycogen.** They lack the ultrastructural features of secretory cells, a fact which strongly suggests their **nonsecretory nature.**

Functional Considerations Two hormones are stored and released by the neurohypophysis, i.e., **vasopressin,** also called the antidiuretic hormone **(ADH),** and **oxytocin** (Gk., rapid birth). The hormones are **transported as granules along axons** to the pars nervosa to be stored largely in the Herring bodies. They are released on demand from the nerve endings and eventually reach the blood capillaries. Each hormone has a binding carrier protein called **neurophysin.** This protein enables the granules to carry more hormones because it reduces the osmotic pressure within the granules as they descend into the posterior lobe.

Oxytocin stimulates **smooth muscle contraction,** especially the musculature of the uterus during parturition and coitus. It also causes **contraction of the myoepithelial cells** surrounding the alveoli and alveolar ducts of the lactating mammary gland. Such action results in the triggering of the milk ejection reflex activated by the suckling action of the infant.

In large doses, the second hormone, vasopressin, **increases blood pressure** by causing contraction of the muscular walls of the small arteries. However, its principal function is its action as a **powerful antidiuretic,** which suppresses urine production (hence its other name, the antidiuretic hormone, **ADH).** An increase of osmotic pressure of the blood plasma is the stimulus for the release of ADH. The hormone acts to greatly **increase the permeability to water** of the distal convoluting tubules and the collecting tubules of the kidney. The immediate result is that water is resorbed by the tubules, and the urine is concentrated and becomes acidic.

A deficiency of ADH results usually from lesions, such as tumors, in the hypothalamus that replace the neurosecretory cells. The end result is the disorder called **diabetes insipidis,** a condition characterized by the excretion of tremendous amounts of very dilute, nonsweet urine (5–15/l per day). This is accompanied by an intense thirst that is relieved by drinking very large quantities of fluids. (Table 21.1 is a summary of hypophyseal dysfunctions.)

Blood Supply

Like all endocrine glands, the **hypophysis** has a **profuse blood supply** that is essential for the synthesis and delivery of its many hormones. It is supplied by two groups of arteries, namely, the superior and posterior **hypophyseal arteries,** which are all directly or indirectly branches of the internal carotid arteries. The **two inferior hypophyseal arteries** are the chief blood supply to the pars nervosa. A larger group, comprised of several **superior hypophyseal arteries,** feeds an extensive capillary network in the stalk and pars

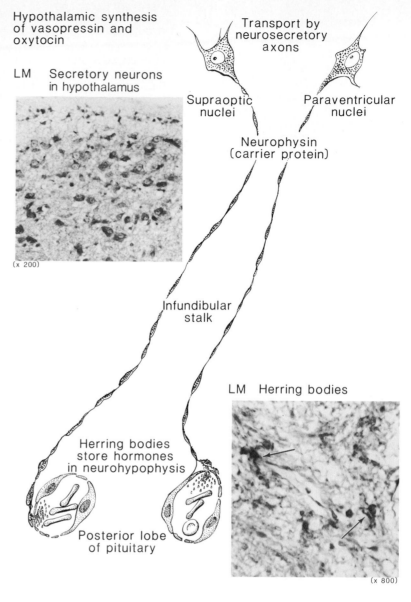

Synthesis, transport, storage and release of hormones :

Hypothalamic synthesis of vasopressin and oxytocin

Transport by neurosecretory axons

LM   Secretory neurons in hypothalamus

Supraoptic nuclei

Paraventricular nuclei

Neurophysin (carrier protein)

(x 200)

Infundibular stalk

LM   Herring bodies

Herring bodies store hormones in neurohypophysis

Posterior lobe of pituitary

(x 800)

Hormones released on demand from neurohypophysis

Vasopressin

► contracts smooth muscle of blood vessels increasing blood pressure

► increases osmotic pressure of blood plasma, H_2O absorbed, concentrating and acidifying urine

Oxytocin

► stimulates uterine smooth muscle contractions during parturition and coitus

► stimulates myoepithelial cells in mammary gland to expel milk

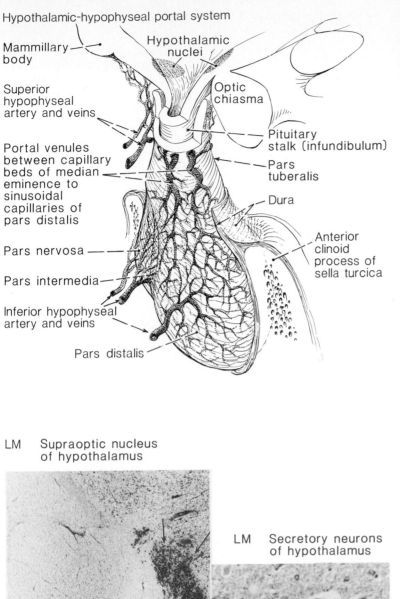

Hypothalamic-hypophyseal portal system

Mammillary body

Hypothalamic nuclei

Superior hypophyseal artery and veins

Optic chiasma

Portal venules between capillary beds of median eminence to sinusoidal capillaries of pars distalis

Pituitary stalk (infundibulum)

Pars tuberalis

Dura

Pars nervosa

Anterior clinoid process of sella turcica

Pars intermedia

Inferior hypophyseal artery and veins

Pars distalis

LM   Supraoptic nucleus of hypothalamus

Optic chiasma

(x 15)

LM   Secretory neurons of hypothalamus

(x 200)

tuberalis. Some of these capillary groups extend superiorly to penetrate the median eminence of the hypothalamus. Capillary beds (**the primary plexus**) of this region and the upper part of the stalk are drained by rather large, **wide venules** that descend in the stalk to supply the sinusoidal capillaries of the pars distalis (**the secondary plexus**). These venules are called **portal veins** because they carry blood between two capillary beds. These two sets of capillaries and the venous vessels connecting them are called the hypothalamic-hypophyseal portal system, or simply the **hypophyseal portal system.**

Except for a small contribution from the inferior hypophyseal arteries, the **anterior lobe** receives no direct arterial blood; it **is dependent upon the portal system** for oxygen and nutrients. Also, it is the portal system that provides the **pathways** for the specific **releasing hormones** of the hypophysis that reach the anterior pituitary, where they initiate the synthesis and/or trigger release of the various pituitary hormones.

As the branches of the paired inferior hypophyseal arteries enter the **pars nervosa,** they break up into an extensive capillary bed. These capillaries, however, do not form a portal system.

The venous drainage of the pituitary is accomplished by short, **wide venules** that drain the capillary beds of all subdivisions. As these vessels reach the periphery of the gland, they run in the **capsule.** They empty into nearby **dural sinuses,** especially the large **cavernous sinus,** an expanded dilation of dura mater on each side of the hypophyseal fossa that houses the pituitary.

HYPOTHALAMUS—THE CONTROLLER OF THE PITUITARY

The hypothalamus occupies only a small area at the base of the brain, posterior to the optic chiasma, and includes the infundibulum and the mammillary bodies. It has a very important role in the **control of pituitary secretions.** Attached to the brain by the stalk (infundibulum), the pituitary has extensive **neural and vascular connections** with the **hypothalamus** that are utilized for communication between the two organs.

Although the pituitary synthesizes a considerable number of hormones, their release or inhibition is triggered by signals from the **hypothalamus.** This statement rests upon the observation that if the **neural and vascular connections** between these two structures are **disrupted,** the **hormonal secretion rates drop** to very low levels and, for some hormones, even to zero. Thus the **control of hypophyseal secretions** rests with the **hypothalamus.**

7657

The pars nervosa functions as a **temporary reservoir** for the neurosecretions of the hypothalamus, **oxytocin and vasopressin**. These hormones are produced by neurosecretory cells (neurons) whose cell bodies are located in the **supraoptic and paraventricular nuclei of the hypothalamus.** The neurosecretory materials (granules) are manufactured in the endoplasmic reticulum, packaged in the Golgi apparatus, and as membrane-bound, **dense core vesicles,** they move along the axons. The axons travel down the nerve tract in the stalk **to terminate** in bulblike terminations **near capillaries.**

Clusters of the granules collect in dilations along the axons (**Herring bodies**) and in their bulbous endings. These aggregates stain selectively with the Gomori method. It is at the bulblike terminals that the **granules (hormones) are released** in response to a stimulus from the **hypothalamus.** These granules disappear in conditions of intense thirst, parturition, or various types of stress.

In contrast, hormones from the **pars distalis** of the pituitary are controlled by a series of **releasing and inhibitory factors** (hormones) synthesized by neurons in unidentified loci (nuclei) within the hypothalamus. Unlike the pars nervosa, the pars distalis **does not have nervous connections** with the hypothalamus. Instead the releasing and inhibiting factors pass to the anterior pituitary by way of a **portal venous system,** discussed earlier (p. 441).

Eventually it should be expected that one releasing factor and one inhibiting factor will be discovered for each hypophyseal hormone. Currently, six releasing and two inhibitory peptide factors have been identified arising from certain areas of the mammalian hypothalamus. They were discussed on p. 437.

In the pars intermedia, the principal hormone produced is **MSH**—melanocyte-stimulating hormone. Other possible hormones include β-endorphin and ACTH. Also only a single releasing factor has been identified, i.e., MRF—melanocyte-stimulating hormone releasing factor. All releasing factors of the hypothalamus appear to be peptides of comparatively low molecular weights.

Thus these neurosecretory cells forge a link between the two great integrating mechanisms of the body, namely, the nervous and endocrine systems. (For a summary of this chapter, see Table 21.2.)

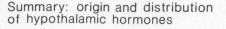

Summary: origin and distribution of hypothalamic hormones

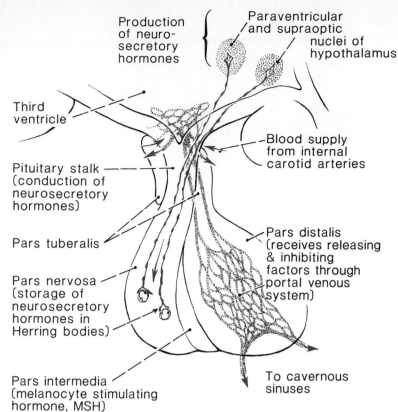

Production of neuro-secretory hormones

Paraventricular and supraoptic nuclei of hypothalamus

Third ventricle

Blood supply from internal carotid arteries

Pituitary stalk (conduction of neurosecretory hormones)

Pars tuberalis

Pars distalis (receives releasing & inhibiting factors through portal venous system)

Pars nervosa (storage of neurosecretory hormones in Herring bodies)

Pars intermedia (melanocyte stimulating hormone, MSH)

To cavernous sinuses

Table 21.1 *CLINICAL EFFECTS OF HYPOPHYSEAL DYSFUNCTIONS*

CLINICAL DIAGNOSIS	HORMONE IMPLICATED	CLINICAL APPEARANCE	REASON FOR DYSFUNCTION	TREATMENT
Pituitary dwarfism	Growth (GH)	Body proportions normal but juvenile in size (3–4 ft tall) and in sexual development	Lack or absence of growth hormone; may result from congenital absence, or destruction of pars distalis by disease or tumor	GH administration before fusion of epiphyses of long bones
Giantism	GH	Very large, tall (7.5–10 ft) individuals with fairly normal body proportions, except limbs unusually long	Excessive secretion of GH *before* puberty, i.e., before closure of epiphyses; usually caused by tumor of pars distalis	Early removal of tumor (hypophysectomy)
Acromegaly	GH	Large body with disproportionate growth of bones of face, esp. mandible, and hands and feet; skin and lips thicken; deep wrinkles over nose, forehead, and scalp	Same as giantism except hypersecretion of GH occurs *after* puberty, when epiphyses are fused and skeletal growth has ceased	Early hypophysectomy
Cushing's syndrome	Adrenocorticotropic (ACTH)	Obesity of upper trunk, esp. "buffalo hump" on back of neck; moon-shaped face that is flushed, edematous, often with acne, and in females, excessive facial hair (hirsutism)	Excessive amounts of the ACTH often produced by pituitary tumor; causes hypertrophy of adrenal cortices which produce an excess of cortisol and androgens; adrenocortical tumors produce similar symptoms	Pituitary irradiation and/or adrenalectomy
Simmond's disease (panhypopituitarism)	All hormones of pars distalis diminished or lacking	Dwarfism if condition develops before puberty; if after puberty the patient shows marked wasting and profound weakness	Usually a tumor causes partial or complete destruction of the pars distalis, resulting in hyposecretion of related hormones which cause secondary atrophy of thyroid, gonads, and adrenal cortices	Multiple hormonal replacement therapy, esp. cortisone
Diabetes insipidus	Antidiuretic (ADH)	Normal appearance; symptoms include, polyuria (production of very dilute urine) and polydipsea (excessive thirst)	Damage to hypothalamus, esp. supraoptic nucleus	Parenteral administration of ADH
Inappropriate ADH syndrome	ADH	Fairly normal appearance; lethargy, weight gain, general body edema, with marked sodium deficiency in plasma	Often due to a hypothalamic tumor that causes an excessive, continual release of ADH; thus the patient excretes a small quantity of hypertonic urine with high levels of sodium	

Table 21.2 *SUMMARY OF HISTOLOGY OF PITUITARY (HYPOPHYSIS) AND HYPOTHALAMUS*

| LOCATION | CELL TYPES | | HORMONE | TARGET TISSUE OR ORGAN | NATURE OF HORMONE | GRANULE SIZE (nm) |
	GENERAL	SPECIFIC				
Pituitary ● Pars distalis	Acidophil	Somatotroph	Somatotropin (STH) or growth hormone (GSH)	Especially muscle and bone	Protein	300–400
	Acidophil	Mammotroph	Prolactin	Breast	Protein	550–700
	Basophil	Gonadotrophs Folliculo-trophic	Follicle stimulating (FSH)	Ovary and testis	Glycoprotein	150–200
	Basophil	Luteotrophic	Luteinizing (LH)	Ovary (corpus luteum)	Glycoprotein	150–200
	—	—	Interstitial cell stimulating (ICSH) (probably same as LH)	Testis	Glycoprotein	150–200
	Basophil or perhaps chromophobe	Corticotroph (APUD)	Adrenocorticotropin (ACTH)	Adrenal cortex	Polypeptide	200–250
	Basophil	Thyrotroph	Thyroid stimulating (TSH)	Thyroid	Glycoprotein	130–150
● Pars intermedia	Basophil	Melanotroph (APUD)	Melanocyte stimulating (MSH)	Skin of lower animals	Polypeptide	200–300
● Pars nervosa	Neuroglia	Pituicyte	None			
Hypothalamus	Neurosecretory neurons	Neurons in paraventricular nuclei	Oxytocin	Smooth muscle, especially uterus	Polypeptide	100–300
		Neurons in supraoptic nuclei	Vasopressin (antidiuretic hormone, ADH)	Renal collecting tubules; arterioles	Polypeptide	100–300
		Neurons in tuberal nuclei	Six releasing factors (RF)	Pars distalis	Peptide	—
			Two known inhibiting factors (IF); others probably present	Pars distalis	Peptide	—

POSITIVE STAINING REACTION	FUNCTIONS
Orange G	Stimulates general growth; promotes protein synthesis, especially in bones and muscles; influences carbohydrate and lipid metabolism
Orange G	Initiates and regulates lactation; promotes mammary development
PAS	Stimulates late development of follicles in ovary and seminiferous tubules in testis
PAS	Stimulates corpus luteum development and progesterone secretion; necessary for ovulation and secretion of estrogen
PAS	Stimulates Leydig cells to produce testosterone
PAS	Stimulates synthesis of adrenocortical steroid hormones
PAS and aldehyde fuchsin	Controls thyroxine production and release
PAS and aldehyde fuchsin	Stimulates melanocyte expansion
	Storage and release of neurohormones of hypothalamus, i.e., oxytocin and vasopressin
Gomori	Stimulates contraction of uterine walls during parturition; also causes milk ejection by stimulating myoepithelial cells of mammary alveoli
Gomori	Increases water absorption of renal collecting tubules; also constricts arterioles to increase blood pressure
	Causes release of anterior pituitary hormones
	Inhibits release of anterior pituitary hormones

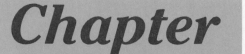

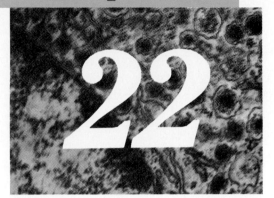

ENDOCRINE SYSTEM II—
ADRENAL, THYROID,
PARATHYROID, AND PINEAL

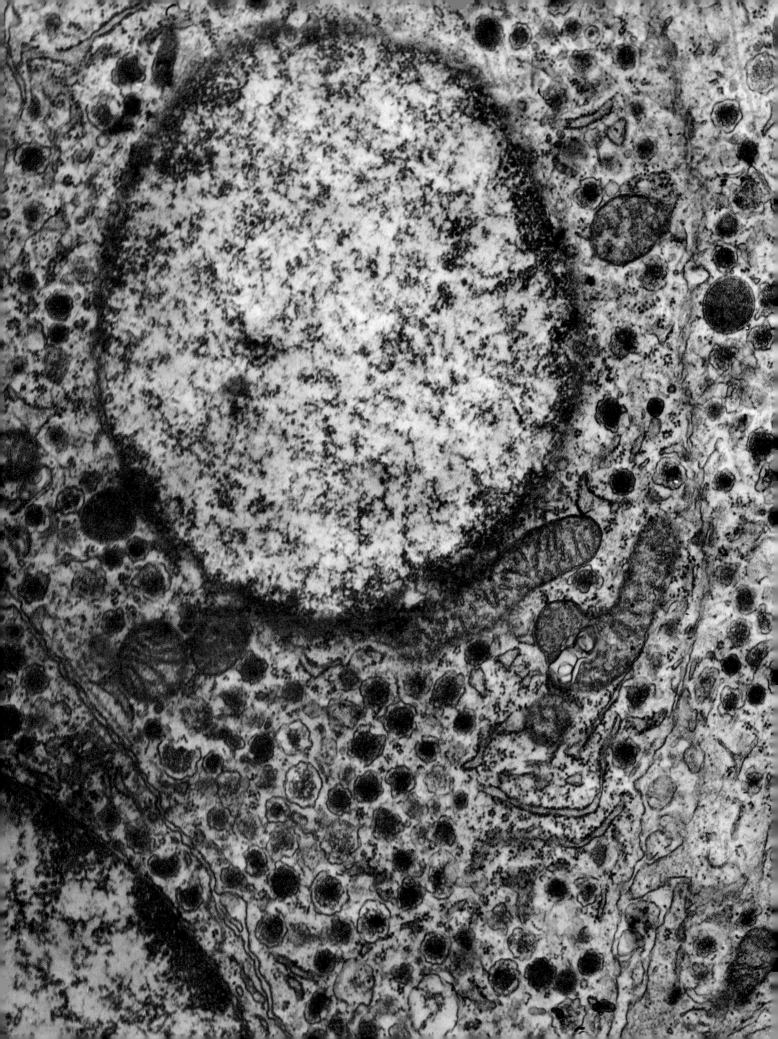

OBJECTIVES

TO EVALUATE THE DIFFERENCES AND SIMILARITIES OF THE ORIGIN, STRUCTURE, AND FUNCTIONS OF THESE ENDOCRINE ORGANS BY:

1. Documenting the concept that the adrenal gland is two separate endocrine organs, linked together by a common capsule and blood supply.

2. Identifying the various hormones synthesized by the adrenal and the clinical disorders that arise from malfunction of these substances.

3. Comparing the thyroid and parathyroid as to their origins, morphology, and the life-threatening diseases which result from their dysfunctions.

4. Critically examining the data that support the concept that the pineal, in certain animals, is a functional endocrine gland.

ADRENAL GLAND

An adrenal (suprarenal) gland is closely applied to the superior pole of each kidney. They resemble cocked hats or helmets tilted medially on the kidneys. These flattened, pyramidal glands actually consist of **two separate endocrine organs,** enclosed in a common capsule. The larger, outermost organ, the **cortex,** completely surrounds the smaller organ, the **medulla.** They are linked by a common blood supply but they are distinct embryonically and functionally.

Development

The cortex is derived from **mesodermal cells** of the peritoneum that lie adjacent to the early developing renal tubules. This anatomical relationship will remain throughout life, hence the name **adrenal** (L. ad, near) or suprarenal (L. supra, above).

The medulla is **ectodermal** in origin. Neural crest cells, which give rise to the sympathetic nervous system, also migrate into the adrenal anlage to invade the cortical tissue and form the medulla. Although these cells have synapses with sympathetic fibers, they do not form nerve processes but are secretory, epithelial cells. When exposed to chrome salts during histological procedures, they stain a yellow–brown color, hence they are called **chromaffin cells.** Cells of both the cortex and medulla develop in clusters or cords of cells adjacent to capillaries and sinusoids, typical of endocrine glands.

Blood Supply

The adrenals are highly vascular organs supplied by numerous arteries of comparatively large size. They arise from three sources: (1) from the **aorta,** as the middle adrenal arteries; (2) from the **inferior phrenic artery,** as the superior adrenal arteries; and (3) from the **renal arteries,** as the inferior adrenal arteries. All branches penetrate the **capsule** and immediately break up into a plexus of arteries. From this plexus emerge **three sets of branches.** The first series supplies the **capsule.** The second group consists of straight sinusoidal capillaries that percolate through the **parenchyma** of the cortex. The third set, the medullary arterioles, bypasses the cortex by following the connective tissue trabeculae to supply only the **medulla.** Upon entering the medulla these arterioles and the cortical sinusoidal capillaries terminate in a rich, sinusoidal capillary bed. Thus the cells of the **medulla have a dual blood supply:** a supply of fresh arterial blood, as well as blood rich in hormones secreted by the cells of the cortex. These secretions, the adrenocorticosteroids, influence the synthesis of epinephrine and norepinephrine in the medulla.

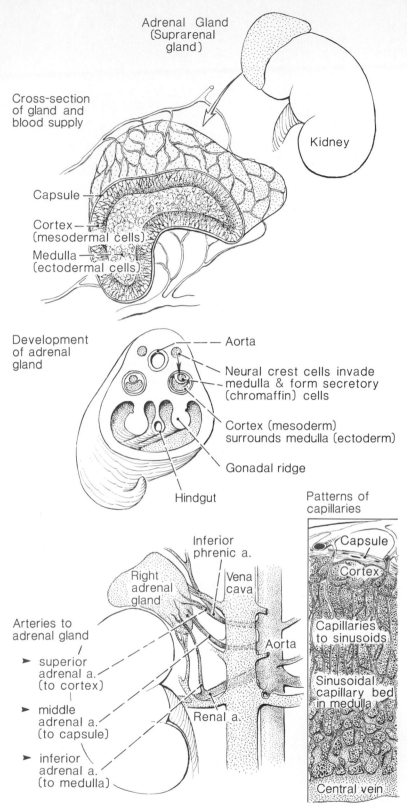

Adrenal Gland (Suprarenal gland)

Kidney

Cross-section of gland and blood supply

Capsule

Cortex (mesodermal cells)

Medulla (ectodermal cells)

Development of adrenal gland

Aorta

Neural crest cells invade medulla & form secretory (chromaffin) cells

Cortex (mesoderm) surrounds medulla (ectoderm)

Gonadal ridge

Hindgut

Patterns of capillaries

Capsule

Cortex

Capillaries to sinusoids

Sinusoidal capillary bed in medulla

Central vein

Inferior phrenic a.

Right adrenal gland

Vena cava

Aorta

Arteries to adrenal gland

► superior adrenal a. (to cortex)

► middle adrenal a. (to capsule)

► inferior adrenal a. (to medulla)

Renal a.

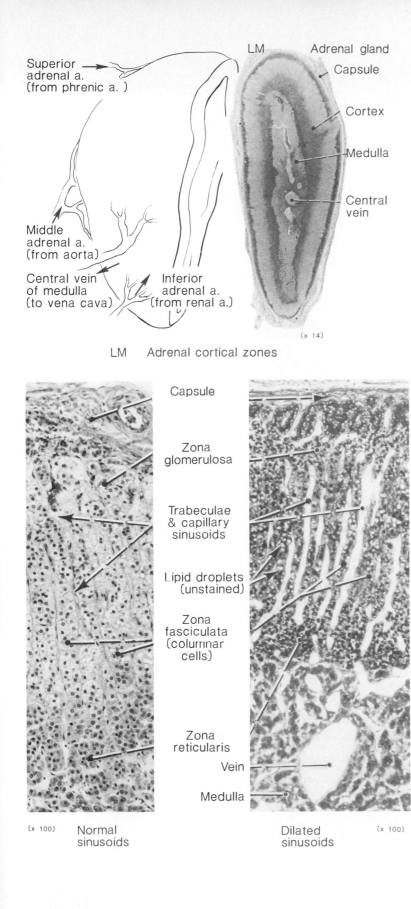

Superior adrenal a. (from phrenic a.)

Middle adrenal a. (from aorta)

Central vein of medulla (to vena cava)

Inferior adrenal a. (from renal a.)

LM   Adrenal gland
Capsule
Cortex
Medulla
Central vein

(× 14)

LM   Adrenal cortical zones

Capsule

Zona glomerulosa

Trabeculae & capillary sinusoids

Lipid droplets (unstained)

Zona fasciculata (columnar cells)

Zona reticularis

Vein

Medulla

(× 100)   Normal sinusoids

Dilated sinusoids   (× 100)

Venous blood from the capsule is drained into small veins which follow the arteries that penetrate the capsule. Blood from the other two sets of arteries empties into the **veins of the medulla.** These coalesce to form the **central veins** of the medulla that exits at the hilum of the gland. Note that there is **no venous system or lymphatics in the cortex.**

Nerve Supply

The sympathetic (splanchnic) nerves richly supply the adrenals. As they pierce the capsule to enter the cortex, most of them immediately traverse the cortex to enter the medulla; only a few pass to the **cortical cells.** In the **medulla,** the nerves terminate on the medullary cells. Recall that these cells are derived from neural crest cells and are homologs of the postganglionic neurons of the sympathetic nervous system. Therefore the **medullary cells respond like neurons,** forming synapses with the axons of the incoming nerves. Interspersed among the medullary cells are a few typical **ganglion cells.** There is no parasympathetic innervation to the medulla.

Cortex

CAPSULE A rather robust, collagenous capsule surrounds the gland, closely applied to the cortex. Thin **trabeculae** from the inner surface of the capsule penetrate the cortex to reach the medulla. They consist largely of **reticular fibers.** Between the trabeculae, the cells of the large central zone of the cortex are arranged into radial columns.

ZONES The cortex is normally divided into **three concentric zones,** differentiated by the arrangement and morphology of their secretory cells. They are named, from the capsule inward, **zona glomerulosa** (cells in clusters; L. glomus, a ball), **zona fasciculata** (cells in columns; L. fascis, a bundle), and **zona reticularis** (cells form a network; L. rete, a net). In humans, the demarcations of the zones are often poorly defined; nonetheless they are recognizable. The **cell arrangement** of one zone is **continuous** with the cells in the adjacent zones.

Zona Glomerulosa Immediately beneath the capsule is the rather **thin zona glomerulosa** that occupies 10–15% of the entire cortical volume. It contains **columnar cells arranged in rounded clusters** separated by delicate trabeculae containing sinusoidal capillaries.

EM studies reveal that the most diagnostic feature of the cytoplasm is the **abundance of sER,** which nearly fills the cells and forms a network of interconnecting tubules. In contrast, profiles of rER are very limited and most of the ribosomes are free within the cytoplasm. Many of the ribosomes are arranged as rosettes of **polyribosomes.** The numerous, elongated **mitochondria** have either broad or flat cristae. The Golgi complex has stacks of cisternae with small vesicles. A few, small, scattered lipid droplets are also present.

Zona Fasciculata The large, middle area, the **zona fasciculata,** occupies about **75–78%** of the adrenal cortex. Its **cuboidal cells** are arranged in **narrow columns,** often only one cell thick, directed perpendicular to the capsule. The cords of cells are separated by thin, reticular connective tissue septa containing **capillary sinusoids.** Thus essentially every secretory cell abuts onto a sinusoid.

The most conspicuous feature of the zone is the abundance of **large, fat droplets** that often fill the cells. During routine histologic procedures, the lipids are removed, giving the cells a highly vacuolated or foamy appearance. Hence these cells are often called **spongiocytes.**

Under the TEM, the numerous, **large mitochondria** in the zona fasciculata are unusual because of their **spherical shape** and their short, **tubular cristae.** The rER is more prominent, while the abundant sER is about the same amount as in the zona glomerulosa. The irregular cell membrane has a few, short microvilli in those areas not adjacent to other cells. The intercellular space of these cells is about 20 nm. In limited areas where the cell membranes are much closer together, they form gap junctions.

Zona Reticularis This is the thinnest and **innermost zone,** encompassing about 7–10% of the entire cortex. As its name implies, it consists of an irregular, branching **network of cords of cells.** They are interspersed with wide, sinusoidal capillaries. The secretory cells are smaller than the adjacent zona fasciculata cells and the cytoplasm is not vacuolated.

Histological features of the cells are similar to the zona fasciculata but differ in that: (1) The **lipid droplets** are greatly reduced in number. (2) The **mitochondria** are more elongated with fewer tubular cristae. (3) The cells are smaller and their nuclei stain more intensely. (4) **Lipofuscin** pigment granules are prominent. (5) **Light and dark secretory cells** are present.

FUNCTIONS Functions of the adrenal cortex are reflected in the ultrastructure of the parenchymal cells. These features are similar to other **steroid-secreting cells,** i.e., the interstitial cells of the testis and the corpus luteum of the ovary. They include (1) the unique, spherical mitochondria with **tubular cristae,** (2) an abundance of **sER,** and (3) many **lipid droplets.** The cells of the adrenal cortex synthesize various hormones of this nature, i.e., mineralocorticoids, glucocorticoids, and sex hormones.

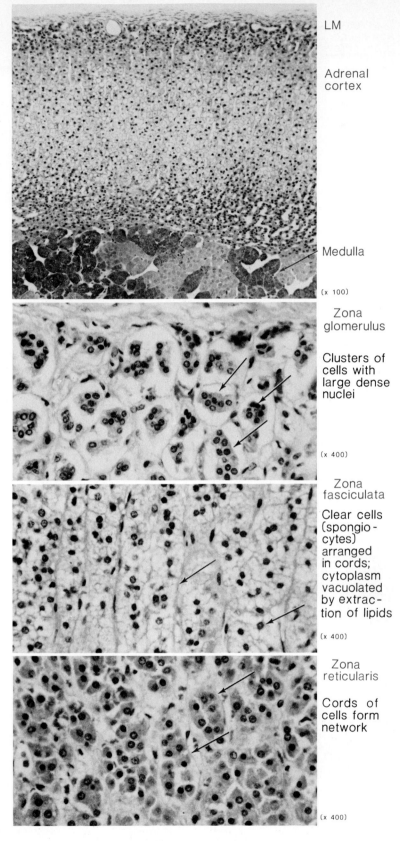

LM

Adrenal cortex

Medulla

(x 100)

Zona glomerulus

Clusters of cells with large dense nuclei

(x 400)

Zona fasciculata

Clear cells (spongiocytes) arranged in cords; cytoplasm vacuolated by extraction of lipids

(x 400)

Zona reticularis

Cords of cells form network

(x 400)

Functions of Adrenal Gland

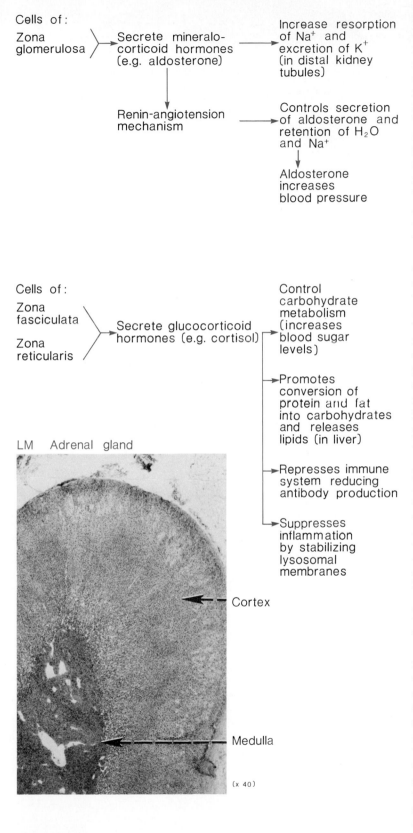

Cells of:
Zona glomerulosa → Secrete mineralo-corticoid hormones (e.g. aldosterone) → Increase resorption of Na$^+$ and excretion of K$^+$ (in distal kidney tubules)

↓

Renin-angiotension mechanism → Controls secretion of aldosterone and retention of H$_2$O and Na$^+$

Aldosterone increases blood pressure

Cells of:
Zona fasciculata
Zona reticularis → Secrete glucocorticoid hormones (e.g. cortisol) → Control carbohydrate metabolism (increases blood sugar levels)

→ Promotes conversion of protein and fat into carbohydrates and releases lipids (in liver)

→ Represses immune system reducing antibody production

→ Suppresses inflammation by stabilizing lysosomal membranes

LM   Adrenal gland

Cortex

Medulla

(x 40)

Cells of the zona glomerulosa secrete **mineralocorticoid hormones**. The most important is **aldosterone.** Acting on the distal tubules of the kidneys, its principal function is to promote the **increase** of the rate of **sodium resorption** from the glomerular filtrate and simultaneously to **increase potassium excretion** by the kidneys. It acts in a similar manner to decrease the sodium levels in the saliva, sweat, and GI tract secretions. Through the **renin-angiotensin mechanism,** the secretion of aldosterone is controlled. This hormone causes retention of large amounts of water and sodium, thus resulting in an **increase of fluid** in the circulation which contributes significantly to an **increase in blood pressure** (see Chapter 20). Aldosterone secretion appears to be independent of the adrenocorticotropic hormone (ACTH) of the pituitary.

Zona fasciculata and zona reticularis may be considered as a single functional unit. They secrete **glucocorticoid hormones**. The most important is **cortisol** (hydrocortisone), which represents about 95% of the glucocorticoid activity in the body. As the name glucocorticoid suggests, its hormones, especially cortisol, are involved in carbohydrate metabolism, especially in **increasing blood sugar** levels. Cortisol also promotes, to a lesser degree, protein and fat metabolism by increasing the **conversion of proteins in the liver into carbohydrates** and the release of lipids. In other words, glucocorticoids act as catabolic hormones.

Another function of **glucocorticoids** is to **repress the immune system** by inhibiting DNA synthesis. This **arrests mitosis** and is especially evident in **lymphoid tissues**. Administration of cortisol causes a sharp reduction in size of the spleen, thymus, and lymph nodes. Concurrently there is a marked reduction in antibody production which produces a profound **immunosuppressive effect.** Patients receiving organ or tissue transplants are maintained on massive levels of glucocorticoids to **suppress the immune system** which normally would cause the body to reject these **foreign transplants.**

Cortisol also has the capacity to **suppress inflammation.** It is this anti-inflammatory effect that enables the patient on cortisol **to cope with stress** arising from heat, cold, and certain diseases, such as rheumatoid arthritis, rheumatic fever, and acute glomerulonephritis, all characterized by severe local inflammation. Its mechanism of action is obscure; however, it may be that the glucocorticoids **stabilize the membranes of lysosomes** so that they do not rupture easily. Recall that intracellular lysosomes contain large amounts of hydrolytic enzymes capable of destroying tissues. The membrane-stabilizing effect may account for the anti-inflammatory effect of cortisol.

Glucocorticoid secretions are controlled by the hypothalamus through the action of **ACTH.** By this pathway, stimuli involving **stress promote release of glucocorticoids,** which causes adjustments in the metabolism of the body to meet stressful situations.

A third group of adrenal hormones are the **steroid sex hormones,** chiefly weak androgens. There is evidence that the zona reticularis is the principal site of secretion. Because the hormones are **relatively impotent,** they usually have little effect on normal physiologic processes. However, an **adrenal tumor** or a defect in an enzyme system in the cortex may cause the androgens to be produced in larger quantities, causing **exaggeration of male sex characteristics** in boys, and **virilism** (development of masculine physical traits), in women.

Adrenal Medulla

The adrenal medulla is much smaller than the cortex. It is only about 10% of the total weight of the gland. Its **parenchyma** consists of ovoid, or polyhedral, **chromaffin cells** arranged in clusters or thick cords separated by wide sinusoids and supported by a fine reticular network. Unlike the cortical cells whose cytoplasm is acidophilic, the **granular cytoplasm** of the medullary cells is strongly **basophilic** and its **granules stain yellow-brown** when exposed to chrome salts, hence the term chromaffin cells. The nuclei are larger and stain more deeply than those of the cortical cells. A nucleolus is usually very prominent in each nucleus. Perhaps the most **diagnostic feature** of the adrenal medulla is the presence of the large, central, **medullary vein** or veins that drain the entire adrenal gland.

Histochemical techniques and TEM studies reveal **two cell populations in the medulla.** About 80% of the cells **synthesize epinephrine** (adrenalin) and the remainder of the cells **produce norepinephrine.** The most obvious EM feature in both cell types is the abundance of electron-dense, **membrane-bound granules,** about 150–350 nm in diameter. The norepinephrine granules have **greater electron density** than the epinephrine granules. Other ultrastructural features are typical of most non-protein-synthesizing cells, such as limited rER (L-A, plate 39).

FUNCTIONS Perhaps the most unique physiological aspect of the hormones of the adrenal medulla is that they are so widespread, affecting, to some degree, every tissue of the body. Unlike the hormones of the cortex, the secretions of the medulla, epinephrine and norepinephrine, do not have a single target organ or tissue but **stimulate many organs and tissues simultaneously.** Release of these hormones into the bloodstream is **controlled by the sympathetic nervous system.** **Under stressful conditions,** a huge surge of epi-

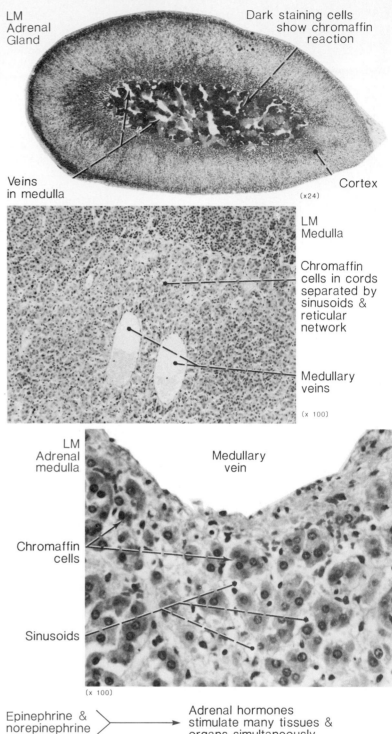

LM Adrenal Gland

Dark staining cells show chromaffin reaction

Veins in medulla

Cortex

(×24)

LM Medulla

Chromaffin cells in cords separated by sinusoids & reticular network

Medullary veins

(× 100)

LM Adrenal medulla

Medullary vein

Chromaffin cells

Sinusoids

(× 100)

Epinephrine & norepinephrine

Provide sympathetic control under stress

Adrenal hormones stimulate many tissues & organs simultaneously

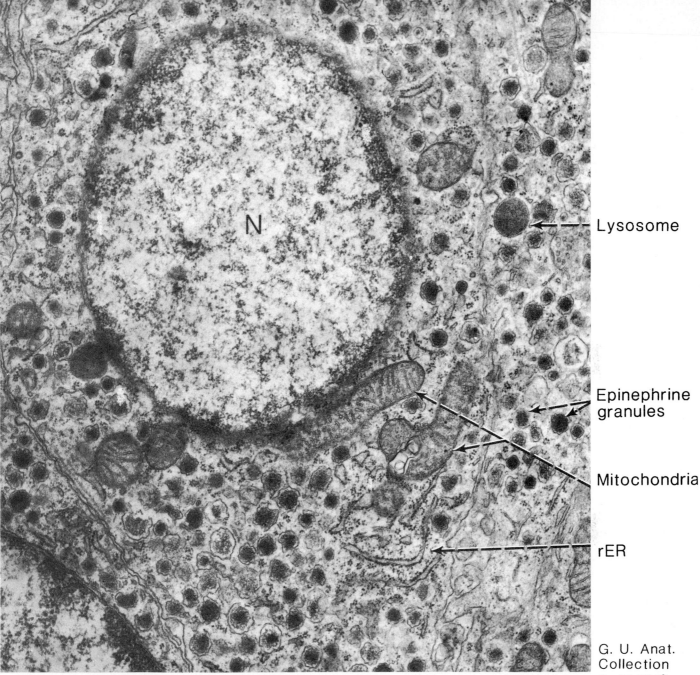

N

Lysosome

Epinephrine granules

Mitochondria

rER

G. U. Anat.
Collection
(x 30,000)

Electron micrograph of chromaffin cells of the adrenal medulla, which synthesize epinephrine. Their most distinctive EM features are the many membrane-bound, secretory granules. They vary in diameter from 150 to 350 nm and have a central core of uneven density, creating light to dark granules. In response to stress, these granules move to the surface of the cell where they are discharged into capillaries that abut onto the cell membrane. The rER is limited while free ribosomes and polyribosomes are abundant. Typical elongated mitochondria with prominent cristae are plentiful. The large spherical nucleus contains mostly euchromatin with only a thin peripheral rim of heterochromatin. Noreprinephrine secretory cells closely resemble the epinephrine variety except that the granules are less uniform in size and shape, and have a much denser core, often eccentric in position.

8231

nephrine and/or **norepinephrine** is released. These conditions are familiar to all of us. They include pain, cold, heat, fear, anoxia, excitement, and other stressful situations.

The immediate responses to stress are the **increase in heart rate and cardiac output.** These responses result in an increase in blood pressure, which is further augmented by vasoconstriction of arteries to the skin and the abdominal region. The **respiration rate is increased** and breathing facilitated by the dilation of the respiratory passageways. The metabolic responses to stress are the **breakdown of glycogen to glucose** in the liver and muscle, and the mobilization of free fatty acids from fat depots, which provide an immediate energy source for "fight-and-flight" situations.

CHROMAFFIN SYSTEM Recall that chromaffin cells have an affinity for chrome salts, such as potassium dichromate, a component of several widely used, tissue fixatives. To qualify for inclusion in the **chromaffin system,** cells must meet the following criteria: (1) They are derived from neuroectoderm (neural crest cells). (2) They give a positive chromaffin reaction. (3) They have a profuse blood supply. (4) They secrete epinephrine and/or norepinephrine.

The largest concentration of these cells is in the **adrenal medulla.** Other masses are found in the **paraganglia.** These are clusters of epithelial cells derived from neural crest cells that are associated with autonomic ganglia. Other groups are found along the aorta where the largest group is called **aortic chromaffin bodies** (of Zuckerkrandl). They all have a profuse blood supply.

THYROID GLAND

Aristotle called the thyroid gland the **globus hystericus,** because individuals with enlarged thyroids (toxic goiter) were prone to episodes of hysteria. Later the structure was designated the **thyroid gland** because of the fancied resemblance of its two pear-shaped lobes to warrior shields (Gk. thyreos, shieldlike).

The thyroid can be indistinctly seen and felt as two, flattened **swellings** (lobes) below the **larynx.** They are molded to the sides of the **trachea** from the second to the sixth tracheal cartilages. Despite its name, the thyroid has little contact with the thyroid cartilage except at the apices of the two lobes that embrace the cartilage inferiorly. The **isthmus** is a narrow band of thyroid tissue connecting the lobes at the level of the second and third tracheal rings. The tough, outer **capsule** is continuous with a connective tissue investment of the trachea and larynx. Therefore in swallowing, the thyroid moves with these organs.

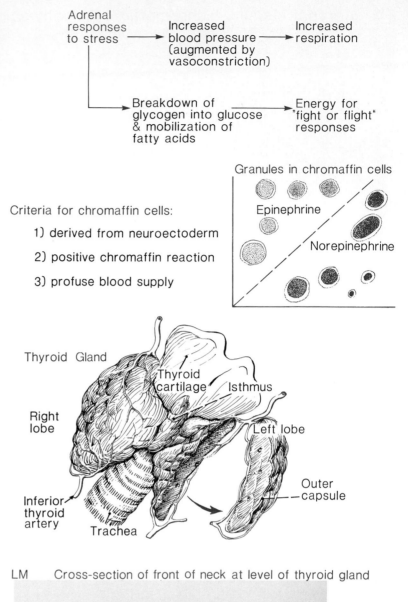

Adrenal responses to stress → Increased blood pressure (augmented by vasoconstriction) → Increased respiration

Breakdown of glycogen into glucose & mobilization of fatty acids → Energy for "fight or flight" responses

Criteria for chromaffin cells:

1) derived from neuroectoderm

2) positive chromaffin reaction

3) profuse blood supply

Granules in chromaffin cells

Epinephrine

Norepinephrine

Thyroid Gland

Thyroid cartilage   Isthmus

Right lobe

Left lobe

Outer capsule

Inferior thyroid artery

Trachea

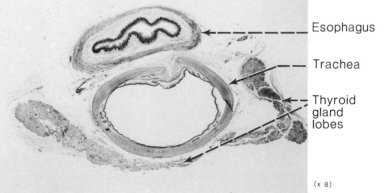

LM   Cross-section of front of neck at level of thyroid gland

Esophagus

Trachea

Thyroid gland lobes

(x 8)

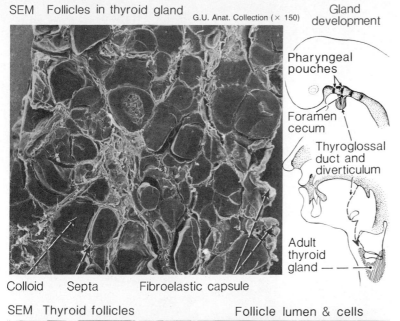

SEM Follicles in thyroid gland G.U. Anat. Collection (× 150)

Gland development

Pharyngeal pouches

Foramen cecum

Thyroglossal duct and diverticulum

Adult thyroid gland ---

Colloid Septa Fibroelastic capsule

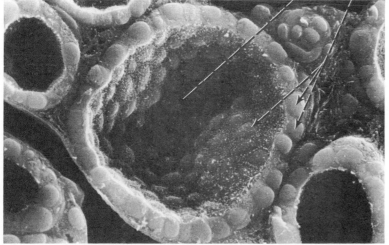

SEM Thyroid follicles

Follicle lumen & cells

K. Tanaka & T. Fujita (x 1900)

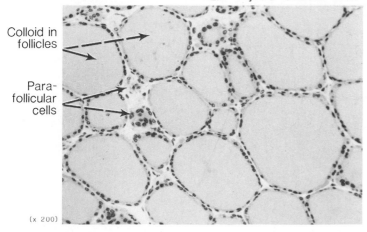

LM Thyroid follicular cells

Colloid in follicles

Para-follicular cells

(x 200)

Origin

The thyroid develops as a median **endodermal downgrowth** at the base of the tongue. In the adult, the telltale evidence of its origin is a prominent depression, the **foramen cecum,** at the back of the tongue. During embryonic development, the thyroid descends inferiorly to its adult position in the lower neck.

A transitory structure, the **thyroglossal duct,** which connects the developing gland to its point of origin, later **solidifies and disappears** in early fetal life. Occasionally the descent of the gland is arrested and the thyroid develops within the base of the tongue. Also cysts and bits of thyroid tissue may be strewn along the path of the duct as **accessory thyroids.** The most constant of these structures is a superior extension of the isthmus called the **pyramidal lobe.** The aberrant cysts may enlarge, rupture, and drain, as **fistulae,** along the sides of the neck. Normally, however, the thyroglossal duct completely disappears, leaving the thyroid to develop as a ductless gland.

Histological Features

A delicate fibroelastic capsule sends septa into the gland to divide it into poorly defined lobules, each composed of several follicles.

The structural unit of the thyroid is the spherical or elongated **follicle.** Its basal lamina rests on a fine connective tissue stroma that is richly laced with capillaries. The follicles vary in size from 0.02 to 0.1 mm in diameter, depending on the functional activity of the gland. Their most conspicuous feature is the viscous, homogeneous **colloid** that fills them. It stains basophilic in actively secreting follicles and lightly eosinophilic in inactive follicles.

The cells lining the follicle are called **follicular cells.** They are usually lightly basophilic, **simple cuboidal cells** with prominent, round nuclei. The shape of these cells changes to **simple squamous** if the follicle is in an inactive, **storage state,** or to **simple columnar** during periods of intensely **active hormone synthesis.** Therefore the height of the epithelium of the follicle is an accurate indicator of the functional state of the gland. These follicular cells rest on a delicate basal lamina surrounded by capillaries and are ultimately responsible for the synthesis of the hormone, **thyroxin** (L-A, plate 30).

The ultrastructure of the follicular cell suggests a cell that is involved in the **synthesis release, and resorption of proteins.** It has a well-developed Golgi apparatus in the supranuclear position, abundant rough endoplasmic reticulum, apical vesicles, free ribosomes, many lysosomes, secretory granules, and considerable luminal microvilli. It has only a few dispersed mitochondria, pinocytotic vesicles, and colloid droplets.

7867

A second, much smaller population of cells is the **parafollicular (or calcitonin) cells.** These are **APUD cells** of neural crest origin. They may occur in small clusters between the follicles or as single cells enclosed within the basal lamina of follicular cells. In either location, they are never in contact with the follicular colloid and therefore **do not contain colloid granules.** These clear, poorly stained cells vary widely in shape and have large, pale, eccentrically located nuclei. Their most distinctive TEM features are (1) the presence of many small, membrane-bound, **dense secretory granules,** 100–180 nm in diameter, believed to contain the hormone calcitonin; and (2) abundant, closely packed, **elongated mitochondria.**

The primary effect of **calcitonin** (thyrocalcitonin) is to **reduce the concentration of calcium salts** in the blood by the inhibition of bone resorption.

Histophysiology

The production of the hormone **thyroxin** has a rather complicated pathway that is divided into two phases. The **first phase** involves the basic ingredients, **amino acids and iodide,** that leave the blood capillaries to enter the cytoplasm of the follicular cell at its basal plasmalemma. Synthesis of the **thyroglobulin precursors** and the sugar mannose occurs on the **rER.** The other larger carbohydrate moiety, **galactose,** is supplied by the **Golgi apparatus,** to form an uniodinated molecule of **thyroglobulin.** By exocytosis, the molecule is released into the **colloid** within the lumen of the follicle.

Simultaneously **iodide** and **thyroperoxidase,** the latter an enzyme of the follicular cells, are transversing the same pathways as the proteins to be incorporated into the colloid mass. By this enzyme, iodide is oxidized into **iodine,** which then unites with thyroglobulin, the storage form of the thyroid hormone.

The **second phase** of thyroid hormone production is the resorption of thyroglobulin by the follicular cells and its breakdown into two active hormones, **tetraiodothyronine (T_4) or thyroxin,** and **triiodothyronine (T_3).** Responding to the release of thyroid-stimulating hormone (**TSH**) by the anterior hypophysis, the **thyroglobulin,** contained within tiny colloid droplets, **is resorbed** by the follicular cells by endocytosis. As the droplet enters the cell, it is attacked by acid proteases in lysosomes. The **proteases** cleave the thyroglobulin molecule into two active thyroid hormones. These diffuse through the basal plasmalemma to enter the **blood and lymph capillaries.** Thyroxin (T_4) is the most abundant of these hormones, providing about 90% of the total hormone, yet T_3 is more potent and acts more rapidly.

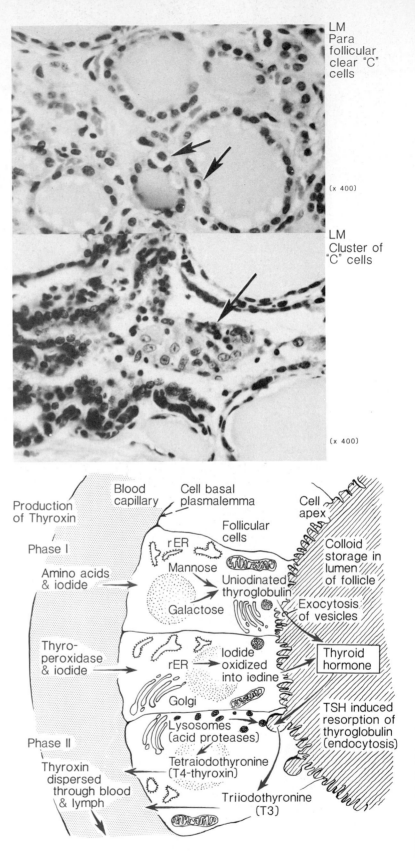

LM
Para
follicular
clear "C"
cells

(x 400)

LM
Cluster of
"C" cells

(x 400)

7846

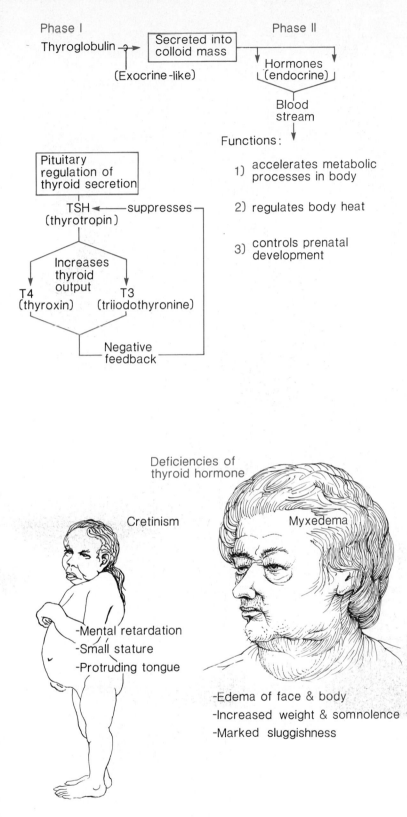

Thyroid hormone functions:

Phase I

Thyroglobulin ⟶ Secreted into colloid mass
(Exocrine-like)

Phase II

Hormones (endocrine)

Blood stream

Functions:

1) accelerates metabolic processes in body

2) regulates body heat

3) controls prenatal development

Pituitary regulation of thyroid secretion

TSH (thyrotropin) ⟵ suppresses

Increases thyroid output

T4 (thyroxin)   T3 (triiodothyronine)

Negative feedback

Deficiencies of thyroid hormone

Cretinism

Myxedema

-Mental retardation
-Small stature
-Protruding tongue

-Edema of face & body
-Increased weight & somnolence
-Marked sluggishness

The two-phased thyroid hormone synthesis is somewhat of a paradox for an endocrine gland. Observe that the **first phase** has an exocrinelike function, i.e., thyroglobulin is secreted apically into the colloid mass. Yet the **second phase** is a true **endocrine function**, i.e., the thyroglobulin is broken down into two active hormones that are released basally into the bloodstream in a typical endocrine fashion.

Functions of Thyroid Hormones

Thyroid hormones greatly **accelerate** the **general metabolic processes** of the body, which increases the basal metabolic rate (**BMR**). Hence an abnormally high BMR probably reflects a hyperactive thyroid. The thyroid is also involved in **heat regulation** in the body.

Through the synergistic action of other hormones, especially the growth hormone, the thyroid hormones **control the prenatal development** of the tissues of the body, especially the muscular, skeletal, nervous, and reproductive tissues. A deficiency of thyroxin in the fetus causes these tissues to remain immature and incapable of normal postnatal functions. The thyroid also is involved in many specific metabolic processes, e.g., the rate of protein, carbohydrate, and fat metabolism. Also it acts to increase blood flow, heart rate, and blood pressure.

The regulation of thyroid hormone secretion is largely by the pituitary through the **thyroid-stimulating hormone (TSH)**, also called **thyrotropin.** It acts specifically to **increase the secretion of thyroxin** (T_4) and **triiodothyronine** (T_3) by the thyroid gland. This pituitary-thyroid axis forms a **feedback circuit** so that an increase of level of thyroid hormones in the bloodstream acts to **suppress TSH output** and the level of thyroid hormone production is subsequently reduced.

Thyroid Disorders

In infancy and childhood, a deficiency of thyroid hormones (hypothyroidism) causes a condition called **cretinism.** It is characterized by mental retardation, dwarfed stature, large protruding tongue, dry skin, and an obese, stocky build. If a cretin is treated with thyroid extracts shortly after birth, the infant usually returns to fairly normal growth patterns.

Severe hypothyroidism in the adult is called **myxedema** (Gk. myxa, mucous; oiedema, swelling). This is an appropriate name because an individual with hypothyroidism has marked puffiness (**edema**) of the face, especially about the eyes, and general body edema. Other symptoms include considerable increase in weight, marked somnolence, i.e., sleeping 14–18 h/day, mental torpor, extreme muscular sluggishness, decreased cardiac output, slow heart rate, poor hair growth, and dry scaly skin.

Hypothyroidism may also be precipitated by a **dietary iodine deficiency,** usually endemic, which interferes with the synthesis of thyroid hormones. Such a reduction of T_3 and T_4 triggers an overproduction of TSH by the anterior pituitary, which in turn causes **hypertrophy of the thyroid follicular cells.** The overstimulated cells produce large amounts of thyroglobulin (colloid) but very small quantities of thyroid hormones. With hypertrophy of the follicular cells and the massive distension of the follicles with colloid, the thyroid gland is increased in size severalfold, typical of **nontoxic colloid goiter.**

Toxic goiter is caused by an **overactive thyroid** not necessarily associated with iodine deficiency. Rather, it results from an **excess of TSH,** which stimulates an overproduction of T_3 and T_4. Such a condition results in the enlargement of the thyroid gland two or three times its normal size, and the patient's **BMR is sharply increased.** Other symptoms include an intolerance for heat which is accompanied by profuse sweating, severe weight loss, muscular weakness, extreme fatigue, and psychic disorders, including severe nervousness. Most individuals develop a most dramatic symptom, a marked protrusion of the eyeballs called **exophthalmos.** This pop-eyed condition is caused by edema of the extracellular spaces behind the eyeball. Treatment with injection of radioactive iodine will inactivate the hyperactive follicular cells, hormone production is reduced, and most symptoms will subside, except the exophthalmos which often persists throughout life.

PARATHYROID

As late as the 1890s complete thyroidectomies usually resulted in death from asphyxia (lack of oxygen), caused by spasms of the laryngeal and thoracic muscles, a major symptom of **tetany.** In 1892 the French physiologist Gley demonstrated that the **removal** of the four small oval glands, the **parathyroids,** located behind the thyroid, usually embedded in the thyroid capsule, was the cause of the **tetanic seizures** and not the removal of the thyroid per se. Therefore, conservation of the normal parathyroids is now a cardinal principle in thyroid surgery and partial, rather than complete, thyroidectomies are planned accordingly. Thus the life-threatening tetany is prevented.

Origin

The two inferior parathyroids develop from the **third pharyngeal pouch** in the embryo and the two superior glands from the lowest (**fourth**) **pouch.** The third pouch is also the site of the origin of the thymus gland, and the inferior parathyroids migrate inferiorly with it. Normally the parathyroids break away from the thymus at the lower pole of the thyroid and do not migrate into the upper chest region.

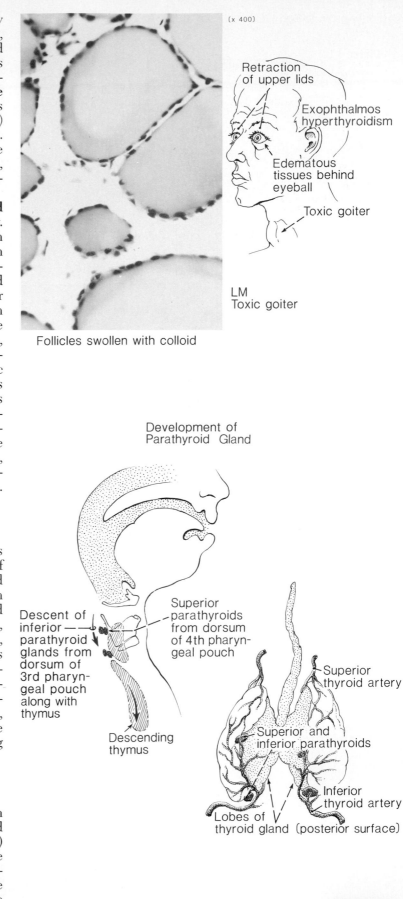

(x 400)

LM
Toxic goiter

Follicles swollen with colloid

Development of Parathyroid Gland

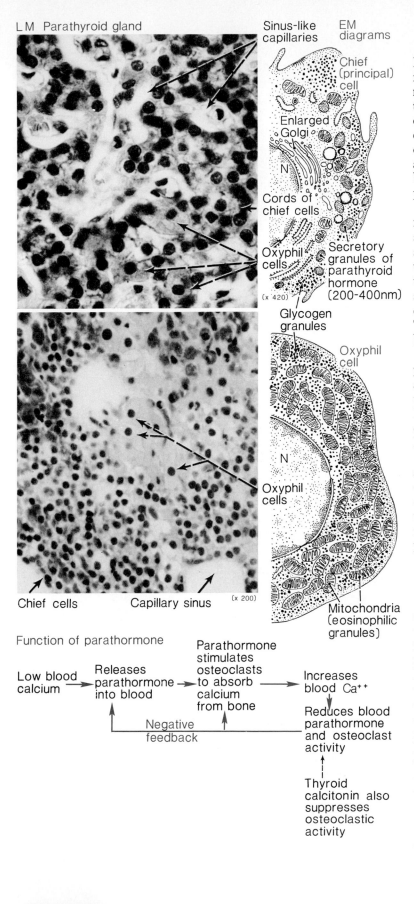

LM Parathyroid gland

Sinus-like capillaries

EM diagrams

Chief (principal) cell

Enlarged Golgi

N

Cords of chief cells

Oxyphil cells

Secretory granules of parathyroid hormone (200-400nm)

(x 420)

Glycogen granules

Oxyphil cell

N

Oxyphil cells

Chief cells

Capillary sinus

(x 200)

Mitochondria (eosinophilic granules)

Function of parathormone

Low blood calcium → Releases parathormone into blood → Parathormone stimulates osteoclasts to absorb calcium from bone → Increases blood Ca⁺⁺ → Reduces blood parathormone and osteoclast activity

Negative feedback

Thyroid calcitonin also suppresses osteoclastic activity

Histological Features

A thin, fibrous capsule surrounds each gland. It sends delicate septa into the gland to divide it into incomplete, poorly defined lobules. The **parenchyma** of the gland consists of two populations of cells profusely supplied with **sinusoidal capillaries**. The most numerous cell type is the **chief or principal cell**. These are small, cuboidal cells with relatively large, dark nuclei. The cells are arranged in clumps or cords. The cells either border on a capillary or are nearby. Their cytoplasm is pale and slightly eosinophilic.

TEM studies of actively secreting chief cells reveal a prominent **enlarged Golgi body**, rER, small oval mitochondria, and an abundance of small dense, membrane-bound **secretory granules** 200–400 nm in diameter, located at or near the cell membrane. In the **inactive chief cells** are several small Golgi bodies and considerable accumulation of **glycogen and lipofuscin granules**. The parathyroid hormone (**PTH**) is synthesized by the chief cells.

The other, less numerous cell type, is the **oxyphil or acidophil cells**. They do not occur in all animals and, in humans, perhaps do not appear until puberty. They increase in number with age. Initially they are scattered singly among the chief cells. In later life they often form rather large clusters.

Oxyphils are larger than chief cells. They have a **smaller, more condensed nucleus** and the abundant cytoplasm has a large number of very fine, **eosinophilic granules**. EM micrographs reveal these granules to be **mitochondria** with prominent cristae. There is no known function for oxyphils.

Function

A lowering of blood calcium causes the release of the parathyroid hormone (parathormone) into the bloodstream. The hormone stimulates the rate of **activity of osteoclasts** to absorb the calcified matrix of bone and also causes a rapid proliferation of new osteoclasts. The osteolytic activity of the osteoclasts **increases the blood calcium** to normal levels. Finally hormone production is suppressed, followed by the diminished activity of the osteoclasts. Recall that the hormone **calcitonin** of the thyroid is an **antagonist to parathormone** by suppressing the action of osteoclasts.

Parathyroid Disorders

Hypoparathyroidism is a pathological condition resulting in a **decrease of calcium ions** and an **increase of phosphate ions** in the blood. When the blood calcium level drops from a normal of 10 mg/100 ml to about 6 mg/100 ml, the symptoms of **tetany** appear. Due to the hyperexcitability of the peripheral nervous system, **muscle spasms** ensue. Especially sensitive are the laryngeal muscles. Spasms of these muscles obstruct respiration, the usual cause of death in tetany. Administration of calcium or parathormone terminates the spasms.

Hyperparathyroidism is usually caused by a **tumor** of one or more of the parathyroid glands. This condition causes intense **osteoclastic activity** in the bones, resulting in **elevation of blood calcium** and a weakening of the bone by extensive **decalcification**. The bone is replaced by fibrous connective tissue and multiple cysts, a condition called **osteitis fibrosa cystica**. Also calcium is deposited in larger arteries and kidneys. Removal of the offending tumor usually corrects the condition.

Like the hormone calcitonin of the thyroid, the parathyroid hormone is **regulated directly by the blood calcium levels** and not by the nervous system or the pituitary gland. **No pituitary tropic hormones** are known to exist for the follicular cells of the thyroid, the oxyphils of the parathyroid, or the cells of the adrenal medulla.

PINEAL GLAND (EPIPHYSIS CEREBRI)

The small, cone-shaped pineal gland has been the subject of much speculation among anatomists since the time of Galen (130–200 A.D.). Centuries later the controversy was still continuing when the French philosopher Descartes (1629) described the pineal gland as "the seat of the soul." Only recently has its morphology been fully described and its functions tentatively established.

Development

During the second embryonic month the pineal gland begins to develop as a **dorsal diverticulum** (outpocketing) of the roof of the primitive brain, **the diencephalon**. The walls of the outpocketing thicken to eventually occlude its lumen, except at its base where it persists in the adult as the **pineal recess**. Still attached to the base of the brain, the developing pineal solidifies with the proliferation of two types of cells, **secretory cells**, the **pinealocytes**, and **interstitial (neuroglial) cells**. The latter type gives rise to a thin capsule and septa that penetrate the gland to divide it into incomplete lobules.

Histological Features

Light microscopy of the pineal tissue reveals three useful features for organ identification.

1. The **concretions** are small grains of "brain sand" or **corpora arenacea** that are especially numerous in older individuals.

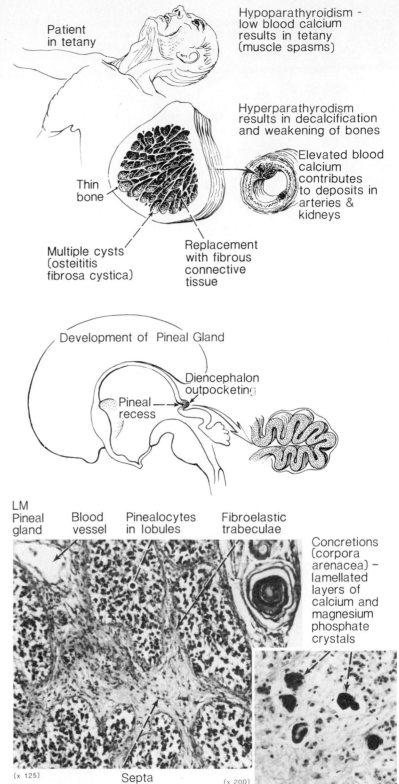

Patient in tetany

Hypoparathyroidism – low blood calcium results in tetany (muscle spasms)

Hyperparathyrodism results in decalcification and weakening of bones

Elevated blood calcium contributes to deposits in arteries & kidneys

Thin bone

Multiple cysts (osteititis fibrosa cystica)

Replacement with fibrous connective tissue

Development of Pineal Gland

Diencephalon outpocketing

Pineal recess

LM Pineal gland

Blood vessel

Pinealocytes in lobules

Fibroelastic trabeculae

Concretions (corpora arenacea) – lamellated layers of calcium and magnesium phosphate crystals

(x 125)

Septa

(x 200)

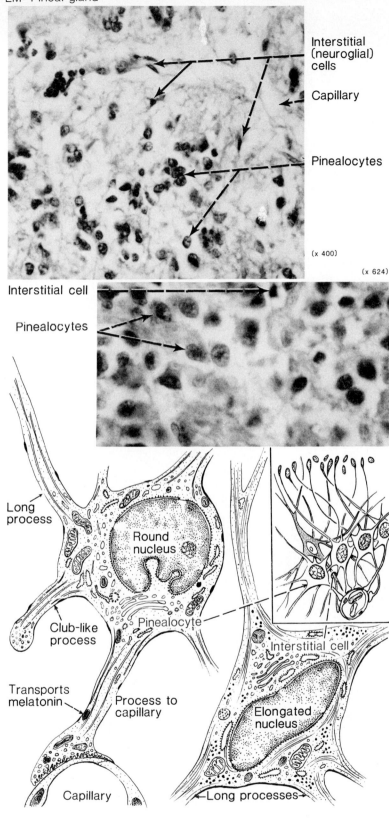

Interstitial (neuroglial) cells

Capillary

Pinealocytes

(x 400)

(x 624)

Interstitial cell

Pinealocytes

Long process

Round nucleus

Club-like process

Pinealocyte

Transports melatonin

Process to capillary

Capillary

Elongated nucleus

Interstitial cell

Long processes

2. The gland is incompletely divided into **lobes** by irregular fibroelastic **trabeculae** and incomplete **septa** derived from the capsule. The larger trabeculae convey blood vessels that pierce the capsule to extend deep into the gland. The more delicate septa are largely reticular fibers that support uneven clusters of parenchymal cells and their rich capillary plexuses.

3. The third diagnostic feature is the **nucleus of the pinealocyte.** It is a large, polymorphic organelle that has infoldings or lobulations. It has one or more prominent nucleoli and an abundance of peripheral, dense chromatin.

Pinealocytes

Pinealocytes or pineal parenchymal cells constitute most of the gland. With special silver impregnation techniques, they resemble greatly **modified neurons** with many branched, clublike processes. They often extend into a well-developed perivascular space to terminate on capillaries. EM observations show cytoplasm with **extensive sER,** an **abundance of microtubules,** and **free ribosomes.** Other features include limited profiles of rER, a rather well-developed Golgi complex, and numerous polymorphic mitochondria. The cells secrete the hormone melatonin, which is synthesized from the biogenic amine **serotonin.**

Interstitial Cells

The basophilic interstitial or **neuroglial** cell has an **elongated nucleus** that is deeper staining than those of the pinealocytes. These cells are found chiefly dispersed among the clumps of pinealocytes and capillary beds. They may have **long, protoplasmic processes** with many **fine filaments** (5–6 nm in diameter). These processes surround the pinealocytes as well as sympathetic nerve fibers and other processes. Microtubules are scarce. Mitochondria are smaller and less numerous than those of the parenchymal cells. From fine structural observations, the interstitial cell has been identified as a type of **astrocyte.**

Functions

Since most research on the pineal has involved nonprimates, its functions in man remain uncertain. However, in **lower animals** its activities include: (1) **regulating the reproductive system,** particularly in animals that are seasonal breeders; (2) moderating the timing of various **circadian and diurnal rhythms** in many birds and some reptiles, in response to daily variations in periods of light and darkness; and (3) the **melatonin synthesized** in darkness promotes blanching of the skin in amphibians and reptiles by the aggregations of the melanosomes in melanocytes. It has little known effect on mammalian melanocytes. (Table 22.1 is a summary of the chapter.)

7699

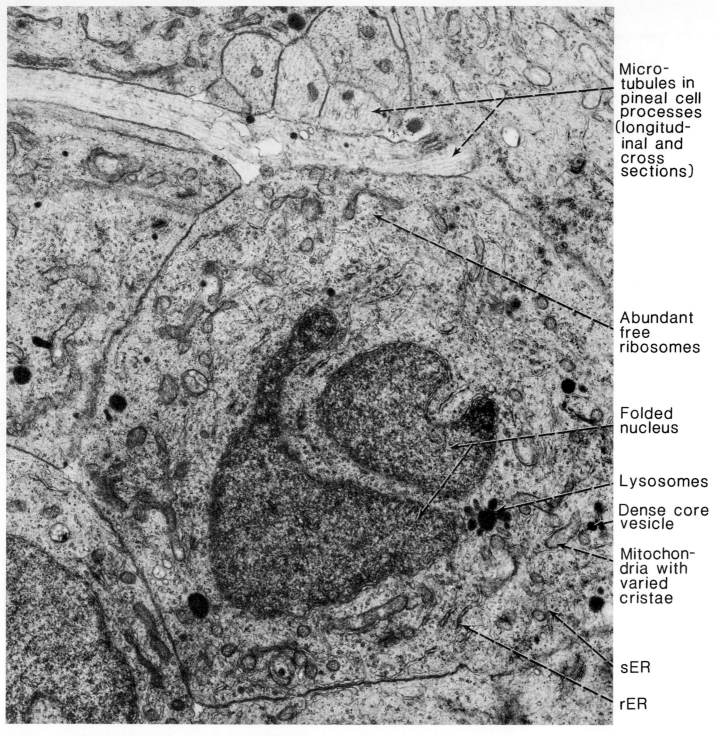

Micro-
tubules in
pineal cell
processes
(longitud-
inal and
cross
sections)

Abundant
free
ribosomes

Folded
nucleus

Lysosomes

Dense core
vesicle

Mitochon-
dria with
varied
cristae

sER

rER

Electron micrograph of parenchymal cells of the pineal gland. One of the cells displays the typical large, deeply creased or folded nucleus with abundant heterochromatin. The cytoplasm contains many polymorphic mitochondria with varied membranous and tubular cristae, considerable sER but limited rER, abundant free ribosomes, many arranged in rosettes, and an array of various electron-dense lysosomes, lipid bodies, and dense core vesicles. At the top of the field are several cross sections and one longitudinal section of cytoplasmic processes of pinealocytes. These projections contain many microtubules and microfilaments, a few small mitochondria, several smooth-surfaced clear vesicles, and an occasional dense core vesicle.

Table 22.1 *SUMMARY OF THYROID, PARATHYROID, ADRENAL, AND PINEAL GLANDS*

GLAND	CELL TYPE(S)	HORMONE(S)	TARGET ORGAN OR TISSUE	NATURE OF HORMONE	FUNCTIONS
Thyroid	Follicular	Thyroxin and triiodothyronine	All tissues and organs	Amino acid	Stimulates general oxidative metabolism, growth and development
	Parafollicular (C-cells) (APUD)	Calcitonin	Bone	Polypeptide	Inhibits excessive blood calcium
Parathyroid	Principal (Chief)	Parathormone	Bone	Polypeptide	Synthesizes hormone which raises blood calcium levels by action on osteoclasts
	Oxyphil	Unknown but may secrete traces of parathormone	Probably bone	Unknown	These cells may be senile chief cells that still secrete some hormone
Adrenal ● Cortex	Zona glomerulosa	Mineralocorticoids, e.g., aldosterone	Collecting tubules of kidney	Steroid	Regulates sodium retention and potassium loss by kidneys
	Zona fasciculata	Glucocorticoids, e.g., cortisol	Most all tissues and organs	Steroid	Responds to stress; is an anti-inflammatory agent; helps regulate lipid, protein, and carbohydrate metabolism
	Zona reticularis	Sex hormones, e.g., androgens	Testis	Steroid	Augments testicular hormonal secretions
● Medulla	Epinephrine cells	Epinephrine	Cardiac and smooth muscle	Biogenic amine	Responds to stress by augmenting cardiovascular functions; increases O_2 consumption and pulse rate; blood sugar levels raised by mobilization of glycogen
	Norepinephrine cells	Norepinephrine	Arterioles	Biogenic amine	Stimulates vasoconstriction; is a neurotransmitter at sympathetic nerve terminals
Pineal (epiphysis cerebri)	Pinealocytes	Melatonin	Melanocytes; also possibly gonads, hypothalamus, and pituitary	Biogenic amine	Regulates circadian and diurnal rhythms; controls dispersion of pigment in skin of reptiles and amphibians
		Seratonin	Arterioles	Biogenic amine	Vasoconstrictor; excitatory transmitter in CNS; is the precursor of melatonin
	Interstitial	None			Support cells; a type of astrocyte

Chapter

23

MALE REPRODUCTIVE SYSTEM

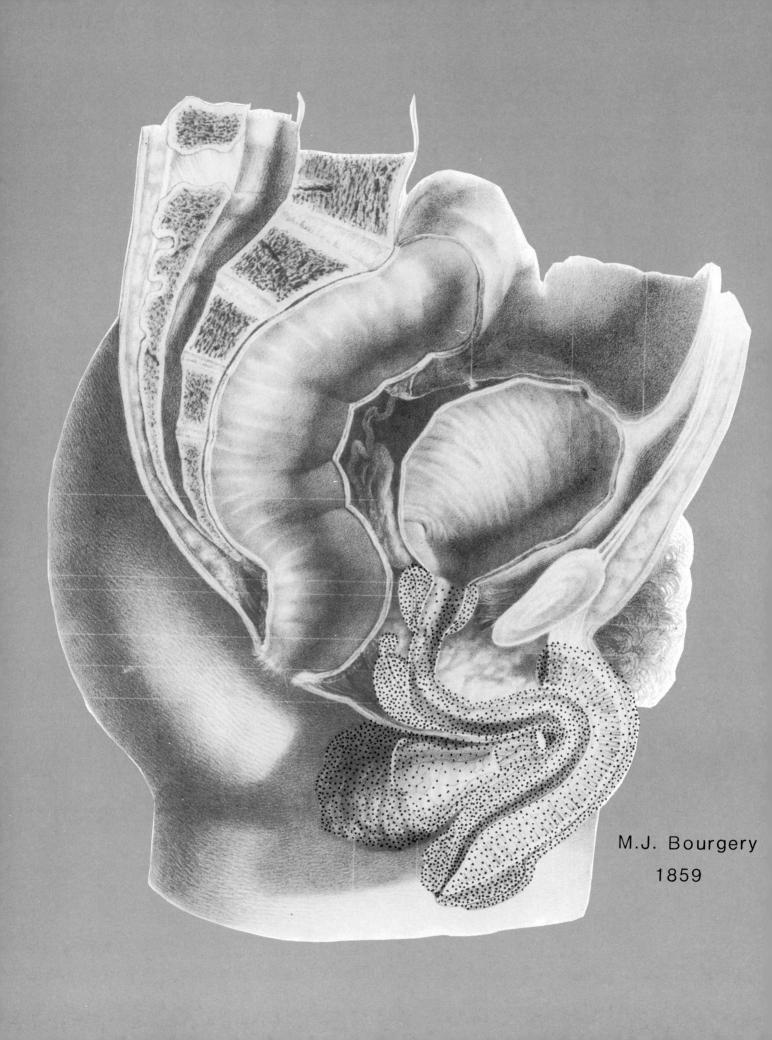

M.J. Bourgery
1859

AFTER STUDYING THIS CHAPTER ONE SHOULD BE ABLE TO:

1. Assess the essentiality of this system to the survival of the species versus the survival of the individual.

2. Compare the support and sex cells of the seminiferous tubules as to size, location, morphology, function, and chromosome number.

3. Differentiate between meiosis and mitosis, spermatogenesis and spermiogenesis, and Sertoli and Leydig cells.

4. List in correct sequence the segments of the male genital duct system and describe their distinctive histological features and functions.

5. Extrapolate from the histology of the prostate, seminal vesicles, and bulbourethral glands, the functions of their secretions as components of the semen.

Reproduction is the most essential of life's processes, for it makes possible the continuity of the species. Without it, a species would become extinct in one generation. Therefore, fundamental to any type of life is its ability to reproduce itself. In the one-celled ameba this vital function is accomplished by dividing into two essentially identical cells which, on maturation, can repeat the process. However, as the phylogenetic scale is ascended, the process of reproduction becomes more complex to ensure the survival of the germ cells and the offspring, regardless of hostile environments or the harsh life-style of the parents.

In man and other mammals, these **reproductive processes** include the production of male and female sex cells (gametogenesis), sexual intercourse followed by fertilization, pregnancy, parturition, and lactation. All of these stages are **controlled by a variety of hormones,** mostly synthesized by the gonads and pituitary. These hormones differ from most other endocrine secretions in that they make more certain the **survival** of the species, yet they are not essential for the survival of the individual.

Sexual development begins in the embryo and continues in the fetus. After birth, there is a quiescent period that lasts until **puberty.** At this time, triggered by the production of various **sex hormones,** sexual development rapidly proceeds until normal, physical, sexual maturity is generally achieved in **late adolescence.**

COMPONENTS

The various components of the male reproductive system may be separated into **four functional groups:** (1) The two cytogenic male **gonads or testes,** located in the scrotum, produce spermatozoa in the seminiferous tubules. In addition, the male sex hormone, **testosterone,** is secreted by **interstitial cells** lying between the seminiferous tubules. (2) A series of paired, **excurrent ducts** are conduits to transport sperm outside the body. They may also **add secretions** to the sperm mass (**semen**) that provide nutrients for the sperm as well as lubricants to facilitate their passage. Proceeding from the seminiferous tubules distally, these **ducts** include the straight ducts (tubuli recti), rete testis, efferent ducts (ductuli efferentes), ductus epididymis, ductus or vas deferens, ejaculatory ducts, and the unpaired urethra. (3) Three **accessory exocrine glands** add their secretions to the semen. They are the unpaired **prostate,** the paired **seminal vesicles,** and the paired **bulbourethral glands.** (4) The **penis** is the organ of copulation.

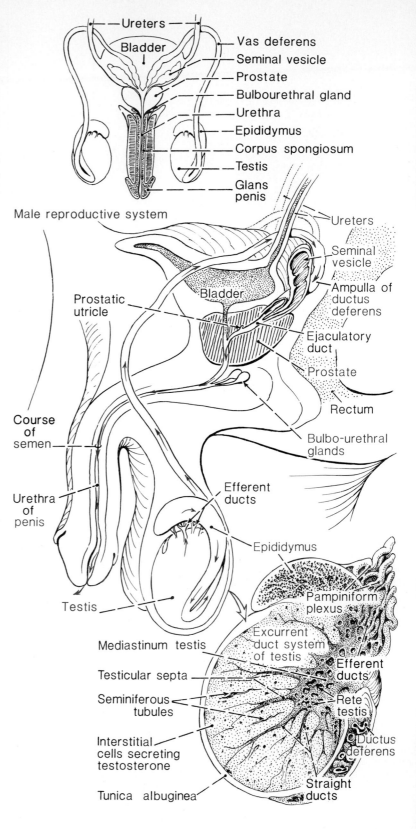

Male reproductive system

17411

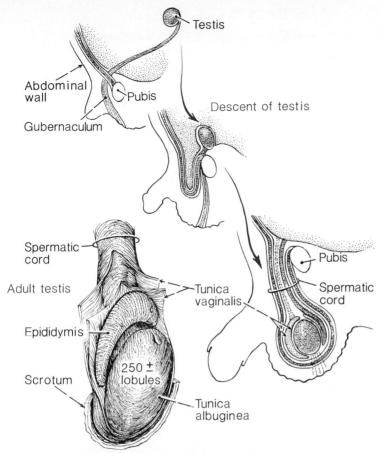

Testis

Abdominal wall

Gubernaculum

Pubis

Descent of testis

Spermatic cord

Adult testis

Tunica vaginalis

Pubis

Spermatic cord

Epididymis

Scrotum

250 ± lobules

Tunica albuginea

LM   Seminiferous tubule (spermatogenesis)

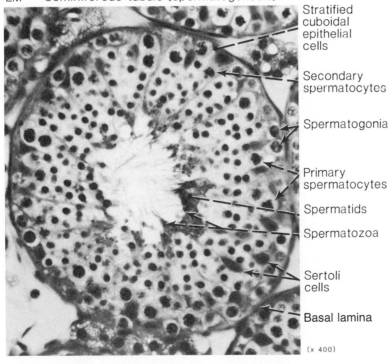

Stratified cuboidal epithelial cells

Secondary spermatocytes

Spermatogonia

Primary spermatocytes

Spermatids

Spermatozoa

Sertoli cells

Basal lamina

(x 400)

TESTES

During fetal development, the **testes develop** in the **upper abdominal cavity** associated with the kidneys and their ducts. During the last month of gestation each **testis descends** in an irregular course along the posterior abdominal cavity to eventually reach the **scrotum**. Enroute it is attached to a partially investing layer of the peritoneum, which forms a double-layered, serous sac, called the **tunica vaginalis,** which encloses the testis except for a slight depression on its posterior surface. Thus the testis lies in a serous cavity which allows it to move freely within the scrotum.

The inner layer of the sac is closely adherent to a robust, collagenous capsule, the **tunica albuginea.** Over the convex surface of the testis, the tunica albuginea gives off thin **septa** that penetrate and converge toward a slight depression on the posterior surface of the testis, called the **mediastinum testis.** These septa divide the organ into about 250 lobules. Each lobe contains one to four highly coiled loops, the **seminiferous tubules,** that house the developing sperm cells (gametes).

Seminiferous Tubules

The seminiferous tubules are enclosed in a fibrous capsule and lined with four to five layers of complex seminiferous epithelial cells, with the basal cells resting on a prominent basal lamina. These consist of two types of cells, **sex cells** and **support (Sertoli) cells.** The most numerous and conspicuous are the **spermatogenic** (sex) cells in various states of sperm development. The most basal of these cells are the spermatogonia, followed by primary spermatocytes, secondary spermatocytes, and bordering the lumen of the tubules are the spermatids and the spermatozoa.

Spermatogenesis and Meiosis

The process by which the sex cells differentiate to produce the highly specialized spermatozoa is called **spermatogenesis.** These changes are initiated directly by testosterone and indirectly by the follicle-stimulating hormone (**FSH**) of the anterior pituitary. The process involves the following specific stages of development of these spermatogenic cells.

1. The basal **spermatogonia** are primitive stem cells with a **diploid** number of chromosomes. They are ovoid or spherical in shape, about 10–20 µm in diameter, and rest on the basal

lamina of the seminiferous tubule. Two types of spermatogonia can be identified. The less numerous and **smaller type A reproduce** themselves for several generations and are committed to the production of additional **spermatogonia.**

2. The more abundant and **larger type B cells** are the **stem cells** for the subsequent **male sex cells.** They undergo mitosis, move away from the basal lamina, increase in size, and are now recognized as primary spermatocytes.

3. **Primary spermatocytes** are the **largest** of the sex cells and occupy roughly the central area of the epithelial layers. They divide by a unique type of cell division, called **meiosis,** which involves two cell divisions. The **first division** halves the diploid number of chromosomes in man, **from 46 to the haploid number of 23.** This is accomplished by the **separation** in metaphase I of each pair of homologous chromosomes which, in anaphase, migrate to opposite poles of the mitotic spindle. Thus in telophase, the **cell divides into two sex cells** (gametes), each with only a **haploid number of chromosomes.** (Recall that in mitosis each chromosome splits longitudinally to form two identical chromosomes. Thus each daughter cell receives the normal diploid number of chromosomes.)

Also, during the extended prophase of the first meiotic division, there is a mechanism for the **exchange of parts** of homologous chromosomes. This process is called **"crossing over" or chiasma** formation and results in chromosomes genetically different from those in the ancestral cell. Thus this random exchange of genetic information between chromosomes, plus the assortment of maternally and paternally derived chromosomes, **assures the infinite variety of offspring,** all essentially different from each other.

4. The product of the first meiotic division is the **haploid secondary spermatocyte.** It lies nearer to the lumen and is about half the size of its immediate precursor cell, the primary spermatocyte. Because its life-span is only a few hours, secondary spermatocytes are **seldom seen** in histological sections. They almost immediately undergo the **second meiotic division** to produce spermatids.

5. The spermatids are either round or elongated (condensing) cells. They are mostly **luminal in position, smallest** of the immature sex cells, and have a small, dense-staining nucleus. The dramatic transformation of a spermatid into a mobile, slender, **mature spermatozoon** with a long flagellum, is called **spermiogenesis.**

6. Spermiogenesis is the last stage of spermatogenesis. It involves a series of extensive changes in which the **spermatid,** a typical cell, becomes a very atypical cell, the **spermatozoon.**

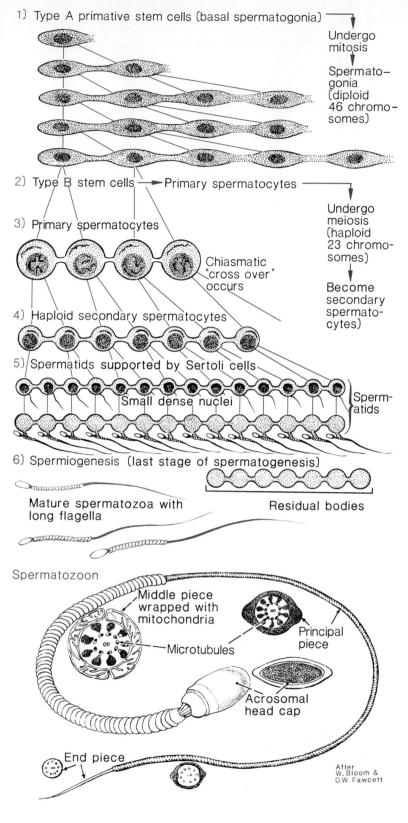

Process of Spermatogenesis

1) Type A primitive stem cells (basal spermatogonia) — Undergo mitosis → Spermatogonia (diploid 46 chromosomes)

2) Type B stem cells → Primary spermatocytes — Undergo meiosis (haploid 23 chromosomes) → Become secondary spermatocytes)

3) Primary spermatocytes — Chiasmatic "cross over" occurs

4) Haploid secondary spermatocytes

5) Spermatids supported by Sertoli cells — Small dense nuclei — Spermatids

6) Spermiogenesis (last stage of spermatogenesis) — Residual bodies

Mature spermatozoa with long flagella

Spermatozoon

Middle piece wrapped with mitochondria
Microtubules
Principal piece
Acrosomal head cap
End piece

After W. Bloom & D.W. Fawcett

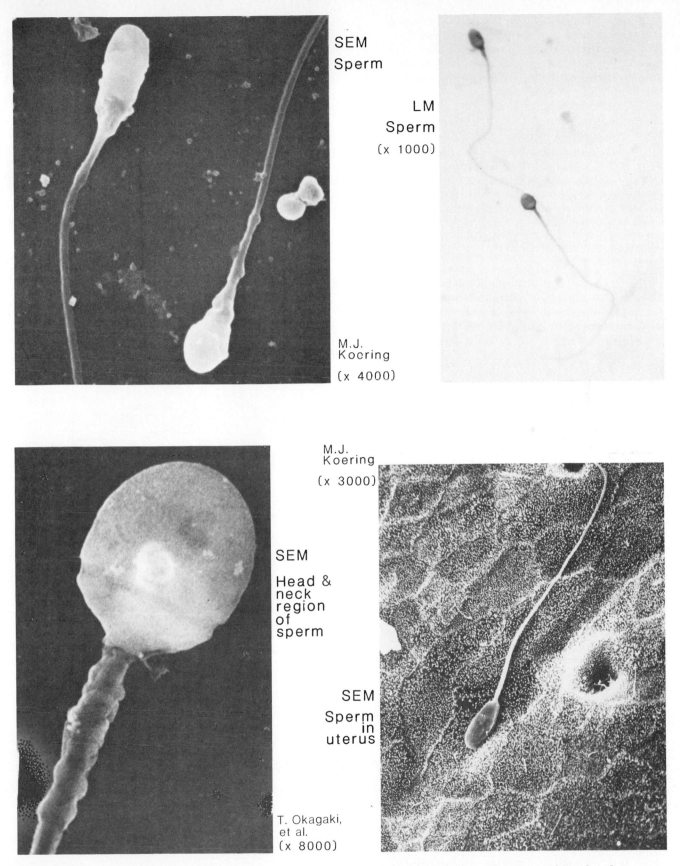

SEM
Sperm

LM
Sperm
(x 1000)

M.J.
Koering
(x 4000)

M.J.
Koering
(x 3000)

SEM
Head &
neck
region
of
sperm

SEM
Sperm
in
uterus

T. Okagaki,
et al.
(x 8000)

SEM micrographs of mature human spermatozoa (about 60 μm long) reveal head and tail regions. The tail is further divided into a narrow neck, middle, principal, and end pieces.

17656

These stages are: (a) the synthesis by the Golgi apparatus of a large vesicle, the **acrosomal vesicle.** It is filled with carbohydrates for the nourishment of the spermatozoon and with hydrolytic enzymes which will function in the penetration of the ovum by the sperm in fertilization. (b) The vesicle becomes associated with the distal pole of the elongating nucleus. The vesicle is now called the **acrosomal cap.** (c) On the opposite pole of the condensing nucleus, one of the **centrioles** elongates to form the **flagellum,** which is structurally similar to a cilium, i.e., it has nine doublets plus two central pairs of microtubules. However, unlike a cilium, the flagellum has nine, outer, dense fibers running longitudinally outside of the microtubules. (d) **Mitochondria** from the cell body migrate distally to form a **sheath** around the proximal portion of the newly formed flagellum. (e) The maturation phase consists principally of the pinching off and the **phagocytosis** of excess spermatid cytoplasm by the **Sertoli cells.** These excess bits of cytoplasm are called **residual bodies.** During all of these stages, the head of the spermatozoon is held in the apical cytoplasm of a Sertoli cell. Thus the Sertoli cell is often called a **nurse cell** because it protects and nourishes the nutrient-poor spermatozoon.

Interstitial (Leydig) Cells

Between the seminiferous tubules lie clusters of large, ovoid, epithelioid cells, the **interstitial cells (of Leydig),** associated with abundant capillary plexuses. Their extensive, lightly eosinophilic cytoplasm has **lipid droplets** and, in the elderly, variable amounts of yellow **lipochrome pigments.** Elongated **crystals** (of Reinke) are also common in the aged.

EM micrographs reveal cytoplasmic organelles characteristic of **steroid-secreting cells,** e.g., many mitochondria with **tubular cristae** and abundant sER. The principal steroid hormone produced is **testosterone.** It is responsible for the development and maintenance of **male secondary sexual characteristics,** the integrity of the seminiferous epithelium, and the control of spermatogenesis.

Blood Vessels, Lymphatics, and Nerves

The thin, **testicular artery,** a branch of the aorta, furnishes the principal blood supply to the testis. Its branches pierce the tunica albuginea to form a vascular area, the **tunica vasculosa.** Blood vessels in the tunic follow the septal walls to supply the **lobules** by ending in networks of **nonfenestrated capillaries.**

The veins emerge mostly at the **mediastinum** to form the extensive, dense, **pampiniform plexus,** which becomes the major component of the **spermatic cord.** The plexus gives rise to the testicular vein. Of passing interest is the intimate relationship of the pampiniform plexus with the

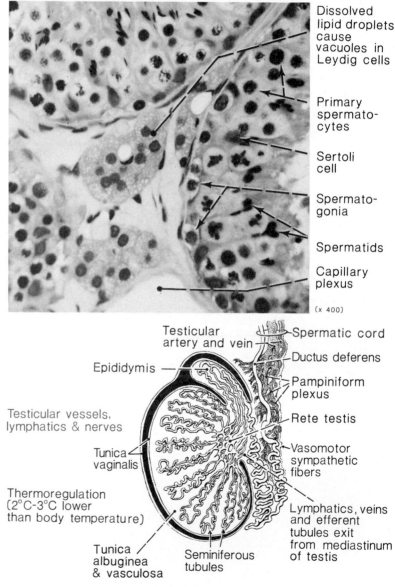

Stages in Spermiogenesis

a) Acrosomal vesicles (nourishment for spermatozoa and sperm penetration of ovum)

b) Acrosomal head cap

c) Flagellum evolves from one centriole

d) Mitochondria form sheath around proximal flagellum

e) Maturation phase of spermatid (phagocytosis of excess spermatid cytoplasm)

Microtubules

LM   Interstitial cells (of Leydig)

Dissolved lipid droplets cause vacuoles in Leydig cells

Primary spermatocytes

Sertoli cell

Spermatogonia

Spermatids

Capillary plexus

(x 400)

Testicular artery and vein — Spermatic cord

Epididymis — Ductus deferens

Pampiniform plexus

Rete testis

Testicular vessels, lymphatics & nerves

Vasomotor sympathetic fibers

Tunica vaginalis

Thermoregulation (2°C-3°C lower than body temperature)

Lymphatics, veins and efferent tubules exit from mediastinum of testis

Tunica albuginea & vasculosa

Seminiferous tubules

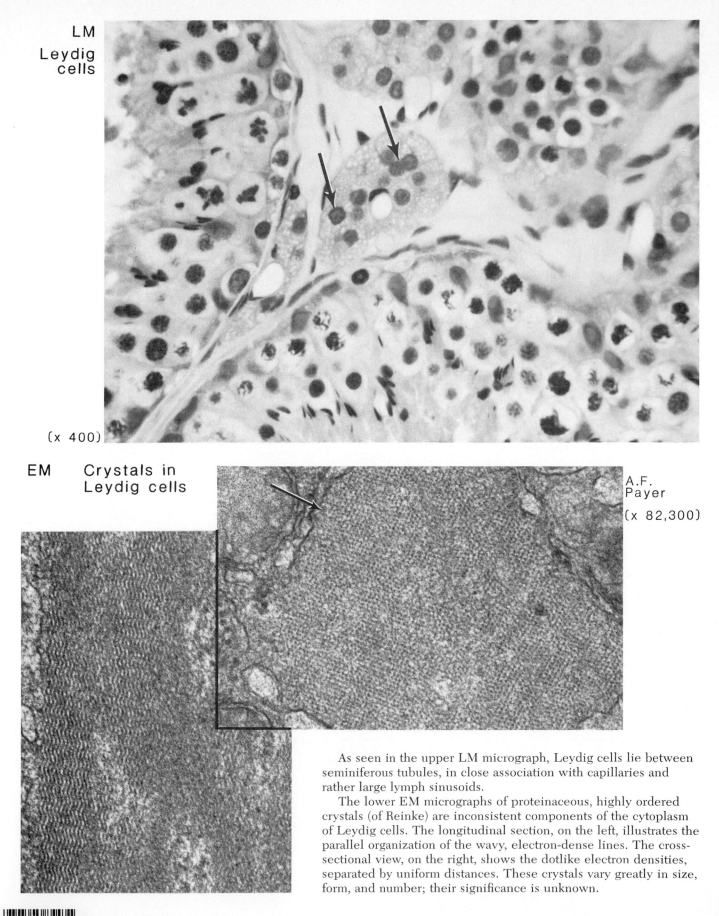

LM
Leydig
cells

(x 400)

EM   Crystals in
     Leydig cells

A.F.
Payer

(x 82,300)

As seen in the upper LM micrograph, Leydig cells lie between seminiferous tubules, in close association with capillaries and rather large lymph sinusoids.

The lower EM micrographs of proteinaceous, highly ordered crystals (of Reinke) are inconsistent components of the cytoplasm of Leydig cells. The longitudinal section, on the left, illustrates the parallel organization of the wavy, electron-dense lines. The cross-sectional view, on the right, shows the dotlike electron densities, separated by uniform distances. These crystals vary greatly in size, form, and number; their significance is unknown.

17474

extensively convoluted testicular artery. The plexus acts as a **thermoregulatory device** for lowering the temperature of the arterial blood before it reaches the testis. For spermatogenesis to proceed normally, the temperature in the scrotum must be 2°C to 3°C lower than the body temperature.

The numerous **lymphatics** of the seminiferous tubules exit at the mediastinum, in company with blood vessels. The **nerves** that enter the testis at the mediastinum are mostly **vasomotor sympathetic fibers,** which ramify around blood vessels. Blood vessels and nerves do not penetrate the basal lamina of the seminiferous epithelium.

MALE GENITAL EXCURRENT DUCTS

The extensive genital duct system begins with the straight tubules or tubuli recti (the terminations of the seminiferous tubules) and ends in the dilated tip of the penile urethra. Along its course the **accessory genital glands,** i.e., the prostate, seminal vesicles, and bulbourethral glands, empty their secretions into the duct system. Together with the spermatozoa, this semifluid mass is called the **semen or seminal fluid.**

Tubuli Recti

The seminiferous tubules end abruptly as tubuli recti (straight tubules) at the apices of the pyramidal-shaped lobules located in the mediastinum testis. The **spermiogenic cells disappear,** leaving only Sertoli cells as a single row of cuboidal epithelium lining the lumen.

Rete Testis

The rete testis is an extensive, anastomosing **network of open spaces** or channels within the mediastinum testis. A single layer of **cuboidal** or **squamous cells,** with prominent dark-staining nuclei, line the empty channels. Some of the cells have a single cilium which aids in the forward movement of the sperm. The epithelial layer has a **prominent basal lamina** that rests on a **highly vascular,** connective tissue layer devoid of muscle fibers.

Ductuli Efferentes

Extending from the rete testis to the head of the epididymis are 10–15 delicate, twisting tubules, the **ductuli efferentes (efferent ducts).** The lumen is characteristically **uneven or scalloped** due to the presence of groups of tall, **ciliated, columnar cells** alternating with shorter, **secretory cells.** The latter nonciliated cells possess many apical microvilli that absorb some of the fluid surrounding the sperm.

Each duct is surrounded by a basal lamina internal to the thin band of **circular smooth muscle fibers.** Note that in the efferent ducts, smooth muscle is first seen in the genital duct system.

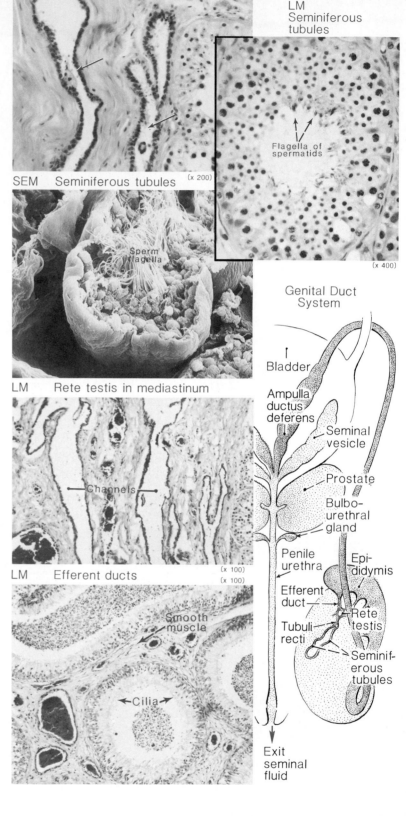

LM   Tubuli recti

LM Seminiferous tubules

Flagella of spermatids

(x 400)

SEM   Seminiferous tubules   (x 200)

Sperm flagella

LM   Rete testis in mediastinum

Channels

LM   Efferent ducts   (x 100) (x 100)

Smooth muscle

Cilia

Genital Duct System

Bladder

Ampulla ductus deferens

Seminal vesicle

Prostate

Bulbo-urethral gland

Penile urethra

Efferent duct

Tubuli recti

Epi-didymis

Rete testis

Seminiferous tubules

Exit seminal fluid

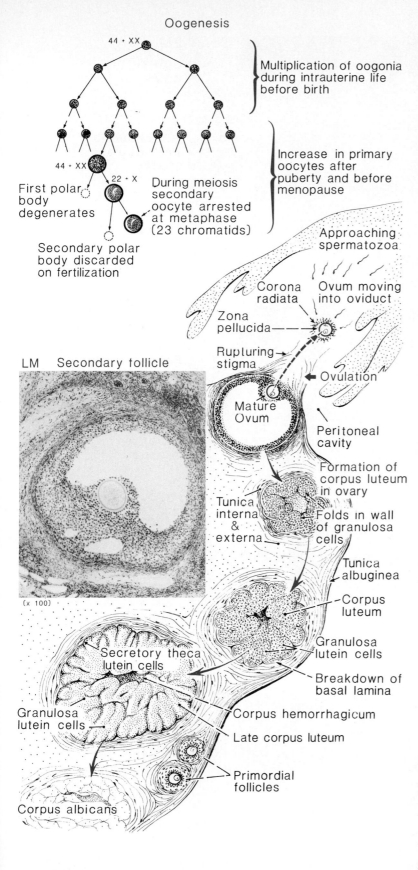

Oogenesis

44 + XX

Multiplication of oogonia during intrauterine life before birth

44 + XX

Increase in primary oocytes after puberty and before menopause

22 + X

First polar body degenerates

During meiosis secondary oocyte arrested at metaphase (23 chromatids)

Secondary polar body discarded on fertilization

Approaching spermatozoa

Corona radiata

Ovum moving into oviduct

Zona pellucida

Rupturing stigma

Ovulation

Mature Ovum

Peritoneal cavity

Formation of corpus luteum in ovary

Tunica interna & externa

Folds in wall of granulosa cells

Tunica albuginea

Corpus luteum

Granulosa lutein cells

Breakdown of basal lamina

Corpus hemorrhagicum

Late corpus luteum

Primordial follicles

Secretory theca lutein cells

Granulosa lutein cells

Corpus albicans

LM   Secondary follicle

(x 100)

The second meiotic division of the secondary oocyte is **arrested at metaphase.** Somewhat similar to mitosis, it will be completed only after fertilization, when the 23 chromosomes split longitudinally. The two identical chromatids in each chromosome separate and move, in anaphase, toward opposite poles. Thus, each daughter cell receives **23 chromatids (called chromosomes when meiosis is completed).** Again, one cell is large and functional, a **secondary oocyte;** the other, a tiny **second polar body,** is discarded.

Ovulation usually occurs on approximately the **fourteenth day** of the menstrual cycle. Its exact cause is obscure, however, it is triggered by the luteinizing hormone. Heightened **intrafollicular pressure** from the increased amount of liquor folliculi is usually given as the reason. Yet, measurements of the pressure just prior to rupture of the follicle shows no significant increase. Nevertheless, as a prelude to ovulation, a **thinning out** of the components of the **wall** of the ovary occurs.

The weakened cortical region immediately develops a small, transparent conical projection, the **stigma.** Within a few minutes, the membrane covering the **stigma ruptures and the mature ovum,** surrounded by the zona pellucida, corona radiata, and other granulosa cells, **is released and ovulation has occurred.** The ovum (secondary oocyte) is swept into the **peritoneal cavity** near the entrance of the oviduct. **Ciliary action** of the lining cells of the oviduct sets up a fluid current that normally wisks the ovum into the **lumen of the oviduct** for fertilization, which must occur within the next 24 h.

SEQUELS OF FOLLICLES

The eventual fate of an ovarian follicle is to transform into one or more **temporary structures or sequels.** These include the temporary corpus luteum (L. corpus, body; luteum, yellow), which later becomes the more permanent corpus albicans; various stages of atretic follicles before they become fibrous scars; and the transitory interstitial gland.

Corpus Luteum

Upon rupture of the follicle, its walls collapse inward, forming folds or pleats. Caught within these folds are the remaining granulosa cells that formerly lined the follicle. They are transformed directly into cords of large, clear, secretory cells, the **granulosa lutein cells.** These cells have abundant **lipid droplets** and **yellow lipochrome granules,** which give the yellow color to the fresh gland. Simultaneously, the **disintegration** of the basal lamina between the granulosa cells and the theca allows for **invasion into the area of blood vessels,** connective tissue cells and **theca interna cells.**

16179

Corpus lutein cells

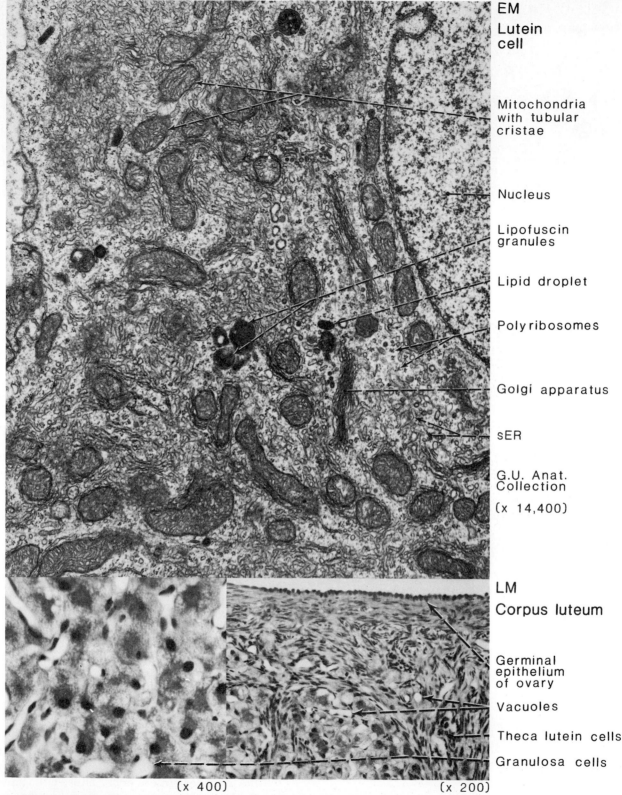

EM

Lutein cell

Mitochondria with tubular cristae

Nucleus

Lipofuscin granules

Lipid droplet

Polyribosomes

Golgi apparatus

sER

G.U. Anat. Collection

(x 14,400)

LM

Corpus luteum

Germinal epithelium of ovary

Vacuoles

Theca lutein cells

Granulosa cells

(x 400)   (x 200)

The upper electron micrograph of a granulosa lutein cell shows extensive smooth endoplasmic reticulum with limited rER. The abundant pleomorphic mitochondria are typical of steroid-producing cells. The cytoplasm also contains numerous lipid droplets, several Golgi complexes, lipofuscin pigment granules, and many free ribosomes and polyribosomes.

The lower photomicrographs contrast the microscopic features of the theca and granulosa lutein cells of the corpus luteum, on the right, with the higher magnification of the theca lutein cells on the left.

16137

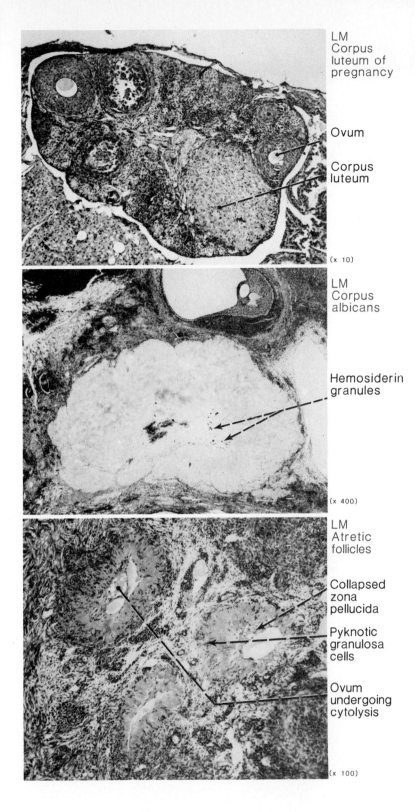

LM
Corpus
luteum of
pregnancy

Ovum

Corpus
luteum

(x 10)

LM
Corpus
albicans

Hemosiderin
granules

(x 400)

LM
Atretic
follicles

Collapsed
zona
pellucida

Pyknotic
granulosa
cells

Ovum
undergoing
cytolysis

(x 100)

If the ovum is not fertilized, the **corpus luteum of menstruation** (corpus luteum spurium) persists for about 10–14 days before it undergoes involution. The granulosa lutein cells degenerate and the amount of lipochrome pigment increases, giving the body a distinct yellow color in the fresh state. Eventually, the moribund cells are replaced by a dense connective tissue scar, the **corpus albicans.**

If pregnancy occurs, the **corpus luteum of pregnancy** (corpus luteum verum) enlarges to 1–3 cm in diameter and is functional for about six months before it begins to undergo involution. However, it continues to secrete **progesterone** until parturition, when the cells undergo rapid degeneration. They are replaced by a large, long-lasting **corpus albicans,** which persists as a fibrous scar for months or even years before it finally disappears.

TEM studies of a functional corpus luteum reveal organelles typical of **steroid-secreting cells,** e.g., an abundance of mitochondria with **tubular cristae,** many profiles of **sER,** fewer profiles of rER, many lipid droplets, and abundant lipofuscin pigment granules.

Corpus Albicans

The morphological end product (sequel) of the **degenerating corpus luteum** is an irregular, pale, relatively acellular scar, the **corpus albicans** (L. albicans, white). It resembles other connective tissue scars in the ovary, the advanced **atretic follicles.** However, the corpus albicans can be distinguished because: (1) it has **fewer cells,** which are flattened fibroblasts; (2) it is usually a **larger structure;** and (3) it may contain **hemosiderin granules.** This pigment results from the breakdown of hemoglobin of red blood cells that formed the corpus hemorrhagicum. Normally, no hemosiderin is found in atretic follicles.

Atretic Follicles

Atresia of the ovarian follicles occurs in **all stages of follicular development.** During late fetal and early postnatal life, many primordial follicles begin to mature but very few, perhaps only 400 of the 400,000 follicles present at birth, mature and ovulate.

The initial sign of **atresia** in the **primary follicle** is that the oocyte is shrunken, irregular, and undergoing cytolysis. Next, the granulosa cells become smaller, pyknotic, and separate from each other and undergo autolysis.

In the secondary or antral follicles, similar changes occur. In addition, loose **granulosa cells invade the antrum.** The basal lamina between the granulosa cells and the theca interna becomes hyalinized, thickened, and folded. It is known as the eosinophilic **glassy membrane.**

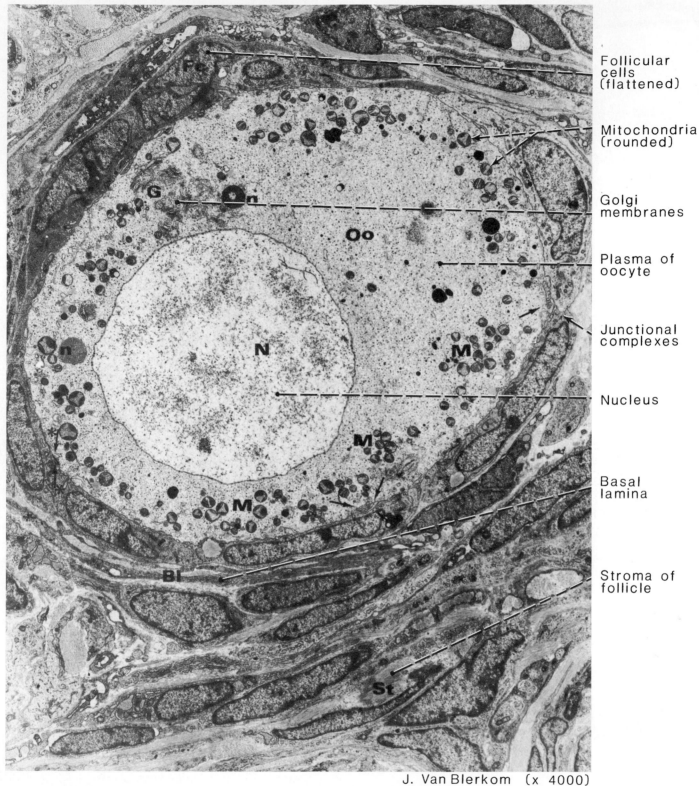

Follicular
cells
(flattened)

Mitochondria
(rounded)

Golgi
membranes

Plasma of
oocyte

Junctional
complexes

Nucleus

Basal
lamina

Stroma of
follicle

J. Van Blerkom   (x 4000)

Portrayed in this transmission electron micrograph is a unilaminar (primordial) follicle of an estrous rabbit. Its most prominent feature is an ovum or oocyte (Oo) containing a large, spherical nucleus (N) with finely dispersed chromatin and usually one or more nucleoli. Immediately surrounding the ovum is a single layer of flattened follicular cells (Fc), resting on a prominent basal lamina (Bl). The cytoplasm of the ovum contains many characteristic small, round mitochondria (M) with typical cristae. A well-developed Golgi apparatus (G) is located near the nucleus.

16011

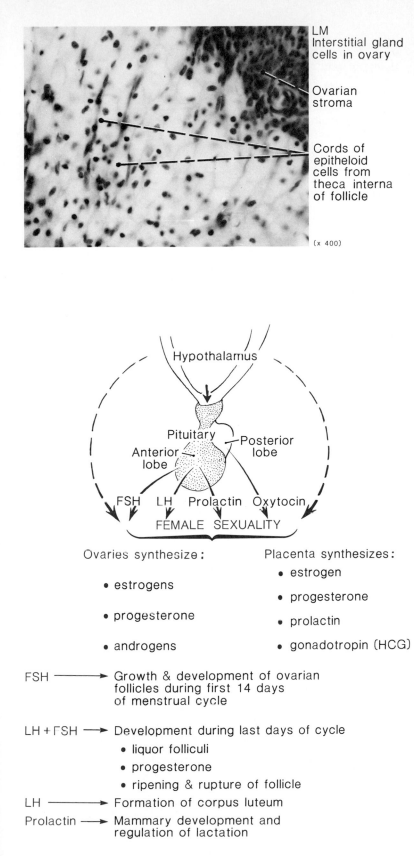

LM
Interstitial gland
cells in ovary

Ovarian
stroma

Cords of
epitheloid
cells from
theca interna
of follicle

(x 400)

Hypothalamus

Pituitary

Anterior
lobe

Posterior
lobe

FSH   LH   Prolactin   Oxytocin
FEMALE SEXUALITY

Ovaries synthesize:

- estrogens

- progesterone

- androgens

Placenta synthesizes:

- estrogen

- progesterone

- prolactin

- gonadotropin (HCG)

FSH ⟶ Growth & development of ovarian
follicles during first 14 days
of menstrual cycle

LH + FSH ⟶ Development during last days of cycle
- liquor folliculi
- progesterone
- ripening & rupture of follicle

LH ⟶ Formation of corpus luteum

Prolactin ⟶ Mammary development and
regulation of lactation

In addition to the above changes, the mature Graafian follicle shows additional modifications. The **theca interna cells** enlarge, become epithelioid, and are arranged in vascularized cords of cells that grow into the collapsed cavity of the atretic follicle, similar to a developing corpus luteum. These cells may give rise to the **interstitial gland** (Table 24.1).

Interstitial Gland

Cords of large epithelioid cells (**interstitial gland**) are often found in the stroma of ovaries of mammals; they are especially prominent in rodents. In humans, they are most abundant during the first year of life and **absent or sparse in the adult.** Since these cells probably arise from the theca interna cells of the atretic follicles, they would be most abundant when atresia is most frequent, i.e., the first postnatal year. They are **remnants of atretic follicles,** dispersed throughout the cortex of the ovary.

Since interstitial cells resemble luteal cells cytologically, some authorities believe they provide **estrogen** for the growth and development of the secondary sex characteristics during the prepubertal period. Other investigators believe these cells may be a source of ovarian **testosterone** and, therefore, perhaps are comparable to the interstitial cells of the testes.

HORMONAL CONTROL

Hormones of the pituitary, ovary, hypothalamus, and placenta all **influence the development of the female sex characteristics.** Principal endocrine secretions from the pituitary include **FSH, LH, and prolactin** from the anterior lobe, and **oxytocin** released from the posterior lobe. Within the ovary, estrogens, progesterone, and limited amounts of androgens, especially testosterone, are synthesized. The **hypothalamus** controls the pituitary and produces **releasing factors** (hormones) that determine when and what hormones will be released into the bloodstream. During late pregnancy, the **placenta,** by its own synthesis, greatly augments the ovarian output of estrogen and progesterone, and, to a lesser degree, the pituitary output of prolactin and gonadotropin, the latter by producing human **chorionic gonadotropin (HCG).**

Pituitary Hormones

FSH is responsible for the **growth and maturation of ovarian follicles,** especially during the first 14 days of the menstrual cycle. **LH,** in conjunction with FSH, controls the final burst of development, characterized by increase in the liquor folliculi, production of **progesterone,** final ripening of the egg, and rupture of the mature follicle. The subsequent **formation of the corpus luteum** is under the precise control of LH.

Ovarian Hormones

The ovarian hormone **estrogen** is produced principally by the **granulosa cells** and the cells of the **theca interna** of the maturing follicle, with some contribution from the cells of the corpus luteum. It functions to stimulate growth and **maturation of follicles** and causes growth of the lining (**endometrium**) of the uterus. **Estrogen** is produced throughout the 28-day sexual cycle but reaches **its peak at day 14, at ovulation.** The high level of estrogen in the blood acts as a negative feedback on centers in the hypothalamus, which **inhibits the release of FSH** from the pituitary. Simultaneously, the high estrogen levels have the opposite effect on cells in the hypothalamus that **produce the LH releasing factor,** resulting in a flood of LH at mid-cycle, which **initiates ovulation** and the beginning of corpus luteum formation.

At or shortly before ovulation, high levels of LH signal the **granulosa lutein cells** to begin the synthesis of **progesterone.** As the amount of progesterone rises, it exerts a negative feedback on certain cells of the hypothalamus. The result is that **gonadotropin-releasing factors are reduced,** the high level of LH in the blood subsides, the corpus luteum is no longer maintained, and the **synthesis of progesterone is arrested.** With the decline of the corpus luteum, the inhibition over the pituitary is negated, FSH is secreted again, and the cycle is repeated.

The prime function of progesterone is to act on the uterine mucosa, specifically to initiate and **maintain the secretory (luteal) stage.** It also acts on the pituitary to **inhibit FSH production.**

Hypothalamic Hormones

Oxytocin, produced by neurosecretory neurons in the **hypothalamus,** is stored in the posterior lobe of the pituitary. This hormone stimulates **contraction of the uterine walls** during parturition and causes **ejection of milk** by stimulating the myoepithelial cells of the mammary alveoli.

Various releasing and inhibiting hormones are synthesized in special nuclei in the hypothalamus. They control the levels of anterior pituitary hormones in the bloodstream. Vasopressin, an antidiuretic hormone (ADH), is also secreted by cells of the hypothalamus. However, it exerts no known influence on the female reproduction system.

Placental Hormones

The placenta synthesizes certain hormones that **maintain the uterine mucosa** so it can continue to nourish and protect the developing fetus. These hormones include estrogen, progesterone, human chorionic gonadotropin (HCG), and human chorionic somatomammotropin (HCS).

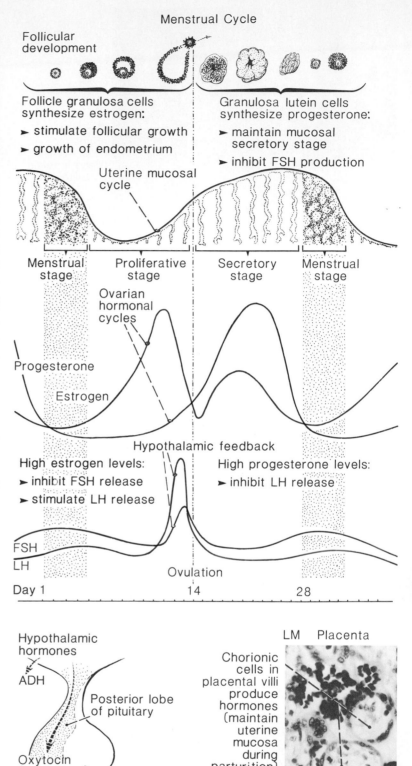

Menstrual Cycle

Follicular development

Follicle granulosa cells synthesize estrogen:
► stimulate follicular growth
► growth of endometrium

Granulosa lutein cells synthesize progesterone:
► maintain mucosal secretory stage
► inhibit FSH production

Uterine mucosal cycle

Menstrual stage | Proliferative stage | Secretory stage | Menstrual stage

Ovarian hormonal cycles

Progesterone

Estrogen

Hypothalamic feedback

High estrogen levels:
► inhibit FSH release
► stimulate LH release

High progesterone levels:
► inhibit LH release

FSH
LH

Ovulation

Day 1   14   28

Hypothalamic hormones

ADH

Posterior lobe of pituitary

Oxytocin (in storage)

Stimulates uterine contractions and mammary alveoli constrictions

LM   Placenta

Chorionic cells in placental villi produce hormones (maintain uterine mucosa during parturition)

(x 400)

Layers separating ovarian surface and oocyte

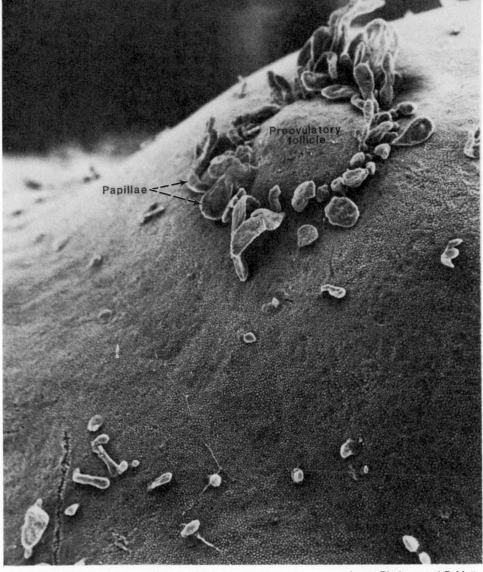

Preovulatory follicle

Papillae

J. van Blerkom and P. Motta

As you examine the above SEM view of the outer surface of the ovary, try to visualize the several layers of cells, or their products, that lie between the ovarian surface and the underlying ovum. These layers, not in proper sequence, are theca externa, germinal epithelium, corona radiata, basal lamina, antrum, tunica albuginea, theca interna, and zona pellucida.

Now list these layers in their proper order, according to information in this chapter.

Table 24.1 *OVARIAN FOLLICLES AND THEIR SEQUELAE*

TYPE OF FOLLICLE OR SEQUEL	LOCATION	HISTOLOGIC FEATURES	
		LM	EM
Primordial or unilaminar	In cortex next to fibrous tunica albuginea	Oocyte is about 25 μm in diameter and surrounded by layer of flat follicular cells; has large nucleus and nucleolus	Limited ooplasm contains large Golgi complex, many round mitochondria, few rER profiles, abundant free ribosomes, a centrosome and sparse lipid granules
Primary or multilaminar	In cortex	Oocyte increases to 50–80 μm in diameter; layers of cuboidal follicular cells fill greatly enlarged follicle; zona pellucida develops between oocyte and follicular cells; outer c.t. layer develops into theca interna and externa	In oocyte, mitochondria and Golgi complexes more abundant; annulate lamellae often present; the mitotically active follicular cells have many free ribosomes and rER profiles; mitochondria, lysosomes and lipid droplets are scarce
Secondary or antral	In cortex but migrates toward medulla	Embedded in cumulus ooporus the oocyte enlarges to 125–150 μm; follicle expands (0.2 mm) with pools of liquor folliculi coalescing to form an antrum; follicle filled with layers of cuboidal follicular cells, the stratum granulosum	Similar to primary follicle
Mature or graafian	From medulla follicle moves to edge of ovary, causing bulging and thinning of ovarian wall, prior to ovulation	Attains adult size (>10 mm); first reduction division of primary oocyte completed with first polar body released; follicle ruptures, releasing secondary oocyte with haploid (1N) chromosomes	Compared to primary follicle, the oocyte has more lysosomes, lipid droplets, and ribosomes; mitochondria are less numerous; follicular cells show fewer mitoses and have junctional complexes; theca interna has many free ribosomes, mitochondria and abundant rER
Atretic	In cortex	Follicles may undergo atresia at any stage; nuclei of oocyte and granulosal cells become pyknotic and degenerate; macrophages, fibroblasts, and granulosal cells invade antrum; thickened basement membrane produces glassy membrane; follicle becomes fibrous scar	Degenerating follicular cells have large accumulation of lysosomes and lipid droplets
Corpus luteum	In cortex and medulla	Enlarged granulosa and theca interna cells are arranged in folded cords; they contain abundant lipofuscin pigment and lipid droplets; the former impart a pale, yellow color to the fresh gland; the latter, a vacuolated appearance to the cells	Has characteristics of steroid secretory gland, e.g., fenestrated capillaries, abundant lipid droplets; many mitochondria with unique tubular cristae and many profiles of sER
Corpus albicans	In cortex and medulla	An irregularly folded white scar of collagenous c.t., the hyaline remnant of a corpus luteum	

ENDOCRINE SECRETIONS	HORMONES ACTING ON STRUCTURE	FUNCTIONS	SEQUELS
None	FSH	Oocytes proliferate by mitosis; some become mature gametes; others undergo atresia; meiosis arrested in gametes (primary oocytes)	Primary follicle
Theca interna cells begin to secrete estrogen	FSH	Nourishes and promotes maturation of oocytes; synthesis of estrogen begins in theca interna, recently differentiated by action of FSH which also promotes hypertrophy and proliferation of follicular cells	Secondary follicle
Estrogen	FSH and LH	Maintains high levels of estrogen production which controls development of endometrium, breasts, and genitalia; FSH stimulates secretion of liquor folliculi	Mature follicle
Estrogen and limited progesterone	LH and FSH	After first meiotic division is completed, second division begins (secondary oocyte); high levels of estrogen inhibit FSH release, while increasing LH levels in blood; also promotes duct development in mammae	Atretic follicle or corpus luteum
Traces of estrogen	None	None	Fibrous scar
Primarily progesterone; limited estrogen	LH and HCG	Synthesis of progesterone maintains uterine mucosa for reception of embryo; develops alveoli in mammae; prevents ovulation	Corpus albicans
None	None	None	Hyaline scar

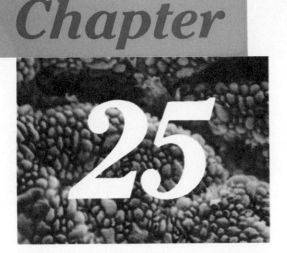

Chapter

25

FEMALE REPRODUCTIVE SYSTEM II—GENITAL TRACT AND OTHER ORGANS OF PREGNANCY

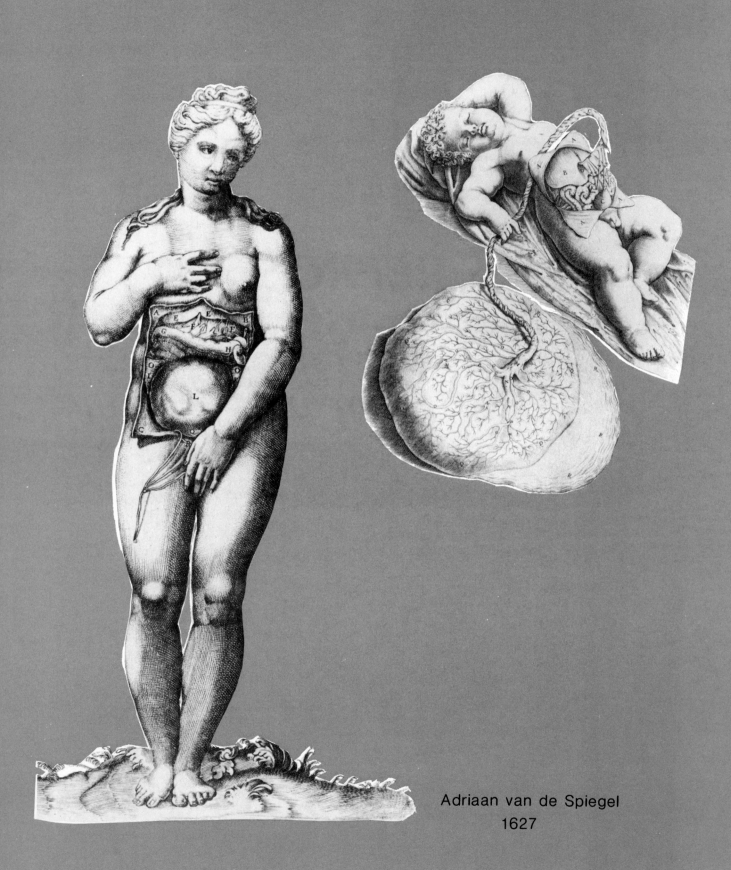

Adriaan van de Spiegel
1627

AFTER STUDYING THIS CHAPTER, ONE SHOULD BE ABLE TO:

1. Explain how ovarian and pituitary hormones control the menstrual cycle and also trigger parturition.

2. Describe the histology of the cyclic changes in the uterus during menstruation and pregnancy.

3. Explain the fetal and maternal components of the placenta and their functions.

4. Compare the histology of the components of the external genitalia in the female with their homologs in the male.

5. Describe the structure and functions of the mammary gland, including the mechanism of milk release.

The female genital tract includes the two oviducts, uterus, cervix, and vagina.

OVIDUCT

The upper segment of the tract, the **oviduct (uterine or fallopian tube),** is the common passageway for the downward migration of the ova and the upward movement of the spermatozoa. Regarding this movement, Blandau (1973) comments: "Only this statement can be made with certainty. Mature eggs are ovulated, mature spermatozoa capable of fertilizing them reach the ampulla (of the oviduct), and under a suitable environment, union of these cells is accomplished—. There is no other tubular system in which cells of such different dimensions are transported in opposite directions in a limited period of time."

These remarkable bilateral tubes extend from the region of the ovaries to the uterus. They provide a **suitable milieu for fertilization** to occur and for the resulting zygote to develop into the morula stage. After about three days, the **morula** is washed into the cavity of the uterus by the ciliary action of the cells lining the oviduct.

Segments

Grossly and histologically, the oviduct is divided into four segments or regions. From lateral to medial, they are as follows: (1) The **infundibulum** is the flared, trumpet-shaped upper extremity which opens into the peritoneal cavity. The mucosa of its open end is extremely folded and fringed with many tapering processes (folds), called **fimbria,** which are often engorged with blood. This open end is potentially dangerous since it always provides an entry for infection to enter the abdominal cavity. (2) The **ampulla** is the continuation of the infundibulum. It is a thin-walled, dilated, tortuous tube with complex mucosal folds that almost fill its lumen. It is about half the length of the oviduct (7–8 cm). (3) The **isthmus,** continuous with the ampulla, is a narrow, thick-walled segment that connects with the uterus. It constitutes about one third of the oviduct. (4) The **interstitial (intramural)** segment is the continuation of the isthmus through the wall of the uterus. It opens onto the inner mucosal surface of the uterus at a small opening called the uterine ostium.

The lumen of the oviduct diminishes sharply (8 mm to 1 mm) as it approaches the uterus. Conversely, the wall of the oviduct thickens progressively in the same direction.

Histological Features

Like most hollow viscera, the wall of the oviduct consists of three layers, a complex inner mucosa, an intermediate muscularis of several layers of smooth muscle, and an outer serosa.

MUCOSA The **mucosal lining** is thrown into

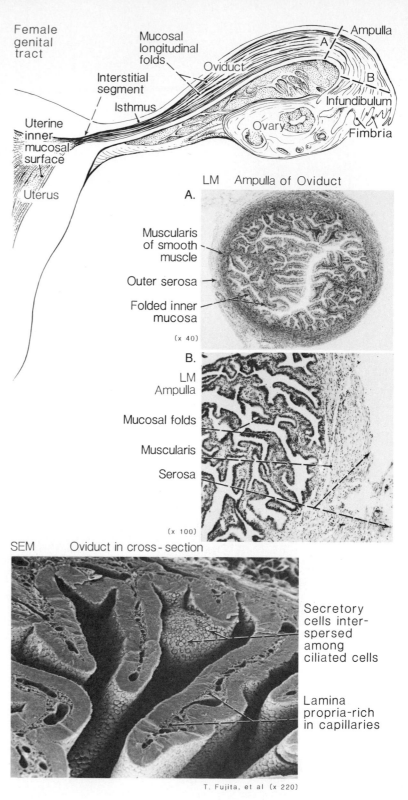

Female genital tract

Mucosal longitudinal folds

Interstitial segment

Isthmus

Oviduct

Ampulla

A

B

Infundibulum

Fimbria

Ovary

Uterine inner mucosal surface

Uterus

LM   Ampulla of Oviduct

A.

Muscularis of smooth muscle

Outer serosa

Folded inner mucosa

(x 40)

B.

LM Ampulla

Mucosal folds

Muscularis

Serosa

(x 100)

SEM   Oviduct in cross-section

Secretory cells interspersed among ciliated cells

Lamina propria-rich in capillaries

T. Fujita, et al (x 220)

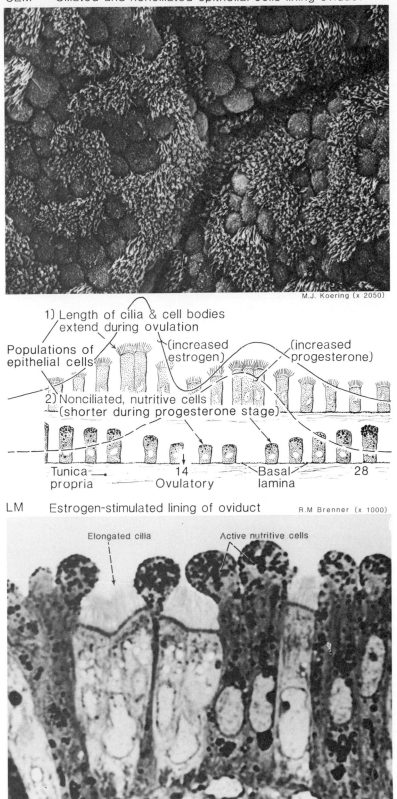

M.J. Koering (x 2050)

1) Length of cilia & cell bodies extend during ovulation

Populations of epithelial cells   (increased estrogen)   (increased progesterone)

2) Nonciliated, nutritive cells (shorter during progesterone stage)

Tunica propria — 14 Ovulatory — Basal lamina — 28

LM   Estrogen-stimulated lining of oviduct   R.M Brenner (x 1000)

Elongated cilia   Active nutritive cells

many fields. The epithelium lining the folds is simple columnar, with two populations of cells: (1) **ciliated cells** with spherical nuclei and cilia that beat toward the uterus, and (2) the less numerous, **nonciliated peg cells** have larger, ovoid nuclei. The nonciliated cells are assumed to be **nutritive,** mucoid, secretory cells, possibly involved in creating a favorable environment for the survival of the male and female gametes and for their eventual union. In some species, these cells secrete some, but not all, components of egg shell.

The epithelium appears to be under hormonal control. The **ciliated cells** increase in height during high estrogen levels, such as during the proliferative (follicular) stage of the uterus. They reach their **maximum height at ovulation,** while the nonciliated cells are shorter during the secretory (progesterone) stage of the uterus. Furthermore, **estrogens** are critical for the genesis and maintenance of the **cilia.** In postmenopausal women, the oviductal epithelium is a low columnar type with few cilia. If these women are given sustained estrogen treatments, the epithelium returns to the reproductive stage, with abundant cilia.

The **tunica propria** has spindle-shaped stromal cells, connective tissue cells and fibers, and leukocytes. A delicate basal lamina is present but no muscularis mucosae, hence, no submucosa.

In case of a **tubal pregnancy,** i.e., an embryo is implanted in the mucosa of the oviduct instead of the uterus, the **stromal cells** enlarge, become epithelioid, and are transformed into **decidual cells.** These cells are capable of nourishing and temporarily sustaining the embryo, similar to the maternal decidual component of the placenta.

MUSCULARIS Although the **muscularis** is usually described as having an inner circular and outer longitudinal layer of smooth muscle, only the **inner circular layer is well developed.** In fact, there is no distinct boundary between them, except possibly near its union with the uterus where the muscularis is thickest. It is thinnest in the infundibulum and the ampulla.

SEROSA The serosa is usually a thin layer of connective tissue covered by **mesothelium** (peritoneum). Within the connective tissue layer, blood vessels supply the muscularis and also form a plexus beneath the mesothelium. The nerves also form a plexus, supplying motor impulses to the muscularis and sensory stimuli to the mesothelium (L–A, plates 24 and 29).

Fertilization

Fertilization usually occurs in the **ampulla.** Just before ovulation occurs, the **infundibulum** and its fimbria reflexly **move toward the ovary** and partially enclose it. The ovum, surrounded by the zona pellucida, corona radiata, and cumulus, is then released and swept into the open

16620

mouth of the oviduct by currents set up by the action of the ciliated cells that line the fimbria and infundibulum. Once inside the lumen of the ampulla, the movement of the ovum is greatly slowed by the labyrinth of **mucosal folds** that practically fill the lumen. While trapped in this maze, the egg is most likely to be **fertilized.**

When penetrated by a spermatozoon, probably by enzymatic action and/or membrane fusion, the ovum completes its **second meiotic division** that has been arrested since ovulation. The male and female nuclei unite to give the resulting **zygote a diploid (46) number of chromosomes.** The dividing zygote forms a rounded mass of cells, the **morula.** After 2–3 days in the oviduct, the morula passes into the lumen of the uterus where it **becomes embedded** in the highly vascular, nutrient-rich uterine mucosal lining, the **endometrium.**

UTERUS

In the human, the uterus lies like an **inverted pear** in the pelvis. The oviducts pierce its wall at the superior, widest region, the body. The uppermost, dome-shaped part of the uterus is the **fundus.** The lower, narrow region, the **cervix,** opens into the upper part of the vagina.

Body and Fundus

The thick wall of the body and fundus of the uterus consist of three layers: a thin outer layer, the **perimetrium** (serosa); a middle, dense, robust, muscular layer, the **myometrium;** and an inner, glandular, spongy mucosa, the **endometrium,** that lines the uterine cavity.

ENDOMETRIUM Within the expansive endometrium the following important events occur: (1) It is the normal locale for the **implantation** of the morula and the blastocyst stages of the early embryo. (2) It is the usual site for the development of the **placenta.** (3) It is the location of the **glandular and vascular changes** associated with the menstrual cycle.

The **endometrium** consists of **simple columnar epithelium with or without cilia,** a wide tunica propria housing **extensive mucosal glands,** and the endometrial stroma. The layer extends from the free luminal surface to the underlying muscle bundles of the myometrium. It is divided into a basal one third, the **lamina (stratum) basalis,** and the luminal two thirds, the **lamina (stratum) functionalis.** During **menstruation,** the functional zone degenerates while most of the basal layer remains intact. It will regenerate the new mucosa for the next menstrual cycle.

Below the epithelium is a **basal lamina,** which separates it from the loose connective tissue stroma of the tunica propria. In the **tunica pro-**

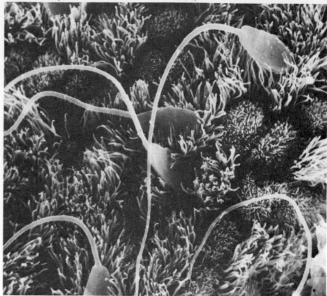

SEM   Sperm in uterus of rabbit

P. Motta & J. Van Blerkom (x 4200)

Fertilization & implantation of ovum

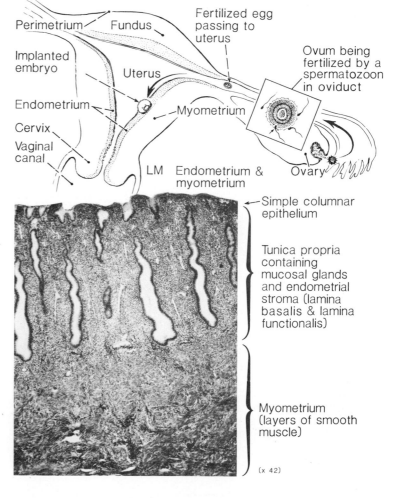

Perimetrium

Fundus

Fertilized egg passing to uterus

Implanted embryo

Uterus

Ovum being fertilized by a spermatozoon in oviduct

Endometrium

Myometrium

Cervix

Vaginal canal

LM   Endometrium & myometrium

Ovary

Simple columnar epithelium

Tunica propria containing mucosal glands and endometrial stroma (lamina basalis & lamina functionalis)

Myometrium (layers of smooth muscle)

(x 42)

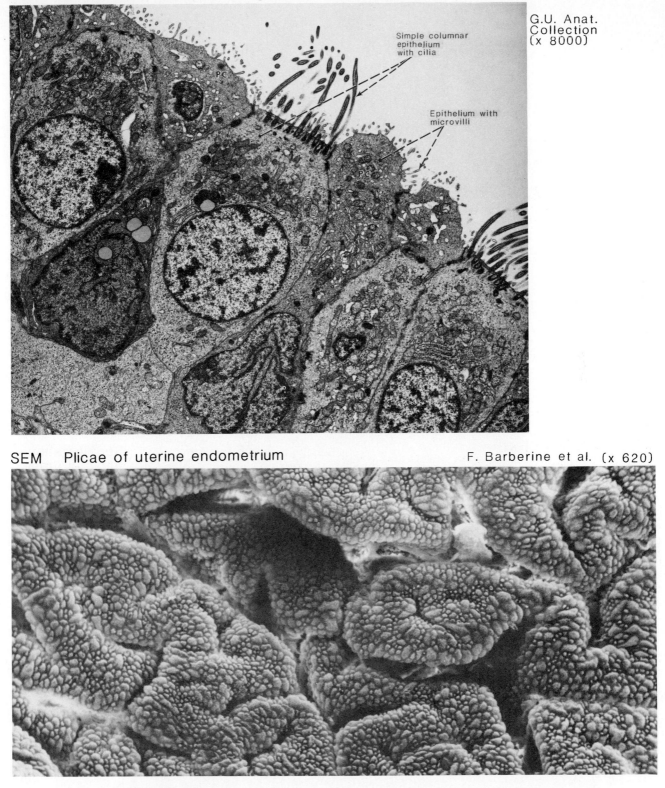

G.U. Anat.
Collection
(x 8000)

Simple columnar
epithelium
with cilia

Epithelium with
microvilli

SEM   Plicae of uterine endometrium   F. Barberine et al. (x 620)

The upper TEM micrograph shows the simple columnar epithelium lining the uterine tube. Two types of cells are present, the slightly elevated peg (Pc) or secretory cell whose apical surface has many microvilli. The other cell type is ciliated and has, in the terminal web, a row of electron-dense basal bodies at the base of the cilia. Mitochondria are abundant in the supranuclear cytoplasm.

The lower SEM micrograph is a view of the mucosa in the rabbit uterus, which discloses extensive plicae and infoldings of the endometrium.

16606

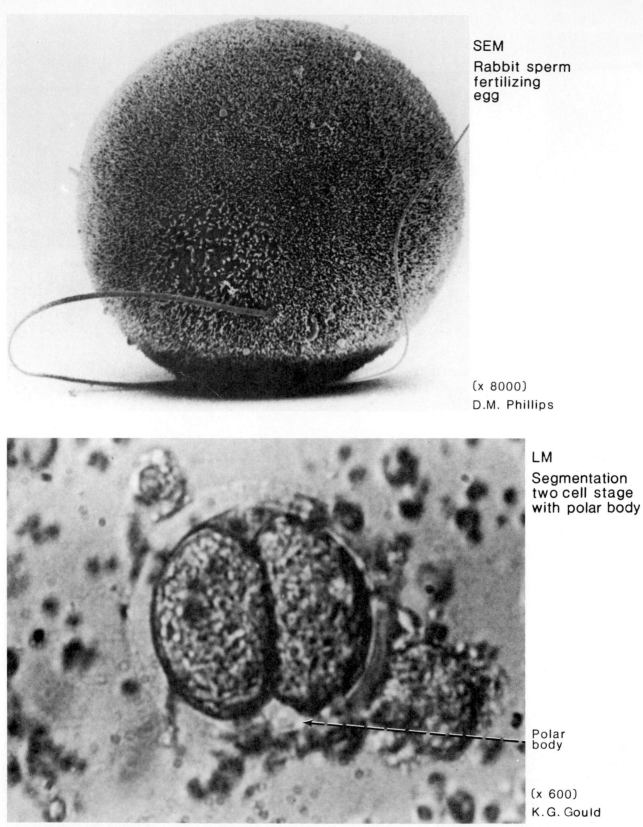

SEM
Rabbit sperm
fertilizing
egg

(x 8000)
D.M. Phillips

LM
Segmentation
two cell stage
with polar body

Polar
body

(x 600)
K.G. Gould

Shown in the upper photograph is a newly ovulated rabbit ovum still surrounded by
the corona radiata of adhering granulosa cells. With invasion of the area by sperm, the
cells of the corona radiata are dispersed, allowing sperm to reach the zona pellucida.

The lower LM micrograph reveals a two-cell stage of the zygote of a squirrel monkey,
following in vitro fertilization. The zona pellucida still surrounds the blastomeres (cells),
while scattered granulosa cells are found in the area; some are in clusters clinging to the
zona pellucida. The second polar body is located between the two blastomeres,
surrounded by the zona pellucida.

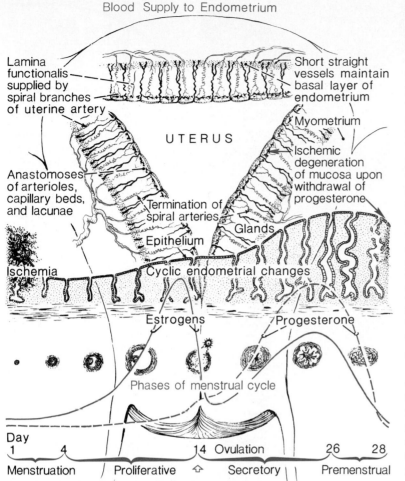

Blood Supply to Endometrium

Lamina functionalis supplied by spiral branches of uterine artery

Short straight vessels maintain basal layer of endometrium

Myometrium

UTERUS

Ischemic degeneration of mucosa upon withdrawal of progesterone

Anastomoses of arterioles, capillary beds, and lacunae

Termination of spiral arteries

Glands

Ischemia

Epithelium

Cyclic endometrial changes

Estrogens

Progesterone

Phases of menstrual cycle

Day
1   4   14 Ovulation   26   28

Menstruation | Proliferative ⇧ Secretory | | Premenstrual

LM   Late proliferative endometrium

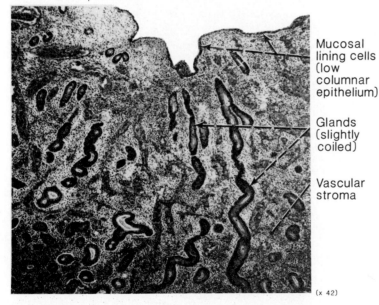

Mucosal lining cells (low columnar epithelium)

Glands (slightly coiled)

Vascular stroma

(× 42)

pria, reticular fibers predominate among the stellate or fusiform mesenchymal stromal cells and the wandering macrophages and leukocytes. There is no muscularis mucosae.

Blood Supply To understand how, in each month in the pubescent female, the lamina functionalis becomes engorged with blood and fluid, sloughs off, and later regenerates, an understanding of its blood supply is essential.

Branches of the **uterine artery** pass from the myometrium into the basal layer to provide a unique vascular system for the next menstrual cycle or pregnancy. Within the myometrium, these branches supply the muscle layers. They divide into short, **straight arteries** that nourish the **basal layer,** and the **spiral (helicine) branches** that supply the **functional layer.** The spiral arteries terminate in **arterioles** that freely anastomose before forming capillary beds and lacunae. The latter are thin-walled, dilated vessels of varying sizes. **Venules** form a network in this region, also with dilations, called **collecting lacunae.** The veins drain into a venous plexus at the junction of the basalis and the myometrium.

Upon withdrawal of the hormone progesterone during the late stages of the menstrual cycle, the **spiral arteries constrict** periodically, rendering the functional layer hypoxic and finally **ischemic.** The ischemia results in degeneration of the engorged mucosa as well as the coiled arteries. However, the straight arteries, supplying the **basalis layer,** are not subject to hormonal control and therefore **remain mostly intact** and functional.

Cyclic Endometrial Changes The cyclic changes in the endometrium are associated with the **menstrual cycle** of sexually mature women, which usually occupies about 28 days. These changes prepare the **endometrium** for implantation and nourishment of the **embryo.** If implantation occurs, the endometrium is arrested in the **secretory phase** until parturition. If implantation does not occur, blood vessels rupture, the **menstrual flow begins,** and the mucosal layer sloughs off.

Phases of the Menstrual Cycle The days of a cycle are reckoned from the first day of the menstrual flow. **Menstruation** usually lasts from **three to five days.** Repair of the mucosa then begins, the **proliferative stage,** and continues until midcycle (14th–15th day), when **ovulation occurs.** Following ovulation, the **secretory phase** of the cycle begins and lasts until about day 26 or 27 when the short premenstrual (**ischemic) phase** occurs just before menstruation.

The histological changes are more easily understood if they are described beginning with the first day of the tissue repair process, i.e., immediately after the menstrual flow. These changes are grouped into four phases or stages.

1. The **proliferative stage** (also called the follicular, estrogenic, or reparative phase) lasts from day 5 to day 14 or 15. Under the stimulus of **estrogen, regeneration and growth** of the endometrium occurs, increasing from 1 mm to 4–5 mm in thickness. Many mitotic figures are present in the epithelium, which grows over the raw surface of the recently denuded mucosa. The **epithelial cells** are initially **low columnar** but gradually increase in height. At first the **glands are short and straight,** but as the mucosa thickens they gradually increase in length and finally become slightly folded. Simultaneously, blood vessels from the myometrium penetrate the new growth and produce a **highly vascular stroma.**

2. The **secretory or luteal** phase begins immediately after ovulation on day 14 or 15 and continues until day 26 or 27. The major changes occur in the **stratum functionalis;** the basalis remains essentially unchanged. The endometrium continues to thicken (6–7 mm). However, the most striking feature is that the **glands** become dilated, sacculated, **coiled, and filled with secretory materials,** largely glycogen and mucus. The stroma is swollen with fluid, and the **coiled arteries** increase in length and complexity. The principal hormone producing these changes is **progesterone,** which is being synthesized in the corpus luteum.

3. The **premenstrual or ischemic** stage occurs at day 26 or 27. The **coiled arteries** begin to **constrict periodically,** triggered principally by the reduction of progesterone. This causes episodes of **hypoxia and anoxia in the stratum functionalis,** resulting in a blanching of the area and a **stasis of blood** in the capillaries. The uterine glands cease to secrete, the endometrium is reduced in thickness by extensive water loss, and the tissues of the functionalis become ischemic.

4. The **menstrual phase** is ushered in by a sudden release of the contraction of the coiled arteries, resulting in a **rush of blood** into the previously closed arterioles and capillaries. The weakened ischemic walls of these **vessels rupture,** flooding the stroma with blood, which separates the epithelium from the stroma. The detached epithelium, uncoagulated blood, glandular secretions, and degenerating endometrial cells are shed into the uterine cavity as the **menses.** Gradually the flow tapers off, usually ceasing after three to five days. About 35 ml of bloody fluid is lost during a normal menstrual period.

Recall that the basal layer of the endometrium is relatively **unaffected by menstruation,** since it has its own independent blood supply, the straight arteries. These arteries are not interrupted during menstruation. Thus, the **basal layer** remains **capable of regenerating** a new **stratum functionalis** (Table 25.1).

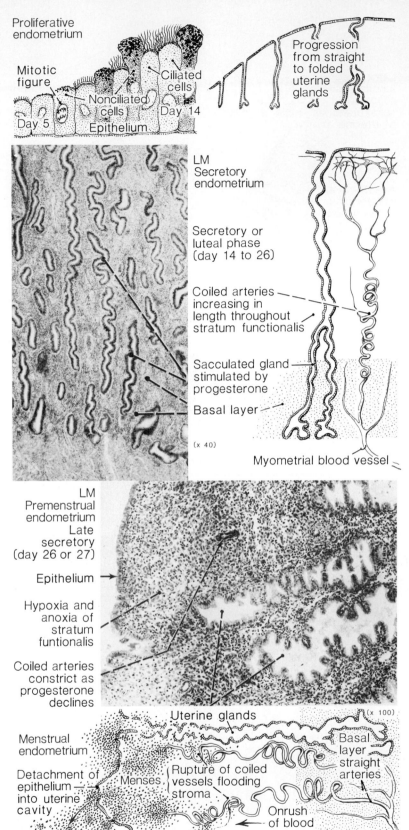

Proliferative endometrium

Mitotic figure

Ciliated cells

Nonciliated cells

Day 5

Epithelium

Day 14

Progression from straight to folded uterine glands

LM Secretory endometrium

Secretory or luteal phase (day 14 to 26)

Coiled arteries increasing in length throughout stratum functionalis

Sacculated gland stimulated by progesterone

Basal layer

(x 40)

Myometrial blood vessel

LM Premenstrual endometrium Late secretory (day 26 or 27)

Epithelium

Hypoxia and anoxia of stratum funtionalis

Coiled arteries constrict as progesterone declines

(x 100)

Uterine glands

Menstrual endometrium

Detachment of epithelium into uterine cavity

Menses

Rupture of coiled vessels flooding stroma

Basal layer straight arteries

Onrush of blood

17005

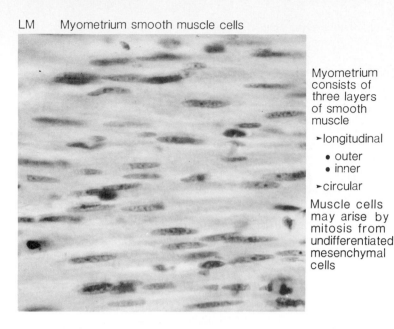

Myometrium consists of three layers of smooth muscle

➤ longitudinal
• outer
• inner

➤ circular

Muscle cells may arise by mitosis from undifferentiated mesenchymal cells

MYOMETRIUM Most of the thick wall of the uterus is the **myometrium,** composed of three poorly delineated layers of smooth muscle, about 15 to 20 mm thick. The thin outer and inner layers are mostly longitudinal or oblique fibers, while the thicker **central layer** is predominantly **circular smooth muscle fibers.** Because this circular layer contains many large blood vessels, it is also called the **stratum vascularis.**

Smooth muscle cells of the uterus are unique in that they **undergo hypertrophy and hyperplasia** during pregnancy. For example, in the nonpregnant uterus, the muscle cells are about 40–60 μm long, while during pregnancy, they reach 500–600 μm in length. Likewise, smooth muscle fibers increase in number in pregnancy. They may arise by mitosis from **preexisting fibers** or from **undifferentiated mesenchymal cells** held over from early developmental stages. Nowhere else in the adult body do these phenomena occur in smooth muscle.

The hormone **oxytocin,** synthesized in the hypothalamus and stored in the neurohypophysis, stimulates the **uterine muscles to contract.** Therefore, the hormone is used clinically to induce labor and to speed up delivery. Also, uterine contractions of the gravid uterus are increased by injections of **prostaglandins.** Concentration of these substances in the blood increases during parturition, suggesting that prostaglandins may initiate the onset of labor.

PERIMETRIUM The perimetrium is the thin, outermost layer of the uterus. It is a **serosal layer** that differs little from the serosa of other abdominal and pelvic organs. It contains blood and lymph vessels, nerves, and sympathetic ganglia. It covers the fundus and body of the uterus and the upper part of the cervix. Histologically, it is a single layer of **mesothelium** resting on a thin layer of connective tissue. It is continuous on each side with the peritoneal layer of the broad ligament of the uterus.

CERVIX

The tapering, almost cylindrical, inferior part of the uterus is the **cervix.** It is divided into an upper portion, the cervical canal, and a lower vaginal portion that projects into the vagina. Although the layers are continuous with the uterus, their histological components vary considerably.

The **cervical canal** differs from the body of the uterus in that: (1) Its **wall** consists largely of **dense collagenous and elastic fibers** with only about 15% of the wall being smooth muscle. (2) The **mucosa** contains very **complex mucous glands** and deep branching folds, called **plicae palmatae.** These glands may become occluded and form cysts. The **mucosa does not participate in menstruation,** perhaps because it is not supplied with spiral arteries as is the functional layer of the endometrium. However, the **glands** undergo

Uterus

Perimetrium (outermost serosal layer)

Oxytocin induces muscular contraction

Longitudinal oblique and circular smooth muscle fibers

Vascularis layer

Uterine blood supply

Dense collagenous and elastic fibers

Plicae palmatae with mucous glands

Canal

Vaginal wall

Cervix

Mucous plug

External os

Transition to stratified squamous epithelium

Vaginal canal

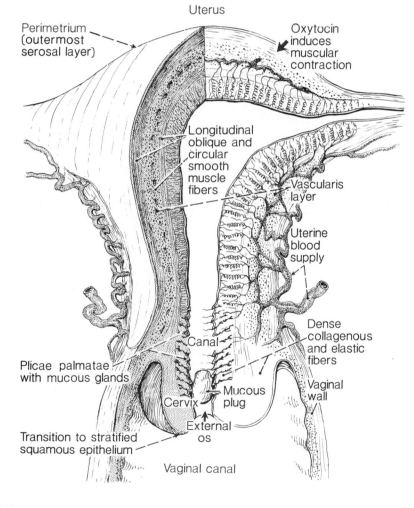

17278

some changes during menstruation, e.g., their secretion is thin and watery during the proliferative (estrogenic) phase. It becomes copious at ovulation and the consistency of egg whites, useful signs for determining the time of ovulation. During pregnancy, it forms a semisolid mucous plug that prevents the passage of sperm, microorganisms, and other materials from entering the uterus from the vagina. (3) Although the cervix does not enlarge during pregnancy, it undergoes tremendous **dilation during parturition.** (4) The columnar epithelium changes abruptly to stratified squamous, nonkeratinized epithelium just above the external os, the external opening of the cervix.

VAGINA

The vagina is a fibromuscular, collapsed tube that connects the uterus to the exterior of the body. As part of the birth canal, it is tremendously dilated during parturition. Its wall follows the pattern of the female genital tract, consisting of a mucosa, a muscularis, and an adventitia (L–A, plate 17).

Mucosa

Longitudinal folds of the mucosa extend throughout the anterior and posterior surfaces of the relaxed vagina. **Stratified squamous,** nonkeratinized epithelium lines its cavity. While the epithelium does not undergo typical menstrual changes, it does **undergo minor cyclic changes** during the sex cycle. Under the influence of estrogen during the proliferative stage, there is a slight keratinization of the lining cells, which stain acidiphilic. These cells store considerable **glycogen,** which is released into the vaginal lumen when the surface cells are exfoliated. There are no glands in the mucosa.

The **tunica propria** contains many elastic fibers, a few small lymph nodules, and various leukocytes. It has a rather **extensive venous plexus** that is engorged with blood during sexual stimulation. The plexus is also the source of tissue fluid that seeps through the epithelium into the lumen of the vagina during copulation. Together with secretions from the cervical and vestibular glands, this fluid provides lubrication of the vaginal lumen during sexual intercourse.

Muscularis

Two poorly defined smooth muscle layers comprise the muscularis. The fibers of the thin inner layer are oriented circularly, while those of the outer, thicker layer are situated longitudinally and are **continuous with the myometrium** of the uterus. Encircling the entrance of the vagina is a **weak sphincter** of skeletal muscle fibers.

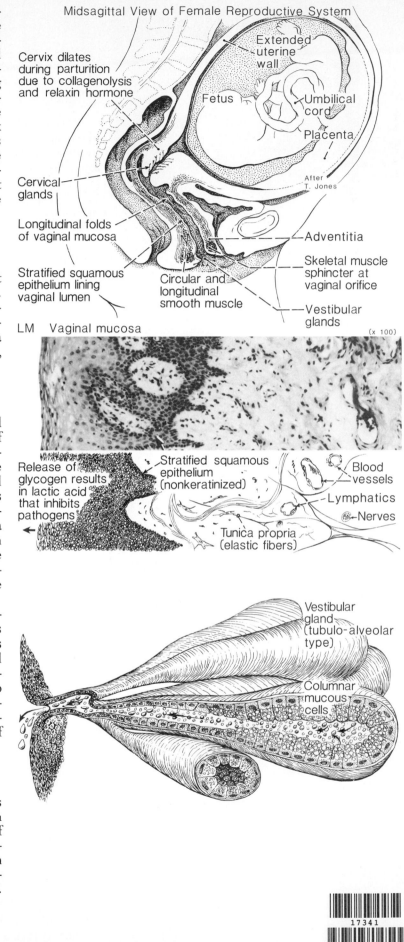

Midsagittal View of Female Reproductive System

Cervix dilates during parturition due to collagenolysis and relaxin hormone

Extended uterine wall

Fetus

Umbilical cord

Placenta

After T. Jones

Cervical glands

Longitudinal folds of vaginal mucosa

Adventitia

Stratified squamous epithelium lining vaginal lumen

Circular and longitudinal smooth muscle

Skeletal muscle sphincter at vaginal orifice

Vestibular glands

LM   Vaginal mucosa   (x 100)

Release of glycogen results in lactic acid that inhibits pathogens

Stratified squamous epithelium (nonkeratinized)

Blood vessels

Lymphatics

Nerves

Tunica propria (elastic fibers)

Vestibular gland (tubulo-alveolar type)

Columnar mucous cells

17341

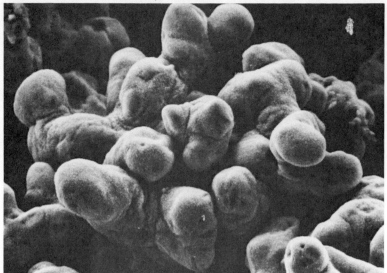

SEM   Chorionic villi in placenta   K. Tanaka (x 300)

LM   Trophoblastic cells in placental villi

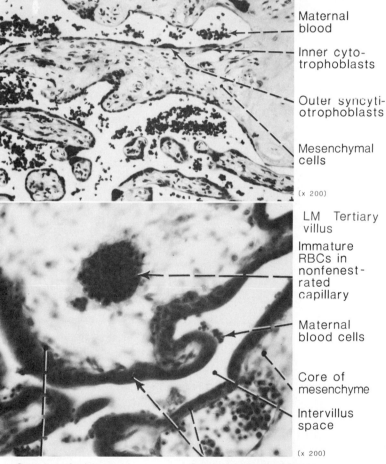

Maternal
blood

Inner cyto-
trophoblasts

Outer syncyti-
otrophoblasts

Mesenchymal
cells

(x 200)

LM Tertiary
villus

Immature
RBCs in
nonfenest-
rated
capillary

Maternal
blood cells

Core of
mesenchyme

Intervillus
space

(x 200)

Cytotrophoblasts   Syncytiotrophoblasts
                          (fused cell boundaries)

Adventitia

A dense connective tissue layer, the **adventitia,** surrounds the vagina and blends with adjacent organs. It has considerable elastic tissue. Blood vessels, nerves, and lymphatics traverse this region to supply the inner layers of the vagina (Table 25.2).

PLACENTA

The transitory placenta is the only organ in the body derived from two separate individuals, i.e., the mother and the unborn young. The embryonic fetal contribution is the **chorionic plate** (sac) and its branching villi, while the maternal component is the modified **stratum basalis** of the endometrium, the decidua basalis, in which the embryo is implanted.

Embryonic/Fetal Component

As the **trophoblastic (nutritive) cells** of the embryonic blastocyst proliferate, they develop into two distinct layers, an inner layer of light-staining cells with distinct boundaries, the **cytotrophoblast** (Gk. cyto, cell; trophe, nutritive; blast, germ, offspring), and an outer, darker-staining layer without cell boundaries, called the **syncytiotrophoblast** (Gk. syn, together). The latter term indicates that the cells are fused together to form a multinucleated mass of protoplasm without cell boundaries, i.e., a **syncytium.**

The cells in the cytotrophoblastic layer proliferate, producing cells that fuse with the syncytiotrophoblast. A layer of mesenchymal cells forms beneath the cytotrophoblast to comprise the **chorion.** Extending from the chorion (chorionic plate) are solid cords of cytotrophoblast, the **primary chorionic villi.** As mesenchyme invades the central core of a villus, it is converted into a **secondary villus.** When embryonic blood vessels enter the central zone, the villus becomes a **tertiary or mature** chorionic villus. All villi extend into the intervillus space, which is filled with maternal blood.

Chorionic villi are also classified as free or anchored. An **anchored villus** passes from the chorionic plate to fuse with the stratum basalis. **Free villi** are branches from the anchoring villi that float freely in the intervillus space. Histologically, anchoring and free villi are essentially the same, differing only in size and site of origin.

A typical villus consists, from outside inward, of (1) a row of basophilic **syncytiotrophoblasts** with small dark nuclei, limited sER, and microvilli on the intervillus space surface. In older villi, the nuclei are often found in clusters, called **syncytial knots.** (2) The **inner cytotrophoblasts** are a layer of light-staining, well-defined, irregular cells that rest on a basal lamina. With time, the cells decrease in number so that during the last half of pregnancy, the layer disappears.

Maternal Component

As stated earlier, the **decidua basalis** of the endometrium is the maternal part of the placenta. The spiral arteries that pass through the decidua basalis are the source of blood that floods the intervillus space. There is virtually **no mixture of fetal and maternal blood.** However, near termination of pregnancy, the wall of the tertiary villi is very thin due to the loss of the cytotrophoblastic layer and the capillaries are very close to the **intervillus space,** separated only by the syncytiotrophoblastic layer. Rupture at delivery of these capillaries will allow some mixing of fetal and maternal blood.

Terminal Placenta

At parturition the placenta is delivered as part of the afterbirth. It is a **thick, spherical disk,** about 15–25 cm in diameter and 3 cm in thickness. When viewed from the maternal side, 15–20 lobules or **cotyledons** comprise the placenta. These are formed from projections of decidual septa between the large, anchoring villi. Since the septa do not reach the chorionic plate, the **maternal blood** flows freely between the cotyledons.

Functions of the Placenta

Although the maternal and fetal vascular systems are in very close proximity, normally they do not communicate. They are separated by an efficient **placental barrier** composed exclusively of fetal tissues. This barrier consists of four layers: (1) the endothelial lining of the fetal vessels, (2) the connective tissue of the core of the villus, (3) the cytotrophoblastic layer, and (4) the outermost syncytiotrophoblastic layer, or syncytium. Gases (CO_2 and O_2), hormones, nutrients, humoral antibodies (IgG), metabolic waste products and, unfortunately, certain harmful drugs and viruses, **traverse the barrier.** Therefore, the placenta acts as a fetal **kidney, lung,** and **digestive system.** Especially in late pregnancy it also is a **major endocrine organ,** synthesizing chorionic hormones, e.g., human chorionic gonadotropin (HCG) and human chorionic somatomammotropin (HCS).

UMBILICAL CORD

Extending from the fetal umbilicus to the placenta is the **umbilical cord,** the lifeline connecting the fetus to the mother. It carries **oxygenated blood** from the placenta into the general circulation of the fetus **via the umbilical vein.** Partially **deoxygenated** blood is returned to the placenta by way of the **two umbilical arteries** for reoxygenation.

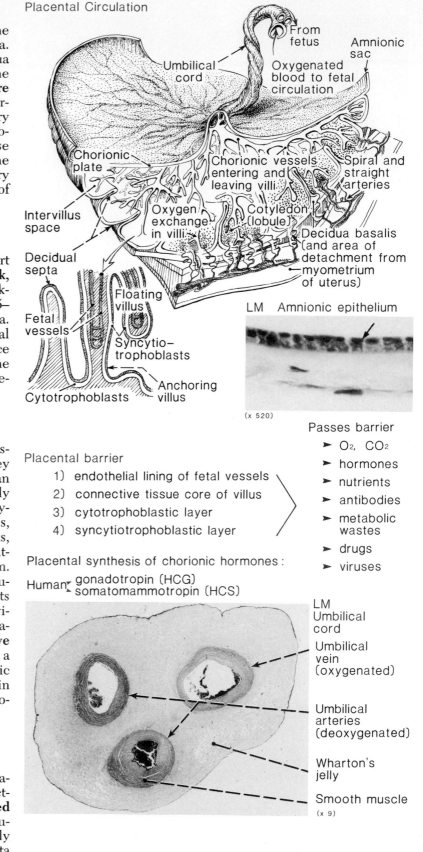

Placental Circulation

From fetus
Umbilical cord
Amnionic sac
Oxygenated blood to fetal circulation
Chorionic plate
Chorionic vessels entering and leaving villi
Spiral and straight arteries
Intervillus space
Oxygen exchange in villi
Cotyledon (lobule)
Decidua basalis (and area of detachment from myometrium of uterus)
Decidual septa
Floating villus
Fetal vessels
Syncytio-trophoblasts
Anchoring villus
Cytotrophoblasts

LM Amnionic epithelium
(x 520)

Placental barrier
1) endothelial lining of fetal vessels
2) connective tissue core of villus
3) cytotrophoblastic layer
4) syncytiotrophoblastic layer

Passes barrier
➤ O_2, CO_2
➤ hormones
➤ nutrients
➤ antibodies
➤ metabolic wastes
➤ drugs
➤ viruses

Placental synthesis of chorionic hormones:
Human ⌐ gonadotropin (HCG)
       ⌐ somatomammotropin (HCS)

LM Umbilical cord
Umbilical vein (oxygenated)
Umbilical arteries (deoxygenated)
Wharton's jelly
Smooth muscle
(x 9)

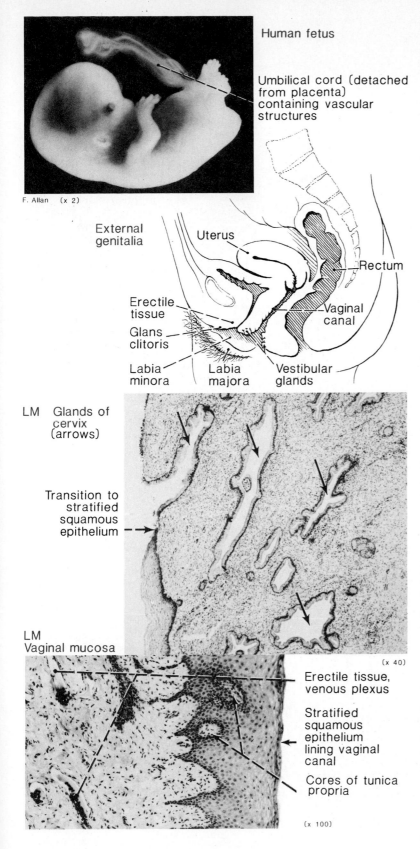

Human fetus

F. Allan (x 2)

Umbilical cord (detached from placenta) containing vascular structures

External genitalia

Uterus

Rectum

Erectile tissue

Glans clitoris

Vaginal canal

Labia minora

Labia majora

Vestibular glands

LM Glands of cervix (arrows)

Transition to stratified squamous epithelium

(x 40)

LM Vaginal mucosa

Erectile tissue, venous plexus

Stratified squamous epithelium lining vaginal canal

Cores of tunica propria

(x 100)

The tortuous umbilical cord is enveloped by the **amniotic sac** and covered by a single layer of epithelium that becomes stratified late in pregnancy. In cross section, it reveals a gelatinous mass of mucous connective tissue (**Wharton's jelly**), including abundant collagenous fibers that enclose the three umbilical blood vessels. They are **two arteries** with an outer circular coat of smooth muscle and a thicker longitudinal layer. These arteries contain no internal elastic lamina, and the adventitia has been replaced by mucous connective tissue. The **single vein** has a larger lumen, yet resembles the arteries because it has a thick muscular wall. The vein has no valves or vasa vasorum.

EXTERNAL GENITALIA (VULVA)

The female external genitalia, also called the **vulva** (L. vulva, covering of womb), consist of the labia majora and minora, the clitoris, and the vestibular (Bartholin's) glands.

Labia Majora

The labia majora are two prominent elongated folds of skin covering considerable amounts of areolar connective tissue and fat. They extend back between the thighs, **concealing the other genital structures.** The skin over the exposed surfaces resembles that of its homolog, the scrotum, i.e., **melanin pigmentation,** sparse, coarse, hairs, and prominent sebaceous glands.

Labia Minora

The labia minora are two thin, **hairless folds of skin,** deeply placed beneath the shelter of the labia majora. The skin covers a **highly vascular core** of connective tissue. Prominent sebaceous glands, not associated with hair follicles, open on both sides of the labium.

Clitoris

The clitoris resembles its homolog, the penis, by the presence of **erectile tissue** in the two small **corpora cavernosa** and a poorly shaped glans **clitoris.** It is covered by a thin layer of stratified squamous epithelium superficial to a highly vascular stroma. It is well supplied with specialized sensory nerve endings.

Vestibular Glands

The space at the entrance of the vagina, bordered by the labia, is the **vestibule.** Located in the lateral walls of the vestibule is a pair of large mucous glands, the **vestibular (Bartholin's) glands.** They are **tubuloacinar glands,** lined with simple columnar cells that **secrete a lubricating mucus** during sexual stimulation.

16711

MAMMARY GLANDS

The apocrine mammary glands are **modified sweat glands.** Their development is similar to, and their structure resembles, the sweat glands of mammals.

Each mammary gland is actually a collection of 10–20 entirely separate glands (**lobes**), arranged in a radial fashion around the nipple. Each lobe has a **lactiferous duct** that widens into a **sinus** before it opens on the summit of the nipple. The **parenchymal tissue** consists of a series of **ducts and acini (alveoli)** lined with simple cuboidal or low columnar epithelium. The acini and ducts are partially surrounded by **myoepithelial cells.** The stroma of the lobe is loose connective tissue, infiltrated with abundant adipose cells and collagen fibers (L—A, plate 30).

Variations in the Female Breast

Great changes in the breast occur during development and the phases of the female reproductive life. Briefly, these **variations** are:

1. In the embryo, the mammary glands begin development as solid epithelial **downgrowths of the epidermis** into the underlying mesenchyme. These cords of cells branch as they penetrate deeper into the vascular stroma. In late fetal life, a poorly shaped nipple forms with a few smooth muscle fibers. It is often depressed during infancy.

2. The two weeks after birth is a period of great activity. The solid **cords of cells** become **channelized,** more branched, and develop dilated extremities. The breast is distended with dilated blood vessels. Some of the glandular cells may secrete a **milky fluid** (often called witch's milk) that can be expressed at the nipple. Such an observation is not surprising since the hormones acting on the mother's breast to produce milk act also on the neonatal mammary gland.

3. With the passing of this short, active period, the blood supply is reduced and the **gland becomes quiescent** until puberty. In the case of the male breast, the gland remains inactive.

4. In the presence of **estrogen** at the onset of puberty, the female **breast resumes activity.** The **ducts lengthen and branch** profusely. Connective tissue elements proliferate, especially adipose cells. Increased levels of **progesterone stimulate acini to develop** on the ends of the ducts. Additional smooth muscle fibers are found in the stroma of the nipple.

5. During **early pregnancy,** estrogen and progesterone promote a more **extensive duct development.** In **late pregnancy,** full **acinar development** occurs, at the expense of the stromal tissue. At full term the lobes are filled with distended acini with limited stroma.

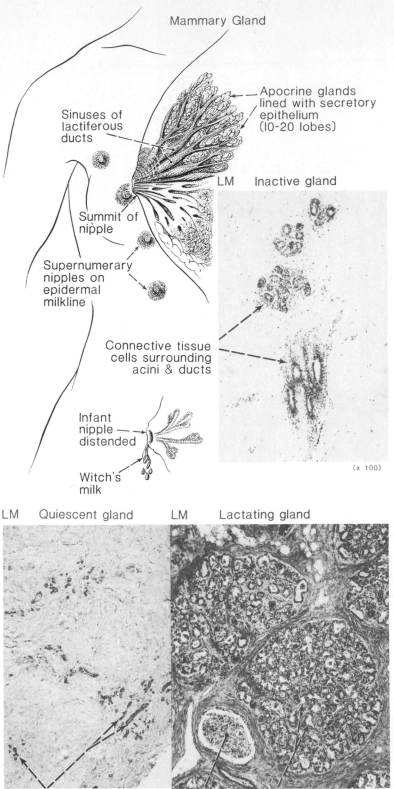

Mammary Gland

Sinuses of lactiferous ducts

Apocrine glands lined with secretory epithelium (10-20 lobes)

LM   Inactive gland

Summit of nipple

Supernumerary nipples on epidermal milkline

Connective tissue cells surrounding acini & ducts

Infant nipple distended

Witch's milk

(x 100)

LM   Quiescent gland

LM   Lactating gland

Collapsed acini and ducts   (x 40)

Duct   Distended acini (increased hormones)   (x 40)

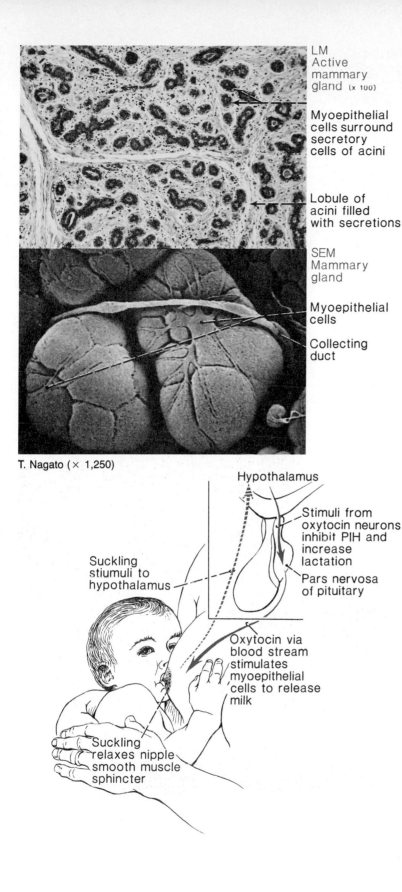

LM
Active
mammary
gland (× 100)

Myoepithelial
cells surround
secretory
cells of acini

Lobule of
acini filled
with secretions

SEM
Mammary
gland

Myoepithelial
cells

Collecting
duct

T. Nagato (× 1,250)

Hypothalamus

Stimuli from
oxytocin neurons
inhibit PIH and
increase
lactation

Pars nervosa
of pituitary

Suckling
stiumuli to
hypothalamus

Oxytocin via
blood stream
stimulates
myoepithelial
cells to release
milk

Suckling
relaxes nipple
smooth muscle
sphincter

6. Upon parturition the placental hormones are withdrawn and the final stages of milk production occur. **Hormones** of the pituitary (prolactin, ACTH, growth hormone, and oxytocin), and of the placenta (chorionic hormones, estrogen, and progesterone) **promote secretory activity** in the cells of the acini. Protein-rich **colostrum** is secreted first, followed on about the second day by the production of **milk.** Histological examination of a lactating breast reveals different acini at different phases of milk production, e.g., some acini are distended with milk, others are being filled, while others are empty, with the milk already discharged into the ducts.

7. If the mammary glands are not emptied regularly, the milk accumulates, the secretions slow, **lactation is arrested,** and the **gland involutes.** With regression of the acini and the retraction of the duct system, the interlobular connective tissue, especially **adipose cells, increases** and replaces most of the epithelial elements. The gland does not return entirely to the pregravid state, since some dilated ducts and a few acini persist, often with coagulated secretions in their lumens.

8. After **menopause,** the **duct system and acini** regress further and **may become cystic.** The cysts are usually benign but may become malignant under certain conditions. Connective tissue fibers increase.

9. Finally, in **senile involution,** the breast is reduced to a bag of adipose tissue with a few small epithelium-lined cysts, remnants of the once extensive milk production system.

Mechanisms of Milk Release

The act of suckling is the stimulus for the release of milk, called the **milk ejection or letdown factor.** Suckling, acting on nervous receptors in the nipple, causes afferent impulses to stimulate the oxytocin neurons in the hypothalamus. This stimulation causes the **release of oxytocin** from the terminations of these nerve fibers in the pars nervosa of the pituitary. Oxytocin stimulates **contraction of the myoepithelial cells** surrounding the ducts and acini, causing **milk to be expressed** toward the nipple.

Simultaneously, these same afferent impulses suppress the release of prolactin-inhibiting hormone (**PIH**). Such inhibition frees **prolactin,** which **stimulates lactation** during nursing. Also, the afferent impulses may cause relaxation of the circular muscle cells in the nipple. These fibers act as **sphincters** to close off the lactiferous ducts between nursing periods. When the sphincters are closed, the milk is not propelled into the lactiferous sinuses and the infant cannot nurse properly. Perhaps ocytocin also relaxes the sphincters, which allows the letdown of the milk to occur during suckling.

Table 25.1 *CYCLIC CHANGES IN THE HUMAN ENDOMETRIUM*

STAGE	DAYS OF MENSTRUAL CYCLE	THICKNESS OF MUCOSA (mm)	EPITHELIUM	GLANDS IN LAMINA PROPRIA	BLOOD VESSELS	HORMONES ACTING ON ENDOMETRIUM
Prepubertal		>2	Simple columnar cells	Many simple tubular glands that open onto surface of endometrium	Abundant straight and coiled arteries	Low levels of FSH and LH are secreted, beginning at about 8th year
Proliferative (follicular)	5th–15th	1–3	Low to tall simple columnar cells, some with cilia; glycogen in basal pole of cells; mitoses often present	More numerous, longer, tubular glands, often slightly dilated; mitoses frequent; have mucoid secretion	Short arteries extend through stratum basalis; capillaries supply stratum functionalis; venules drain both areas	Principally estrogen
Secretory (luteal)	15th–27th	3–5	More mitoses, esp. in stratum functionalis; cells lose glycogen deposits; luminal cells form blebs which detach and blend with secretions	Become greatly coiled and diluted; secrete mucus and glycogen into wide lumina; tissue edematous from tissue fluid entering endometrial stroma	Coiled arteries longer and more spiral; may extend to surface of mucosa; basilar arteries show little change	Principally progesterone
Premenstrual (ischemic)	27th–28th	5–6	Mitoses arrested; cells ischemic and cease secretory activities	Lumina of glands collapse, expelling contents; tissue becomes ischemic; leukocytosis widespread	Constriction of coiled arterioles causes ischemia; sudden release of contraction results in rupture of blood vessels and menstrual flow begins	Reduction in progesterone, some increase in FSH
Menstrual (menses)	1st–5th	0.1–5	Desquamated cells swept into uterine cavity as part of menses	As components of the eroding endometrium, the collapsed glands and surrounding stroma are shed with the menstrual flow	Coiled arteries are lost with menses; basilar arterioles remain functional to permit renewal of stratum functionalis	Slight increase in FSH and LH
Pregnancy (gravid)		5–6	Maintains features of secretory phase	Similar to secretory stage with continued growth of glands and stroma	Continue to function as in secretory stage	LH and HCG
Postmenopausal (senile)		>1	Flattened, atrophic lining cells	Simple tubular, nonproliferative, nonsecretory glands lined with squamous, atrophic cells	Only rudimentary stratum basalis remains	None

Table 25.2 *SUMMARY OF HISTOLOGY OF FEMALE GENITAL TRACT*

ORGAN	EPITHELIUM	LAMINA PROPRIA	GLANDS	MUSCULARIS (SMOOTH MUSCLE)	SEROSA OR ADVENTITIA
Oviduct	Simple columnar; some cells ciliated, others secretory	Spindle-shaped stromal cells and lymphocytes; abundant lymph and blood vessels	None	Well-developed inner circular layer; outer longitudinal layer, less robust	Serosa with many blood and nerve plexuses
Uterus • Body and fundus	Same as above	Stellate stromal cells, WBC, and macrophages enmeshed with reticular fibers; many tubular glands, lymph and blood vessels	Abundant simple tubular in proliferative stage; dilated coiled tubular in secretory phase	Inner layer mostly longitudinal fibers; thick middle layer predominantly circular and oblique fibers; outer layer mostly longitudinal fibers	Serosa on fundic and posterior surfaces of body
• Cervix	Same as above in cervical canal region; changes to stratified squamous in vaginal portion	Dense cellular connective tissue	Very complex, branched tubulo-alveolar mucous type	Fewer fascicles, mostly circular	Adventitia
Vagina	Nonkeratinized stratified squamous with abundant glycogen	Abundant elastic fibers; few, small lymph nodules and vessels; extensive venous and nerve plexuses	None	Thicker outer longitudinal layer; thinner inner circular layer; few circular skeletal muscle fibers form sphincter at orifice	Adventitia; elastic fibers prominent; many blood and lymph vessels, and nerves

Chapter

26

ORGANS OF SPECIAL SENSE— EYE AND EAR

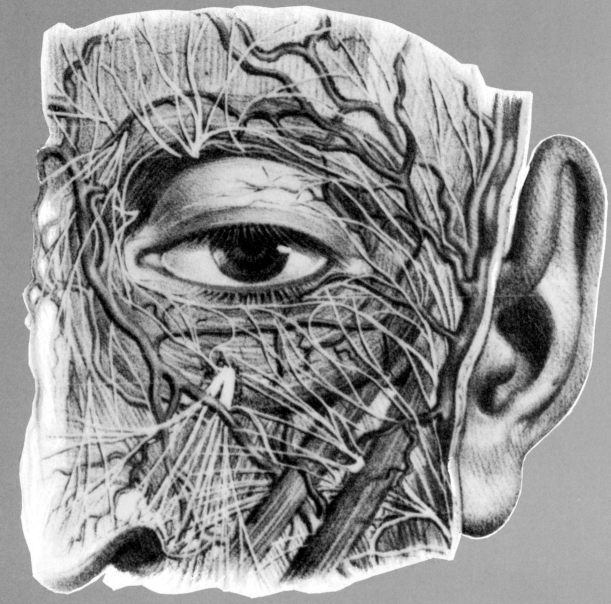

M.J. Bourgery
1854

OBJECTIVES

THIS CHAPTER WILL PROVIDE INFORMATION FOR THE STUDENT TO:

1. Document the unique role of neuroepithelial cells in the reception of the various special senses.

2. Describe the various layers of the eye and explain how the components of each layer are essential for normal vision.

3. Tabulate the cellular constituents of the layers of the retina and indicate how light rays affect them.

4. Analyze how each of the various contents of the eyeball contributes to the focusing mechanism of the eye.

5. Sketch the pathway sound waves travel to reach the neuroepithelium of the organ of Corti.

6. Contrast the structure and functions of the bony and membranous labyrinths of the inner ear.

7. Deduce from their histological structure and location in the inner ear, how each component of the vestibular apparatus contributes to our sense of balance.

The special sense organs contain **neuroepithelial receptor cells** that are limited to specialized regions of the organ. These cells are associated with the special sensations of smell (olfactory epithelium), taste (taste buds), hearing (organ of Corti), equilibrium (semicircular canals, utricle, and saccule), and sight (rod and cone cells). The olfactory and gustatory nerve endings have been discussed with the nasal and oral cavities, respectively. The receptors for sight, hearing, and balance require special treatment and are dealt with in this chapter.

EYE

The eye is the unexcelled sense organ. It is truly our window on the world around us. It alerts us to the first faint stirrings of danger or to the fleeting hues of a rainbow. Housed securely in their deep **bony orbits,** the eyes are well protected from external injury. Surrounded by an ample layer of fat, they are cushioned against injury from violent head movements. Two moist **eyelids** intermittently sweep across the exposed surfaces of each eye, preventing damage from dehydration. All the while, 12 delicate **extrinsic muscles,** six attached to each eye, are contracting in near-perfect synchronization to direct our gaze upon the object of our interest, suspicion, or alarm.

Development of the Eye

In the embryo of about four weeks, the two eyes begin as paired out-pocketings from the forebrain, called the **optic vesicles.** The vesicles are joined with the brain by the **optic stalk,** which becomes the **optic nerve.** The larger distal part of the vesicle develops into the **optic bulb,** which becomes deeply indented on its outer surface, transforming the bulb into a two-walled **optic cup,** the future **retina.** The thinner, outer (posterior) wall is pigmented while the thicker, inner layer of cells becomes the complex, multilayered, light-sensitive part of the retina.

Simultaneously, bilateral thickenings of the surface (skin) ectoderm develop lateral to the developing optic cup. These thickenings are the **lens placodes,** which soon invaginate and separate from the ectoderm. Each detached placode (vesicle) comes to lie within the optic cup where it develops into the definitive **lens.** As the optic and lens vesicles differentiate, the loose mesenchyme of the head region condenses around them to form a two-layered, fibrous **capsule.** The inner layer develops into the highly vascular, pigmented **choroid coat.** It differentiates into the choroid, ciliary body, and pigmented iris. The outer layer surrounds the eye as the tough, fibrous **sclerocorneal coat.**

Layers or Tunics

The wall of the eyeball consists of **three layers or tunics.** They are: (1) the outer, fibrous supportive layer (tunica fibrosa); (2) a middle vascular layer (tunica vasculosa or uvea), and (3) an inner internal layer (tunica interna).

OUTER FIBROUS LAYER The outer layer, the **tunica fibrosa,** is a dense, fibrous connective tissue sheet that gives shape to the eyeball. It has two regions, the robust, opaque, **thick sclera,** which covers about 5/6 of the posterior and lateral surfaces of the orbit, and the **transparent cornea,** occupying the anterior 1/6 of the fibrous tunic.

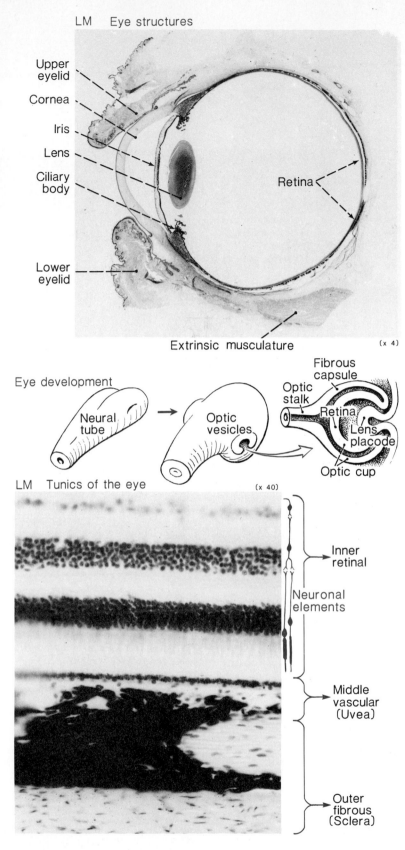

LM   Eye structures

Upper eyelid
Cornea
Iris
Lens
Ciliary body
Lower eyelid
Retina
Extrinsic musculature   (x 4)

Eye development

Neural tube → Optic vesicles →

Fibrous capsule
Optic stalk
Retina
Lens placode
Optic cup

LM   Tunics of the eye   (x 40)

Inner retinal
Neuronal elements
Middle vascular (Uvea)
Outer fibrous (Sclera)

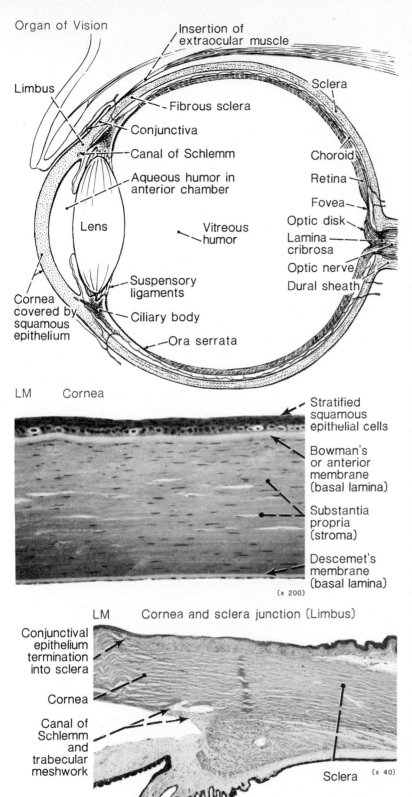

Organ of Vision

Insertion of extraocular muscle

Limbus

Sclera

Fibrous sclera

Conjunctiva

Canal of Schlemm

Choroid

Aqueous humor in anterior chamber

Retina

Fovea

Optic disk

Lens

Vitreous humor

Lamina cribrosa

Optic nerve

Dural sheath

Cornea covered by squamous epithelium

Suspensory ligaments

Ciliary body

Ora serrata

LM   Cornea

Stratified squamous epithelial cells

Bowman's or anterior membrane (basal lamina)

Substantia propria (stroma)

Descemet's membrane (basal lamina)

(x 200)

LM   Cornea and sclera junction (Limbus)

Conjunctival epithelium termination into sclera

Cornea

Canal of Schlemm and trabecular meshwork

Sclera   (x 40)

Ciliary body

SCLERA The extensive, fibrous sclera is opaque, white in color, and about 0.3–1.0 mm thick. It consists of interlacing bundles of **collagenous and elastic fibers,** which run roughly parallel to the outer surface of the sclera. The exposed surface of the sclera is covered by the **conjunctiva,** a delicate **mucous membrane** that also lines the eyelids. Anteriorly, the sclera is continuous with the cornea at a region termed the **limbus.** Near this junction, embedded in the tunica fibrosa, is an irregular, endothelium-lined canal, the **canal of Schlemm,** which completely encircles the margins of the cornea. It functions as an escape route for **aqueous humor,** which eventually reaches the venous circulation.

Also near the limbus are the insertions of the **extraocular skeletal muscles** that move the eyeball. Posteriorly, the unexposed regions of the sclera are continuous with the dural sheath of the **optic nerve.** Here the sclera is perforated by many small openings through which bundles of optic nerve fibers pass. This sievelike area is the **lamina cribrosa.**

CORNEA The transparent, avascular cornea occupies the slightly bulging anterior ⅙ of the outer coat. It is about the same thickness as the sclera (0.5–1.0 mm). Covering its outer surface are four to six layers of nonkeratinized **squamous epithelial cells.** The layers are uniform in thickness, and the superficial cells are constantly being shed; turnover time is about one week. They **regenerate rapidly** following an abrasion. Between these surface cells are numerous, **free nerve endings** mediating the exquisite pain we experience from a foreign object abrading the cornea.

The uniformity of the thickness of the cornea and the evenness of its outer epithelial surface are major factors that create and maintain the **transparency** of the cornea. The corneal epithelium rests on a thick (8–12 μm), homogeneous, basal lamina, termed **Bowman's membrane,** or the anterior membrane. It is sharply delineated by the PAS reaction.

The large central area of the cornea beneath the epithelium is the **substantia propria,** or **stroma,** which constitutes about 90% of the total thickness of the cornea. It is a tough, fibrous structure consisting of layers of **collagen lamellae** that run parallel to the corneal surface, with flattened fibroblasts between them. The transparency of the cornea depends on the uniform, small size of its collagen fibers and the uniform arrangement of the lamellae.

Covering the posterior surface of the substantia propria is **Descemet's membrane.** This is thinner (5–10 μm) than Bowman's anterior membrane. It consists of fine, uniform, collagenous fibers and considerable **elastic fibers;** therefore it stains selectively with elastin stains. On the posterior surface of Descemet's membrane is a layer of simple, squamous epithelium, inappropriately called **endothelium.** The cells are in contact with the aqueous humor and limit the extent of the cornea posteriorly.

The **limbus** is the junction zone (about 1 mm wide) between the sclera and cornea. Here, the corneal epithelium loses its regular cellular arrangement and is replaced by **conjunctival epithelium.** The highly regular, corneal fibers become disarranged as the irregular, typical collagen fibers of the sclera. This zone has a **plexus** of circularly arranged, anastomosing **blood vessels,** whose capillaries do not normally extend beyond the corneal margin. Descemet's membrane disappears, but the simple squamous epithelium of the cornea is continuous over the first part of the sclera.

MIDDLE VASCULAR LAYER (TUNICA VASCULOSA OR UVEA) In the entire posterior half of the eye, the highly vascularized middle coat is present only as the **choroid,** a very vascular, pigmented layer. However, at its anterior edge it becomes a thickened, wedge-shaped structure, the **ciliary body,** with numerous projections into the vitreous humor, called the **ciliary processes.** From the ciliary body, a thin, circular diaphragm, the **iris,** extends across the anterior chamber with the **pupil** at its center. Since all the parts are continuous structures, they are **subject to infections** that spread readily from one structure to another.

Choroid The choroid (Gk. chorion, a covering) is a **highly vascular, brownish-pigmented layer** about 0.1–0.2 mm thick located between the sclera and the retina. It extends anteriorly to the ciliary body and posteriorly to cover the posterior half of the eye. It has three layers. Its outermost layer, next to the sclera, is avascular and called the **epichoroid layer.** It consists mostly of **laminae of elastic fibers** with a liberal scattering of **pigment cells.** The **middle, or vessel, layer** has loose connective tissue with multiple branches of the **ciliary arteries and veins. Many pigment cells** are also present. The **inner layer** is a capillary network called the **choriocapillaris.** These are fenestrated capillaries that arise from the larger blood vessels in the adjacent middle layer. They are the **largest capillaries** in the body, equaling the diameter of sinusoids. They are the source of oxygen and nutrients for the rods and cones and the retinal pigment cells.

Interposed between these retinal pigment cells and the capillaries of the choriocapillaris is the **glassy membrane (of Bruch).** This is composed of a homogeneous **basement membrane,** a product of the retinal pigment cells, and an elastic and collagenous component from the choroid. When exposed to bright light, this membrane reflects the light, causing the eyes to appear to glow in the dark.

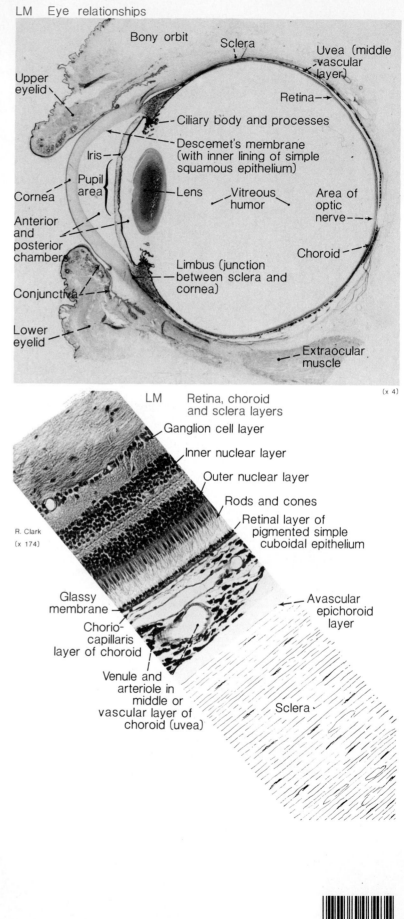

LM   Eye relationships

Bony orbit
Sclera
Uvea (middle vascular layer)
Retina
Upper eyelid
Ciliary body and processes
Descemet's membrane (with inner lining of simple squamous epithelium)
Iris
Pupil area
Lens
Vitreous humor
Area of optic nerve
Cornea
Anterior and posterior chambers
Conjunctiva
Limbus (junction between sclera and cornea)
Choroid
Lower eyelid
Extraocular muscle

(x 4)

LM   Retina, choroid and sclera layers
Ganglion cell layer
Inner nuclear layer
Outer nuclear layer
Rods and cones
Retinal layer of pigmented simple cuboidal epithelium
R. Clark
(x 174)
Glassy membrane
Chorio-capillaris layer of choroid
Venule and arteriole in middle or vascular layer of choroid (uvea)
Avascular epichoroid layer
Sclera

18475

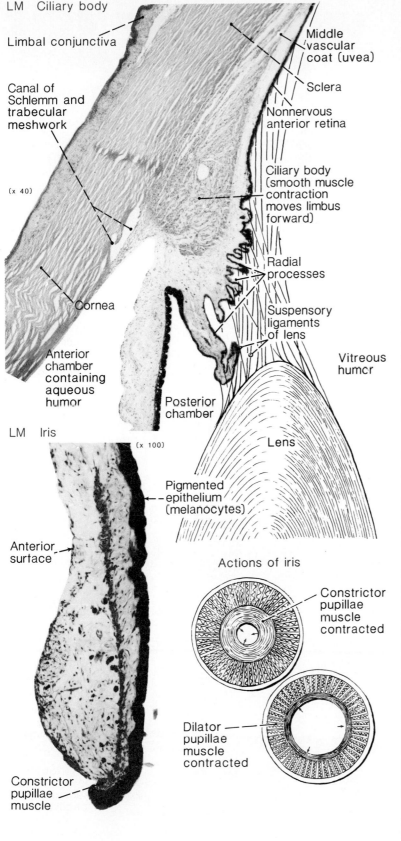

LM Ciliary body

Limbal conjunctiva

Canal of
Schlemm and
trabecular
meshwork

(x 40)

Cornea

Anterior
chamber
containing
aqueous
humor

Middle
vascular
coat (uvea)

Sclera

Nonnervous
anterior retina

Ciliary body
(smooth muscle
contraction
moves limbus
forward)

Radial
processes

Suspensory
ligaments
of lens

Vitreous
humor

Posterior
chamber

Lens

Pigmented
epithelium
(melanocytes)

LM   Iris

(x 100)

Anterior
surface

Constrictor
pupillae
muscle

Actions of iris

Constrictor
pupillae
muscle
contracted

Dilator
pupillae
muscle
contracted

Ciliary Body and Processes The ciliary body is the **muscular,** intermediate portion of the **middle coat (uvea).** It extends from the base of the iris to the anterior edge of the photosensitive part of the retina. It is formed by the gradual thickening of the anterior part of the choroid. The widest part of the enlargement is at the **limbus,** where it is seen as the **wedge-shaped ciliary body** with a fringe of irregular, **radial processes** projecting into the vitreous humor. (Note that in a three-dimensional view, the **ciliary body is a ring of tissue** with a thin outer edge where it joins the choroid, and a much thicker inner edge, where it joins the iris.) The bulk of the structure is occupied by a mass of smooth muscle, the **ciliary muscle.** Upon contraction of the muscle, the ciliary body moves forward, the tension on the suspensory ligament of the lens decreases, and the lens increases its curvature, thus **changing the focus for near vision.**

The ciliary body and its processes are covered by the nonnervous anterior part of the retina. Here the cellular layers are reduced to two layers of **cuboidal epithelium.** The **outer layer** is a continuation of the **pigment cells of the retina,** while the cells of the **inner layer** are **nonpigmented.** These latter cells are the forward extension of the nonphotosensitive inner cell layers of the retina.

Iris The iris is the most anterior part of the uvea. Acting as a perforated curtain or diaphragm, it **separates the anterior and posterior chambers,** except at the pupil. As a continuation of the **ciliary body,** it has essentially the same histological structure. The central mass of the iris is loose connective tissue **stroma,** similar to the choroid.

The iris is **highly vascular and pigmented.** It is populated by many melanocytes, fibroblasts, and some smooth muscle cells. Its **anterior surface** is grooved with a number of **concentric folds.** A single layer of **flat cells covers the surface,** but in the crypts of the folds the cells are absent. Although these discontinuous cells appear to be epithelial, they are probably flattened fibroblasts and melanocytes. In contrast, the **posterior surface** is covered with two layers of cuboidal cells, the continuation of the two layers that cover the ciliary body. However, the **superficial layer,** which is nonpigmented in the ciliary body, **is pigmented** in the iris. The **deeper layer,** pigmented in the ciliary body, is composed of many **nonpigmented, myoepithelial cells** and a few smooth muscle cells.

There are two arrangements of smooth muscle fibers that form the dilator and constrictor pupillae muscles. The radially arranged **dilator muscle fibers** are located on the **periphery of the iris.** When its fibers are stimulated by sympathetic impulses, the **pupil is dilated.** The circu-

18573

larly arranged pupillary **sphincter muscle** forms a circle of smooth muscle near the **free margin of the pupil.** Upon parasympathetic stimulation, the muscle contracts, the **pupil is narrowed,** and the amount of light entering the eye is reduced.

The color of the iris is determined by the number of **pigmented cells in the stroma.** If melanocytes are abundant, the person has brown eyes; if scanty, blue eyes. Variations in the number of cells between these extremes produce green, grey, or other varieties of eye color. Therefore, **eye color** is determined by the **amount of melanin pigment.**

RETINA Recall that in the development of the eye, all retinal cells arise from two cellular layers, derived from the invaginating optic vesicle. The **outer layer becomes the nonphotoreceptive,** pigmented cells of the retinal pigmented epithelium, the outer layer of the ciliary epithelium, and the posterior region of the iris, as described earlier. This region is often referred to as the **nonnervous retina.**

The posterior part of the **retina (pars optica)** extends from the optic nerve (optic disk) to the posterior border of the ciliary body, where the nervous retina ends on a wavy line, the **ora serrata.** The cells of the **inner layer** differentiate into a multilayered, **light-sensitive epithelium** consisting of two limiting membranes and three neurons in synaptic series, i.e., photoreceptor **rod and cone cells,** interposed **bipolar cells,** and **ganglion cells,** whose axons form the optic nerve.

Layers of the Retina Except for minor variations in certain regions, the retina consists of **ten histologically distinct layers.** All but the outermost layer belong to the light-sensitive nervous retina. The layers are numbered from the outside inward (towards the center of the eyeball).

1. **Layer of pigmented epithelium.** A simple layer of **cuboidal, pigmented cells** is closely attached to the choroid. Basally, its cells rest on **Bruch's membrane.** On its inner surface, each cell sends several, slender, pigmented **cytoplasmic projections** between the outer processes of the rods and cones. Such an arrangement provides only a loose attachment. It is along this plane that the **retinal cells separate** in the clinical condition of **detached retina.** It is also the original cleft between the inner and outer layers of the invaginating optic vesicle. These **pigmented cells synthesize melanin,** absorb light rays, and prevent their scattering. They are also **phagocytic cells** that ingest the discarded tips of the retinal rod cells, as discussed later.

2. **Layer of rods and cones.** Note that this is not a true cellular layer, since it consists only of the **light-sensitive processes of the rods and**

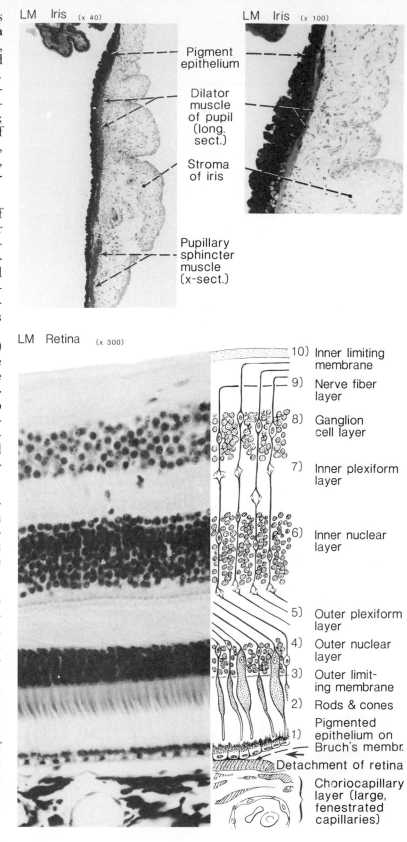

LM Iris (x 40)

Pigment epithelium

Dilator muscle of pupil (long. sect.)

Stroma of iris

Pupillary sphincter muscle (x-sect.)

LM Iris (x 100)

LM Retina (x 300)

10) Inner limiting membrane
9) Nerve fiber layer
8) Ganglion cell layer
7) Inner plexiform layer
6) Inner nuclear layer
5) Outer plexiform layer
4) Outer nuclear layer
3) Outer limiting membrane
2) Rods & cones
1) Pigmented epithelium on Bruch's membr.
Detachment of retina
Choriocapillary layer (large, fenestrated capillaries)

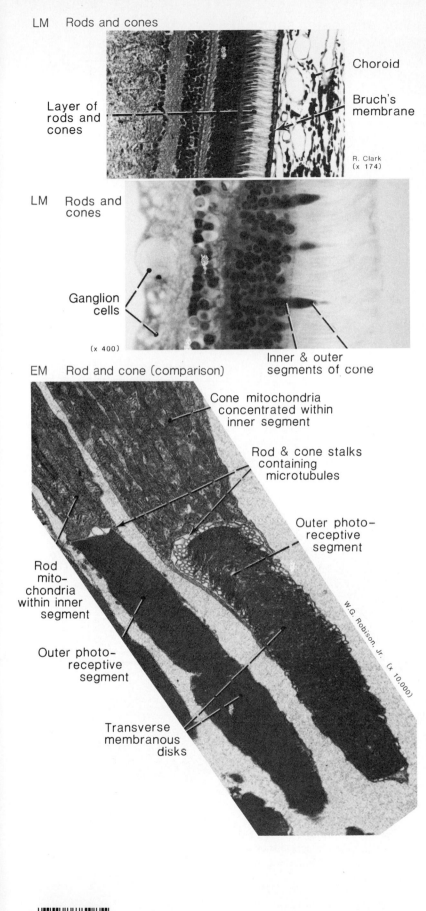

LM   Rods and cones

Layer of
rods and
cones

Choroid

Bruch's
membrane

R. Clark
(x 174)

LM   Rods and
      cones

Ganglion
cells

(x 400)

Inner & outer
segments of cone

EM   Rod and cone (comparison)

Cone mitochondria
concentrated within
inner segment

Rod & cone stalks
containing
microtubules

Outer photo-
receptive
segment

Rod
mito-
chondria
within
inner
segment

Outer photo-
receptive
segment

Transverse
membranous
disks

W.G. Robison, Jr. (x 10,000)

cones, whose nuclei are located in the adjacent nuclear layer. These processes are photoreceptors, upon which sight is completely dependent.

These **photoreceptors** are named from their shape. The more numerous, **slender, narrow processes are the rods,** while the less abundant, broad-based, **tapering projections are the cones.** The tip (**outer segment**) of each of these processes is embedded in the fingerlike projections of the **pigment layer,** while their base (**inner segment**) is attached to the **visual cell body** by a short stalk composed of nine doublets of microtubules, similar to a cilium.

The outer segments contain **photoreceptor substances.** The **rods** contain the visual pigment, **rhodopsin,** also called **visual purple,** which has a low threshold of stimulation by light. Therefore, rods are **activated by dim light,** e.g., night vision and peripheral vision. In the **cones,** the principal visual pigment is **iodopsin** which responds to **high light intensity** and functions for **visual acuity and color perception.** Other visual pigments in the cones make possible the perception of various colors.

Ultrastructurally, a **rod outer segment** contains, within the plasmalemma, a series of uniform, flattened, **laminated disks** formed from many infoldings of the plasma membrane, which contain the **rhodopsin.** Upon exposure to light, the rhodopsin molecule **changes its configuration.** This photochemical reaction results in the **hyperpolarization** of the rod plasmalemma. This change in electrical potential is transmitted to the dendrites of the bipolar cells where the axons of the rod cells synapse. Immediately **after light stimulation, the rhodopsin is reconstituted,** and the process is repeated upon the next exposure to light.

The **membranous disks** of the outer segment of the rods are **constantly being replenished at the base** of the process, and **shed at its extremity.** This is accomplished by proteins synthesized in the inner segment, which are transported to the bases of the outer segments. Here **new disks are formed** by an infolding of the cell membrane. Thus, the disks are constantly replaced outward, and the **older disks** are continuously cast off and **phagocytized** by the pigment epithelium.

The fine structure of the cones is similar to the rods, with the following exceptions.

a. The **cone disks are not sloughed,** or phagocytized by the pigment epithelial cells, although they are invested by these cells.

b. The spaces between the disks communicate with the outside of the cell. In other words, the membranous **disks are continuous with the plasma membrane.**

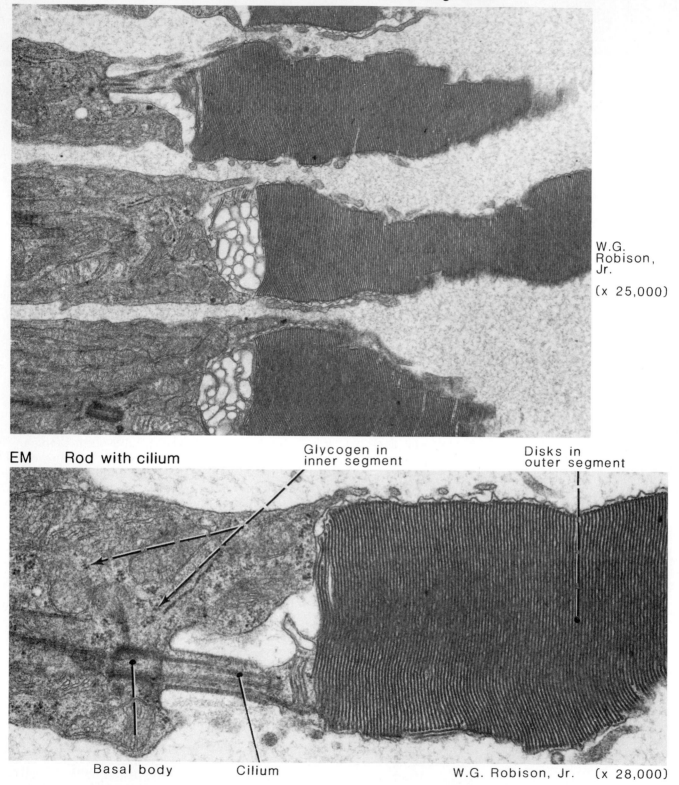

W.G.
Robison,
Jr.

(x 25,000)

EM   Rod with cilium   Glycogen in
inner segment   Disks in
outer segment

Basal body   Cilium   W.G. Robison, Jr.   (x 28,000)

Upper view: Electron micrograph of a row of rod photosensitive cells. The junctional
area between the outer and inner segments of the upper cell shows a modified
connecting cilium. Section of this area of the other cells does not traverse the plane of
the connecting cilia but does show numerous vesicles.

Lower view: Higher magnification of a rod junctional area reveals the basal body of a
cilium, rod cell plasma membrane enclosing the cilium, membranous disks, and glycogen
particles interspersed among mitochondria in the inner segment.

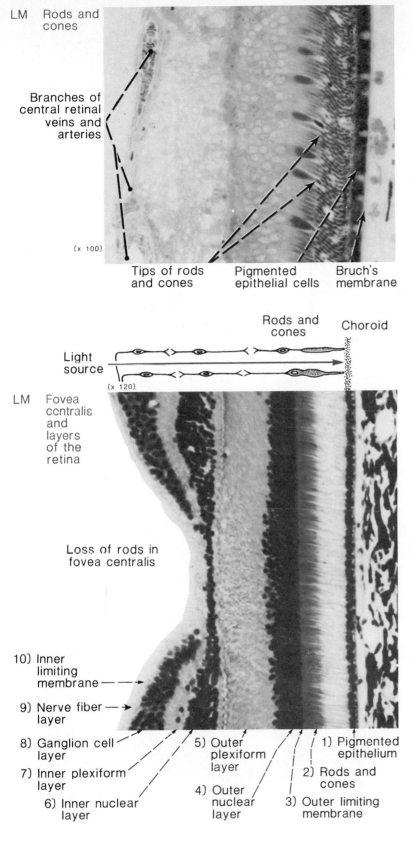

LM Rods and
    cones

Branches of
central retinal
veins and
arteries

(x 100)

Tips of rods   Pigmented   Bruch's
and cones   epithelial cells   membrane

Rods and
cones   Choroid

Light
source

(x 120)

LM Fovea
    centralis
    and
    layers
    of the
    retina

Loss of rods in
fovea centralis

10) Inner
    limiting
    membrane

9) Nerve fiber
   layer

8) Ganglion cell
   layer

7) Inner plexiform
   layer

6) Inner nuclear
   layer

5) Outer
   plexiform
   layer

4) Outer
   nuclear
   layer

1) Pigmented
   epithelium

2) Rods and
   cones

3) Outer limiting
   membrane

c. Cones contain **several visual pigments,** each responsive to either green, red, or blue light. (Rods have only rhodopsin.)

d. In cones, the **disks are uneven in size,** i.e., wider near the base and progressively narrower near the extremity.

e. Cones **synapse one-to-one** with bipolar neurons, while several rods may synapse on a single bipolar cell, a condition called **summation.**

3. **Outer limiting membrane.** Actually this is not a membrane but a narrow **zone of junctional complexes** between certain glial (Müller) cells and the adjoining rod and cone cells.

4. **Outer nuclear layer.** Contains the closely packed **nuclei and cell bodies** of the rods and cones.

5. **Outer plexiform layer.** A broad, **synaptic zone** where axons of rod and cone cells synapse with the dendrites of the bipolar cells. Horizontal neurons also synapse here.

6. **Inner nuclear layer.** Similar to, but thinner than, the outer nuclear layer. It is crowded with **nuclei and cell bodies of the bipolar cells.** It also contains a few horizontal neurons and amacrine neurons (which lack axons), and the nuclei of Müller (glial) cells.

7. **Inner plexiform layer.** The zone where axons of **bipolar cells synapse** with the profusely branched dendrites of the **ganglion cells.** Also integrative connections of ganglionic and amacrine neurons occur here.

8. **Ganglion cell layer.** Contains the **large ganglion cell bodies** (10–30 μm), a few scattered glial cells, and retinal blood vessels.

9. **Nerve fiber layer.** Consists largely of **unmyelinated axons of ganglion cells** arranged in nerve bundles that lie parallel to the inner surface of the retina. They converge on the optic papilla (disk) to form the **optic nerve.** Between the bundles are glial cells, e.g., astrocytes and Müller cells.

10. **Inner limiting membrane.** Formed by the bulbous **end processes of Müller cells and their basal laminae.** These cells are the **chief supporting cells** of the retina (Table 26.1).

Retinal Modifications The relative thickness of the retinal layers accounts for several **regional differences** in the retina. The most prominent is an **oval-shaped depression** about 1.5 mm in diameter near the posterior pole of the eye, the **macula lutea** (yellow spot), so-called because of its yellow color in gross specimens. In the center of the depression, the inner retinal layers have been displaced, creating a small pit about 0.5 mm in diameter, called the **fovea centralis.** In this area, all of the photoreceptors are tightly packed, slender **cones.** Because of the thinning out of the internal retinal layers and the absence of blood vessels, the light rays fall directly on the cones, producing the area of **greatest visual acuity and sharpest color discrimination.**

Another retinal modification is the **optic papilla (disk)** or blind spot. This is where the optic nerve fibers from all parts of the retina congregate to exit the eyeball. This area has **no photoreceptors** and is, therefore, a blind spot. It is also where retinal blood vessels enter and leave the eye, especially the **central retinal artery and veins,** which course through the optic nerve.

Contents of the Eyeball

AQUEOUS HUMOR The aqueous humor is a **clear, lymphlike fluid** that is elaborated by the nonpigmented **ciliary epithelium** covering the ciliary body and the ciliary processes. Its production is similar to the synthesis of cerebrospinal fluid by the choroid plexuses in the brain. The aqueous humor **flows continuously** from the posterior chamber into the anterior chamber through the pupil, where it circulates primarily toward the angle of the anterior chamber. Here the fluid passes at a constant rate through the **trabecular meshwork** into a rather large, irregular vessel, the **canal of Schlemm,** which empties into the veins of the sclera.

Blockage of the exit route for the aqueous humor results in high intraocular pressure, clinically known as **glaucoma.** If left untreated, the pressure will cause damage to the optic nerve, resulting in varying degrees of blindness.

LENS AND ITS CAPSULE Recall that the lens develops from surface (skin) ectoderm opposite the optic cup. The early lens separates from this layer and becomes suspended in the opening of the optic cup, where it is anchored. In the fully developed eye, the lens is an **elastic, biconvex, transparent body** enclosed in a transparent capsule of basal lamina. The lens lies behind the iris, next to the vitreous body. It is about 10 mm in diameter and varies from 3.5 to 5.0 mm in thickness. Its posterior surface is more convex, than the anterior surface. Beneath the anterior half of the capsule is a layer of simple cuboidal cells, called the **lens epithelium.** No such layer is present beneath the posterior capsule.

It is the lens epithelial cells that undergo mitotic division and differentiate into **lens fiber cells.** These cells elongate, accumulate large amounts of protein, and lose their nuclei in the process of becoming **mature lens fibers.** In spite of its dense, proteinaceous nature, the lens is remarkably transparent through life. However, in the elderly, **opacities (cataracts)** may occur and vision is dimmed or lost. Surgical removal of the clouded lens, followed by implantation of a plastic lens, or use of heavy corrective lenses, usually restores vision.

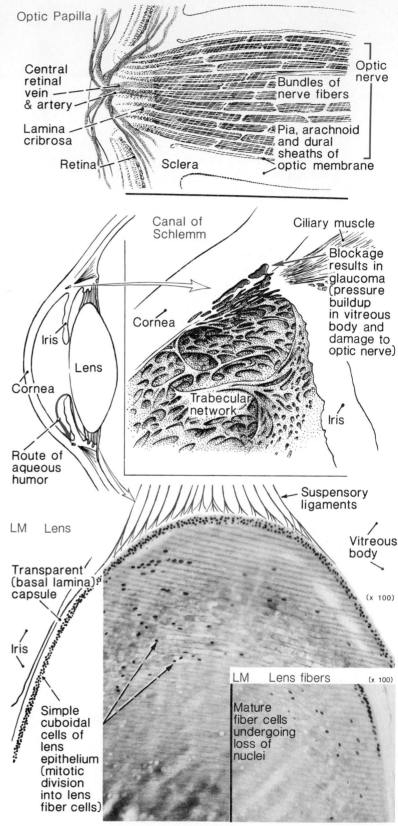

NERVE		
FIBERS	CELLS	FUNCTION(S)
Free nerve endings (pain)	None	Principal area of light refraction
Posterior ciliary nerves; also bundles of optic nerve fibers which penetrate sclera posteriorly at lamina cribrosa	None	Provides insertions for extraocular muscles; maintains shape and rigidity of eyeball
Ciliary nerves	Autonomic ganglia	Provides nutrients and O_2 to retina
Many fibers from ciliary ganglion interlace with muscle fibers; sympathetic fibers pass to walls of blood vessels	None	Vascular stroma produces aqueous humor; ciliary muscle controls focal adjustments of lens
Autonomic fibers among muscle for reflex control	None	As a diaphragm controls amount of light entering eye
None	None	Synthesize melanin; absorb light and prevent its scattering; phagocytize discarded tips of retinal rods
None	Rods—long cylindrical outer segment of bipolar cells; cones—shorter, tapering, conical, outer segments	Rods sensitive to low light levels; cones respond to brighter light intensity and color vision
Axons extend into outer plexiform layer	Cell bodies and nuclei of rods and cones cells	First neurons of three neuron visual pathway
Synapses of axons of rods and cones with dendrites of bipolar cells	Occasional horizontal cells	Synaptic region for first and second neurons of vision pathway

Table 26.1 *(continued)*

STRUCTURE	LOCATION	EPITHELIUM	CONNECTIVE TISSUE	MUSCLE
● Inner nuclear	Innermost broad dense, nuclear zone	None	Glial cells, e.g., astrocytes, microglia, Müller cells	None
● Inner plexiform	Clear area between bipolar and ganglion cell layers	None	Same as above	None
● Ganglion cells	Innermost nuclear layer	None	Same as above	None
● Nerve fiber	Innermost fibrous layer	None	Same as above	None
● Inner limiting	Rests on optic nerve fibers	Heavy basement membrane, inner surface flat; outer surface (next to optic nerve) uneven	None	None

NERVE		
FIBERS	CELLS	FUNCTION(S)
Axons and dendrites of bipolar cells	Bipolar, horizontal and amacrine neurons	Shelter and nourish bipolar neurons
Synapses of axons of bipolar cells with dendrites of ganglion cells	None	Synaptic region for second and third visual neurons
Axons and dendrites interlace to form meshwork	Usually several rows of large ganglion cells	Third order neurons of visual pathway
Axons form unmyelinated optic nerve fibers that parallel retinal surface	None	Origin of optic nerve for transmission of light-sensitive impulses
None	None	Forms inner boundary of retina

Table 26.2 *SUMMARY OF STRUCTURES OF THE EAR*

STRUCTURE	LOCATION	ENVIRONMENT	EPITHELIUM
EXTERNAL EAR			
Auricle	Side of head	Air	Stratified squamous (thin skin)
External auditory meatus	Extends from auricle to eardrum	Air	Stratified squamous associated with hair and wax glands
Tympanic membrane (eardrum)	Medial termination of external auditory meatus	Air	Stratified squamous (thin skin) externally; simple cuboidal internally
MIDDLE EAR			
Tympanic cavity	Between inner surface of eardrum and wall of internal ear	Air	Lined with simple cuboidal
Auditory (eustachian) tube	Between tympanic cavity and nasopharynx	Air	Proximally, simple cuboidal; distally, respiratory epithelium
Auditory ossicles	Form bridge between eardrum and oval window	Air	Covered by simple cuboidal
Oval window	Medial superior wall of tympanic cavity, next to scala vestibuli	Air on outer surface; perilymph on inner surface	Simple cuboidal over footplate of stapes which covers membrane of oval window
Round window	Medial inferior wall of tympanic cavity next to scala tympani	Same as above	Simple cuboidal covers outer membranous surface
INNER EAR			
Bony labyrinth	Petrous portion of temporal bone	Inner surface immersed in perilymph	None
Membranous labyrinth	Within bony labyrinth	Outer surface bathed in perilymph; lumen filled with endolymph	Lined with simple squamous with small areas of neuroepithelium

CONNECTIVE TISSUE	NERVOUS TISSUE	FUNCTION(S)
Elastic cartilage	Sensory nerves	Receives sound waves and directs them towards meatus
Distally, elastic cartilage; proximally, bone	Same as above	Transmits sound waves to eardrum
Fibroelastic central core	Motor nerve to tensor tympani muscle and sensory nerves	Vibrates on same frequency as sound waves; transfers vibrations to malleus
Loose areolar beneath epithelium	Motor nerve to stapedius muscle, also sensory nerves	Houses auditory ossicles; communicates with nasopharynx via auditory tube
Same as above	Sensory nerves	Allows for equalization of ambient air with air in tympanic cavity
Periosteum beneath epithelium; bone	Same as above	Transmits vibrations of eardrum to oval window
Stapes fixed to window by annular ligament of elastic fibers	Same as above	Receives vibrations from stapes and transforms them into fluid waves in scala vestibuli
Fibrous membrane	Same as above	By outward movements, it dissipates the fluid sound waves in scala tympani
Compact bone	Same as above	Contains the membranous labyrinth
Walls of fibrous connective tissue	Patches of sensory hair cells	Houses the organ of hearing (cochlea) and the organs of equilibration (utricle, saccule, and semicircular canals)

Table 26.2   (continued)

STRUCTURE	LOCATION	ENVIRONMENT	EPITHELIUM
INNER EAR			
Vestibule	Central, irregular cavity of osseous labyrinth	Perilymph	Simple squamous
● Utricle and saccule	Vestibule	Submerged in perilymph; lumen contains endolymph	Simple squamous
● Semicircular canals	Superior and posterior to vestibule in osseous labyrinth	Same as above	Simple squamous
Cochlea	Anterior and medial to vestibule in bony labyrinth	Perilymph and endolymph	Mostly simple squamous and some simple cuboidal
● Scala vestibuli	Above spiral lamina of modiolus	Perilymph	Simple squamous
● Scala tympani	Below spiral lamina	Perilymph	Simple squamous
● Scala media	Between scalae vestibuli and tympani	Endolymph	Simple squamous
● Organ of Corti	Floor of scala media; rests on basilar membrane	Endolymph	Neuroepithelium (hair cells); cuboidal and columnar support cells (pillar and phalangeal)

CONNECTIVE TISSUE	NERVOUS TISSUE	FUNCTION(S)
Periosteum	Vestibular nerve (equilibrium)	Contains sense organs responsible for maintaining of balance and orientation
Subepithelial layer of loose connective tissue	A site of origin of vestibular nerve; small regions (maculae) of receptor hair cells with otoliths	Hair cells in maculae stimulated by linear acceleration and gravity
Same as above	A site of origin of vesticular nerve; in ampullae, hair cells in cristae void of otoliths	Hair cells respond to rotational acceleration of head in any plane
Periosteum	Origin of auditory nerve; sensory hair cells in organ of Corti	Houses nervous and supportive cells involved in hearing
Periosteum	Sensory nerves	Transmits fluid waves to scala media, or to scala tympani through helicotrema, or both
Periosteum	Sensory nerves	Transmits fluid waves to round window where pressure waves are dissipated
Externally fibrous connective tissue	Axons of auditory nerve; hair cells in organ of Corti	Houses the organ of Corti
Subepithelial loose connective tissue	Auditory nerve arises from nerve endings terminating on inner and outer hair cells	Is the organ of hearing; hair cells convert fluid waves into electrical impulses which are interpreted by the brain as sound

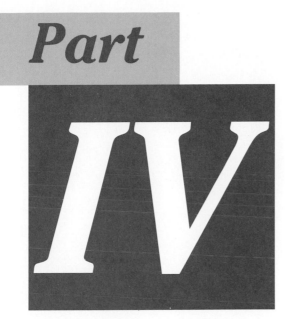

Part

IV

TOOLS FOR LEARNING

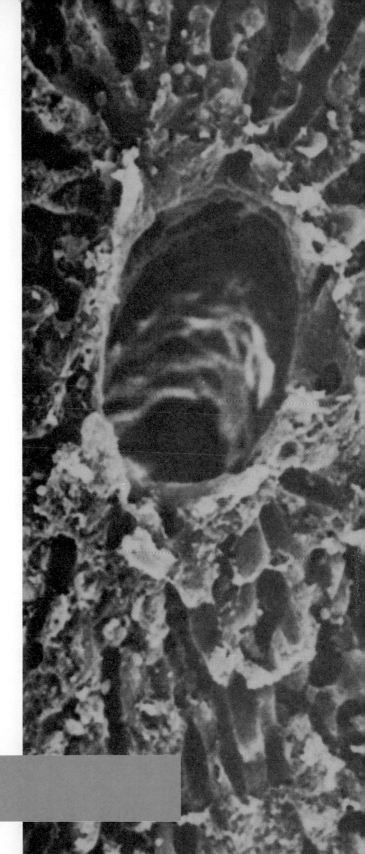

Chapter

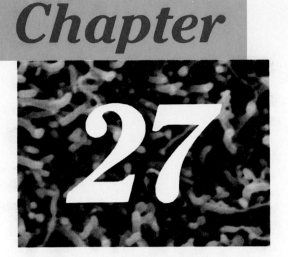

27

MICROSCOPY

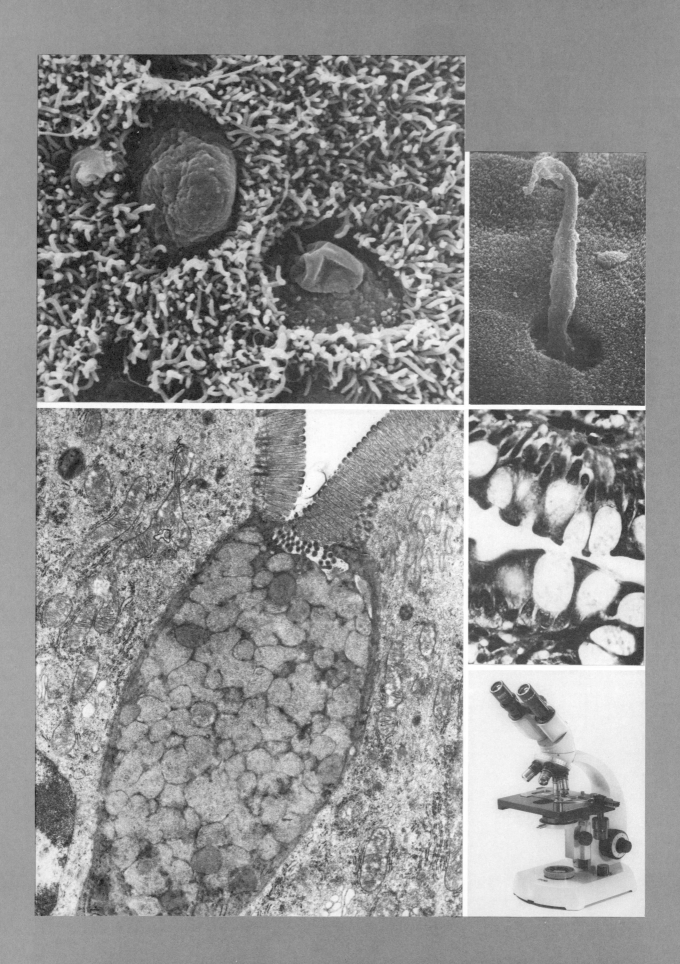

OBJECTIVES

BY STUDYING THIS CHAPTER, THE STUDENT SHOULD:

1. Understand the advantages and limitations of the various types of microscopes used in histology.

2. Gain the ability to interpret correctly data from both light and electron microscopic micrographs.

3. Understand the various methods used to prepare fresh tissues for microscopic and ultramicroscopic study.

4. Realize the advantages of staining tissues before they are examined microscopically.

MICROSCOPES

The primary tool of the histologist is the microscope. Several types are available for examination of biological material, whether dead or living, stained or unstained, thick or thin. Microscopes are grouped according to the type of light they use. For example, **visual light** is used in the conventional bright field optical microscope, including several modifications, e.g., phase contrast, dark field, polarizing, and interference microscopes. Those instruments using **invisible radiation** include the electron, x-ray, and ultraviolet microscopes.

As important as its capacity to magnify may be, perhaps the microscope's greatest value is its ability to resolve detail, i.e., a capacity for a lens system to separate clearly two points close together. Thus, the **resolving power** of a lens is the least distance between two objects that can be detected as two and not a single object. The limit of resolution of the best light microscope is about 0.1–0.2 μm.

Light (Bright Field) Microscope

The conventional compound light microscope is essentially **two sets of magnifying lenses** aided by a condenser lens beneath the microscopic stage. The condenser lens modifies and concentrates the light into a bright light beam that illuminates the object to be studied. The modified beam enters the **objective lens system,** the first set of magnifying lenses, where a magnified image of the specimen is formed. As the image passes through the second set of lenses in the **ocular** (eyepiece), further magnification occurs. The total **magnification** of the specimen is simply the product of these lens systems. For example, if the objective lens is 40× and the ocular system is 10×, the magnification of the specimen is 400×.

Since most cells and tissues are essentially colorless, they all appear about the same under the light microscope. However, if they are appropriately **stained,** various structures appear lighter or darker in density, as well as variously colored.

Phase Contrast Microscope

When it is desirable to study **unstained** cells, particularly **living cells,** a **phase contrast** microscope may be used. This is a modified light microscope that produces visual images from quite transparent objects. This is possible because the various cell organelles have **different refractive indices.** By definition, the refractive index is the speed of a light wave passing through an object, expressed in relation to air, which has an arbitrary value of 1.0. As light waves traverse a living cell, they will be refracted or slowed down if they pass through an organelle, such as a nucleus or mitochondrion. The waves will emerge from

Resolving power

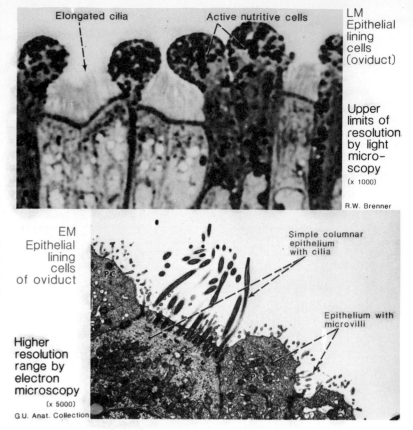

Elongated cilia   Active nutritive cells

LM
Epithelial lining cells (oviduct)

Upper limits of resolution by light microscopy
(x 1000)

R.W. Brenner

EM
Epithelial lining cells of oviduct

Simple columnar epithelium with cilia

Epithelium with microvilli

Higher resolution range by electron microscopy
(x 5000)

G.U. Anat. Collection

Magnification principles of the light microscope

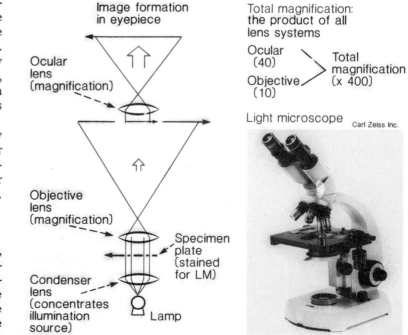

Image formation in eyepiece

Ocular lens (magnification)

Objective lens (magnification)

Condenser lens (concentrates illumination source)

Specimen plate (stained for LM)

Lamp

Total magnification: the product of all lens systems

Ocular (40)
Objective (10)
Total magnification (x 400)

Light microscope

Carl Zeiss Inc.

Principles of phase contrast microscopy

► Optical plate retards intensity of defracted rays, thus converting phase differences into amplitude differences (light and dark)

► Rays defracted by cell structures emerge out-of-phase with nondefracted rays

► Light is concentrated and patterned then directed through specimen

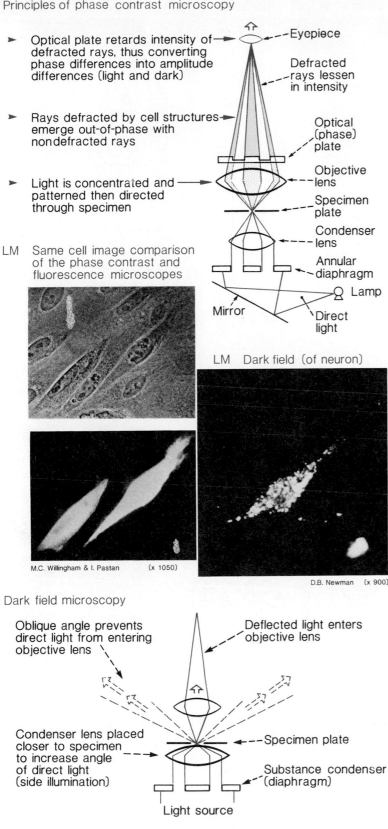

- Eyepiece
- Defracted rays lessen in intensity
- Optical (phase) plate
- Objective lens
- Specimen plate
- Condenser lens
- Annular diaphragm
- Lamp
- Mirror
- Direct light

LM   Same cell image comparison of the phase contrast and fluorescence microscopes

M.C. Willingham & I. Pastan   (x 1050)

LM   Dark field (of neuron)

D.B. Newman   (x 900)

Dark field microscopy

Oblique angle prevents direct light from entering objective lens

Deflected light enters objective lens

Condenser lens placed closer to specimen to increase angle of direct light (side illumination)

- Specimen plate
- Substance condenser (diaphragm)
- Light source

the cell at **different times or phases,** that is, they emerge out-of-phase with each other.

The phase microscope is equipped with optical plates in the objective and condenser lenses that convert phase differences into **amplitude differences.** This special equipment reveals, in terms of brightness, all points of diversions of light waves traversing any organelle or inclusion of the cell. In this way, a detailed pattern is formed of a structure whose lack of contrast would make it invisible under the bright field microscope.

Interference Microscope

The interference microscope is a more precise version of the phase microscope. It differs from the phase type by utilizing **two separate beams of light;** one passes through the specimen, the other does not. The two light beams are combined in the image plane. How these **beams interfere** with each other gives a **measure of density** (thickness) of various regions. Since the optical density and phase retardation are in proportion to the tissue mass, the mass of the various cell components can be calculated.

Dark Field Microscope

Unstained, living specimens can also be visualized in a **dark field microscope.** As its name suggests, it is a method of illumination whereby the specimen is made to **appear luminous against a dark field.** Its effectiveness depends on a special substage condenser that excludes the central beam of light from entering the condenser. Instead the object is illuminated by rays of **light that strike the specimen from the side.** If there are moving organisms of greater refractive index than the surrounding media, such as protozoa or bacteria, they will deflect light into the objective and appear as self-luminous objects against a dark background. An example of this interesting phenomenon is the clinical identification, by dark field examination, of the slender, corkscrew **spirochete microorganisms of syphilis.**

Fluorescence Microscope

This is another variation of the light microscope, but in this instrument **ultraviolet light** is used to illuminate the specimen. If the tissue contains molecules that absorb this invisible light, they may emit visual light at higher wavelengths, i.e., they **fluoresce.** The fluorescence may occur naturally within the cell (**endogenous**) or may result from an application of fluorescent dyes (**exogenous**), which tags or labels certain molecules or other components of the specimen. The fluorescence microscope is perhaps the most precise instrument for locating specific proteins within fresh or fixed tissues, such as **antigen-antibody complexes.**

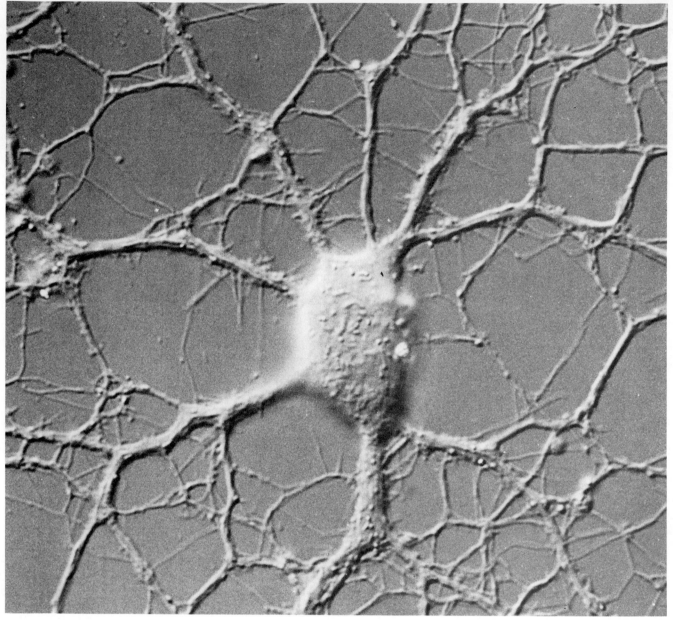

B. Kachar, T. Behar, and M. Dubois-Dalcq   (x 1,800)

A cultured oligodendrocyte from a neonatal rat optic nerve. Differential interference contrast microscopy reveals a limited three-dimensional view of eight main cellular processes with many small lateral projections. These processes form an intrinsic, symmetrical network covering an area of about 100 μm in diameter.

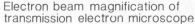

Electron beam magnification of
transmission electron microscope

Heated tungsten
filament (cathode)

Anode

Condenser
(electro-
magnetic coils)

Specimen plate

Objective
(electromagnetic
coils)

Projection
(electromagnetic
coils)

Image forms on
fluorescent screen or
photographic plate

Carl Zeiss Inc.

Electron microscope

Scanning electron microscope (SEM)

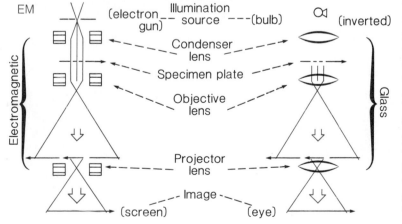

Liver lobule
M.J. Koering

Electron
beam

Condenser
and
objective
lenses

Secondary
electrons
deflected off
treated
areas of
specimen
(light areas)

Transmitted
electrons
(dark areas)

Image
formed
on video
amplifier

Comparisons between electron and light microscopes

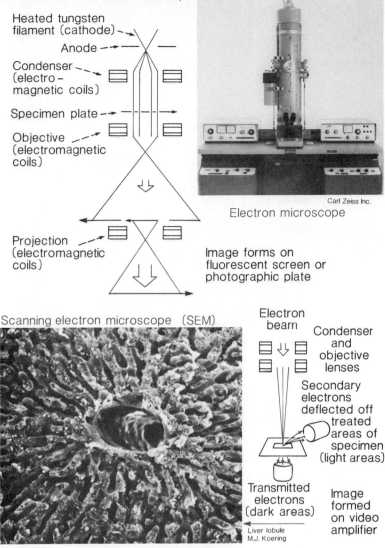

EM

Electromagnetic

(electron gun)

Illumination
source

(bulb)

Condenser
lens

Specimen plate

Objective
lens

Projector
lens

Image

(screen)

(inverted)

Glass

(eye)

Transmission Electron Microscope (TEM)

Limited by the wavelengths of visual light, the resolution of the light microscope has remained essentially unchanged for nearly a century at about 0.2 μm. However, using the **wavelength of electrons,** the electron microscope has an effective reproducible resolution of biological objects of 0.2 nm, about a thousand times better resolution than the best light microscope.

The design of the TEM is similar to the conventional bright field microscope except that it is much larger, inverted, and uses a beam of **electrons instead of visual light.** The electrons are generated by a **heated tungsten filament** (a cathode) situated on top of a vacuum cylinder. The electrons are then **accelerated by high voltage** to a nearby anode, which is a metal plate with a very small aperature (about 30 μm). It is through this opening that the beam of electrons passes down into the cylinder. Situated at intervals within the column are three sets of **electromagnetic coils which focus the electron beam,** analogous to glass lenses focusing the light beam in the light microscope. After passing the first coil (condenser lens), the electron beam passes through the very **thin specimen (about 40–80 nm thick)** held in vacuum. The electrons are focused by the second set of coils (objective lens) to form an **enlarged image** similar to an image formed in the light microscope. This image is further enlarged by the projection coils that project the image either onto a fluorescent screen or onto a photographic plate.

Scanning Electron Microscope (SEM)

To obtain three-dimensional images of a specimen, the scanning electron microscope is used. This is similar to the TEM but is smaller and in some ways less sophisticated. Before the specimen can be studied with the SEM, it must be fixed, dried, and coated with a thin layer of heavy metal (gold or platinum) evaporated onto it in a vacuum, known as **shadowing.** Instead of the electron beam passing through the tissue as in the TEM, the **beam is reflected** from the surface of the coated specimen. As the tissue is scanned by a focused beam of electrons, **secondary electrons** are excited and emerge from the various parts of the surfaces of the specimen. These electrons are converted into an image on a cathode ray tube which may be viewed directly or photographed. Dark shadows and bright highlights appear on the screen in **three dimensions,** since the amount of electron gathering is dependent on the relative angle of the electronic beam to the tissue surface.

With the resolution of the SEM of only about 10 nm and an effective magnification of less than 20,000, this instrument is usually used to study **intact cells,** small sections of organs, and small organisms.

IDENTIFICATION OF TISSUES AND ORGANS

Skill in the identification and interpretation of histological sections should be acquired early in your study. A major problem is that we are usually viewing sections of a **three-dimensional object in two dimensions** only. We must quickly learn how to mentally reconstruct the image of a mass of cells from very thin, flat sections with very little depth.

Furthermore, the **fourth dimension, time,** is also missing from our microscopic picture. We have only a snapshot, a single static image of what was happening in the cell or tissue at the instant of fixation. We have arrested, at a point in time, the dynamic flow of the cellular processes, yielding only **fragments of information** about the cell's morphology and function. It is analogous to reading a single page from a book. We cannot know the content of the book from a single page, but it is at least a beginning.

Examining Light Microscopic Sections

A few sequential procedures for examining microscopic sections are suggested.

1. Recall the basic gross anatomy of the structure. What can you expect to see of this organ in this tiny fragment? If it has a **lumen, epithelium** will probably line it. If it is a solid structure, some pattern of blood vessels, connective tissue, special arrangements of the parenchymal cells, etc., probably exists. Even before you have microscopically examined the slide, you have probably already formed in your mind a **tentative three-dimensional concept** of the organ.

2. Hold the slide to the light to gain some idea of the tissue's general shape, density, staining reactions, and whether or not you are dealing with a single organ or tissue, or several. This procedure is called "grossing" the slide, i.e., viewing it with the **unaided eye.**

3. With a hand lens or an **inverted eyepiece** (ocular) of your microscope, examine the slide to identify any semigross features that will give you clues as to what the organ may be.

4. Now examine the tissue under a light microscope with four objectives, starting with the **scanning (4×)** lens and gradually proceeding to the higher objectives. Under the low-power objective (10×) you will be able to identify most types of tissues, organs, and their relationships.

5. Since most cellular details are indistinct at low power, now switch to the **high-dry objective (40×)** and these finer features can be clearly seen, especially **nuclear details.** You will use high-dry and **oil immersion (100×)** objectives to verify morphological details, which are only suggested at lower magnification.

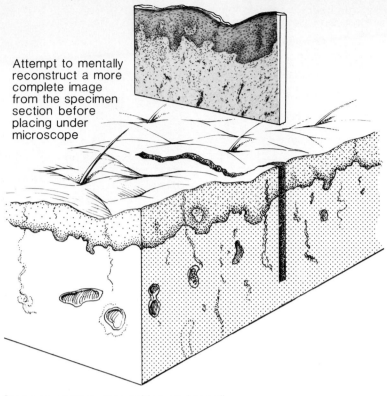

Attempt to mentally reconstruct a more complete image from the specimen section before placing under microscope

Steps to pattern recognition and recall in morphological studies

1) Think of larger structure and its significant characteristics

Stomach e.g.

➤ folds ➤ mucous cells

➤ villi ➤ microvilli

2) Grossing the slide: preliminary examination of specimen (with unaided eye)

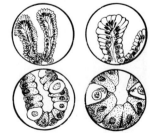

3) Look for significant features on specimen

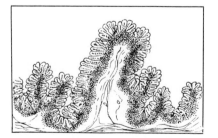

4) Use succeedingly higher objective lenses

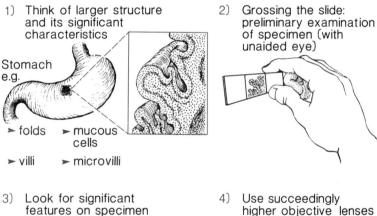

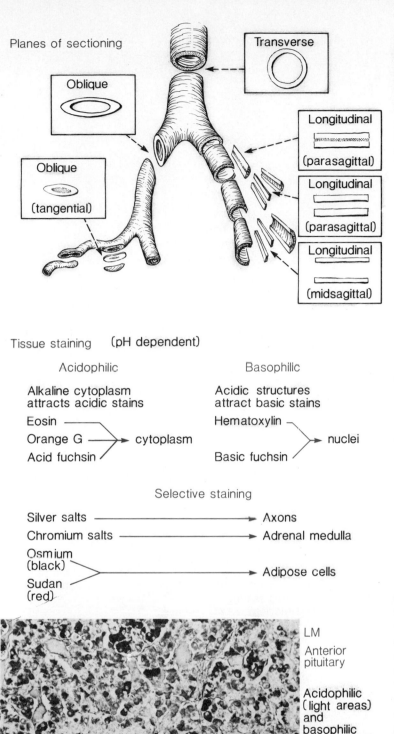

Planes of sectioning

Transverse

Oblique

Longitudinal
(parasagittal)

Oblique
(tangential)

Longitudinal
(parasagittal)

Longitudinal
(midsagittal)

Tissue staining   (pH dependent)

Acidophilic

Alkaline cytoplasm
attracts acidic stains

Eosin
Orange G → cytoplasm
Acid fuchsin

Basophilic

Acidic structures
attract basic stains

Hematoxylin
→ nuclei
Basic fuchsin

Selective staining

Silver salts ————————→ Axons
Chromium salts ———————→ Adrenal medulla
Osmium (black)
Sudan (red) → Adipose cells

LM

Anterior
pituitary

Acidophilic
(light areas)
and
basophilic
(dark areas)
stained cells

(x 208)

By following the above procedures, one quickly learns to identify histological structures by their unique, **morphological patterns**, even under various magnifications and bizarre staining reactions. As we develop this skill of **pattern recognition** in problem solving, our identification of a structure may be almost instantaneous. Such **pattern recall** is also very important in other scientific disciplines, such as histopathology and microbiology.

Planes of Sectioning

Following the above suggestions will help but will not solve your problem of mentally reconstructing a three-dimensional image of the organ. You must also know how to interpret the various **planes of sectioning** of the organ or tissue found in your preparation. Examine carefully the adjacent figures which show various planes of sectioning of several common objects. Likewise, in histology, similar objects or structures, e.g., vessels, ducts, nerves, muscles, etc., are cut in several planes. These **similar structures** appear quite **dissimilar** when they are sectioned in transverse, longitudinal, or oblique planes. When you grasp these three-dimensional concepts, the often static, two-dimensional histology then becomes a vital, dynamic, three-dimensional science.

Staining of Tissues

Perhaps the greatest aid in interpretation of tissues is the use of various **staining techniques.** Except for pigments, all cellular organelles, inclusions, and the cells themselves, are colorless and usually indistinguishable under the LM, unless they have been stained.

There are basically two types of stains, **basophilic and acidophilic. Acid-containing structures,** such as nuclei, are stained a deep blue or purple by basophilic dyes because they have an **affinity for basic stains,** e.g., hematoxylin, basic fuchsin, etc. The affinity of nuclei for these basic dyes is due to their high level of nucleic acids, i.e., DNA and RNA. The cytoplasm stains acidophilic because of its higher pH value. In other words, **alkaline substances** or solutions **attract acid dyes,** such as eosin, orange G, acid fuchsin, etc. Most cellular constituents are selectively basophilic or acidophilic depending on their **pH values.** They become identifiable as distinct entities because of these staining reactions.

Those cellular components that do not react to acidic or basic dyes may stain selectively with other materials. For example, nerve **axons** take up **silver salts** and are therefore said to be argyrophilic or argentophilic. Certain cells in the adrenal medulla stain **brown with chromium salts** and give a chromaffin reaction. Adipose cells have an affinity for **osmium** and stain black.

PREPARATION OF MICROSCOPIC SECTIONS

Paraffin Method for Light Microscopy

To correctly interpret a stained histological slide, one should first understand the various basic processes involved in its preparation; otherwise, one may have greater difficulty in deciding whether some variation in structure or staining is due to unusual physiological or pathological conditions or artifacts from improper histological methods. Such **artifacts** include shrinkage, poor preservation, postmortem changes, folds, wrinkles, and tears in the tissue. The basics of the pertinent procedures for the **paraffin method** are now briefly described.

Tissue Procurement

Great care should be taken in obtaining the tissue. Of cardinal importance is that the tissue must be **fresh,** procured as soon as possible after death. Often this time interval must be only a few minutes, because with cessation of circulation **tissue autolysis** sets in almost immediately, especially in the digestive tract. With a very sharp razor blade or scalpel, a small block of tissue, perhaps a 5-mm cube or less, is removed.

Fixation

The fresh tissue block is immediately submerged in a chemical solution called **fixative,** whose function is to preserve the protoplasm with all of its components in place, i.e., they are "fixed" in their normal position. To accomplish this objective, chemical fixatives must **penetrate the tissue quickly and thoroughly.** Because fixatives are usually precipitants, coagulants, or cross-linking agents, the cellular **proteins** are immediately denatured and **hardened** in position. Simultaneously, the cellular **enzymes are largely inactivated,** so no tissue putrefaction occurs and the integrity of the cell structure is maintained. In addition to the preservation of the framework of the cells, fixation **increases the affinity** of the denatured protoplasm for various stains. Incomplete fixation causes many artifacts, and even good fixation causes **shrinkage** of proteins, especially near the nucleus and between cell boundaries. The most commonly used fixative is **10% formalin** buffered to neutral pH.

Dehydration

Because most widely used fixatives are aqueous solutions, the **water must be removed** before the tissue can be infiltrated with paraffin wax. This is accomplished by passing the tissue block through a series of progressively higher concentrations of an organic solvent (usually ethyl alcohol), until no water remains, i.e., **dehydration is complete.** This procedure facilitates the embedding of the tissue in melted paraffin.

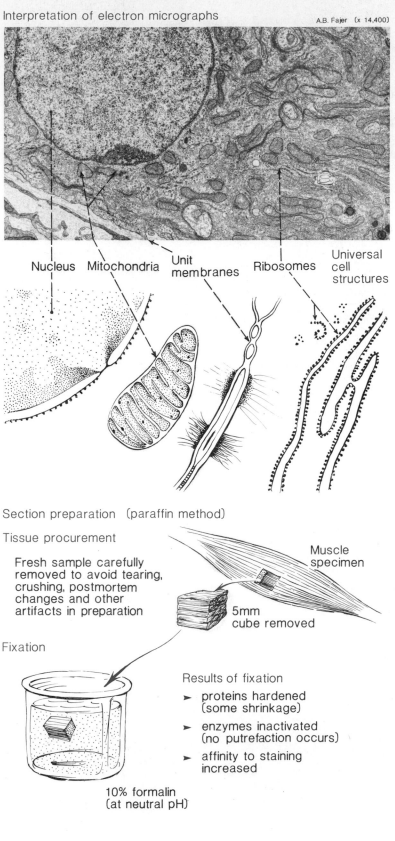

Interpretation of electron micrographs

A.B. Fajer (x 14,400)

Nucleus Mitochondria Unit membranes Ribosomes Universal cell structures

Section preparation (paraffin method)

Tissue procurement

Fresh sample carefully removed to avoid tearing, crushing, postmortem changes and other artifacts in preparation

Muscle specimen

5mm cube removed

Fixation

Results of fixation
- proteins hardened (some shrinkage)
- enzymes inactivated (no putrefaction occurs)
- affinity to staining increased

10% formalin (at neutral pH)

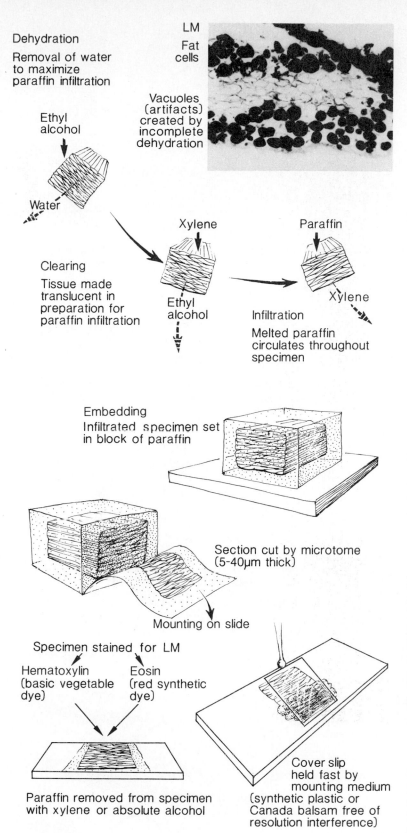

Dehydration

Removal of water to maximize paraffin infiltration

Ethyl alcohol

Water

LM

Fat cells

Vacuoles (artifacts) created by incomplete dehydration

Clearing

Tissue made translucent in preparation for paraffin infiltration

Xylene

Ethyl alcohol

Infiltration

Melted paraffin circulates throughout specimen

Paraffin

Xylene

Embedding

Infiltrated specimen set in block of paraffin

Section cut by microtome (5-40μm thick)

Mounting on slide

Specimen stained for LM

Hematoxylin (basic vegetable dye)

Eosin (red synthetic dye)

Paraffin removed from specimen with xylene or absolute alcohol

Cover slip held fast by mounting medium (synthetic plastic or Canada balsam free of resolution interference)

Clearing

The tissue is next "cleared," that is, made **translucent**, by immersing it in a clearing agent such as the organic solvent, **xylene**, which is miscible in both paraffin and alcohol. This procedure prepares the tissue so it can be rapidly **infiltrated by melted paraffin.**

Infiltration

The "cleared" block is now placed in a container of **melted paraffin** and placed in an oven, set at the melting point of paraffin, for several hours. The tissue remains in the melted wax until all of the **xylene is replaced by paraffin.** The step is called infiltration.

Embedding

When the tissue is completely infiltrated with wax, the block is transferred to another container of melted paraffin which is allowed to harden. The specimen block is trimmed and firmly secured to a metal block, which is mounted on a microtome, a slicing instrument, for sectioning.

Sectioning

The **microtome** is equipped with an advance mechanism sensitive enough to advance the tissue block in **intervals of 1 μm.** Thus, thin sections are usually cut ranging from 5 to 40 μm in thickness. Here again artifacts arise, e.g., tearing, wrinkling, and overlapping of tissues.

Staining

Before sections can be stained they must be attached to a microscopic glass slide and the paraffin removed, usually by xylene or infrequently by absolute alcohol. For light microscopy the most common stain is a combination of the weak **basic,** vegetable dye, **hematoxylin,** and the red, synthetic dye, **eosin.** The latter stains the cytoplasm various shades of red, or eosinophilic, while the nucleus is stained blue to purple, or basophilic, with hemotoxylin.

Mounting

For permanent preservation of a stained section, the tissue is covered by a drop of mounting medium and then covered by a thin glass wafer, called a **cover slip.** The medium may be a solution of synthetic plastic or Canada balsam, both of which harden upon evaporation. They have the **same refractive index** as glass and therefore do not interfere with the resolution of objects by the light microscope.

PLASTIC METHOD

For the past century, tissue specimens destined for light microscopy have been embedded in paraffin. Although this method has served the pathologist and the histologist well, it is flawed by its inability to preserve satisfactorily cytological detail. This deficiency is due primarily to the relative thickness (4–7 μm) of the paraffin sections.

During the early 1950s, microscopists became increasingly aware of the superior quality of microscopic slides prepared from **plastic embedded specimens,** a method formerly used exclusively in electron microscopy. Since plastic embedding **preserves tissue structures** much more faithfully than the paraffin method, the tissues have **less distortion** and therefore greatly enhance the diagnostic ability of the microscopist.

With a few modifications, the procedures for preparing plastic sections are quite similar to the paraffin method. These **modifications** include:

1. **Smaller specimen size** (13 × 11 mm as compared to 30 × 20 mm for paraffin embedding).

2. Formalin and/or **glutaraldehyde** as fixatives.

3. Glycol methacrylate or **epoxy resins** for embedding media.

4. Plastic rotary or **ultramicrotomes** and glass knives, for sectioning.

5. Sections are **very thin** (0.5–1.5 μm as compared to 4–7 μm for paraffin sections).

6. **Staining limited** to certain stains, e.g., H and E, PAS, toluidine blue.

PREPARATION OF ULTRAMICROSCOPIC SECTIONS

For transmission electron microscopy the rationale for tissue preparation is similar to light microscopy. These procedures include fixation, embedment, sectioning, and to a very limited extent, "staining." The differences are: (1) Two fixatives are usually used, i.e., **glutaraldehyde** followed by **osmium tetroxide,** which produce a fine coagulum of proteins with minimal structural distortion and the preservation of lipid structures. (2) Dehydration by organic solvents is followed by embedding in hard **acrylic or epoxy resins.** (3) Sectioning of the hardened resin block is accomplished by an **ultramicrotome** ca-

Preparation differences for paraffin, plastic, and ultramicroscopic methods of sectioning

		Paraffin	Plastic	Ultramicroscopic
1)	Specimen size	30 X 20 mm	13 X 11 mm	13 X 11 mm
2)	Fixatives	Formalin	Formalin and/or glutaraldehyde	Glutaraldehyde or osmium tetraoxide
3)	Embedding	Paraffin	Glycol methacrylate Epoxy resins	Hard acrylic or epoxy resins
4)	Sectioning tools	Microtome	Ultramicrotome Glass knives	Ultramicrotome with diamond knife or fractured plate glass
5)	Section thickness	4-7 μm	0.5-1.5 μm	50-100 nm
6)	Staining	Basophilic, acidophilic or other selective staining	Limited to: H & E, PAS, toluidine blue	Limited to salts of heavy metals

Resolution effects of plastic and paraffin methods

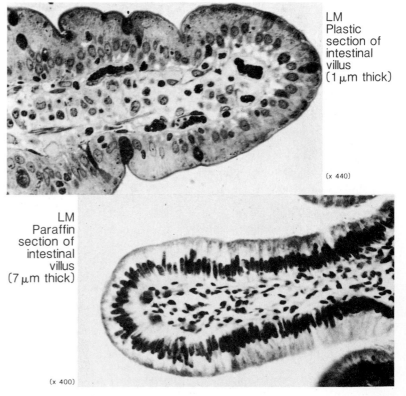

LM Plastic section of intestinal villus (1 μm thick)

(x 440)

LM Paraffin section of intestinal villus (7 μm thick)

(x 400)

Principles of freeze fracture method

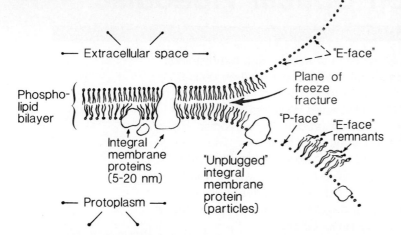

EM   Freeze fracture replica

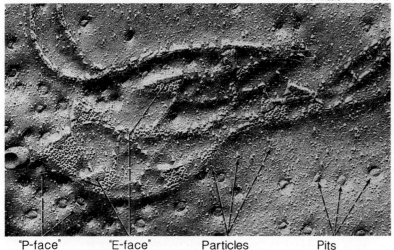

J.J. Anders (x 135,000)

"P-face"   "E-face"   Particles   Pits

Microscope categories

Visible light

► light (bright field)
► phase contrast
► dark field
► polarizing
► interference

Invisible radiation

► electron (transmission)
► x-ray
► ultra-violet
► scanning

pable of cutting very thin **sections 50–100 nm** thick with a diamond knife or the fractured edge of plate glass. (4) Staining, in the conventional color sense, does not exist. However, when sections are exposed to salts of heavy metals, such as **uranyl acetate and lead hydroxide,** they are deposited on certain regions or organelles, imparting various **degrees of density** to these structures. Thus, light (electron-lucent) and dark (electron-dense) images can be registered photographically as black, white, or shades of grey.

Freeze Fracture

A transmission electron microscopic technique in wide use is freeze fracture, a method that provides a view of the three-dimensional contours of cells and organelles and reveals the internal structure of their membranes.

The value of the freeze-fracture technique is derived from the fact that the plane of fracture through frozen tissue tends to follow the hydrophobic interiors of lipid bilayers of membranes. Broad expanses of cell membrane are thus exposed on the fracture face, separated by areas where the fracture plane cracked through organelles and their membranes, cytoplasm, or extracellular space. The exposed membrane surface in a freeze-fracture replica is either the interior (i.e., hydrophobic) surface of one of the two leaflets adjacent to extracellular space (the "**E face**"), or the outward-directed face of the leaflet adjacent to protoplasm (the "**P face**"). On the adjacent freeze-fracture replica, the E and P faces are exposed. On the P face, the well-spaced, spheroid depressions are called pits. As seen in TEM micrographs, they are probably identified as vacuoles or caveolae.

Interpretation and Electron Micrographs

A first step in learning to make sense of electron micrographs is to learn to identify a small number of structures that are **universally present** in biological tissues. The most common and readily identifiable structures are nuclei, mitochondria, membranes, microtubules, and the ribosomes of rough endoplasmic reticulum. If one learns the **diagnostic features** of each of these organelles, then one can identify them in any of their various guises. They can then be used as internal gauges to assess the relative **magnification** of virtually any electron micrograph of biological tissue and the probable **identity** of other less common organelles.

A Visual Data Base on Optical Videodisc

The barcodes printed in this book allow users to supplement the histologic information contained in the book with visual information stored on optical videodisc. Full color images of tissue sections (over 2500 in number) have been stored on videodisc by Dr. Frank D. Allan of George Washington University.

To facilitate access to the photomicrographs stored on the videodisc, disc frame numbers are sandwiched between two types of barcodes. The barcode systems used are "interleaved 2 of 5" and the alphanumeric "code 3 of 9." The barcodes in the book can be read by inexpensive barcode scanner wands. For further information on the barcode approach, including hardware and user-supported shareware (software), write to the developer of this systems design: David S. Lyons, P.O. Box 1177, Oak Park, Illinois 60304.

Instructors using this book may also want to use the Textual Data Base available with the videodisc developed by Dr. Allan. This was accomplished in collaboration with the staff at the Lister Hill National Center for Biomedical Communications, National Library of Medicine.

For information on purchasing the optical videodisc, titled *Human Light Microscopy,* and for obtaining software on the Textual Data Base, write to the distributors of the disc and software:

Health Sciences Center for Educational Resources
SB-56
University of Washington
Seattle, Washington 98195

REFERENCES

Chapter 1: Cytoplasmic Organelles and Inclusions

Alberts B, Bray D, Lewis I, Raff M, Roberts K, Watson JD: Molecular Biology of the Cell. New York, Garland, 1983.

Bretscher MS: The molecules of the cell membrane. Sci Am 253:100, 1985.

DeDuve C: Microbodies in the living cell. Sci Am 248:74, 1983.

Farquhar MG, Palade GE: The Golgi apparatus (complex) (1954–1981): Artifact to center stage. J Cell Biol 91:77s, 1981.

Fawcett D: The Cell, ed 2. Philadelphia, WB Saunders, 1981.

Holtzmann E: Lysosomes: A Survey. New York, Springer-Verlag, 1976.

Hooke R: Micrographia: Or Some Physiological Descriptions of Minute Bodies Made by Magnifying Glasses, with Observations and Inquiries Thereupon. J. Martyn and J. Allestry, London (facsimile edition, Culture et Civilization, Brussels), 1665.

Krstić RV: Ultrastructure of the Mammalian Cell. Berlin, Springer-Verlag, 1979.

Lake JA: The ribosome. Sci Am 245:84, 1981.

Lentz TL: Cell Fine Structure: An Atlas of Drawings and Whole-Cell Structure. Philadelphia, WB Saunders, 1971.

Luft JH: The structure and properties of the cell surface coat. Int Rev Cytol 45:291, 1976.

Osborn M, Weber K: Intermediate filaments: Cell-type-specific markers in differentiation and pathology. Cell 31:303, 1982.

Porter KR: The cytomatrix: A short history of its study. J Cell Biol 99 (No. 1, Part 2):3s, 1984.

Rothman J: The compartmental organization of the Golgi apparatus. Sci Am 253:74, 1985.

Singer SJ, Nicolson GL: The fluid mosaic model of the structure of cell membranes. Science 175:720, 1972.

Whittaker PA, Danks SM: Mitochondria: Structure, Function, and Assembly. New York, Longman, 1979.

Chapter 2: The Nucleus and Its Organelles

Alberts B, Bray D, Lewis J, Raff M, Roberts K, Watson JD: Molecular Biology of the Cell. New York, Garland, 1983, pp. 385–435.

Goessens G: Nucleolar structure. Int Rev Cytol 87:107, 1984.

Igo-Kemenes T, Horz W, Zachu HG: Chromatin. Annu Rev Biochem 51:89, 1982.

Inoue S: Cell division and the mitotic spindle. J Cell Biol 91:131s, 1981.

John B, Lewis KR: The meiotic mechanism. In Oxford Biology Readers. JJ Head, (ed.). Oxford, Oxford University Press, 1976.

Jordan EG: The Nucleolus, ed 2. Oxford, Oxford University Press, 1978.

Kornberg RD, Klug A: The nucleosome. Sci Am 244:52, 1981.

Lloyd D, Poole PK, Edwards SW: The Cell Division Cycle. New York, Academic Press, 1982.

Pickett-Heaps JD, Tippit DH, Porter KR: Rethinking mitosis. Cell 29:729, 1982.

Wischnitzer S: The nuclear envelope: Its ultrastructure and functional significance. Endeavour 33:137, 1974.

Chapter 3: Primary Tissues

Bourne GH (ed.): The Structure and Function of Muscle, Vols 1–3. New York, Academic Press, 1960.

Bourne GH (ed.): Structure and Function of Nervous Tissue, Vols 1–5. New York, Academic Press, 1972.

Clark WE, Le Gros: The Tissues of the Body, ed 6. Oxford, Clarendon Press, 1975.

Huddart H: The Comparative Structure and Function of Muscle. Oxford, Pergamon Press, 1975.

Jackson SF: Connective tissue cells. In The Cell, Vol 6. J Brachet and AE Mirsky (eds.). New York, Academic Press, 1964, p. 387.

Leblond CP, Walker BE: Renewal of cell populations. Physiol Rev 36:255, 1956.

Peters A, Palay SL, Webster HF: The Fine Structure of the Nervous System. Philadelphia, WB Saunders, 1976.

Ragan C (ed.): Connective Tissues. 3rd Conf. Josiah Macy, Jr., Foundation, New York, 1953.

Simons K, Fuller SD: Cell surface polarity in epithelia. Annu Rev Cell Biol 1:243, 1985.

Chapter 4: Epithelium

Alberts B, Bray D, Lewis J, Raff M, Roberts K, Watson JD: Cell junctions. *In* Molecular Biology of the Cell. New York, Garland, 1983, p. 682.

Berridge MJ, Oschman JL: Transporting Epithelia. New York, Academic Press, 1972.

Bridgman PC, Reese TS: The structure of cytoplasm in directly frozen cultured cells. I. Filamentous meshworks and the cytoplasmic ground substance. J Cell Biol 99:1655, 1984.

Farquhar MG, Palade GE: Junctional complexes in various epithelia. J Cell Biol 17:375, 1963.

Fawcett D: The Cell, ed 2. Philadelphia, WB Saunders, 1981.

Gilula NB: Junctions between Cells. *In* Cell Communication. RP Cox (ed.). New York, Wiley, 1974.

Hertzberg EL, Lawrence TS, Gilula NB: Gap junctional communication. Annu Rev Physiol 43:479, 1981.

Hirokawa N, Tilney LG, Fujiwara K, Heuser JE: Organization of actin, myosin, and intermediate filaments in the brush border of intestinal epithelial cells. J Cell Biol 94:425, 1982.

Hull BE, Staehelin LA: The terminal web: A reevaluation of its structure and function. J Cell Biol 81:67, 1979.

Porter KR, Tucker JB: The ground substance of the living cell. Sci Am 244:57, 1981.

Simons K, Fuller SD: Cell surface polarity in epithelia. Annu Rev Cell Biol 1:243, 1985.

Staehelin LA, Hull B: Junctions between living cells. Sci Am 238:140, 1978.

Chapter 5: Specializations of Epithelia—Glands, Serous and Mucous Membranes

Baron MA: Structure of the intestinal peritoneum in man. Am J Anat 69:439, 1941.

Cunningham RS: The physiology of the serous membranes. Physiol Rev 6:242, 1926.

Odor DL: Observations of the rat mesothelium with the electron and phase microscopes. Am J Anat 95:433, 1954.

Puumala RH: Morphologic comparison of the parietal and the visceral peritoneal epithelium in fetus and adult. Anat Rec 68:327, 1937.

Chapter 6: Connective Tissue

Alberts B, Bray D, Lewis J, Raff M, Roberts K, Watson JD: The extracellular matrix. *In* Molecular Biology of the Cell. New York, Garland, 1983, p. 692.

Angel A, Hollenberg CH, Roncari DAK (eds.): The Adipocyte and Obesity: Cellular and Molecular Mechanisms. New York, Raven Press, 1983.

Aschoff L: Das reticulo-endotheliale System. Ergeb Inn Med und Kinderheilkd 26:1, 1924.

Bornstein P, Sage H: Structurally distinct collagen types. Annu Rev Biochem 49:957, 1980.

Carr I: The Macrophage: A Review of Ultrastructure and Function. New York, Academic Press, 1973.

Fessler JH, Fessler LI: Biosynthesis of procollagen. Annu Rev Biochem 47:129, 1978.

Gabbiani G, Rungger-Brandle E: The fibroblast. *In* Tissue Repair and Regeneration. Handbook of Inflammation, Vol 3. LE Glynn (ed.). Amsterdam, Elsevier/North Holland Biomedical Press, 1981, p. 1.

Hall DA: The Aging of Connective Tissue. New York, Academic Press, 1976.

Hay ED (ed.): Cell Biology of the Extracellular Matrix. New York, Plenum, 1981.

Heathcote JG, Grant ME: The molecular organization of basement membranes. Int Rev Connect Tissue Res 9:191, 1981.

Kleinman HK, Klebe HK, Martin GR: Role of collagenous matrices in the adhesion and growth of cells. J Cell Biol 88:473, 1981.

Montes GS, et al: Histochemical and morphological characterization of reticular fibers. Histochemistry 65:131, 1980.

Nedergaard J, Linburg O: The brown fat cell. Int Rev Cytol 74:310, 1982.

Pearsall NN, Weisser RS: The Macrophage. Philadelphia, Lea & Febiger, 1981.

Riley JF: The Mast Cells. Edinburgh, E&S Livingstone, 1959.

Ross R, Bornstein P: Elastic fibers in the body. Sci Am 224:44, 1971.

Sbarra AJ, Strauss RR: (eds.): The Reticuloendothelial System. *In* Biochemistry and Metabolism. Vol 2, New York: Plenum, 1980.

Chapter 7: Cartilage, Bone, and Joints

Bourne GH (ed.): The Biochemistry and Physiology of Bone, ed 2, 4 vols. New York, Academic Press, 1971–1976.

Fischman DA, Hay ED: Origin of osteoclast from mononuclear leukocytes in regenerating new limbs. Anat Rec 143:329, 1962.

Hall BK (ed.): Cartilage, Vol 1, Structure, Function and Biochemistry. New York, Academic Press, 1983.

Hancox NM: Biology of Bone. London, Cambridge University Press, 1972.

Holtrop ME, King, GJ: The ultrastructure of the osteoclast and its functional implications. Clin Orthop 123:177, 1977.

Jande SS, Belanger JF: The life-cycle of the osteocyte. Clin Orthop 94:281, 1973.

Jones SJ, Boyde A: The migration of osteoblasts. Cell Tissue Res 184:179, 1977.

Jones SJ, Boyde A: Some morphologic observations on osteoclasts. Cell Tissue Res 185:387, 1977.

Kimmel DB, Jee WSS: Bone cell kinetics during longitudinal bone growth in the rat. Calcif Tissue Int 32:123, 1980.

Minns RJ, Stevens FS: The collagen fibril organization in human articular cartilage. J Anat 123:437, 1977.

Owen M: Histogenesis of bone cells. Calcif Tissue Res 25:205, 1978.

Parfitt AM: The actions of parathyroid hormone on bone. Metabolism 25:809, 1976.

Rasmussen H, Bordier P: Vitamin D and bone. Metab Bone Dis Res 1:7, 1978.

Sokoloff L (ed.): The Joints and Synovial Fluid. New York, Academic Press, 1978.

Chapter 8: Circulating Blood and Lymph

Bessis M: Living Blood Cells and Their Ultrastructure. New York, Springer-Verlag, 1973.

Bessis M: Corpuscles. Atlas of Red Blood Cells Shapes. Berlin, Springer-Verlag, 1974.

Bishop C, Surgenor DM (eds.): The Red Blood Cell. New York, Academic Press, 1964.

Cline MJ: The White Cell. Cambridge, MA, Harvard University Press, 1975.

Kincade PW: Formulation of B lymphocytes in fetal and adult life. Adv Immunol 31:177, 1981.

Smith JA: Molecular and cellular properties of eosinophils (a review). Ric Clin Lab 11:181, 1981.

Weissmann G (ed.): The Cell Biology of Inflammation, Handbook of Inflammation, Vol 2. Amsterdam, Elsevier/North Holland Biomedical Press, 1980.

Zucker-Franklin D et al: Atlas of Blood Cells: Function and Pathology, Vols 1 and 2. Philadelphia, Lea & Febiger, 1981.

Chapter 9: Hemopoiesis

Ackerman GA: The human neutrophil myelocyte. A correlated phase and electron microscopic study. Z Zellforsch Mikrosk Anat 121:153, 1971.

Bainton DF, Farquhar MG: Segregation and packaging of granule enzymes in eosinophilic leukocytes. J Cell Biol 45:54, 1970.

Bainton DF, Ullvot JL, Farquhar MG: The development of neutrophilic polymorphonuclear leukocytes in human bone marrow: Origin and content of azurophil and specific granules. J Exp Med 134:907, 1971.

Bessis M: Life Cycle of the Erythrocyte. Sandoz Monographs. Basel, Sandoz Ltd, 1966.

Diggs LW, et al: The Morphology of Human Blood Cells, ed 4. Abbott Laboratories, 1984. Abbott Park, Ill.

Golde DW, Cline MJ: Regulation of granulopoiesis. N Engl J Med 231:1388, 1974.

Lajtha LG: Haemophoietic stem cells: Concepts and definitions. Blood Cells 5:447, 1979.

Metcalf D: Regulation of hemopoiesis. Nouv Rev Fr Hematol 20:521, 1978.

Meuret G: Origin, ontogeny and kinetics of mononuclear phagocytes. Adv Exp Med Biol 73(Part A):71, 1976.

Nichols BA, Bainton DF, Farquhar MG: Differentiation of monocytes: Origin, nature and fate of their azurophil granules. J Cell Biol 50:498, 1971.

Osmond DG: Formation and maturation of bone marrow lymphocytes. J Reticuloendothel Soc 17:99, 1975.

Pennington DG: The cellular biology of megakaryocytes. Blood Cells 5:5, 1979.

Van Furth R: Current view on the mononuclear phagocyte system. Immunobiology 161:178, 1982.

Weiss L: The hematopoietic microenvironment of the bone marrow: An ultrastructural study of the stroma in rats. Anat Rec 186:161, 1976.

Yoffey JM: Transitional cells of haemopoietic tissues: Origin, structure, and developmental potential. Int Rev Cytol 62:311, 1980.

Chapter 10: Muscle Tissue

Alberts B, Bray D, Lewis J, Raff M, Roberts K, Watson JD: Muscle contraction. *In* Molecular Biology of the Cell. New York, Garland, 1983, pp. 550–561.

Bourne GH (ed.): The Structure and Function of Muscle. New York, Academic Press, 1972.

Bülbring E, Bolton TD (eds.): Smooth muscle. Br Med Bull 35:127, 1979.

Campion DR: The muscle satellite cell: A review. Int Rev Cytol 87:225, 1984.

Franzini-Armstrong, C, Peachey LD: Striated muscle: Contractile and control mechanisms. J Cell Biol 88:166, 1981.

Huddart H: The Comparative Structure and Function of Muscle. Oxford, Pergamon Press, 1975.

Huxley HE: The mechanism of muscular contraction. Science 164:1356, 1969.

Sommer JR, Waugh RA: The ultrastructure of the mammalian cardiac muscle cell—with special emphasis on the tubular membrane systems: A review. Am J Pathol 82:192, 1976.

Stratcher A (ed.): Muscle and Nonmuscle Motility, Vol 1. New York, Academic Press, 1963.

Telford IR: Loss of nerve endings in degenerated skeletal muscles of young vitamin E deficient rats. Anat Rec 81:171, 1941.

Telford IR: Experimental Muscular Dystrophies in Animals. A Comparative Study. Springfield, IL, Charles C Thomas, 1971.

Chapter 11: Nervous Tissue

Axelrod J: Neurotransmitters. Sci Am 230:58, 1974.

Bourne GH (ed.): The Structure and Function of Nervous Tissue, Vol 1. New York, Academic Press, 1968.

Bridgman CF, Eldred E: Hypothesis for a pressure-sensitive mechanism in muscle spindles. Science 143:481–482, 1962.

De Robertis EDP: Ultrastructure and cytochemistry of the synaptic region. Science 156:907, 1967.

Friede RL, Samorajski T: The clefts of Schmidt-Lantermann: A quantitative electron microscopic study of their structure in developing and adult sciatic nerves of the rat. Anat Rec 165:89, 1969.

Hubbard JI (ed.): The Peripheral Nervous System. New York, Plenum Press, 1974.

Jacobson M, Hunt RK: The origins of nerve-cell specificity. Sci Am 228:26, 1973.

Landon DN (ed.): The Peripheral Nerve. London, Chapman & Hall, 1976.

Langley JN: The Autonomic Nervous System, Vol 1. Cambridge, UK, Heffer, 1921.

Morell P, Norton WT: Myelin. Sci Am 242:88, 1980.

Ruffini A: Sur un nouvel Organe nerveux terminal et sur la présence des corpuscles Golgi-Mazzoni dans le conjonctif sous-cutané de la pulpe des doigts de l'homme. Arch Ital Biol 21:249, 1894.

Scharrer E: The general significance of the neurosecretory cell. Scientia 46:177, 1952.

Schwartz JH: The transport of substances in nerve cells. Sci Am 242:152, 1980.

Chapter 12: Central Nervous System

Brightman MW, et al: The blood-brain barrier to proteins under normal and pathological conditions. J Neurol Sci 10:215, 1970.

Junqueira LCU, Montes GS, Krisztán RM: The collagen of the vertebrate peripheral nervous system. Cell Tissue Res 202:453, 1979.

Llinas RR: The cortex of the cerebellum. Sci Am 232:56, 1975.

Morales R, Duncan D: Specialized contacts of astrocytes with astrocytes and other cell types in the spinal cord of the cat. Anat Rec 182:255, 1975.

Palay SL, Chan-Palay V: Cerebral Cortex, Cytology and Organization. New York, Springer-Verlag, 1974.

Peters A, Palay S, Webster H: The Fine Structure of the Nervous System: The Neurons and Supporting Cells. Philadelphia, WB Saunders, 1976.

Shepherd GM: Microcircuits in the nervous system. Sci Am 238:93, 1978.

Stevens CF: The neuron. Sci Am 241:55, 1979.

Chapter 13: Circulatory System

Challice CE, Viragh S (eds.): Ultrastructure of the Mammalian Heart. New York, Academic Press, 1973.

Fishman AP: Endothelium. Ann NY Acad Sci 401:1–8, 1982.

Kaley G, Altura BM (eds.): Microcirculation, Vols 1–3. Baltimore, University Park Press, 1977–1978.

Maul GG: Structure and formation of pores in fenestrated capillaries. J Ultrastruct Res 36:768, 1971.

McNutt NS, Fawcett DW: Myocardial ultrastructure.

In The Mammalian Myocardium. GA Langer and TW Brady (eds.). New York, Wiley, 1974, pp. 1–49.

Rhodin JAG: Architecture of the vessel wall. *In* Handbook of Physiology, Section 2: Cardiovascular System, Vol 2. RM Berne (ed.), American Physiological Society, Bethesda, Md. 1980, pp. 1–31.

Ross R: Atherosclerosis: A problem of the biology of arterial wall cells and their interactions with blood components. Arteriosclerosis 1:293, 1981.

Simionescu N, Simionescu M, Palade GE: Recent studies on vascular endothelium. Ann NY Acad Sci 275:64, 1976.

Simionescu N: Cellular aspects of transcapillary exchange. Physiol Rev 63:1536, 1983.

Truex RC: Structural basis of atrial and ventricular conduction. Cardiovasc Clin 6:1, 1974.

Chapter 14: Lymphatic System

Alberts B, Bray D, Lewis J, Raff M, Roberts K, Watson JD: The cellular basis of immunity. *In* Molecular Biology of the Cell. New York, Garland, 1983, pp. 952–963.

Bach JF: Thymic hormones. J Immunopharmacol 1:277, 1979.

Bearman RM, Levine GD, Bensch KG: The ultrastructure of the normal human thymus: A study of 36 cases. Anat Rec 190:755, 1978.

Borkman DB, Cooper MD: Pinocytosis by epithelium associated with lymphoid follicles in the bursa of Fabricius, appendix. and Peyer's patches. An electron microscopic study. Am J Anat 136:455, 1973.

Chen LL, Adams JC, Steinman RM: Anatomy of germinal centers in mouse spleen, with special reference to "follicular dendritic cells." J Cell Biol 77:148, 1978.

Chen LT, Weiss L: Electron microscopy of the red pulp of human spleen. Am J Anat 134:425, 1972.

Chen LT: Microcirculation of the spleen: An open or closed circulation? Science 201:157, 1978.

Fujita T: A scanning electron microscope study of the human spleen. Arch Histol Jpn 37:187, 1974.

Hirasawa Y, Tokuhiro H: Electron microscopic studies on the normal human spleen, especially on the red pulp and the reticuloendothelial cells. Blood 35:201, 1970.

Klaus GGB, et al: The follicular dendritic cell: Its role in antigen presentation in the generation of immunological memory. Immunol Rev 53:3, 1980.

Marrack P, Kappler J: The T cell and its receptor. Sci Am 254:36, 1986.

Pictet R, Orci L, Forssmann WG, Girardier L: An electron microscope study of the perfusion-fixed spleen. I. The splenic circulation and the RES concept. Z Zellforsch Mikrosk Anat 96:372, 1969.

Stevens SK, Weissman IL, Butcher EC: Differences in the migration of B and T lymphocytes: Organ-selective localization in vivo and the role of lymphocyte-endothelial cell recognition. J Immunol 128:844, 1982.

Weiss L: A scanning electron microscopic study of the spleen. Blood 43:665, 1974.

Chapter 15: The Integumentary System

Epstein WL, Maibach HI: Cell renewal in human epidermis. Arch Dermatol 92:462, 1965.

Green H: The keratinocyte as differentiated cell types. Harvey Lect 74:101, 1980.

Guevedo WC Jr: Epidermal melanin units: Melanocyte-keratinocyte interactions. Am Zool 12:35, 1972.

Iggo A: Cutaneous and subcutaneous sense organs. Br Med Bull 33:97, 1977.

Jarrett A (ed.): The Hair Follicle. London, Academic Press, 1977.

Lockhart RD, Hamilton GF, Fyfe FW: Anatomy of the Human Body. Philadelphia, JB Lippincott, 1959.

Matoltsy AG: Desmosomes, filaments and keratohyaline granules: Their role in the stabilization and keratinization of the epidermis. J Invest Dermatol 65:127, 1975.

Millington PF, Wilkinson R: Skin. London, Cambridge University Press, 1983.

Montagna W, Parakkal PF: The Structure and Function of Skin. ed. 3, New York, Academic Press, 1974.

Shelley WB, Lennart J: The Langerhans cell: Its origin, nature and function. Acta Derm Venereol (Stockh) 79:7, 1978.

Strauss JS, Fochi PE, Downing DT: The sebaceous glands: Twenty-five years of progress. J Invest Dermatol 67:90, 1976.

Terzakis JA: The ultrastructure of monkey eccrine sweat glands. Z Zellforsch Mikrosk Anat 64:493, 1964.

Winkelman RK: The Merkel cell system and a comparison between it and the neurosecretory or APUD cell system. J Invest Dermatol 69:41, 1977.

Zaias N, Alvarez J: The formation of the primate nail plate. J Invest Dermatol 51:120, 1968.

Chapter 16: Respiratory System

Andrews PM: A scanning electron microscopic study of the extrapulmonary respiratory tract. Am J Anat 139:399, 1974.

Breeze RG, Wheeldon EB: The cells of the pulmonary airways. Am Rev Respir Dis 116:705, 1977.

Fink BR: The Human Larynx: A Functional Study. New York, Raven, 1975.

Goerke J: Lung surfactant. Biochim Biophys Acta 344:241, 1979.

Graziadei PPC, Monti Graziadei GA: In Handbook of Sensory Physiology, Vol IX: Development of Sensory Systems: Continuous Nerve Cell Renewal in the Olfactory System. M Jacobson (ed.). New York, Springer-Verlag, 1978, p. 55.

Hocking WB, Golde DW: The pulmonary-alveolar macrophage. N Engl J Med 301:580–639, 1979

Miller WS: The Lung, ed 2. Springfield, IL, Charles C Thomas, 1947.

Nagaishi C: Functional Anatomy and Histology of the Lung. Baltimore, University Park Press, 1972.

Stratton JC: The ultrastructure of multilamellar bodies and surfactant in the human lung. Cell Tissue Res 193:219, 1978.

Thurlbeck WM, Abell MR (eds.): The Lung: Structure, Function, and Disease. Baltimore, Williams & Wilkins, 1978.

Weibel ER: Morphological basis of alveolar-capillary gas exchange. Physiol Rev 53:419, 1973.

Weibel ER: The Pathway for Oxygen. Cambridge, Harvard University Press, 1984.

Widdicombe JG, Pack RJ: The Clara cell. Eur J Respir Dis 63:202, 1982.

Chapter 17: Digestive System I—Oral Cavity and Pharynx

Beertsen WM, Brekelmans M, Everts V: The site of collagen resorption in the periodontal ligament of the rodent molar. Anat Rec 192:305, 1978.

Beidler LM, Smallman RL: Renewal of cells with the taste buds. J Cell Biol 27:263, 1965.

Bernard GW: Ultrastructural observations of initial calcification in dentin and enamel. J Ultrastruct Res 41:1, 1972.

Castle JD, Jamieson JD, Palade GE: Radioautographic analysis of the secretory process in the parotid acinar cell of the rabbit. J Cell Biol 53:290, 1972.

Frank RM: Tooth enamel: Current state of the art. J Dent Res 58(B):684, 1979.

Hodgson ES: Taste receptors. Sci Am 204:135, 1961.

Leblond CP, Warshawsky H: Dynamics of enamel formation in the rat incisor tooth. J Dent Res 58(B):950, 1979.

Mjör IA, Fejerskow O: Histology of the Human Tooth, ed 2. Copenhagen, Munksgaard, 1979.

Murray RG: The ultrastructure of taste buds. In The Ultrastructure of Sensory Organs. J Friedmann (ed.). Amsterdam, North Holland, 1973, p. 1.

Ten Cate AR: Oral Histology: Development, Structure and Function. St. Louis, CV Mosby, 1980.

Young, JA, van Lennep EW: The Morphology of Salivary Glands. New York, Academic Press, 1978.

Chapter 18: Digestive System II—Alimentary Canal

Cheng H, Leblond CP: Origin, differentiation and renewal of the four main epithelial cell types in the mouse small intestine. 5. Unitarian theory of the origin of the four epithelial cell types. Am J Anat 141:537, 1974.

Davenport HW: Why the stomach does not digest itself. Sci Am 226:87, 1972.

Erlandsen SL, Parsons JA, Taylor TD: Ultrastructural immunocytochemical localization of lysozyme in the Paneth cells of man. J Histochem Cytochem 22:401, 1974.

Forte JG: Mechanism of gastric H^+ and Cl^- transport. Annu Rev Physiol 42:111, 1980.

Freeman JA: Goblet cell fine structure. Anat Rec 154:121, 1966.

Fujita T, Kobayashi S: Structure and function of gut endocrine cells. Int Rev Cytol (Suppl) No. 6:187, 1977.

Gannon BJ, et al: Mucosal microvascular architecture of the fundus and body of the human stomach. Gastroenterology 86:866, 1984.

Grube D, Forssmann WG: Morphology and function of the entero-endocrine cells. Horm Metab Res 11:589, 1979.

Hapwood D, et al: The electron microscopy of normal human esophageal epithelium. Virchows Arch (Cell Pathol) 26:345, 1978.

Leeson TS, Leeson CR: The fine structure of Brunner's glands in man. J Anat 103:263, 1968.

Moog F: The lining of the small intestine. Sci Am 245:154, 1981.

Pearse AGE: The diffuse neuroendocrine system: Peptides, amines, placodes and the APUD theory. Prog Brain Res 68:25, 1986.

Siten W, Ito S: Mechanisms for rapid epithelialization of the gastric mucosal surface. Annu Rev Physiol 47:217, 1985.

Tagaki T, et al: Scanning electron microscopy on the human gastric mucosa: Fetal, normal and various pathological conditions. Acta Pathol Jpn 24:233, 1974.

Chapter 19: Digestive System III—Pancreas, Liver, and Biliary Tract

Bruni C, Porter KR: The fine structure of the parenchymal cell of the normal rat liver. Am J Pathol 46:691, 1965.

Elias H, Sherrick JC: Morphology of the Liver. New York, Academic Press, 1969.

Howard JG: The origin and immunological significance of the Kupffer cells. In Mononuclear Phagocytes. R VanFurth (ed.). Oxford, Blackwell, 1970.

Motta PM: Three-dimensional architecture of the mammalian liver. A scanning electron microscopic review. In Three Dimensional Microanatomy of Cells and Tissue Surfaces. DJ Allen, PM Motta, and JA DiDio (eds.). New York, Elsevier/North-Holland, 1981, pp. 33–50.

Mueller JC, Jones AL, Long JA: Topographical and subcellular anatomy of the guinea pig gallbladder. Gastroenterology 63:856, 1972.

Rappaport AM: Physioanatomical basis of toxic liver injury. In Toxic Injury of the Liver, Part A. E Farber and MM Fisher (eds.). New York, Marcel Dekker, 1979.

Tanikawa K: Ultrastructural Aspects of the Liver and Its Disorders, ed. 2. Tokyo, Igaku-Shoin, 1979.

Wisse, E, Knook DL (eds.): Kupffer Cells and Other Sinusoidal Cells. New York, Elsevier/North-Holland, 1977.

Chapter 20: Urinary System

Andrews PM, Porter KR: A scanning electron microscopic study of the nephron. Am J Anat 140:81, 1974.

Barajas L: The ultrastructure of the juxtaglomerular apparatus as disclosed by three-dimensional reconstructions from serial sections. The anatomical relationship between the tubular and vascular components. J Ultrastruct Res 33:116, 1970.

Brenner BM, Rector FC (eds.): The Kidney, Vol 1, ed 2. Philadelphia, WB Saunders, 1981.

Christensen JA, Meyers DS, Bohle A: The structure of the human juxtaglomerular apparatus. Arch Pathol Anat Histol 367:83, 1975.

Farquhar MG: The glomerular basement membrane: A selective macromolecular filter. In Cell Biology of Extracellular Matrix. E Hay (ed.). New York, Plenum Press, 1981, p. 417.

Fujita T, Tokunga J, Edanaga M: Scanning electron microscopy of the glomerular filtration membrane in the rat kidney. Cell Tissue Res 166:299, 1976.

Ganong WF: Formation and excretion of urine. Chapter 38 in Review of Medical Physiology, ed 13. Los Altos, CA, Lange, 1987, pp. 581–606.

Harmanci MC, Kachadorian WA, Valtin H, DiScala VA: Antidiuretic hormone-induced intramembranous alterations in mammalian collecting ducts. Am J Physiol 235:F440–F443, 1978.

Hicks, RM: The fine structure of transitional epithelium of the rat ureter. J Cell Biol 26:25, 1965.

Hicks RM: The mammalian urinary bladder: An accommodating organ. Biol Rev 50:215, 1975.

Hicks RM, Ketterer B: Isolation of the plasma membrane of the luminal surface of rat bladder epithelium, and the occurrence of a hexagonal lattice of subunits both in negatively stained whole mounts and in sectional membranes. J Cell Biol 45:542, 1970.

Kokko JP, Rector FC: Countercurrent multiplication system without active transport in the inner medulla. Kidney Int 2:214, 1972.

Kriz W, Lever AF: Renal countercurrent mechanisms: Structure and function. Am Heart J 78:101, 1969.

Michielsen P, Creemers J: The structure and function of the glomerular mesangium. In Ultrastructure of the Kidney. AJ Dalton and F Haguenau (eds.). New York, Academic Press, 1967, p. 57.

Osvaldo L, Latta H: The thin limb of the loop of Henle. J Ultrastruct Res 15:144, 1966.

Smith HW: The Kidney. New York, Oxford University Press, 1969.

Staehelin A, Chlapowski FJ, Bonneville MA: Luminal plasma membrane of the urinary bladder. I. Three-dimensional reconstruction from freeze-etch images. J Cell Biol 53:73, 1972.

Chapter 21: Endocrine System I—Pituitary and Hypothalamus

Bargmann W: Neurosecretion. Int Rev Cytol 19:183, 1966.

Bergland RM, Page RB: Pituitary-brain vascular relations: A new paradigm. Science 204:18, 1979.

Bhatnagar AS (ed.): The Anterior Pituitary Gland. New York, Raven Press, 1983.

Brownstein MJ, Russell JT, Gainer H: Synthesis, transport and release of posterior pituitary hormones. Science 207:373, 1980.

Cross BA, Leng G (eds.): The neurohypophysis: Structure, function and control. Prog Brain Res 60:3, 1982.

Dierickx K, Vandesande F: Immunocytochemical localization of the vasopressinergic and oxytocinergic neurons in the human hypothalamus. Cell Tissue Res 184:15, 1977.

Duello TM, Halmi NS: Ultrastructural immunocytochemical localization of growth hormone and prolactin in human pituitaries. J Clin Endocrinol 49:189, 1979.

Guillemin R, Burgus R: The hormones of the hypothalamus. Sci Am 227 (5):24, 1972.

Hadley ME, Heward CB, Hruby VJ, Sawyer TK, Yang YCS: Biological actions of melanocyte-stimulating hormone. *In* Peptides of the Pars Intermedia. D. Evered, G Lawrenson (eds.). Ciba Foundation Symposium 81. London, Pitman Medical, 1981, pp. 244–262.

Herlant M: The cells of the adenohypophysis and their functional significance. Int Rev Cytol 17:299, 1974.

Holmes RL, Ball JN: The Pituitary Gland: A Comparative Account. Biological Structure and Functional Series, Vol 4. London, Cambridge University Press, 1974.

Morris JF, et al: Structure-function correlation in mammalian neurosecretion. Int Rev Exp Pathol 18:1, 1973.

Reichlin S (ed.): The Neurohypophysis: Physiological and Clinical Aspects. New York, Plenum, 1984.

Seyama S, Pearl GS, Takei Y: Ultrastructural study of the human neurohypophysis. 1. Neurosecretory axons and their dilatations in the pars nervosa. Cell Tissue Res 205:253, 1980.

Tixier-Vidal A, Farquhar MG (eds.): The Anterior Pituitary. New York, Academic Press, 1975.

Chapter 22: Endocrine System II—Adrenal, Thyroid, Parathyroid, and Pineal

Brown WJ, Barajas L, Latta H: The ultrastructure of the human adrenal medulla: With comparative studies of white rat. Anat Rec 169:173, 1971.

Christy NP (ed.): The Human Adrenal Cortex. New York, Harper & Row, 1971.

Coupland RE, Fujita T (eds.): Chromaffin, Enterochromaffin and Related Cells. New York, Elsevier, 1976.

Fetter AW, Capen CC: The ultrastructure of the parathyroid gland of young pigs. Acta Anat (Basel) 75:359, 1970.

Fujita H: Fine structure of the thyroid cell. Int Rev Cytol 40:197, 1975.

Gaillard PJ, Talmage RV, Budy AM (eds.): The Parathyroid Glands. Chicago, University of Chicago Press, 1965.

Gray JK, Cooper CW, Munson PL: Parathyroid hormone, thyrocalcitonin, and the control of mineral metabolism. *In* Endocrine Physiology. SM McCann (ed.). Oxford, Butterworth, 1974, pp. 239–275.

Idelman S: Ultrastructure of the mammalian adrenal cortex. Int Rev Cytol 27:181, 1970.

James VHT (ed.): The Adrenal Gland. New York, Raven Press, 1979.

Johannisson E: The foetal adrenal cortex in the human: Its ultrastructure at different stages of development and in different functional states. Acta Endocrinol (Suppl) (Copenh) 130:1, 1968.

Klinch GH, Oertel JE, Winship I: Ultrastructure of normal human thyroid. Lab Invest 22:2, 1970.

Long JA, Jones AL: Observations on the fine structure of the adrenal cortex of man. Lab Invest 17:355, 1967.

Nunez EA, Gershon MD: Cytophysiology of thyroid parafollicular cells. Int Rev Cytol 52:1, 1978.

Rasmussen H, Pechet MM: Calcitonin. Sci Am 223(4):42, 1970.

Reiter RJ (ed.): The Pineal Gland. New York, Raven Press, 1984.

Tapp E, Huxley M: The histological appearance of the human pineal gland from puberty to old age. J Pathol 108:137, 1972.

Wurtman RJ: The pineal as a neuroendocrine transducer. Hosp Pract 15(1):82, 1980.

Chapter 23: Male Reproductive System

Brandes D: Male Accessory Sex Organs. Structure and Function in Mammals. New York, Academic Press, 1974.

Christensen AK: Leydig cells. *In* Handbook of Physiology: Endocrinology, Vol 5, Sect 7, Male Reproductive System. DW Hamilton and RO Greep (eds.). Washington, DC, American Physiological Association, 1975, pp. 57–94.

Clermont Y: Renewal of spermatogonia in man. Am J Anat 118:509, 1966.

Clermont Y, Hermo L: Spermatogonial stem cells and their behavior in the seminiferous epithelium of rats and monkeys. *In* Stem Cells of Renewing Populations. AB Cairnie, PK Lala, and DG Osmond (eds.). New York, Academic Press, 1976.

Dym M: The fine structure of the monkey Sertoli cell and its role in maintaining the blood-testis barrier. Anat Rec 175:639, 1973.

Dym M: The mammalian rete testes: A morphological examination. Anat Rec 186:493, 1976.

Fawcett DW: The mammalian spermatozoon. Dev Biol 44:394, 1975.

Fawcett DW, Bedford JM (eds.): The Spermatozoon: Maturity, Motility and Surface Properties. Baltimore, Urban & Schwarzenberg, 1979.

Gilula NB, Fawcett DW, Aoki A: Ultrastructural and experimental observations on the Sertoli cell junctions of the mammalian testis. Dev Biol 50:142, 1976.

Holstein AF, Roosen-Runge EC: Atlas of Human Spermatogenesis. Berlin, Grosse Verlag, 1981.

Johnson AD, Gomes WR (eds.): The Testis, Vols 1–4. New York, Academic Press, 1970–1977.

Nagano T, Suzuki F: Freeze-fracture observations on the intercellular functions of Sertoli cells and of Leydig cells in the human testis. Cell Tissue Res 166:37, 1976.

Tindall DJ, Rowley DA, Murthy L, Lipshultz LI, Chang CH: Structure and biochemistry of the Sertoli cell. Int Rev Cytol 94:127, 1985.

Chapter 24: Female Reproductive System I—Ovary

Balboni GC: Histology of the ovary. In The Endocrine Function of the Human Ovary. Proceedings of the Serono Symposia, Vol 7. VHT James, M Serio, and G Giusti (eds.). London, Academic Press, 1976.

Blandau RJ: Biology of eggs and implantation. In Sex and Internal Secretions, Vol 2, ed 3. WC Young (ed.). Baltimore, Williams & Wilkins, 1955, p. 797.

Coutts JRT (ed.): Functional Morphology of the Human Ovary. Lancaster, MTP Press, 1981.

Crisp TM, Dessouky DA, Denys FR: The fine structure of the human corpus luteum of early pregnancy and during the progestational phase of the menstrual cycle. Am J Anat 127:37, 1970.

Dorrington JH, Armstrong DT: Effects of FSH on gonadal functions. Recent Prog Horm Res 35:301, 1979.

Gulyas BJ: Fine structure of the luteal tissue. In Ultrastructure of Endocrine Cells and Tissues. PM Motta (ed.). Dordrecht, Martinus Nijhoff, 1984, pp. 238–254.

Hertig AT, Rock J, Adams EC: A description of 34 human ova within the first 17 days of development. Am J Anat 98:435, 1956.

Johnson MH, Everitt BJ: Essential Reproduction. Oxford, Blackwell, 1980.

Jones RE (ed.): The Vertebrate Ovary. New York, Plenum Press, 1978.

Mossman MH, Koering MJ, Ferry D Jr: Cyclic changes of interstitial gland tissue of the human ovary. Am J Anat 115:235, 1964.

Motta PM, Hafez ESE (eds.): Biology of the Ovary. Dordrecht, Martinus Nijhoff, 1980.

Van Blerkom J, Motta P: The Cellular Basis of Mammalian Reproduction. Baltimore, Urban & Schwarzenberg, 1979.

Weiss G, O'Byrne EM, Steinetz BG: Relaxin: A product of the human corpus luteum of pregnancy. Science 194:948, 1976.

Zuckerman S, Weir BJ (eds.): The Ovary, Vol 1. General Aspects, ed 2. New York, Academic Press, 1977.

Chapter 25: Female Reproductive System II— Genital Tract and Other Organs of Pregnancy

Amorosa EC: Histology of the placenta. Br Med Bull 17:81, 1961.

Banarjee MR: Responses of mammary cells to hormones. Int Rev Cytol 47:1, 1976.

Beaconsfield P, Birdwood G, Beaconsfield R: The placenta. Sci Am 243(2):94, 1980.

Blandau RJ, Moghissi K: The Biology of the Cervix. Chicago, University of Chicago Press, 1973.

Enders AC: Formation of the syncytium from cytotrophoblast in the human placenta. Obstet Gynecol 25:378, 1965.

Finn CA, Porter DG: The Uterus, Handbooks of Reproductive Biology. London, Paul Elek, 1974.

Greep RO (ed.): Handbook of Physiology, Section 7: Endocrinology, Vol II: Female Reproductive System. Washington, DC, American Physiological Society, 1975.

Hafez ESE, Blandau RJ: The Mammalian Oviduct. Chicago, University of Chicago Press, 1969.

Kaufman P, Sen DK, Schweikhart G: Classification of human placental villi. I. Histology. Cell Tissue Res 200:409, 1979.

King BF: Ultrastructure of the non-human primate vaginal mucosa: Epithelial changes during the menstrual cycle and pregnancy. J Ultrastruct Res 82:1, 1983.

Ludwig H, Metzger H: The Human Female Reproductive Tract: A Scanning Electron Microscopic Atlas. New York, Springer-Verlag, 1976.

Nemanic MK, Pitelka DR: A scanning electron microscopic study of the lactating mammary gland. J Cell Biol 48:410, 1971.

Tersakis J: The ultrastructure of normal human first trimester placenta. J Ultrastruct Res 9:268, 1963.

Villee DB: Development of endocrine function in the human placenta and fetus. N Engl J Med 281:473, 1969.

Vorherr H: The Breast: Morphology, Physiology and Lactation. New York, Academic Press, 1974.

Wynn RM (ed.): Biology of the Uterus. New York, Plenum Press, 1977.

Chapter 26: Organs of Special Sense—Eye and Ear

Anderson DH, Fisher SK, Steinberg RH: Mammalian cones: Disc shedding, phagocytosis, and renewal. Invest Ophthalmol Vis Sci 17:117, 1978.

Bothelho SY: Tears and the lacrimal gland. Sci Am 211:78, 1964.

Engström B: Scanning electron microscopy of the inner ear structure of the organ of Corti and its neural pathways. Acta Otolaryngol (Suppl) 319:57, 1974.

Engström H, Ades H, Anderson A: Structural Pattern of the Organ of Corti. Stockholm, Almquist & Wiksell, 1966.

Fine BS, Yanoff M: Ocular Histology, ed 2. New York, Harper & Row, 1979.

Hogan MJ, Alvarado JA, Weddell JE: Histology of the Human Eye. Philadelphia, WB Saunders, 1971.

Hudspeth AJ: The hair cells of the inner ear. Sci Am 248(1):54, 1983.

Jacobs GH: Comparative Color Vision. New York, Academic Press, 1981.

Kimura RS: The ultrastructure of the organ of Corti. Int Rev Cytol 42:173, 1975.

Parker DE: The vestibular apparatus. Sci Am 243(5):118, 1980.

Soudijn ER: Scanning electron microscopy of the organ of Corti. Annu Otol Rhinol Laryngol (Suppl) 86:16, 1976.

Young RW: Visual cells and the concept of renewal. Invest Ophthalmol 15:700, 1976.

Chapter 27: Microscopy

Conn HJ: Biological Stains, ed 9. Baltimore, Williams and Wilkins, 1977.

Everhart TE, Hayes TL: The scanning electron microscope. Sci Am 226:54, 1972.

Hayat MA: Basic electron microscopy technics. J Microsc 123:201, 1981.

James J: Light Microscopic Techniques in Biology and Medicine. The Hague, Martinus Nijhoff, 1976.

Kawamura A Jr (ed.): Florescent Antibody Techniques and Their Application, ed 2. Baltimore University, Park Press, 1977.

Pease DC, Porter KR: Electron microscopy and ultramicrotomy. J Cell Biol 91:287s, 1981.

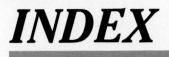

INDEX

Note: Pages with tables are marked "t."

myelination of, 205–207
   in reflex arc, 207–208
Mouth, 329
MSH. *See* Melanocyte-stimulating hormone, 432, 438
Mucigen, 20–21
   droplets, 28–29t
Mucopolysaccharides, 70, 100
Mucoproteins, 21
Mucosa, 84–87
   of alimentary tract, 348–364
      of colon, 363
      of oral cavity, 329
      of small intestine, 355–356
      of stomach, 351
   of female genital tract, 510–519
      of oviduct, 510
      of uterus, 512
      of vagina, 518
   of respiratory system, 309–317
   of urinary passageways, 416–420
Mucous
   connective tissue, 102
   crypts, 80
   glands, 271
   goblet cells, 80
   membranes. *See* Mucosa, 84–87
Mucus, 73
   formation of, 20
   in respiratory system, 309
Multiple sclerosis, demyclination in, 207
Multipolar nerve cells, 52–53, 194
   in spinal gray matter, 227
Multivesicular bodies, 15
Mumps, 337
Muscle, 174–184
   classification of, 57t
   electron microscopy of, 179–186
      of fibers, 51
   functions of, 50–51, 56
   light microscopy of, 174–178
   red and white fibers, 176, 180
   regeneration of, 184–186
   spasms of, 462
   types of, 186–187t
Muscle contraction theory, 182
Muscle motor units, 203
Muscle spindles, 202–203. *See also* Neuromuscular spindles, 176
Muscular
   arteries, 250–251
   dystrophies, 185
Muscularis externa, 312, 349
   of colon, 363
   of esophagus, 350
   of small intestine, 359
   of stomach, 352
Muscularis mucosae, 86, 349
   of esophagus, 349–350
   of large intestine, 361–365
   of reproductive system, female, 510–517
   of respiratory system, 322–323
   of small intestine, 355–356
   of stomach, 351
   of urinary passageways, 416–420
Myelin, 196
   formation, 205–207
Myelinated fibers, 53
Myelin figure, 14, 17

Myelin sheaths, 53, 195, 197
   loss of, 207
Myeloblasts, 165, 185
Myelocytes, 166
Myenteric plexus of Auerbach, 349
Myocardium, 247–249
Myoepithelial cells, 81, 401
   contraction of, 440
Myofibrils, 26–27t, 50, 51, 175, 179
   contraction of, 51
Myofilaments, 174
   thick and thin, 179
Myoglobin, 176
Myometrium, 517
Myosin, 179
   filaments of, 16
      sliding theory of, 182
   strands of, 182
Myxedema, 134, 459

Nails, 300
Nasal
   cavities, 309–311
   infections, 542
   vestibule, 310
Nasopharynx, 312, 342, 542
Nephrons, 399, 402–407
Nerve
   endings, 53, 200–202
   fibers, 53, 226
   growth factor, 213
Nerves, 192. *See also specific nerves*
   degeneration and regeneration of, 211–213
   grafts, 212
   impulses, 54
Nervous systems, 52, 174. *See also* Autonomic nervous system, 213–215; Central nervous system, 223–240; Peripheral nervous system, 192–211
   divisions of, 52, 192
   in homeostasis, 430
Nervous tissue, 52, 192. *See also* Nervous systems
   classification of, 58t
   divisions of, 192
   elements of, 52–54
   function of, 56
   organization of, 52
Neuroblasts, 194
Neuroepithelial receptor cells, 529
Neuroepithelium, 48, 543
Neurofibrils, 26–27t
Neurofilaments, 16, 196
Neuroglandular junction, 197
Neuroglia, 54, 232–235, 463
   astrocytes, 232
   ependymal cells, 238
   oligodendroglia, 233
   microglia or mesoglia, 235
Neurohypophysis, 433, 439–440
Neurokeratin, 205
Neurolemma, 53, 197
   cells of, 212
   sheaths of, 211
   tubes of, 213
Neuroma, 212
Neuromuscular
   junction, 197

spindle, 176. *See also* Muscle spindle, 202–203
Neuron doctrine, 193
Neurons, 62, 194, 242t
   cell processes of, 195–196
      axon, 195
      dendrite, 196
   components of, 52–54
   morphological classification of, 194, 242t
   perikaryon, 194–195
   peripheral, 197–203
      investments, 198
   in spinal cord, 226
   synapses of, 197
Neuropil, 229
Neurophysin, 440
Neurosecretory
   cells, 439
   granules, 294
Neurotransmitters, 53
Neutrophilic granules, 146
Neutrophils, 96, 143, 145–146
Nicolson, G. L., 6
Nipple, 522
Nissl bodies, 194–196, 210
Nodes
   atrioventricular, 246
   lymph, 267
   of Ranvier, 195, 198–199, 205
   sinoatrial, 246
Norepinephrine, 53, 197
   release of, 456
Normoblasts, 163
Nuclear
   bag fibers, 203
   chain fibers, 203
   envelope, 34–35
      in mitosis, 40
      pores, 34
Nucleolonema, 35
Nucleolus, 34–35, 194
   in mitosis, 40
Nucleosome, 36
Nucleus, 5, 34
   in cell cycle, 38–42
   function of, 24
   organelles of, 34–36
   structures of, 36–38
Nutrient canal, 121
Nutrients
   for bone growth, 134
   transported by blood, 50

Oddi, sphincter of, 375
Odontoblasts, 339, 341
Odor receptors, 311
Olfactory
   area, 311
   bulb, 311
   vesicles, 311
Oligodendrocytes, 54, 207, 233–235, 236–237
Oocytes, 492
   release of, 493
Oogenesis, 492
Oogonia, 492
Optic
   nerve, 530, 538
   papilla (disk), 538

Look-alikes
in Histology

Contents

Section I – Color photomicrographs

Section I – Color photomicrographs

Section II–Electron micrographs

PLATE 1 Epithelium

A / Stratified squamous (x 200)
1. Surface cells flattened and dehydrated
2. Basal cuboidal cells become squamous
3. Many cell layers

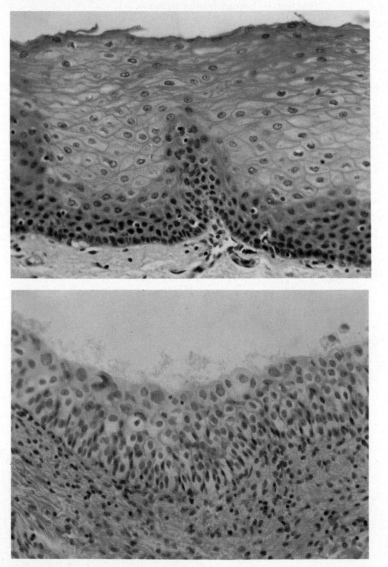

B / Transitional (contracted) (x 200)
1. Large dome-shaped surface cells
2. Cells remain cuboidal or columnar
3. Fewer cell layers

PLATE 2 Cartilage

A / Hyaline (x 162)
1. Homogeneous, slightly basophilic matrix
2. Lacunae often contain two or more cells (cell nests)
3. Lacunae rather evenly spaced and rimmed
   with basophilic matrix

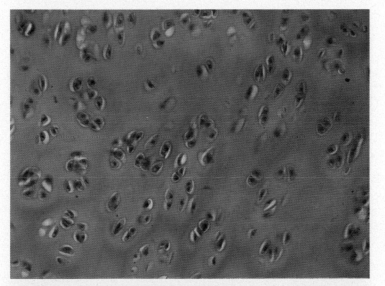

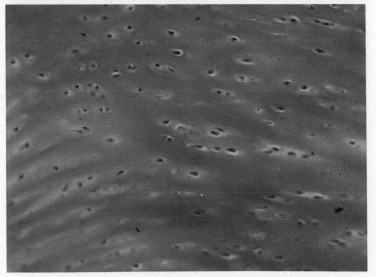

B / Fibrous (x 162)
1. Collagenous fibers in eosinophilic matrix
2. Cells usually in individual lacunae
3. Lacunae more widely spaced and arranged in
   rows or clusters

PLATE 3 **Leukocytes** (Wright's stain)

A / Lymphocyte (large) (x1200)

   1. Round, dark nucleus

   2. Smaller cell (10-12μ)

   3. Less cytoplasm

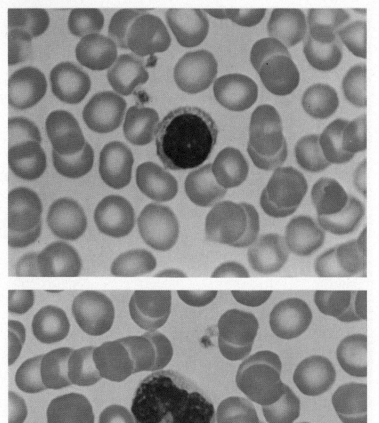

B / Monocyte (x1200)

   1. Indented, lighter-staining, flocculent nucleus

   2. Larger cell (12-15μ)

   3. More cytoplasm

PLATE 4 Muscle

A / Cardiac (x 216)
    1. Central nuclei
    2. Branching fibers
    3. Cross striations faint
    4. Intercalated disks (not shown)

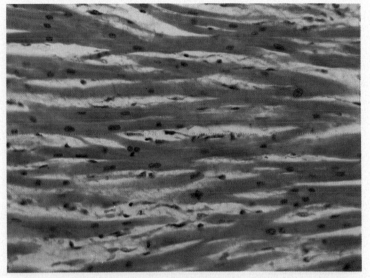

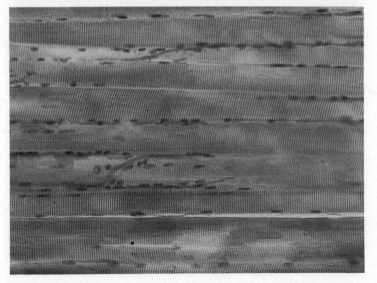

B / Skeletal (x 216)
    1. Peripheral nuclei
    2. Nonbranching fibers
    3. Cross striations prominent

PLATE 5

A / Peripheral nerve (myelinated) (x 248)

1. Uneven distribution of various types
   or shapes of nuclei
2. Spongy network of neurokeratin around central axons
3. Somewhat wavy appearance
4. Nodes of Ranvier

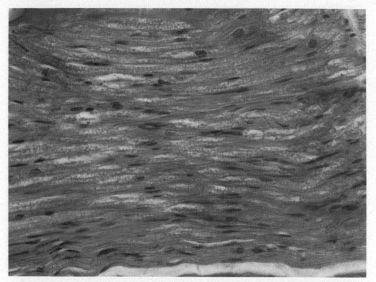

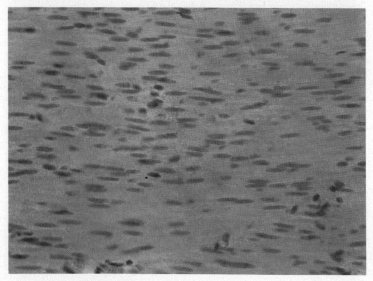

B / Smooth muscle (x 248)

1. Fusiform nuclei quite uniform in
   size and distribution
2. Darker, homogeneous cytoplasm

PLATE 6

A / **Peripheral nerve (myelinated) (x 320)**

1. Several rounded, light-staining neurolemmal nuclei; many dark-staining fibroblast (endoneurial) nuclei
2. Parallel, light-staining fibers
3. "Washed-out," spongy neurokeratin around axis cylinders
4. Blood vessels absent except in larger nerves
5. Nodes of Ranvier

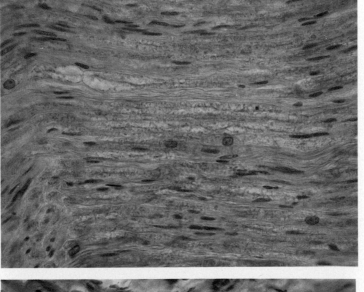

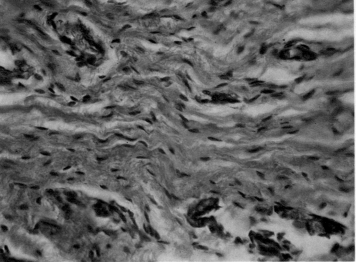

B / **Collagenous fibers (x 320)**

1. Many uniform, dark-staining fibroblast nuclei
2. Uneven, undulating, dark-staining fibers
3. Reduced cytoplasm in fibroblasts
4. Blood vessels usually present

PLATE 7 **Ganglia** (Cajal's silver stain)

A / Spinal (x 200)
 1. Central nuclei
 2. Both large and small cells
 3. Cells unipolar

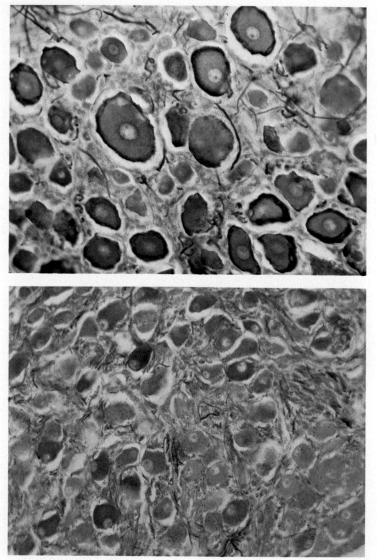

B / Sympathetic (x 200)
 1. Many eccentric nuclei
 2. Only small cells
 3. Cells multipolar
 4. Cells often have pigment

PLATE 8

A / Lymph node (x 336)

1. Medullary cords prominent (not shown)
2. Lymph sinuses prominent
3. Large subcapsular sinus
4. Many lymphoid follicles

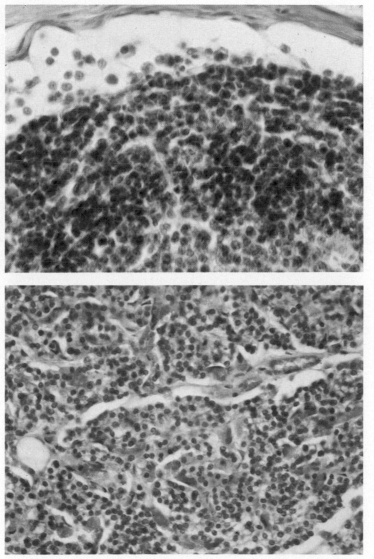

B / Parathyroid (x 336)

1. Chief cells in cords resemble lymphocytes
2. Prominent capillary bed, no lymph sinuses
3. Some oxyphil cells
4. No lymphoid tissue

PLATE 9 **Neuroglia** (del Rio Hortega stains)

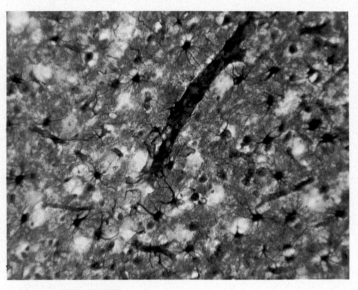

A / Astrocytes (x180)

1. Large, star-shaped cells
2. Many long processes end on capillaries (perivascular feet)
3. Abundant cytoplasm

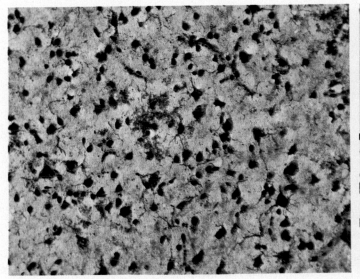

B / Oligodendroglia (x180)
1. Medium-sized angular or oval cells
2. Few, short, beaded processes
3. Less cytoplasm

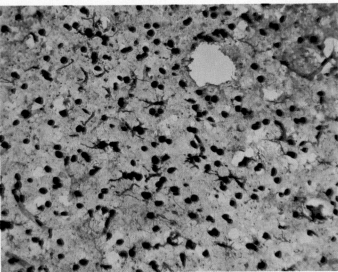

C / Microglia (x180)
1. Small, oval, irregular cells
2. Short, spiny processes
3. Scanty cytoplasm

PLATE 10 **Lymphoid organs**

A / Lymph node (x 44)
1. Thin connective-tissue capsule
2. Cortical sinus
3. Cortex and medulla
4. Medullary cords

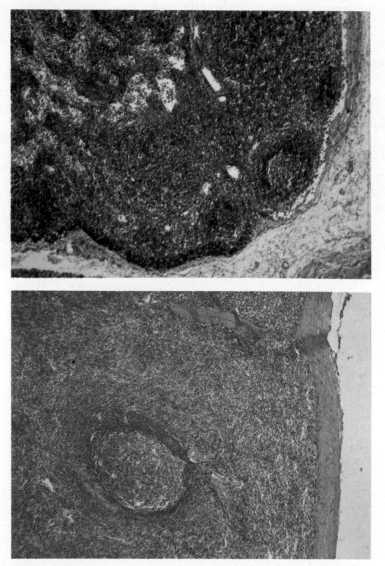

B / Spleen (x 44)
1. Heavy fibromuscular capsule with trabeculae
2. Eccentric central arteries in white pulp
3. No cortex or medulla
4. Red and white pulp

C / Thymus (x 44)

1. Thin connective-tissue capsule
2. Hassall's bodies
3. Medulla and cortex in each lobule
4. Lobules are "blocks" of tissue

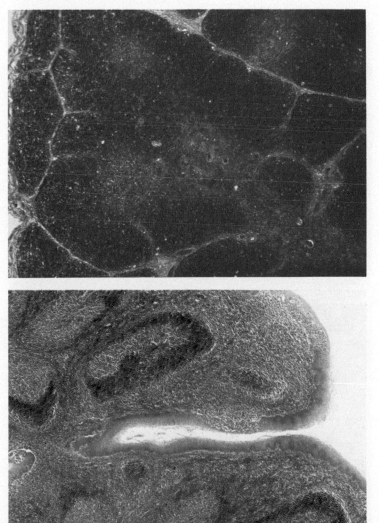

D / Palatine tonsil (x 44)

1. Heavy connective-tissue capsule surrounds base (not shown)
2. Free surface and crypts lined with stratified squamous epithelium
3. Numerous subepithelial lymph nodules

PLATE 11

A / Bronchiole (x100)

  1. Ciliated columnar epithelium
  2. Prominent longitudinal epithelial folds
  3. Empty lumen
  4. Thin circular smooth-muscle layer

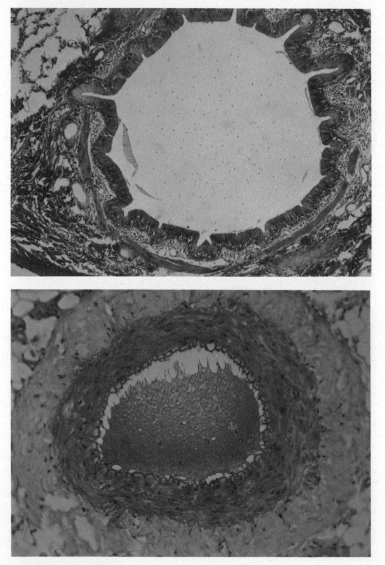

B / Small artery (x100)

  1. Simple squamous epithelium (endothelium)
  2. Delicate wavy folds in endothelium
     due to undulations of underlying internal
     elastic membrane
  3. Lumen may contain blood
  4. Prominent circular smooth-muscle layer

PLATE 12 Tonsils

A / Palatine (x148)

1. Stratified squamous epithelium
   lining crypts
2. Robust capsule at base (not shown)

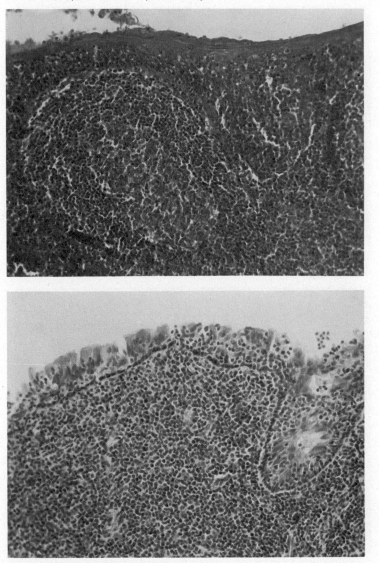

B / Pharyngeal (x148)

1. Pseudostratified columnar ciliated
   epithelium lining crypts
2. Thin capsule (not shown)

PLATE 13 **Salivary glands**

A / Parotid (x 96)

1. All alveoli are serous
2. No demilunes
3. Numerous fat cells

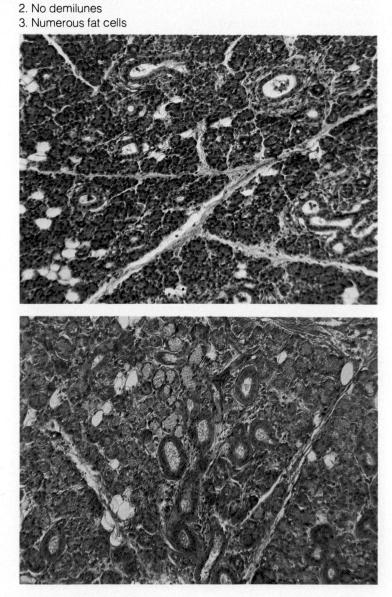

B / Submandibular (x 96)

1. Most alveoli are serous
2. Some mucous alveoli with serous demilunes
3. Some fat cells

PLATE 14 Salivary glands

A / Submandibular (x 96)

1. Alveoli mostly serous, some mucous
2. Serous demilunes on some mucous alveoli
3. Few fat cells

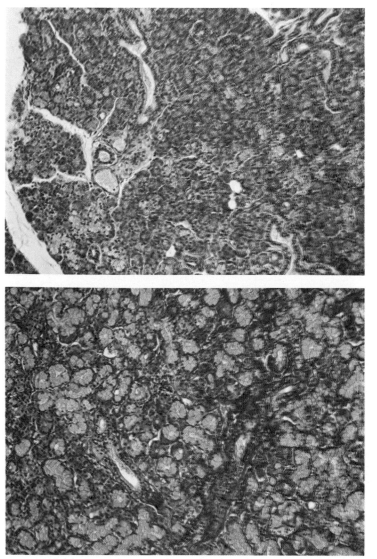

B / Sublingual (x 96)

1. Mucous alveoli equal or exceed serous
   alveoli in number
2. Many mucous alveoli with serous demilunes
3. Occasional fat cell

PLATE 15 Serous glands

A / Pancreas (x 148)

1. All serous acini with pyramidal cells
2. Minute acinar lumina associated with centroacinar cells
3. Few fat cells
4. Islet tissue prominent

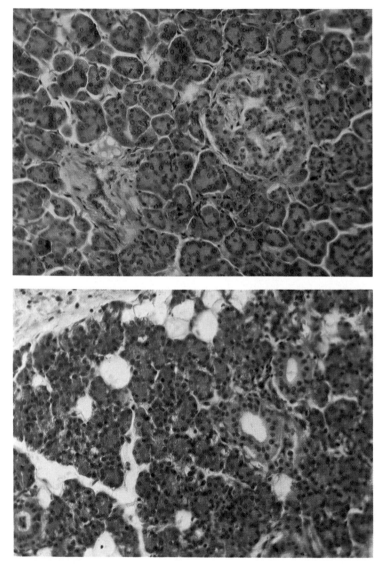

B / Parotid (x 148)

1. All serous acini with pyramidal cells
2. Small acinar lumina—no centroacinar cells
3. Many fat cells

C / Lacrimal (x148)

1. Only serous acini with low columnar cells
2. Conspicuous acinar lumina—
   no centroacinar cells
3. Usually some fat cells

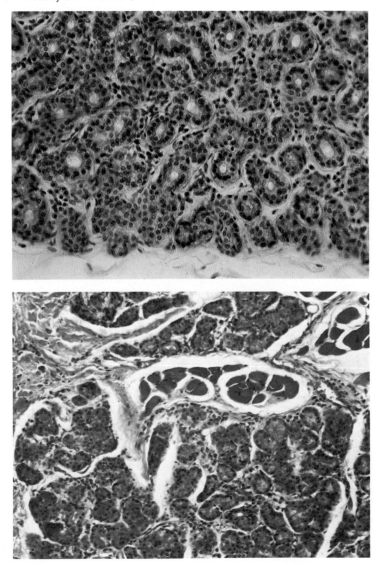

D / Posterior lingual (von Ebner's) (x148)

1. All serous acini
2. Acini extend into skeletal muscle of tongue
3. Poorly developed duct system

PLATE 16

A / Oropharynx–longitudinal section (x 34)

1. Interlacing bundles of skeletal muscle
2. No muscularis mucosae (Replaced by layer
   of elastic fibers)

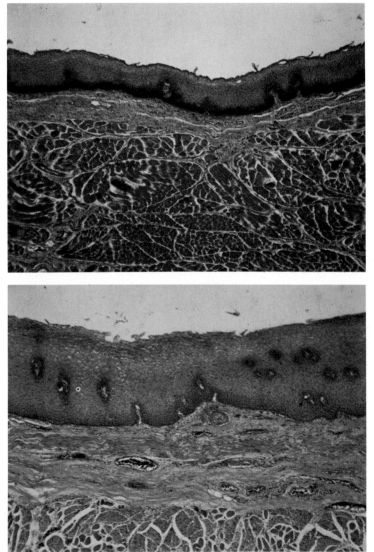

B / Esophagus–longitudinal section (x 34)

1. Outer longitudinal (not shown), inner circular
   layers of either smooth muscle or skeletal muscle
   or both (as shown here)
2. Prominent muscularis mucosae
3. Esophageal glands may be present (not shown)

PLATE 17

A / **Vagina (x 46)**

1. Venous plexuses prominent
2. Many leukocytes, occasional lymph nodule
3. No glands
4. Smooth-muscle fibers
5. Collagenous fibers indistinct

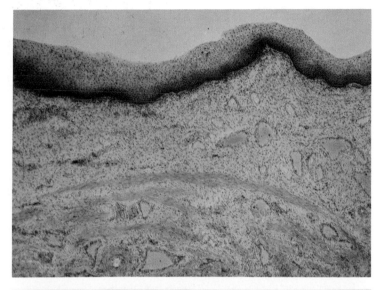

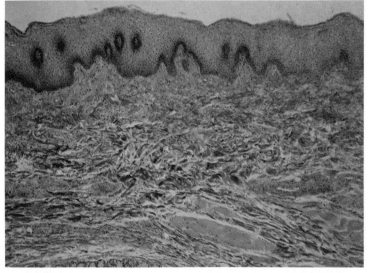

B / **Lip (x 46)**

1. Arteries prominent
2. Few leukocytes
3. Mucous and serous (labial) glands (not shown)
4. Skeletal muscle fibers
5. Collagenous fibers conspicuous

PLATE 18 **Stomach glands**

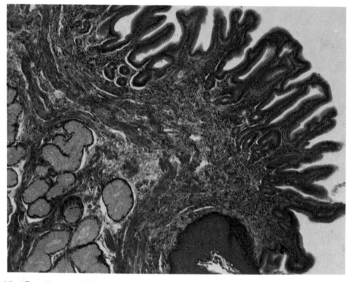

A Cardiac (x 64)
  1. Open gastric pits
  2. Slightly coiled, shallow glands
  3. Only mucous-type cells
  4. Often associated with esophagus

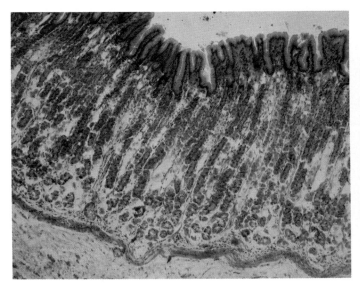

B / Fundic (x 64)

1. Pits narrow and shallow
2. Straight, long, tubular glands
3. Many parietal and chief cells
4. Found in body and fundic regions

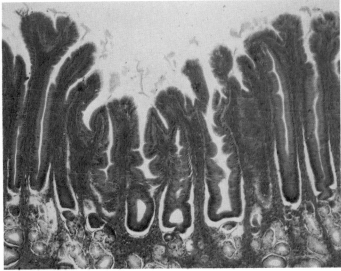

C / Pyloric (x 64)

1. Pits open and deep
2. Quite short, coiled glands
3. Mucous-type cells, few parietal cells
4. May be associated with duodenum

PLATE 19

A / Stomach–esophageal junction (x 52)

1. Simple columnar epithelium lining
   stomach–no goblet cells
2. Cardiac glands empty into wide gastric pits
3. Muscularis mucosae persists across junction
4. Mucous glands in submucosa (not shown)

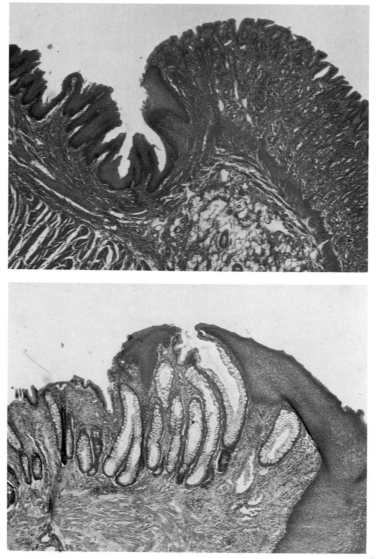

B / Rectoanal junction (x 52)

1. Simple columnar epithelium with many goblet
   cells lining rectum
2. Deep intestinal glands lined mostly with
   goblet cells
3. Muscularis mucosae broken up and lost
   at junction
4. No submucosal glands

PLATE 20

A / Gallbladder (x 34)

1. No true villi; mucosal folds resemble villi
2. No goblet cells (except in neck region)
3. Diverticula (sinuses) present
4. No muscularis mucosae
5. Smooth-muscle layers thin and interlacing

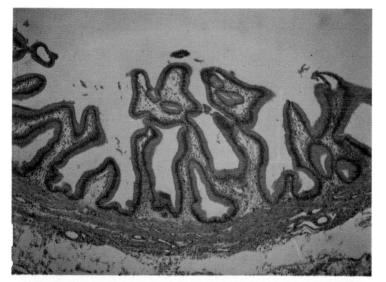

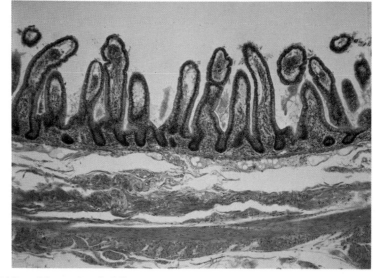

B / Small intestine (x 34)

1. Many villi
2. Abundant goblet cells
3. No diverticula
4. Muscularis mucosae present
5. Two distinct smooth-muscle layers

PLATE 21

A / Duodenum (x16)

    1. Brunner's glands in submucosa
    2. No Peyer's patches, only solitary lymph nodules
       in tunica propria

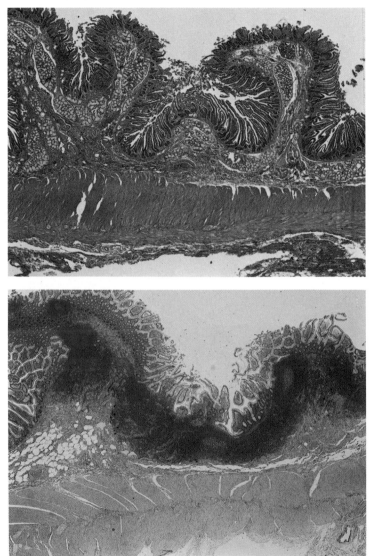

B / Ileum (x16)

    1. No glands in submucosa
    2. Peyer's patches in tunica propria

PLATE 22

A / Anal canal (x 42)

1. Nonkeratinized stratified squamous epithelium—
   becomes keratinized at anus
2. No glands except circumanal (sweat) glands near anus
3. Diffuse lymphoid tissue
4. Prominent venous plexuses—when widely dilated
   called internal hemorrhoids
5. Smooth-muscle layer thickens as internal sphincter

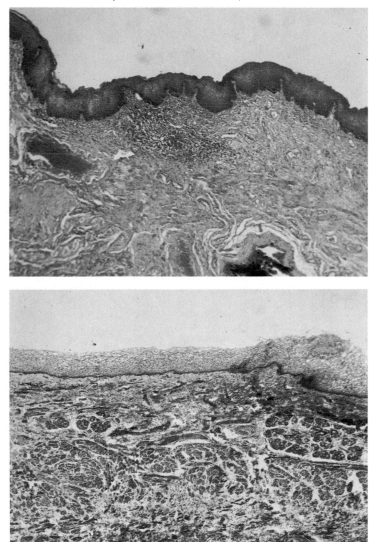

B / Inner lip (x 42)

1. Nonkeratinized stratified squamous epithelium
2. Labial glands—mostly mucous, some serous
3. No lymphoid tissue
4. No obvious venous patterns
5. Skeletal muscle fibers prominent as
   orbicularis oris muscle

PLATE 23

A / Corpus luteum (x 148)

1. No definite capsule
2. Cells arranged in cords
3. Remnant of corpus hemorrhagicum
   may be present (not shown)

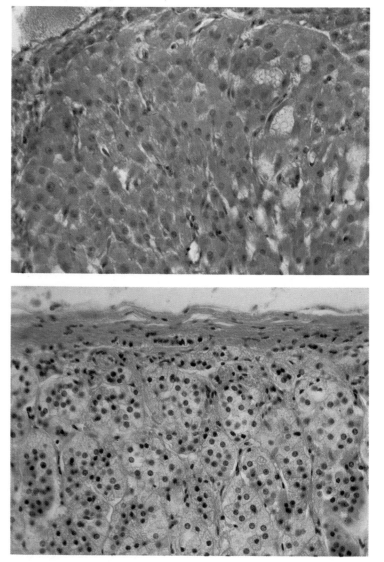

B / Adrenal cortex (x 148)

1. Capsule present
2. Cords of cells in ovoid clusters (zona glomerulosa),
   in parallel columns (zona fasciculata),
   or in network (zona reticularis–not shown)

PLATE 24

A / Seminal vesicle (x 34)

1. Lumen filled with cellular debris
   and secretions
2. Pseudostratified columnar epithelium covers
   branching mucosal folds
3. Interlacing smooth-muscle layers

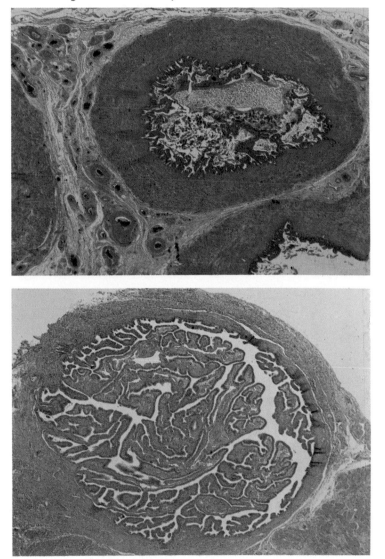

B / Oviduct (ampulla) (x 34)

1. Lumen free from debris
2. Simple columnar epithelium, some cells
   with cilia
3. Greatly folded mucous membrane
4. Inner circular, outer longitudinal
   smooth-muscle layers

PLATE 25

A / Epididymis (x 96)

1. Large circular lumina with clusters of spermatozoa
2. Tall columnar epithelium with tufted stereocilia

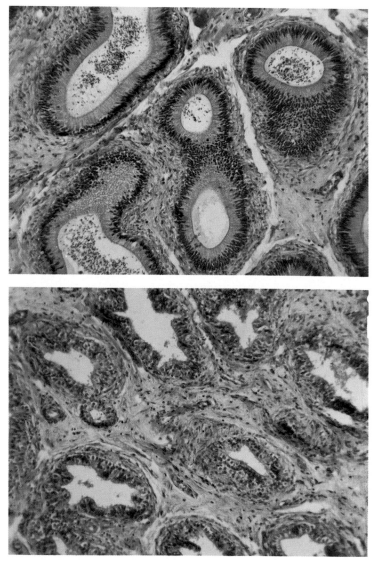

B / Ductuli efferentes testis (x 96)

1. Irregular lumina free from spermatozoa
2. Simple columnar epithelium with patches of cilia

PLATE 26

A / **Prostate (x 64)**

1. Clusters of alveolar-type glands
2. Abundance of smooth muscle
3. Limited secretions and cellular
   debris in lumen
4. Concretions may be present (not shown)

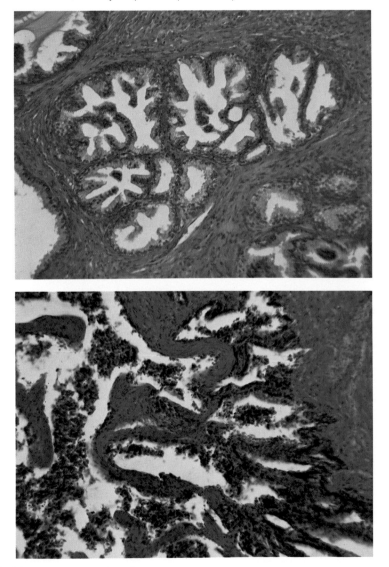

B / **Seminal vesicle (x 64)**

1. Large ductile organ, no alveoli
2. Less smooth muscle
3. Lumen partially filled with secretions
   and debris
4. No concretions
5. Extensive mucosal folds extend into lumen

PLATE 27

A / Bulbourethral gland (x130)

1. Only mucous acini, some of which form cyst-like dilatations
2. Acinar lumina often large and dilated
3. Skeletal muscle fibers in capsule

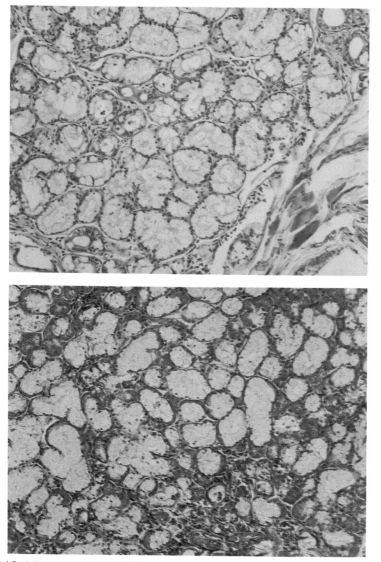

B / Sublingual gland (x130)

1. Some serous acini and demilunes among abundant mucous acini
2. Acinar lumina small and inconspicuous
3. No muscle in capsule

PLATE 28 Urethra

A / Male (penile portion of urethra) (x16)
1. Erectile tissue prominent
2. Muscle absent
3. Urethral glands (of Littré) prominent

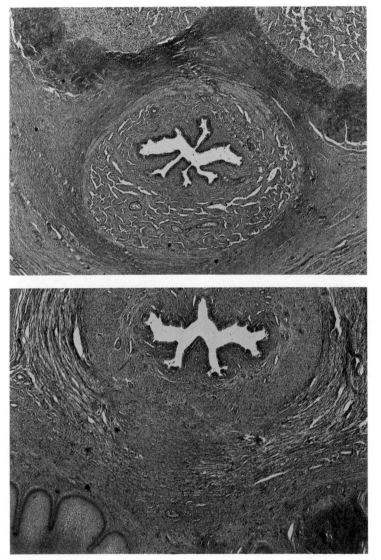

B / Female (x16)
1. No erectile tissue
2. Sphincter muscle usually present
3. Urethral glands scarce

PLATE 29

A / Ureter (x 34)
1. Transitional epithelium
2. Outer circular, inner longitudinal
   smooth-muscle layers

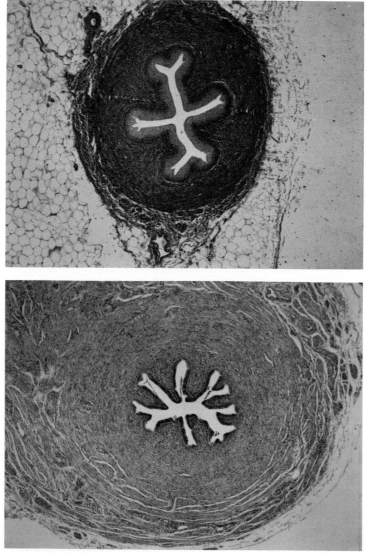

B / Oviduct (isthmus) (x 34)
1. Simple columnar epithelium, some cilia
2. Outer longitudinal, inner circular
   smooth-muscle layers

PLATE 30

A / Thyroid (x 90)

1. Clear hyaline colloid in follicles
2. Vacuoles may be present in colloid
3. No ducts
4. No lobules
5. Islets of parafollicular cells

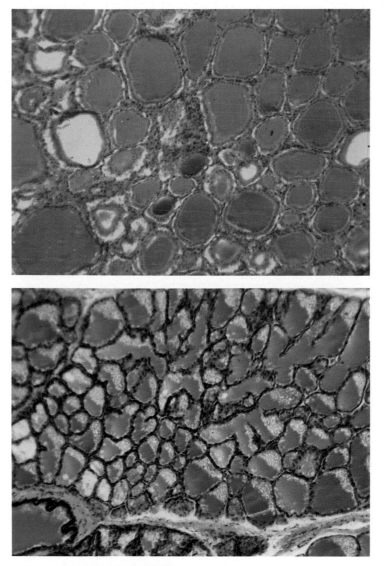

B / Active mammary gland (x 90)

1. Granular or hyaline secretion in
   expanded alveoli
2. Fat droplets (vacuoles) in alveoli and ducts
3. Excretory ducts present
4. Lobulated

PLATE 31

A / Granular (rough) endoplasmic reticulum – human ovary (x 25,500)

1. Outer surface of membranes studded with ribosomes
2. Usually arranged as flattened parallel membranous sacs (cisternae)
3. Cisternae quite uniform in size and shape

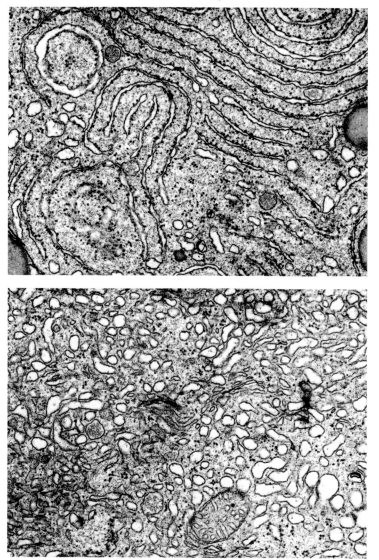

B / Agranular (smooth) endoplasmic reticulum – human ovary (x 25,500)

1. Membranes lack ribosomes
2. Arranged as a network of tubules or whorls
3. Tubule size quite uniform in well-fixed tissue

PLATE 32

A / Golgi apparatus–human ovary (x17,280)

1. Several stacks of flat, membranous saccules or tubules
2. Saccules usually present a discoidal, curved appearance
3. Tubules compressed at their centers but dilated as vesicles peripherally
4. Usually located near center of cell

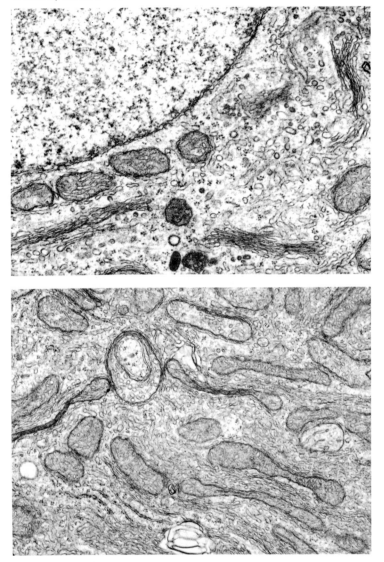

B / Agranular (smooth) endoplasmic reticulum– human ovary (x17,280)

1. Anastomosing network of closely packed membranous vesicles or tubules
2. Present throughout cell

PLATE 33

**A / Pigment granules (melanosomes)
human skin (x17,300)**

 1. In formative stages each granule has several
    very electron-dense, elongated lamellae enclosed
    by a common membrane
 2. Usually spherical

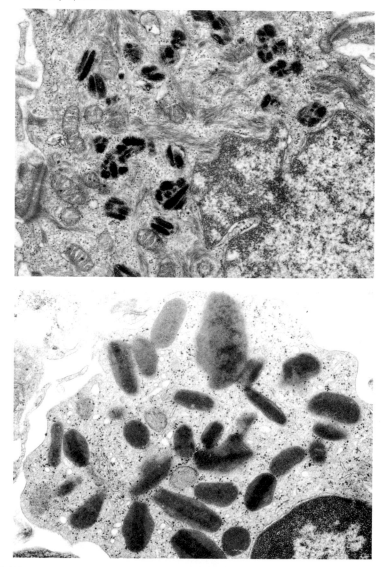

B / Eosinophil granules–guinea pig (x17,000)

 1. Typical granule has an electron-dense
    central band
 2. Oval shaped

PLATE 34

A / **Melanin granules (melanosomes)**
human skin (x19,000)

1. In late formative stages, granules are homogeneous with a very electron-dense core
2. Membrane-bound

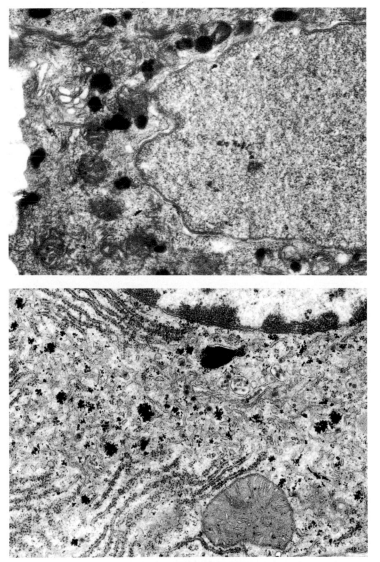

B / **Glycogen granules – rat liver (x 20,000)**

1. Appear either as scattered electron-dense, small (about 30 nm), irregular granules (the beta particles) or as larger (about 90 nm), rosette-like clusters (the alpha particles)
2. Not membrane-bound

PLATE 35

A / Microvilli−small intestine of guinea pig (x 100,000)

1. Core lightly stippled by straight, parallel, fine filaments
2. Prominent filamentous surface coat
3. Average diameter about 90 nm

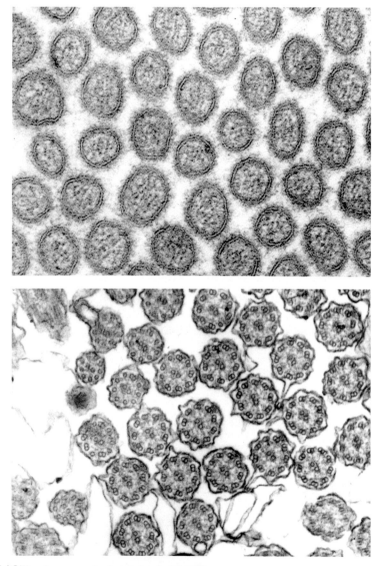

B / Cilia−human uterine tube (x 40,000)

1. Core has an axoneme consisting of two central singlet and nine peripheral doublet microtubules
2. No filamentous surface coat
3. Average diameter about 250 nm; cilia and microvilli *do not* look alike at same magnification

PLATE 36

A / Cilia–human uterine tube (x 8,000)
1. Ciliary process contains longitudinal microtubules –two central surrounded by nine doublets
2. Electron-dense body at base of each cilium
3. Larger diameter

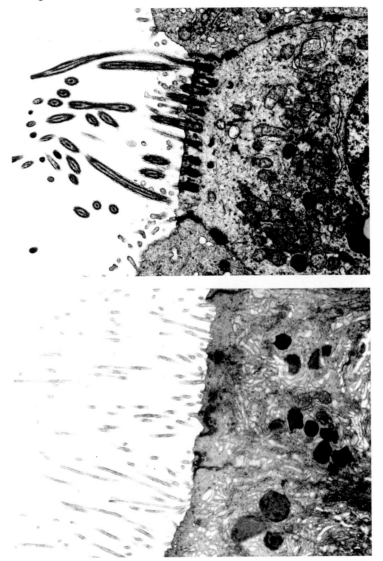

B / Stereocilia–rabbit epididymis (x 7,500)
1. Are long, often branched, microvilli–not true cilia
2. Central core quite homogeneous–contains straight, fine filaments
3. No basal bodies

PLATE 37 Granules

A / Lipid–rhesus monkey ovary (x12,800)

  1. Variable size
  2. Electron density may vary from light to very dark
  3. Distributed randomly throughout cell
  4. Matrix usually homogeneous

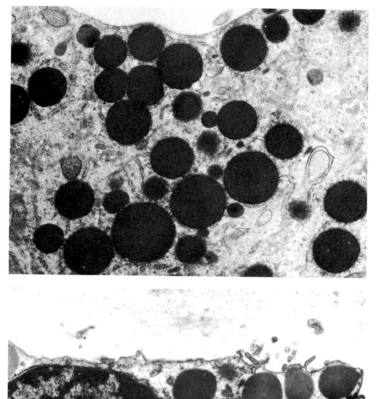

B / Mast cell–rat connective tissue (x12,000)

  1. Some variation in density and size
  2. Finely granular texture (not clearly shown)
  3. Fill entire cell

C / Zymogen—rat pancreas (x 12,000)
1. Generally uniform in size
2. Uniformly electron-dense
3. Tend to collect in apex of cell
4. Homogeneous matrix

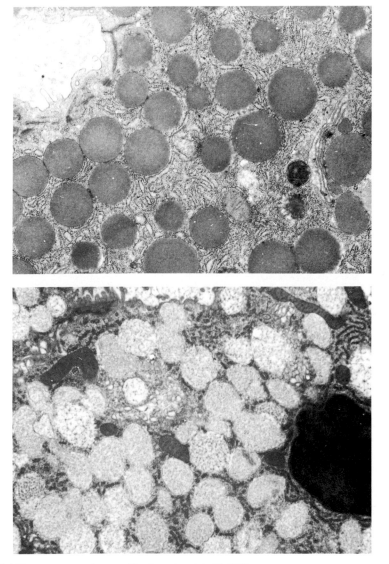

D / Mucus—rat submandibular gland (x 12,000)
1. Quite uniform in size
2. Electron-lucent, some granules confluent
3. Heterogeneous, reticular-like matrix
4. Fill most of cell

PLATE 38

A / Lipid droplets–rat liver (x 50,000)

1. Large droplets in cytoplasm with homogeneous electron-opaque core
2. Periphery more electron opaque due to greater osmophilia at interface
3. Small lipid particles within cisternae of agranular endoplasmic reticulum

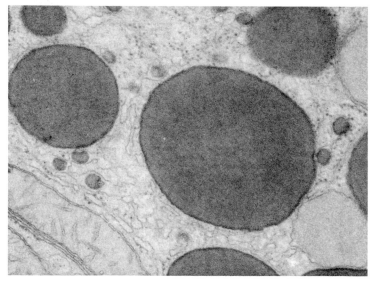

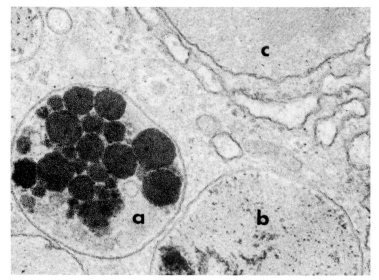

B / Lysosomes–rat liver (x 70,000)

1. Central core heterogeneous–may contain
   (a) small lipid droplets and vesicles,
   (b) fine granules and membrane remnants, or
   (c) an area of crystalloid in electron-lucent matrix
2. Bounded by distinct unit membrane

PLATE 39 Secretions of the adrenal medulla (rat)

A / Epinephrine granules (x 9,000)

1. Less electron-dense core
2. Light and dark granules
3. Even distribution in cell
4. Each granule fills a spherical vesicle

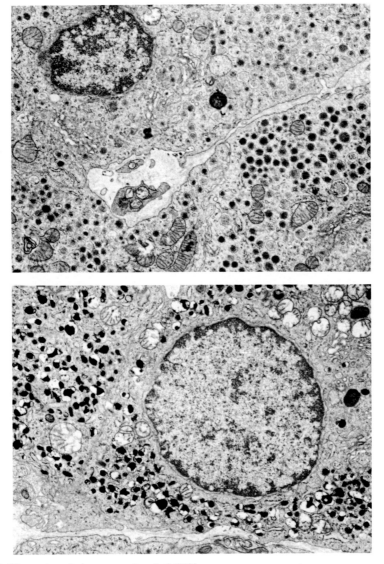

B / Norepinephrine granules (x 9,000)

1. Very electron-dense core – often eccentric
   in position
2. Often in clusters, uneven distribution in cell
3. Size and shape less uniform

PLATE 40 Hypophyseal secretory cells (rat)

A / Mammotroph (luteotroph) (x 7,125)

1. Largest granules (500 to 700 nm)
2. Granules irregular in shape and size, electron dense
3. Granular endoplasmic reticulum well developed

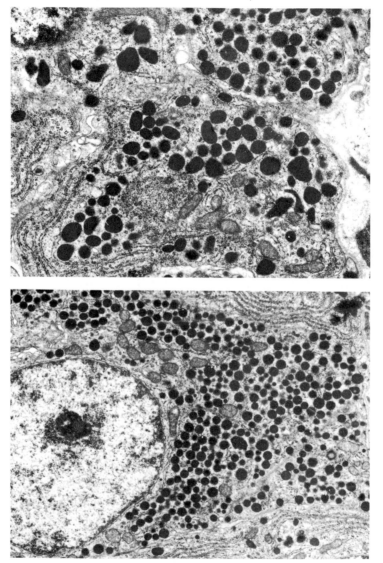

B / Somatotroph (x 7,125)

1. Granules intermediate in size (300 to 400 nm)
2. Numerous, dense, spherical granules
3. Prominent granular endoplasmic reticulum, cisternae parallel to cell surface

C / Gonadotroph (x 7,125)

1. Granules smaller (150 to 250 nm)
2. Spherical, less electron-dense granules, variable in size
3. Granular endoplasmic reticulum often with rounded irregular cisternae (lacunae)

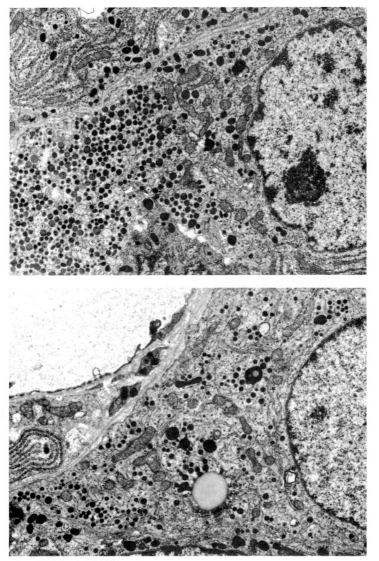

D / Thyrotroph (x 7,125)

1. Smallest granules (120 to 170 nm)
2. Granules frequently congregate at periphery of cell
3. Granular endoplasmic reticulum scanty